DYING IN AMERICA

Improving Quality and Honoring Individual Preferences Near the End of Life

Committee on Approaching Death: Addressing Key End-of-Life Issues

INSTITUTE OF MEDICINE
OF THE NATIONAL ACADEMIES

THE NATIONAL ACADEMIES PRESS
Washington, D.C.
www.nap.edu

THE NATIONAL ACADEMIES PRESS   500 Fifth Street, NW   Washington, DC 20001

NOTICE: The project that is the subject of this report was approved by the Governing Board of the National Research Council, whose members are drawn from the councils of the National Academy of Sciences, the National Academy of Engineering, and the Institute of Medicine. The members of the committee responsible for the report were chosen for their special competences and with regard for appropriate balance.

Any opinions, findings, conclusions, or recommendations expressed in this publication are those of the authors and do not necessarily reflect the views of the organizations or agencies that provided support for the project.

International Standard Book Number-13:   978-0-309-30310-1
International Standard Book Number-10:   0-309-30310-9
Library of Congress Control Number: 2014959553

Additional copies of this report are available for sale from the National Academies Press, 500 Fifth Street, NW, Keck 360, Washington, DC 20001; (800) 624-6242 or (202) 334-3313; http://www.nap.edu.

For more information about the Institute of Medicine, visit the IOM home page at: **www.iom.edu.**

The serpent has been a symbol of long life, healing, and knowledge among almost all cultures and religions since the beginning of recorded history. The serpent adopted as a logotype by the Institute of Medicine is a relief carving from ancient Greece, now held by the Staatliche Museen in Berlin.

Suggested citation: IOM (Institute of Medicine). 2015. *Dying in America: Improving quality and honoring individual preferences near the end of life.* Washington, DC: The National Academies Press.

"Knowing is not enough; we must apply.
Willing is not enough; we must do."
—Goethe

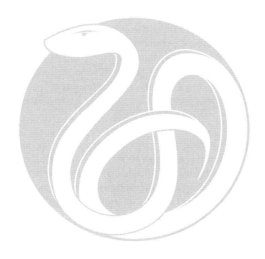

INSTITUTE OF MEDICINE
OF THE NATIONAL ACADEMIES

Advising the Nation. Improving Health.

THE NATIONAL ACADEMIES
Advisers to the Nation on Science, Engineering, and Medicine

STEPHEN G. PAUKER, Professor of Medicine and Psychiatry, Tufts University School of Medicine; Division of Clinical Decision Making, Informatics and Telemedicine, Tufts Medical Center, Boston, Massachusetts

JUDITH R. PERES, Clinical Social Worker and Policy Consultant, Chevy Chase, Maryland

LEONARD D. SCHAEFFER, Judge Robert Maclay Widney Chair and Professor, University of Southern California, Santa Monica

W. JUNE SIMMONS, President and CEO, Partners in Care Foundation, San Fernando, California

CHRISTIAN T. SINCLAIR, Assistant Professor, Division of Palliative Medicine, Department of Internal Medicine, University of Kansas Medical Center, Kansas City, Kansas

JOAN M. TENO, Professor of Health Services, Policy, and Practice, Brown University School of Public Health, Providence, Rhode Island

FERNANDO TORRES-GIL, Professor of Social Work, Professor of Public Policy, and Director of the Center for Policy Research on Aging, Luskin School of Public Affairs, University of California, Los Angeles

JAMES A. TULSKY, Professor of Medicine and Nursing and Chief, Duke Palliative Care, Duke University, Durham, North Carolina

Study Staff

ADRIENNE STITH BUTLER, Senior Program Officer
STEPHANIE H. PINCUS, Scholar-in-Residence
LAUREN SHERN, Associate Program Officer
BRADLEY ECKERT, Research Associate
JIM BANIHASHEMI, Financial Officer
THELMA COX, Administrative Assistant

Consultants

JUDITH A. SALERNO, President and CEO, Susan G. Komen Breast Cancer Foundation
NEIL WEISFELD, Writer
VICTORIA WEISFELD, Writer
RONA BRIERE, Editor

Reviewers

This report has been reviewed in draft form by individuals chosen for their diverse perspectives and technical expertise, in accordance with procedures approved by the National Research Council's Report Review Committee. The purpose of this independent review is to provide candid and critical comments that will assist the institution in making its published report as sound as possible and to ensure that the report meets institutional standards for objectivity, evidence, and responsiveness to the study charge. The review comments and draft manuscript remain confidential to protect the integrity of the deliberative process. We wish to thank the following individuals for their review of this report:

Susan Block, Harvard Medical School
Christine K. Cassel, National Quality Forum
Myra J. Christopher, Center for Practical Bioethics
Don E. Detmer, University of Virginia School of Medicine
Kathleen A. Dracup, University of California, San Francisco, School of Nursing
Alexandra Drane, Eliza Corporation
Thomas Edes, U.S. Department of Veterans Affairs
Betty Ferrell, City of Hope Medical Center
Anita K. Jones, University of Virginia
Judith R. Lave, University of Pittsburgh
Joanne Lynn, Center on Elder Care and Advanced Illness, Altarum Institute
Willard G. Manning, The University of Chicago

Charlie Sabatino, American Bar Association Commission on Law and Aging
Tracy Schroepfer, University of Wisconsin–Madison
Mark D. Smith, California HealthCare Foundation
VJ Periyakoil, Stanford University School of Medicine
James W. Vaupel, Max Planck Institute for Demographic Research
Joanne Wolfe, Children's Hospital Boston

Although the reviewers listed above provided many constructive comments and suggestions, they were not asked to endorse the report's conclusions or recommendations, nor did they see the final draft of the report before its release. The review of this report was overseen by **Bradford H. Gray,** The Urban Institute, and **Donald M. Steinwachs,** Johns Hopkins University. Appointed by the National Research Council and the Institute of Medicine, they were responsible for making certain that an independent examination of this report was carried out in accordance with institutional procedures and that all review comments were carefully considered. Responsibility for the final content of this report rests entirely with the authoring committee and the institution.

Foreword

In spring 2009, bills for what eventually became the Patient Protection and Affordable Care Act were being drafted in the House and Senate. A bipartisan group of representatives sponsored a provision in the House version of the bill that would have authorized Medicare to pay doctors who counsel patients about living wills, advance directives, and options for end-of-life care. AARP endorsed the provision. However, pundits, bloggers, op-ed writers, talk show hosts, and other legislators claimed the provision would lead to government-sponsored euthanasia and heartless "death panels" that would adjudicate who shall live. The administration distanced itself from the proposal, which never found its way into the law.

Still, the specter of death panels had staying power. One 2011 poll of American adults found that 23 percent believed the Affordable Care Act gave government the power to make end-of-life decisions on behalf of seniors, and 36 percent were not sure. When Donald Berwick became commissioner of the Centers for Medicare & Medicaid Services, he attempted to authorize payment for counseling on advance care planning as part of annual wellness visits provided for under the Affordable Care Act. This provision was to go into effect on January 1, 2011. By January 4, the administration had withdrawn this provision. Doctors would still be free to talk with patients about living wills, hospice care, or other end-of-life concerns, but they could not bill Medicare for this service.

The controversy on this topic and the political desire to avoid it do not alter the fact that every person will face the end of life one day, and many have had hard experience with the final days of a parent, a spouse, a child, a sibling, another relative, or a dear friend. At a time when public leaders hesitate to speak on a subject that is profoundly consequential for the health and well-being of all Americans, it is incumbent on others to examine the facts dispassionately, assess what can be done to make those final days better, and promote a reasoned and respectful public discourse on the subject.

With these goals in mind, the Institute of Medicine undertook the study documented in this report. A public-spirited donor, wishing to remain anonymous, came forward to support this study. We are grateful to this donor and to the outstanding and diverse committee, skillful co-chairs, and able staff who produced this comprehensive and compelling report. We hope it will stimulate the personal and public conversations and changes necessary to honor individual preferences and meet everyone's needs at the end of life.

Harvey V. Fineberg, M.D., Ph.D.   Victor J. Dzau, M.D.
Former President, Institute of Medicine   President, Institute of Medicine

Preface

Death is ultimately a deeply personal human experience that evokes different reactions, emotions, and perceptions from individuals, families, and communities throughout the life cycle. The perception of death is different for children, adults seen to be in the prime of life, and those in the later years of life, but it is also highly subjective and deeply personal irrespective of when it occurs along the life journey.

Perceptions and views about death are also influenced by a wide array of social, cultural, economic, geographic, spiritual, and religious beliefs and experiences. While most people have given thought to how they would like to die, many have found it difficult to communicate those views and choices to family and loved ones, and in many cases, family and loved ones have their own perceptions and views about death that can influence discussions about dying. Even when individuals and families are aligned, societal norms, expectations, and requirements are not always concordant with the patient's wishes and choices. No one really knows whether, in the end, the death of a loved one occurred with the dignity that was hoped for, or to what degree the dying experience was marred by pain, fear, and discomfort, emotional or physical.

Unfortunately, the evidence demonstrates that even if one completes an advance directive or has a discussion on the subject with family and loved ones, it tends to be separated from the time of dying by months, years, or even decades. Most people envision their own death as a peaceful and an ideally rapid transition. But with the exception of accidents or trauma or of a few illnesses that almost invariably result in death weeks or months after diagnosis, death comes at the end of a chronic illness or the frailty accompanying old age. Few people really have the opportunity to know when their death will occur.

Even though death is very much part of the cycle of life and the journey to physical dying begins with the inception of living, thinking and talking about one's own death usually remains in the background, at least until its prospect become more probable or imminent. Of course, death can occur without warning, as it does with assaults and trauma, whether accidental or purposeful. Sudden death can also occur with certain illnesses, but death most often is more insidious and the result of a chronic illness or disease. And while it is true that the likelihood of death increases with age, it is also true that death occurs throughout the life cycle. As a discipline, moreover, medicine is filled with examples of faulty predictions offered prospectively, sometimes too tentatively and often too definitively. Humility about the inability to predict the actual time of death is an important attribute for the health care professional regardless of discipline or area of expertise.

As longevity becomes more common and disease leading to early and frequent death becomes less prevalent, it is easy to be lulled into the belief that death may be postponed or, as some prominent figures have forecast, even avoided. To be sure, advances in science and medicine and the burgeoning field of stem cell biology and regenerative medicine offer the prospect of delaying death to a much greater extent than previously thought possible. After all, in just one century, life expectancy in the United States rose from age 47 to 78, and individuals over 90 are now the most rapidly growing (albeit still a small) portion of the population. It appears probable that many children being born today will still be active at the turn of the next century. Still, death will inevitably occur.

While optimism about the prospect of continued life abounds, fears about death—or at least how it can happen or who governs it—can easily be stoked. Witness the impact of the unfortunate (although purposeful) choice of the words "death panels" during the heated debate surrounding the passage of the Patient Protection and Affordable Care Act in August 2009. Those two words conveyed that individual choice in how one faces dying and death could be supplanted by a distant and uncaring bureaucracy. While this fear was unfounded, its very presence and the ease with which it was evoked underscore the sensitivity of the topic of their personal mortality for many Americans, especially the elderly. That 20 percent of the U.S. population will be older than 65 by 2050 further demonstrates the importance of finding ways to improve the quality of the final days of life and honoring individual choices about end-of-life issues and concerns.

The Institute of Medicine (IOM) has played an important role in conversations and policies surrounding end-of-life care. In 1997, the IOM produced the report *Approaching Death: Improving Care at the End of Life*, and in 2003, it extended the conversation to pediatrics in its report *When*

Children Die: Improving Palliative and End-of-Life Care for Children and Their Families. Each of these reports has had a major impact on end-of-life care, and a number of new programs, policies, providers, and systems of care have developed as a consequence. While many of the observations from these two major reports remain relevant, the United States has undergone many changes in its demography, in health care outcomes, and in the costs of health care delivery since these reports were published. Indeed, the past several years have witnessed a heightened focus on health care in this country, on what does and does not work, and on how systems of care vary across the population and differ from those of other developed countries. There is no question that while the cost of care in the United States is the highest in the world, the outcomes of care are not superior to those in other nations in any dimension or metric. And while cost should not by itself drive how high-quality, evidence-based care is delivered, it must be part of the dialogue. This applies to the care provided throughout the life course.

In 2012, the leadership of the IOM determined that another study on the end of life was needed given the intense ongoing dialogue surrounding health care reform in the United States. Dr. Harvey Fineberg, who was then president of the IOM, determined that this study should be conducted by a committee led by co-chairs whose collective expertise bridged the spectrum of the health care debate. One of us (Philip A. Pizzo) has spent decades caring for children and families with catastrophic disease facing the prospect of death. He has also been deeply steeped in biomedical research and the leadership of two major academic medical centers. The other (David M. Walker) has extensive experience in connection with fiscal responsibility and health care policy issues. His leadership experience spans all three major sectors of the U.S. economy. Of course each of us also brought personal history and experiences to the endeavor that resulted in areas of overlap, synergy, and sometimes difference in perspective. Our consensus committee included 19 other members, each with deep expertise related to various aspects of the medical, social, economic, ethical, and spiritual dimensions surrounding death.

Along with our highly competent study director, Dr. Adrienne Stith Butler, the committee held six meetings and hosted numerous discussions by phone, email, and other forms of communication. Those discussions generated both heat and light and gave witness to the strong and sometimes polarizing views that are engaged around the topic of the death and dying of vulnerable patients and families. Understandably, there were times when dialogues and debates seemed to reach an impasse, reflecting the larger public conversation (or the lack thereof) about various dimensions of the end of life. At the same time, those discussions helped sharpen our understanding of the issues involved and ultimately enabled us to reach consensus on conclusions and recommendations that we hope will further shape the national conversation on dying in America.

As committee co-chairs, we owe a deep debt of gratitude to all the committee members for their time, energy, passion, commitment, and diligence. In the end, we share a common goal of improving the individual and highly personal experience of dying in America. We also want to thank the IOM members and staff who provided invaluable support for this study. Dr. Judith Salerno, who was Leonard D. Schaeffer executive officer of the IOM when our work commenced, left the IOM to become CEO of the Susan G. Komen Breast Cancer Foundation. Without missing a beat, she sustained her commitment and dedication to the committee's work, as evidenced by her active and continued participation in committee meetings, discussions, and debates. We also want to thank Dr. Stephanie Pincus for her commitment and important insights, as well as Thelma Cox, Bradley Eckert, and Lauren Shern for their support. In addition, we were the beneficiaries of the writing and insights of Neil and Vicki Weisfeld, who enabled our discussion and debates to be framed in words with substance. Each of these many individuals exceeded expectations and enabled our progress to be sustained and successful. We also want to thank the numerous individuals who provided public testimony in person or in writing. The insights we received were invaluable and helped ground us in reality. It is our hope that this report will capture those insights and ultimately lead to improvements in end-of-life care and the experience of dying for all.

Philip A. Pizzo, *Co-Chair*
David M. Walker, *Co-Chair*
Committee on Approaching Death:
Addressing Key End-of-Life Issues

Acknowledgments

Several individuals and organizations made important contributions to the study committee's process and to this report. The committee wishes to thank these individuals, but recognizes that attempts to identify all and acknowledge their contributions would require more space than is available in this brief section.

To begin, the committee would like to thank the sponsor of this study. Funds for the committee's work were provided by a donor that wishes to remain anonymous. The committee gratefully acknowledges the contributions of the many individuals and organizations that assisted in the conduct of this study. Their perspectives were valuable in understanding critical topics with regard to end-of-life care. The committee thanks those individuals who provided important presentations and oral testimony at its open workshops. Appendix A lists each of these individuals and their affiliations. Written testimony received from hundreds of individuals and organizations also helped the committee understand the experiences of those who are likely approaching death and their family members and caregivers, as well as health care providers, and the perspectives of many stakeholder organizations. Appendix C provides a summary of this input. We would also like to thank the following Institute of Medicine (IOM) staff for their valuable contributions to this study: Jim Banihashemi, Daniel Bethea, Marton Cavani, Laura Harbold DeStefano, Chelsea Frakes, Greta Gorman, Jim Jensen, Nicole Joy, Abbey Meltzer, and Jennifer Walsh. The committee is grateful for the time, effort, and valuable information provided by all of these dedicated individuals and organizations.

The committee would like to thank the authors whose commissioned papers added to the evidence base for this study: Haiden A. Huskamp, Harvard Medical School, and David G. Stevenson, Vanderbilt University School of Medicine; Melissa D. Aldridge and Amy S. Kelley, Icahn School of Medicine at Mount Sinai; and Chris Feudtner, Wenjun Zhong, Jen Faerber, and Dingwei Dai, Children's Hospital of Philadelphia, and James Feinstein, Northwestern University. The committee is also grateful to Bryan Doerries, artistic director for Outside the Wire, and to T. Ryder Smith and Alex Morf, who performed at an event sponsored by the IOM and the committee at the Chautauqua Institution. Great thanks are owed as well to Sherra Babcock, who first extended the invitation for the IOM's participation at the Chautauqua Institution, and George Murphy, who was instrumental in coordinating the logistics of the event. The committee is also grateful to Maureen Valenza from The University of Texas MD Anderson Cancer Center and Mira Engel from the Stanford University School of Medicine, who helped to coordinate the committee's off-site meetings.

Contents

ACRONYMS   xxi

SUMMARY   1

1   INTRODUCTION   21
    Why This Study Is Important Now, 24
    Study Charge and Approach, 25
    Study Scope, 29
    17 Years of Progress, 32
    Dying in America: 2014, 33
    Research Needs, 39
    Summary, 39
    Organization of the Report, 40
    References, 41

2   THE DELIVERY OF PERSON-CENTERED,
    FAMILY-ORIENTED END-OF-LIFE CARE   45
    Review of the Current Situation, 46
    The Palliative Approach, 55
    The Pursuit of Quality in Care Near the End of Life, 74
    The Problem of Prognosis, 87
    Family Caregivers, 92
    Research Needs, 97
    Findings, Conclusions, and Recommendation, 100
    References, 104

3   CLINICIAN-PATIENT COMMUNICATION AND ADVANCE
    CARE PLANNING   117
    Background, 119
    The Current State of Advance Care Planning and
        What It Achieves, 124
    Advance Care Planning and Treatment Preferences Among
        Specific Population Groups, 141
    Elements of Good Communication in Advance Care Planning, 157
    Model Advance Care Planning Initiatives, 172
    A Proposed Life Cycle Model of Advance Care Planning, 185
    Research Needs, 187
    Findings, Conclusions, and Recommendation, 189
    References, 191
    Annex 3-1: Advance Care Planning in the Context of Common
        Serious Conditions, 211
    Annex 3-2: Oregon Physician Orders for Life-Sustaining
        Treatment (POLST) Form, 217

4   PROFESSIONAL EDUCATION AND DEVELOPMENT   221
    Progress and Continuing Needs, 221
    Impediments to Changing the Culture of Care Through
        Education, 225
    Roles and Preparation of Palliative Care Team Members, 237
    Findings, Conclusions, and Recommendation, 250
    References, 253

5   POLICIES AND PAYMENT SYSTEMS TO SUPPORT
    HIGH-QUALITY END-OF-LIFE CARE   263
    The Quality Challenges, 266
    The Cost Challenges, 267
    Financing and Organization of End-of-Life Care, 271
    Perverse Incentives and Program Misalignment, 275
    The Gap Between Services Paid for and What Patients and
        Families Want and Need, 307
    The Changing Health Care System: Financing and
        Organization, 314
    The Need for Greater Transparency and Accountability, 324
    Research Needs, 326
    Findings, Conclusions, and Recommendation, 328
    References, 331

6   PUBLIC EDUCATION AND ENGAGEMENT   345
    The State of Public Knowledge About End-of-Life Care, 347
    The Changing Climate for Discussion of Death and Dying, 352
    Considerations for Public Education and Engagement
        Campaigns, 355
    Controversial Issues, 362
    Recommendation, 370
    References, 371
    Annex 6-1: Selected Public Engagement Campaigns on
        Health-Related Topics, 378

GLOSSARY   385

APPENDIXES
A   Data Sources and Methods   391
B   Recommendations of the Institute of Medicine's Reports
    Approaching Death (1997) and *When Children Die* (2003):
    Progress and Significant Remaining Gaps   407
C   Summary of Written Public Testimony   443
D   Financing Care at the End of Life and the Implications of
    Potential Reforms   455
E   Epidemiology of Serious Illness and High Utilization of
    Health Care   487
F   Pediatric End-of-Life and Palliative Care: Epidemiology and
    Health Service Use   533
G   Committee Biographies   573

Acronyms

AACN	American Association of Colleges of Nursing
AAHPM	American Academy of Hospice and Palliative Medicine
AAMC	Association of American Medical Colleges
ABIM	American Board of Internal Medicine
ABMS	American Board of Medical Specialties
ACA	Patient Protection and Affordable Care Act
ACC	associate certified chaplain
ACE	Aid to Capacity Evaluation
ACGME	Accreditation Council for Graduate Medical Education
ACL	Administration for Community Living
ACO	accountable care organization
ACOVE	Assessing Care of Vulnerable Elders initiative
ADL	activity of daily living
AGS	American Geriatrics Society
AHRQ	Agency for Healthcare Research and Quality
AoA	Administration on Aging
APACHE	Acute Physiology and Chronic Health Evaluation
APC	Association of Professional Chaplains
APHA	American Public Health Association
AP-NORC	Associated Press-National Opinion Research Center
AQC	Alternative Quality Contract
ARRA	American Recovery and Reinvestment Act of 2009
ASHP	American Society of Health-System Pharmacists
ASPE	Assistant Secretary for Planning and Evaluation

BCC	board certified chaplain
BCCI	Board of Chaplaincy Certification Inc.
BCC-PCC	board certified chaplain-palliative care certified
BPCII	Medicare Bundled Payments for Care Improvement Initiative
BPS	Board of Pharmacy Specialties
CAPC	Center to Advance Palliative Care
CARE	Consumer Assessments and Reports of End of Life
CARING	Cancer, Admissions ≥2, Residence in a nursing home, Intensive care unit admit with multiorgan failure, ≥2 Noncancer hospice Guidelines
CBO	Congressional Budget Office
CCC	complex chronic condition
CCCC	Community Conversations on Compassionate Care
CCU	critical care unit
CDC	Centers for Disease Control and Prevention
CHCF	California HealthCare Foundation
CHF	congestive heart failure
CHIP	Children's Health Insurance Program
ChiPACC	Children's Program of All-Inclusive Coordinated Care for Children and Their Families
ChiPPS	Children's International Project on Palliative/Hospice Services
CLASS	Community Living Assistance Services and Supports Act
CMS	Centers for Medicare & Medicaid Services
COPD	chronic obstructive pulmonary disease
CPR	cardiopulmonary resuscitation
C-TraC	Coordinated-Transitional Care
DNR	do not resuscitate
DO	doctor of osteopathy
DRG	diagnosis-related group
ED	emergency department
EHB	essential health benefit
ELNEC	End-of-Life Nursing Education Consortium
EMS	emergency medical services
EMT	emergency medical technician
ENABLE	Educate, Nurture, Advise Before Life Ends intervention
EPEC	Education in Palliative and End-of-life Care Program
EPSDT	Early Periodic Screening, Diagnosis, and Treatment

ER	emergency room
ESRD	end-stage renal disease
FDA	U.S. Food and Drug Administration
FFS	fee-for-service
GDP	gross domestic product
GRACE	Geriatric Resources for Assessment and Care of Elders
HCAT	Hopkins Competency Assessment Test
HCBS	home- and community-based services
HCUP	Healthcare Cost and Utilization Project
HEDIS	Healthcare Effectiveness Data and Information Set
HHS	U.S. Department of Health and Human Services
HIPAA	Health Insurance Portability and Accountability Act
HIS	Hospice Item Set
HITECH	Health Information Technology for Economic and Clinical Health Act
HMDCB	Hospice Medical Director Certification Board
HPM	hospice and palliative medicine
HPNA	Hospice and Palliative Nurses Association
HQRP	Hospice Quality Reporting Program
HRS	Health and Retirement Study
IADL	instrumental activity of daily living
ICD	implantable cardioverter defibrillator or International Classification of Diseases
ICU	intensive care unit
IHI	Institute for Healthcare Improvement
IPPC	Initiative for Pediatric Palliative Care
KFF	The Henry J. Kaiser Family Foundation
KID	Kids' Inpatient Dataset
MA	Medicare Advantage
MEPS	Medical Expenditure Panel Survey
MMA	Medicare Prescription Drug Improvement and Modernization Act of 2003
MOLST	Medical Orders for Life-Sustaining Treatment
MSSP	Medicare Shared Savings Program
NASW	National Association of Social Workers

NBCHPN®	National Board for Certification of Hospice and Palliative Nurses
NCCN	National Comprehensive Cancer Network
NCHS	National Center for Health Statistics
NCI	National Cancer Institute
NCOA	National Council on Aging
NCP	National Consensus Project for Quality Palliative Care
NCQA	National Committee for Quality Assurance
NDS	National Data Set
NEDS	Nationwide Emergency Department Sample
NHDD	National Healthcare Decisions Day
NHPCO	National Hospice and Palliative Care Organization
NIH	National Institutes of Health
NINR	National Institute of Nursing Research
NPCRC	National Palliative Care Research Center
NQF	National Quality Forum
OECD	Organisation for Economic Co-operation and Development
P4P	pay-for-performance
PACE	Program of All-inclusive Care for the Elderly
PACT	Patient Aligned Care Team
PaP	Palliative Prognostic score
PBRN	practice-based research network
PCLC	Palliative Care Leadership Center
PCORI	Patient-Centered Outcomes Research Institute
PCPI	American Medical Association-Physician Consortium for Performance Improvement
PCRC	Palliative Care Research Cooperative Group
PDIA	Project on Death in America
PDQ®	Physician Data Query
PEACE	Prepare, Embrace, Attend, Communicate, Empower Project
PEC	Pediatric Early Care program
PERCS	Program to Enhance Relational and Communication Skills
PHIS	Pediatric Health Information System
PIPS	Prognosis in Palliative Care Study
POLST	Physician Orders for Life-Sustaining Treatment
PPC	pediatric palliative care
PPCN	Pediatric Palliative Care Network
PPD	Premier Perspective Database

QALY	quality-adjusted life-year
QIP	Quality Incentive Program
RWJF	Robert Wood Johnson Foundation
SGR	sustainable growth rate
SNAP	Supplemental Nutrition Assistance Program
SNF	skilled nursing facility
SUPPORT	Study to Understand Prognoses and Preferences for Outcomes and Risks of Treatments
UTD	Understanding Treatment Disclosure
VA	U.S. Department of Veterans Affairs
WHO	World Health Organization

Summary[1]

Health care delivery for people nearing the end of life has changed significantly in the past two decades. Factors such as the increasing number of elderly Americans, structural barriers in access to care for certain populations, and a fragmented health care system present challenges to providing quality care near the end of life. There are, however, opportunities to improve this care, including a better understanding of ways to improve individuals' participation in advance care planning and shared decision making, provisions of the Patient Protection and Affordable Care Act (ACA), and efforts to develop quality measures to enable accountability. In light of these developments, the Institute of Medicine was asked to produce a comprehensive report on the current state of care for people of all ages who may be approaching death. The report focuses specifically on the subset of people with "a serious illness or medical condition who may be approaching death."

For most people, death results from one or more diseases that must be managed carefully over weeks, months, or even years. Ideally, health care harmonizes with social, psychological, and spiritual support as the end of life approaches. To achieve this goal, care near the end of life should be person-centered, family-oriented, and evidence-based. A palliative approach can offer patients near

---

[1]This summary does not include references. Citations for the discussion presented in the summary appear in the subsequent report chapters.

the end of life and their families the best chance of maintaining the highest possible quality of life for the longest possible time. Hospice is an important approach to addressing the palliative care needs of patients with limited life expectancy and their families. One of the greatest remaining challenges is the need for better understanding of the role of palliative care among both the public and professionals across the continuum of care so that hospice and palliative care can achieve their full potential for patients and their families.

As much as people may want and expect to be in control of decisions about their own care throughout their lives, numerous factors can work against realizing that desire. Many people nearing the end of life are not physically or cognitively able to make their own care decisions. It is often difficult to recognize or identify when the end of life is approaching, making clinician-patient communication and advance care planning particularly important. Advance care planning conversations often do not take place because patients, family members, and clinicians each wait for the other to initiate them. Understanding that advance care planning can reduce confusion and guilt among family members forced to make decisions about care can be sufficient motivation for ill individuals to make their wishes clear. Yet even when these important conversations have occurred and family members are confident that they know what the dying person wishes, making those decisions is emotionally difficult, and families need assistance and support in this role.

The education of health professionals who provide care to people nearing the end of life has improved substantially in the past two decades, although serious problems remain. Knowledge gains have not necessarily been transferred to clinicians caring for people with advanced serious illness who are nearing the end of life. In addition, the number of hospice and palliative care specialists is small, which means the need for palliative care also must be met through primary care and through the other clinical specialties that entail care for significant numbers of people nearing the end of life.

A substantial body of evidence shows that improved care for people near the end of life is a goal within the nation's reach. Improving the quality of care for people with advanced serious illness and focusing on their preferences may help stabilize both total health care and social costs over time. In the end-of-life arena, there are opportunities for savings by avoiding acute care services that patients and families do not want and that are unlikely to benefit them. The committee that produced this report believes these savings would free up funding for relevant supporting services—for example, caregiver training, nutrition services, and home safety modifications—that would ensure a better quality of life for people near the end of life and protect and support their families.

More than one-quarter of all adults, including those aged 75 and older, have given little or no thought to their end-of-life wishes, and even fewer have captured these wishes in writing or through conversation. This is the case despite the results of recent polls showing that Americans worry about the potential high costs of care near the end of life and desire not to be a burden—financial or otherwise—on family members. As the baby boom generation ages, public interest in and acceptance of information on death and dying may increase. Key considerations in developing public education and engagement campaigns on this topic include sponsorship and engagement of key stakeholders, selection of target audiences, crafting and testing of messages, and evaluation of results.

The recommendations presented in this report are intended to address the needs of patients and families. They also should assist policy makers, clinicians in various disciplines along with their educational and credentialing bodies, leaders of health care delivery and financing organizations, researchers, public and private funders, religious and community leaders, advocates for better care, journalists, and members of the interested public in learning more about what constitutes good care for people nearing the end of life and the steps necessary to achieve such care for more patients and families. The committee offers five recommendations in the areas of care delivery, clinician-patient communication and advance care planning, professional education and development, policies and payment systems, and public education and engagement, which collectively offer a roadmap for progress in the nation's approach to end-of-life care and management.

Health care delivery for people nearing the end of life has changed markedly since the Institute of Medicine (IOM) published *Approaching Death: Improving Care at the End of Life* (1997) and *When Children Die: Improving Palliative and End-of-Life Care for Children and Their Families* (2003). Among the challenges to providing health care to this population are the following factors:

- the increasing number of elderly Americans, including those with some combination of frailty, significant physical and cognitive disabilities, multiple chronic illnesses, and functional limitations;

- growing cultural diversity of the U.S. population, which makes it ever more important for clinicians to approach all patients as individuals, without assumptions about the care choices they might make;
- structural barriers in access to care that disadvantage certain population groups;
- a mismatch between the services patients and families need most and the services they can readily obtain;
- failure of the availability of palliative care services to keep pace with the growing demand;
- wasteful and costly systemic problems, including perverse financial incentives, a fragmented care delivery system, time pressures that limit communication, and a lack of service coordination across programs; and
- the resulting unsustainable growth in costs of the current health care delivery system over the past several decades.

These challenges are to some extent balanced by new opportunities for improving the delivery of health care near the end of life:

- an increased understanding of ways to improve participation in effective advance care planning and shared decision making among patients and families, including seriously ill children and adolescents, who may be able to participate in end-of-life decision making on their own behalf;
- various provisions of the Patient Protection and Affordable Care Act (ACA) and other system reforms that affect the organization and financing of health services;
- increasing use of communication and health information technologies, including electronic health records;
- growing recognition of and support for the role of caregivers; and
- efforts to develop quality measures to enable accountability.

To translate some of these opportunities into practice will require additional research; however, the greater challenge is to incorporate into practice the currently known evidence-based models of care.

STUDY CHARGE AND APPROACH

In view of these developments, the IOM was charged with conducting a consensus study to produce a comprehensive report on the current state of care for people of all ages who may be approaching death (see Box S-1). To conduct this study, the IOM assembled the 21-member Committee on Approaching Death: Addressing Key End-of-Life Issues, which comprised experts in clinical care, aging and geriatrics, hospice and palliative care, pediatrics, consumer advocacy, spirituality, ethics, communications, clinical decision making, health care financing, law, and public policy. The committee and the IOM recognize that many of the actions and systemic

---

BOX S-1
Study Charge

The Institute of Medicine (IOM) will conduct a consensus study that will produce a comprehensive report on the current state of medical care for persons of all ages with a serious illness or medical condition who may be approaching death and who require coordinated care, appropriate personal communication (or communication with parents or guardians for children), and individual and family support. The committee will assess the delivery of medical care, social, and other supports to both the person approaching death and the family; person-family-provider communication of values, preferences, and beliefs; advance care planning; health care costs, financing, and reimbursement; and education of health professionals, patients, families, employers, and the public at large. The study will also explore approaches to advance the field. Specifically, the committee will:

1. Review progress since the 1997 IOM report *Approaching Death: Improving Care at the End of Life* and the 2003 IOM report *When Children Die: Improving Palliative and End-of-Life Care for Children and Their Families.* The committee will assess major subsequent events and recommendations that have been implemented as well as those that were not implemented along with remaining challenges and opportunities.
2. Evaluate strategies to integrate care of those with serious illness or medical condition who may be approaching death into a person- and family-centered, team-based framework. Demographic shifts, cultural changes, fiscal realities, and the needs of vulnerable populations will be considered as will advances in technology that affect the provision of care in different settings, most notably in the home. Families are a vital component of the health care team, and the financial and other ramifications for families and society will be considered.
3. Develop recommendations for changes in policy, financing mechanisms and payment practices, workforce development, research and measurement, and clinical and supportive care. These recommendations will align care with individual values, preferences, and beliefs and promote high-quality, cost-effective care for persons with serious illness or medical condition who may be approaching death, as well as with their families.
4. Develop a dissemination and communication strategy to promote public engagement understanding, and action. This strategy will need to consider the fears and anxieties surrounding care for patients who may be approaching death as well as functional dependency, aging and death, and cultural diversity in values, preferences and beliefs.

changes that would improve care for people nearing the end of life would also benefit many other patient groups, especially those with advanced serious illnesses, severe chronic conditions, and the functional limitations that come with frailty. However, the committee's charge limited this study's focus specifically to the subset of people with "a serious illness or medical condition who may be approaching death."

This study was supported by a donor that wishes to remain anonymous and whose identity was unknown to the committee. The sponsor played no role in the selection of the committee's co-chairs or members or in its work. To carry out its charge, the committee reviewed evidence that has accumulated since the two earlier IOM studies cited above were produced; conducted public meetings and additional events to gather testimony from interested individuals; held six meetings of its members; and, via an active Web portal, received comments from more than 500 additional individuals. In addition, papers were commissioned on the financing, utilization, and costs of adult and pediatric end-of-life care. (See Appendix A for further discussion of the data sources and methods for this study.)

STUDY FINDINGS AND RECOMMENDATIONS

The recommendations presented in this report are intended to address the needs of patients and their families. They should also assist policy makers, clinicians in various disciplines along with their educational and credentialing bodies, leaders of health care delivery and financing organizations, researchers, public and private funders, religious and community leaders, advocates for better care, journalists, and members of the interested public in learning more about what constitutes good care for people nearing the end of life and the steps necessary to achieve such care for more patients and families. The committee offers five recommendations in the areas of care delivery, clinician-patient communication and advance care planning, professional education and development, policies and payment systems, and public education and engagement, which collectively offer a roadmap for progress in the nation's approach to end-of-life care and management.

The Delivery of Person-Centered, Family-Oriented End-of-Life Care

For most people, and except for those who die suddenly as a consequence of an accident or trauma, death results from one or more diseases that must be managed carefully over weeks, months, or even years, through many ups and downs. Ideally, health care harmonizes with social, psychological, and spiritual support as the end of life approaches. To achieve this goal, care near the end of life should be person-centered, family-oriented, and evidence-based.

A palliative[2] approach can offer patients near the end of life and their families the best chance of maintaining the highest possible quality of life for the longest possible time. The committee defined palliative care for this report as care that provides relief from pain and other symptoms, that supports quality of life, and that is focused on patients with serious advanced illness and their families. Hospice is an important approach to addressing the palliative care needs of patients with limited life expectancy and their families. For people with a terminal illness or at high risk of dying in the near future, hospice is a comprehensive, socially supportive, pain-reducing, and comforting alternative to technologically elaborate, medically centered interventions. It therefore has many features in common with palliative care.

Palliative care can begin early in the course of treatment for any serious illness that requires excellent management of pain or other distressing symptoms, such as difficulty breathing or swallowing, and for patients of any age. It can be provided in conjunction with treatments for cancer, heart disease, or congenital disorders, for example. Palliative care is provided in settings throughout the continuum of care. Often it is provided through hospital-based consultation programs and outside the hospital through hospice programs in the home, nursing home, assisted living facility, or long-term acute care facility; palliative care outpatient clinics are also becoming increasingly prevalent. Besides physician specialists in hospice and palliative medicine, interdisciplinary palliative care teams include specialty advanced practice nurses and registered nurses, social workers, chaplains, pharmacists, rehabilitation therapists, direct care workers, and family members.

A number of specialty professional associations encourage clinicians to counsel patients about palliative care, but too few patients and families receive this help in a timely manner. Palliative care programs and other providers that care for patients nearing the end of life are not currently required to measure and report on the quality of the end-of-life care they provide, nor is there consensus on quality measures. These gaps are a barrier to accountability. Only hospice programs report on the quality of end-of-life care.

As yet, the evidence base is insufficient to enable establishment of a validated list of the core components of quality end-of-life care across all settings and providers. The committee proposes a list of at least 12 such components (see Table S-1). They include frequent assessment of a patient's physical, emotional, social, and spiritual well-being; management of emo-

---

[2]Basic palliative care is provided by clinicians in primary care and various specialties that care for people with advanced serious illness, while specialty palliative care is provided by specialists in hospice and palliative medicine, nursing, social work, chaplaincy, and other palliative care fields.

tional distress; referral to expert-level hospice or palliative care if needed and desired; and regular revision of a care plan and access to services based on the changing needs of the patient and family.

The committee paid special attention to the growing demand for family caregiving. Family caregivers provide a wide range of essential and increasingly complex services for people with advanced serious illnesses and those nearing the end of life. Three in 10 U.S. adults are family caregivers (although this number represents all caregivers, not just those caring for someone near the end of life). This growing unpaid workforce generally is invisible; undertrained; and stressed physically, emotionally, and financially.

When the 1997 IOM report *Approaching Death: Improving Care at the End of Life* was published 17 years ago, hospice was well on its way to achieving mainstream status, and palliative care was in the early stages of development. Now, hospice is in the mainstream, and palliative care is well established in larger hospitals and in the professions of medicine, nursing, social work, and chaplaincy. Even so, one of the greatest remaining challenges is the need for better understanding of the role of palliative care among both the public and professionals across the continuum of care so that hospice and palliative care can achieve their full potential for patients of all ages with serious advanced illness.

TABLE S-1 Proposed Core Components of Quality End-of-Life Care

Component	Rationale
Frequent assessment of the patient's physical, emotional, social, and spiritual well-being	Interventions and assistance must be based on accurately identified needs.
Management of emotional distress	All clinicians should be able to identify distress and direct its initial and basic management. This is part of the definition of palliative care, a basic component of hospice, and clearly of fundamental importance.
Offer referral to expert-level palliative care	People with palliative needs beyond those that can be provided by non-specialist-level clinicians deserve access to appropriate expert-level care.
Offer referral to hospice if the patient has a prognosis of 6 months or less	People who meet the hospice eligibility criteria deserve access to services designed to meet their end-of-life needs.
Management of care and direct contact with patient and family for complex situations by a specialist-level palliative care physician	Care of people with serious illness may require specialist-level palliative care physician management, and effective physician management requires direct examination, contact, and communication.

TABLE S-1 Continued

Component	Rationale
Round-the-clock access to coordinated care and services	Patients in advanced stages of serious illness often require assistance, such as with activities of daily living, medication management, wound care, physical comfort, and psychosocial needs. Round-the-clock access to a consistent point of contact that can coordinate care obviates the need to dial 911 and engage emergency medical services.
Management of pain and other symptoms	All clinicians should be able to identify and direct the initial and basic management of pain and other symptoms. This is part of the definition of palliative care, a basic component of hospice, and clearly of fundamental importance.
Counseling of patient and family	Even patients who are not emotionally distressed face problems in such areas as loss of functioning, prognosis, coping with diverse symptoms, finances, and family dynamics, and family members experience these problems as well, both directly and indirectly.
Family caregiver support	A focus on the family is part of the definition of palliative care; family members and caregivers both participate in the patient's care and require assistance themselves.
Attention to the patient's social context and social needs	Person-centered care requires awareness of patients' perspectives on their social environment and of their needs for social support, including at the time of death. Companionship at the bedside at time of death may be an important part of the psychological, social, and spiritual aspects of end-of-life care for some individuals.
Attention to the patient's spiritual and religious needs	The final phase of life often has a spiritual and religious component, and research shows that spiritual assistance is associated with quality of care.
Regular personalized revision of the care plan and access to services based on the changing needs of the patient and family	Care must be person-centered and fit current circumstances, which may mean that not all the above components will be important or desirable in all cases.

NOTE: The proposed core components of quality end-of-life care listed in this table were developed by the committee. Most of the components relate to one of the domains in the Clinical Practice Guidelines for Quality Palliative Care set forth by the National Consensus Project for Quality Palliative Care.

Recommendation 1. Government health insurers and care delivery programs as well as private health insurers should cover the provision of comprehensive care for individuals with advanced serious illness who are nearing the end of life.

Comprehensive care should

- be seamless, high-quality, integrated, patient-centered, family-oriented, and consistently accessible around the clock;
- consider the evolving physical, emotional, social, and spiritual needs of individuals approaching the end of life, as well as those of their family and/or caregivers;
- be competently delivered by professionals with appropriate expertise and training;
- include coordinated, efficient, and interoperable information transfer across all providers and all settings; and
- be consistent with individuals' values, goals, and informed preferences.

Health care delivery organizations should take the following steps to provide comprehensive care:

- All people with advanced serious illness should have access to skilled palliative care or, when appropriate, hospice care in all settings where they receive care (including health care facilities, the home, and the community).
- Palliative care should encompass access to an interdisciplinary palliative care team, including board-certified hospice and palliative medicine physicians, nurses, social workers, and chaplains, together with other health professionals as needed (including geriatricians). Depending on local resources, access to this team may be on site, via virtual consultation, or by transfer to a setting with these resources and this expertise.
- The full range of care that is delivered should be characterized by transparency and accountability through public reporting of aggregate quality and cost measures for all aspects of the health care system related to end-of-life care. The committee believes that informed individual choices should be honored, including the right to decline medical or social services.

Clinician-Patient Communication and Advance Care Planning

As much as people may want and expect to be in control of decisions about their own care throughout their lives, numerous factors can work against realizing that desire. Many people nearing the end of life are not physically or cognitively able to make their own care decisions. It is often difficult to recognize or identify when the end of life is approaching, making clinician-patient communication and advance care planning particularly important. Advance directives were developed to ensure that the decisions people make when fully able are followed when they can no longer speak for themselves. However, these checkbox-style documents have proven inflexible, inconsistent with subsequent events and decisions, and for various reasons both ineffective and unpopular. Electronic storage of advance directives, statements of wishes, health care proxies, or other relevant material—either in the patient's electronic health record or in an external database—holds promise for addressing a few of the current problems (see also Recommendation 4).

The advance care planning process can start at any age and state of health and should involve family members and clinicians. The discussion centers on life values, goals, and treatment preferences; this knowledge, gained in periodic revisiting of perceptions over time, provides a guide for matching subsequent care decisions with the patient's wishes and becomes increasingly specific as illness progresses. Advance directives (forms) can be useful when they are a component of these more comprehensive discussions, but they must be flexible and give health care agents and clinicians leeway to make decisions based on specific circumstances.

People who capture their care preferences in discussion or writing most commonly choose care that focuses on improving quality of life. However, the vast majority of people have not engaged in an end-of-life discussion with their health care provider or family and do not have an advance directive. People who are younger, poorer, less educated, and nonwhite are less likely to have such a document. Moreover, within all population groups, end-of-life preferences vary widely. Clinicians and even close family members cannot accurately guess or assume what an individual's preferences will be; they must ask the patient—that is, have "the conversation"—and do so as often as necessary.

Advance care planning conversations often do not take place because patients, family members, and clinicians each wait for the other to initiate them. Understanding that advance care planning can reduce the burden of confusion and guilt among family members forced to make decisions about care can be sufficient motivation for ill individuals to make their wishes clear. Yet even when these important conversations have occurred and family members are confident that they know what the dying person wishes, making those decisions is emotionally difficult, and families need assistance and support in this role.

The overall quality of communication between clinicians and patients with advanced illness is poor, particularly with respect to discussing prognosis, dealing with emotional and spiritual concerns, and finding the right balance between hoping for the best and preparing for the worst. Ample evidence documents structural and financial disincentives for having these discussions. In the absence of adequate documented advance care planning, the default decision is to treat a disease or condition, no matter how hopeless or painful. A result of inadequate advance care planning, therefore, can be more intensive treatment, as well as more negative impacts on family members.

Because most people who participate in effective advance care planning choose maximizing independence and quality of life over living longer, advance care planning can potentially save health care costs associated with unnecessary and unwanted interventions. The misrepresentation of the ACA provisions for advance care planning as "death panels" confused many Americans about the benefits and goals of advance care planning, which amount to ensuring that patients' care preferences, insofar as possible, are honored. This caused the national dialogue to turn away from how best to facilitate earlier and more meaningful discussions about end-of-life preferences among individuals, families, and clinicians.

> **Recommendation 2. Professional societies and other organizations that establish quality standards should develop standards for clinician-patient communication and advance care planning that are measurable, actionable, and evidence-based.** These standards should change as needed to reflect the evolving population and health system needs and be consistent with emerging evidence, methods, and technologies. Payers and health care delivery organizations should adopt these standards and their supporting processes, and integrate them into assessments, care plans, and the reporting of health care quality. Payers should tie such standards to reimbursement, and professional societies should adopt policies that facilitate tying the standards to reimbursement, licensing, and credentialing to encourage
>
> - all individuals, including children with the capacity to do so, to have the opportunity to participate actively in their health care decision making throughout their lives and as they approach death, and receive medical and related social services consistent with their values, goals, and informed preferences;
> - clinicians to initiate high-quality conversations about advance care planning, integrate the results of these conversations into the

ongoing care plans of patients, and communicate with other clinicians as requested by the patient; and

- clinicians to continue to revisit advance care planning discussions with their patients because individuals' preferences and circumstances may change over time.

Professional Education and Development

The education of health professionals who provide care to people nearing the end of life has improved substantially since the two previous IOM reports cited above were published, although serious problems remain. Hospice and palliative medicine has become an established medical specialty. Other areas of progress include preparation of more faculty members to teach palliative care, greater inclusion of some palliative care content throughout clinical education, development of the professional infrastructure of palliative care organizations and journals, and expansion of the evidence base.

On the other hand, two important deficiencies persist. First, the knowledge gains have not necessarily been transferred to clinicians caring for people with advanced serious illness and nearing the end of life. Second, the number of hospice and palliative care specialists is small, which means the need for palliative care also must be met through primary care and through the other clinical specialties that entail care for significant numbers of people nearing the end of life (for example, cardiology, oncology, pulmonology, and nephrology).

In the committee's judgment, three deeply ingrained educational patterns obstruct further development of palliative care. First, hospice and palliative care are generally absent from the usual curricula of medical and nursing schools. One way to ensure attention to this topic in the undergraduate curriculum, in graduate training, and among future health professionals would be to add more such content to licensure and certification examinations.

A second negative pattern is the persistence of single-profession education silos. This is problematic because palliative care embraces an interdisciplinary, team-based approach.

A third pattern, most notable among physicians, is the lack of attention to developing clinicians' ability to talk effectively to patients about dying and teaching them to take the time to truly listen to patients' expression of their concerns, values, and goals. Studies have established that physicians can be taught the communication skills needed to provide good end-of-life care, but few medical educators teach these skills. *Approaching Death* (IOM, 1997) and *When Children Die* (IOM, 2003) specify the same four domains of clinical competency in palliative care: scientific and clinical knowledge, interpersonal skills and knowledge, ethical and professional principles, and organizational skills. These domains are as relevant today as they were when those earlier reports were produced.

In addition to physician board certification in hospice and palliative medicine, the fields of nursing, social work, and chaplaincy all have established specialty certification programs in hospice and palliative care, although the number of certified individuals in each of these professions remains small relative to the need. Pharmacists also play important roles in palliative care, although the pharmacy field has no comparable certification program. From time to time, as needed, rehabilitation therapists specializing in occupational therapy, physical therapy, and speech-language pathology become additional members of the palliative care team. At the bedside, vital roles are played by direct care workers—a category that comprises nursing assistants, home health aides, and personal care aides. Finally, and in many ways most important, are family members. Even those who are not fully engaged as caregivers may have considerable day-to-day responsibility for patient management at home and coordination of care across services and among care providers.

> **Recommendation 3. Educational institutions, credentialing bodies, accrediting boards, state regulatory agencies, and health care delivery organizations should establish the appropriate training, certification, and/or licensure requirements to strengthen the palliative care knowledge and skills of all clinicians who care for individuals with advanced serious illness who are nearing the end of life.**

Specifically,

- all clinicians across disciplines and specialties who care for people with advanced serious illness should be competent in basic palliative care, including communication skills, interprofessional collaboration, and symptom management;
- educational institutions and professional societies should provide training in palliative care domains throughout the professional's career;
- accrediting organizations, such as the Accreditation Council for Graduate Medical Education, should require palliative care education and clinical experience in programs for all specialties responsible for managing advanced serious illness (including primary care clinicians);
- certifying bodies, such as the medical, nursing, and social work specialty boards, and health systems should require knowledge, skills, and competency in palliative care;

- state regulatory agencies should include education and training in palliative care in licensure requirements for physicians, nurses, chaplains, social workers, and others who provide health care to those nearing the end of life;
- entities that certify specialty-level health care providers should create pathways to certification that increase the number of health care professionals who pursue specialty-level palliative care training; and
- entities such as health care delivery organizations, academic medical centers, and teaching hospitals that sponsor specialty-level training positions should commit institutional resources to increasing the number of available training positions for specialty-level palliative care.

Policies and Payment Systems to Support High-Quality End-of-Life Care

A substantial body of evidence shows that greatly improved care for people nearing the end of life is a goal within the nation's reach. At the same time, broad agreement exists across the political and ideological spectrum that the United States must take steps to stabilize expenditures on health care over time. In addressing care at the end of life, these goals can be reached in tandem: evidence indicates that improving the quality of care and the availability of services to meet patients' and families' most pressing needs does not have to entail increased expenditures.

Improving quality of care for people with advanced serious illness and focusing on their preferences may help stabilize total health care and social costs over time. In the end-of-life arena, there are opportunities for savings by avoiding acute care services that patients and families do not want and that are unlikely to benefit them. The committee believes these savings would free up funding for relevant supporting services—for example, caregiver training, nutrition services, and home safety modifications—that would ensure a better quality of life for people near the end of life and protect and support their families.

What requires closer examination and reform is how those resources are spent; the ways in which perverse financial incentives distort the current system and impede high-quality care; how geographic variations in expenditures can be reduced; and whether currently funded services are well matched to the values, goals, preferences, diverse cultural differences, expectations, and needs of patients and families, with ample evidence suggesting they are not.

U.S. national health care expenditures totaled $2.8 trillion in 2012, or about 17.2 percent of gross domestic product (GDP). Although the annual increase in health care spending has slowed in recent years, the size of the sector and the possibility of continued future growth remain a significant concern to analysts across the political spectrum. Of particular concern is the likely growth in public spending on health care, a consequence in part of growing numbers of people eligible for Medicare as baby boomers age and for Medicaid as expansions under the ACA are implemented. These two programs are especially important in the end-of-life context because approximately 80 percent of U.S. deaths occur among people covered by Medicare, and Medicaid is the principal payer for long-term services needed by frail elderly individuals. The inefficiencies and payment incentives that have evolved in these two programs create opportunities for savings that, if recovered, could pay for a needed expansion in key supporting services and stabilize the costs of care for these patients.

A major reorientation and restructuring of Medicare, Medicaid, and other health care delivery programs is needed to craft a system of care designed to ensure quality and address the central needs of all people nearing the end of life and their families. Current financial incentives and a lack of more appropriate alternatives drive a reliance on the riskiest and most costly care settings. These incentives should be changed, and positive alternatives should be further developed.

In addition, many of the most urgent needs of these patients and their families are not medical per se and require the design and implementation of affordable support service programs that rigorously target the highest-risk patients and families, and tailor services to specific family needs as they evolve over time.

This approach, the essence of person-centeredness, is fundamental to achieving the efficiency goals of public financing programs: on the one hand, Medicare's efforts to decrease utilization of unnecessary acute care and on the other, Medicaid's attempts to prevent unnecessary use of nursing homes. These goals cannot be met without improving the supporting services that allow families to keep their loved ones safe and well cared for in the setting where the vast majority of seriously ill patients want to be—at home, which for some people may be an assisted living residence, nursing home, or skilled nursing facility.

The U.S. health care system is changing significantly. This fact underscores the need to establish additional accountability and transparency measures so that the effects of these changes—both intended and unintended—on people nearing the end of life can be assessed. Further changes in health care policy and legislation may be required to serve this group of Americans well.

Recommendation 4. Federal, state, and private insurance and health care delivery programs should integrate the financing of medical and

social services to support the provision of quality care consistent with the values, goals, and informed preferences of people with advanced serious illness nearing the end of life. To the extent that additional legislation is necessary to implement this recommendation, the administration should seek and Congress should enact such legislation. In addition, the federal government should require public reporting on quality measures, outcomes, and costs regarding care near the end of life (e.g., in the last year of life) for programs it funds or administers (e.g., Medicare, Medicaid, the U.S. Department of Veterans Affairs). The federal government should encourage all other payment and health care delivery systems to do the same.

Specifically, actions should

- provide financial incentives for
    - medical and social support services that decrease the need for emergency room and acute care services,
    - coordination of care across settings and providers (from hospital to ambulatory settings as well as home and community), and
    - improved shared decision making and advance care planning that reduces the utilization of unnecessary medical services and those not consistent with a patient's goals for care;
- require the use of interoperable electronic health records that incorporate advance care planning to improve communication of individuals' wishes across time, settings, and providers, documenting (1) the designation of a surrogate/decision maker, (2) patient values and beliefs and goals for care, (3) the presence of an advance directive, and (4) the presence of medical orders for life-sustaining treatment for appropriate populations; and
- encourage states to develop and implement a Physician Orders for Life-Sustaining Treatment (POLST) paradigm program in accordance with nationally standardized core requirements.

Medical and social services provided should accord with a person's values, goals, informed preferences, condition, circumstances, and needs, with the expectation that individual service needs and intensity will change over time. High-quality, comprehensive, person-centered, and family-oriented care will help reduce preventable crises that lead to repeated use of 911 calls, emergency department visits, and hospital admissions, and if implemented appropriately, should contribute to stabilizing aggregate societal expenditures for medical and related social services and potentially lowering them over time.

Public Education and Engagement

The IOM's 1997 report *Approaching Death* (p. 270) concludes that "a continuing public discussion is essential to develop a better understanding of the modern experience of dying, the options available to patients and families, and the obligations of communities to those approaching death." Likewise, the IOM's 2003 report *When Children Die* calls for better communication about end-of-life issues in ways that encompass but are somewhat broader than the activities of advance care planning. In the years since these reports were published, the need for public education and engagement concerning end-of-life care has not abated, and it is manifest at several levels:

- at the societal level, to build support for constructive public policy related to the organization and financing of care near the end of life and for institutional and provider practices that ensure that this care is high-quality and sustainable;
- at the community and family levels, to raise public awareness of care options in the final phase of life, the needs of caregivers, and the hallmarks of high-quality care; and
- at the individual level, to motivate and facilitate advance care planning and meaningful conversations with family, caregivers, and clinicians about values, goals, and informed preferences for care.

More than one-quarter of all adults, including those aged 75 and older, have given little or no thought to their end-of-life wishes, and even fewer have captured these wishes in writing or through conversation. This is the case despite the results of recent polls showing Americans harbor several consistent worries about care near the end of life, centered around its potential high costs and the desire not to be a burden—financial or otherwise—on family members.

Expecting people to understand or have meaningful conversations about end-of-life care issues presumes a common vocabulary; however, surveys show people do not understand what palliative care is or what role it plays near the end of life, do not have a clear concept of "caregiver," and may be confused by the various titles assigned by state laws to people who serve as health care agents (such as surrogate decision makers or proxies). Even some clinicians mistakenly confuse palliative care (care oriented toward quality of life for people with serious illnesses) with hospice (a model for delivering palliative care for people in their last months of life).

Events and activities since 1997 have improved the climate for discussions of death and dying, and the topic is not as taboo as it was a few decades ago. As the baby boom generation ages, public interest in and acceptance of information on death and dying may increase. Key considerations in developing public education and engagement campaigns on this topic include sponsorship and engagement of key stakeholders, selection of target audiences, crafting and testing of messages, selection of the media mix, and evaluation. Meanwhile, stories about dying—"good deaths" and bad ones—appear regularly in the news media, in entertainment television programming and movies, in books, and in social media.

Conflicts of values related to end-of-life care can be expected in a heterogeneous nation such as the United States. People's views on serious illness and the end of life, bereavement and loss, and the duties of caregivers are deeply held and vary widely among individuals. While people may differ in their opinions, it is important to disseminate accurate information and evidence so that those opinions are based, to the extent possible, on the facts as they are known and a candid assessment of their limits.

> **Recommendation 5. Civic leaders, public health and other governmental agencies, community-based organizations, faith-based organizations, consumer groups, health care delivery organizations, payers, employers, and professional societies should engage their constituents and provide fact-based information about care of people with advanced serious illness to encourage advance care planning and informed choice based on the needs and values of individuals.**
>
> Specifically, these organizations and groups should
>
> - use appropriate media and other channels to reach their audiences, including underserved populations;
> - provide evidence-based information about care options and informed decision making regarding treatment and care;
> - encourage meaningful dialogue among individuals and their families and caregivers, clergy, and clinicians about values, care goals, and preferences related to advanced serious illness; and
> - dispel misinformation that may impede informed decision making and public support for health system and policy reform regarding care near the end of life.
>
> In addition,
>
> - health care delivery organizations should provide information and materials about care near the end of life as part of their practices to facilitate clinicians' ongoing dialogue with patients, families, and caregivers;

- government agencies and payers should undertake, support, and share communication and behavioral research aimed at assessing public perceptions and actions with respect to end-of-life care, developing and testing effective messages and tailoring them to appropriate audience segments, and measuring progress and results; and
- health care professional societies should prepare educational materials and encourage their members to engage patients and their caregivers and families in advance care planning, including end-of-life discussions and decisions.

All of the above groups should work collaboratively, sharing successful strategies and promising practices across organizations.

CONCLUSION

The committee identified persistent major gaps in care near the end of life that require urgent attention from numerous stakeholder groups. Understanding and perceptions of death and dying vary considerably across the population and are influenced by culture, socioeconomic status, and education, as well as by misinformation and fear. Engaging people in defining their own values, goals, and preferences concerning care at the end of life and ensuring that their care team understands their wishes has proven remarkably elusive and challenging.

While the clinical fields of hospice and palliative care have become more established, the number of specialists in these fields is too small, and too few clinicians in primary and specialty fields that entail caring for individuals with advanced serious illness are proficient in basic palliative care. Often clinicians are reluctant to have honest and direct conversations with patients and families about end-of-life issues. Patients and families face additional difficulties presented by the health care system itself, which does not provide adequate financial or organizational support for the kinds of health care and social services that might truly make a difference to them.

In sum, the committee believes that a patient-centered, family-oriented approach to care near the end of life should be a high national priority and that compassionate, affordable, and effective care for these patients is an achievable goal.

Introduction

Every American has a stake in improving care for people nearing the end of life. For patients and their families, that stake is immediate and personal, and no care decisions are more profound. For the millions of Americans who work with or within the health care sector—clinicians, clergy, other direct care providers, and support staff—the stake is a matter of professional commitment and responsibility. Health system managers, payers, and policy makers also have a professional stake in the provision of end-of-life care that is not only high quality but also affordable and sustainable. All Americans should be able to expect that they and their loved ones will receive the care and services they need at the end of their lives. Meanwhile, the number of Americans with some combination of aging, frailty, dependence, and multiple chronic conditions is rising, placing growing pressure on the health system at every level and on every stakeholder group.

As this report shows, the advances in medicine and health care that today help people survive advanced illnesses and serious injuries have been accompanied by several collateral effects:

- growing frustration among health care professionals at the mismatch between their training and the complex needs of the people they serve;
- a high—and escalating—financial price, which includes costs for interventions that many people near the end of life do not want and that may be unlikely to benefit them; and

- a perception among many Americans that the health care system is not designed to meet their most pressing needs and priorities, many of which involve not medical care but social services.

This study was conducted by the Institute of Medicine (IOM) Committee on Approaching Death: Addressing Key End-of-Life Issues. While opinions vary regarding many dimensions of the nation's health care system, the committee reached the conclusion that substantially higher-quality, compassionate, yet affordable and sustainable care for people with advanced illnesses is a goal within reach. We recognize the broad agreement across many political fronts that the nation must stabilize expenditures on health care. In the end-of-life context, however, we believe that goal must be achieved in tandem with the provision of quality care that offers patients and families both compassion and choice.

This is a challenging agenda; however, this report makes clear that effective, evidence-based strategies for improving care for people nearing the end of life are already known. For the most part, money currently in the health care system can be reallocated to implement those strategies and even add some of the much-needed social supports now unavailable. In short, the committee envisions an approach to care for people near the end of life that is both high quality and compassionate; delivers value to patients, families, and the health system; and is sustainable and affordable.

Much has been written about the high costs of care in the last year of life. Persuasive arguments have been made, however, that it is misleading to look back at these expenditures and attribute them all to "the high cost of dying." Methodologically, it is difficult to define the "end of life"—which, generally entailing acute illness, necessarily involves intense treatment—until the patient has died. People who survive these serious episodes do not appear in these calculations (Neuberg, 2009). Worse, such arguments imply that the sickest and most vulnerable people in society (some of whom will die, but many of whom will not) are somehow unworthy of investment. Moreover, costs of care in the final phase of life vary from one hospital region to another by large amounts. Yet people treated in high-cost locales live no longer than people who are equally ill but whose care costs considerably less (Dartmouth Institute for Health Policy and Clinical Practice, undated; see also Appendix E).

The key question for health care policy makers and analysts, however, should center not on costs, but on whether people nearing the end of life are receiving high-quality, effective health and supporting services and whether the mix of services available to them reflects their needs and preferences. As detailed in this report, evidence suggests a mismatch between the services most readily available to people near the end of life (acute care) and what they most often say they want (supportive services) (Gruneir et al., 2007).

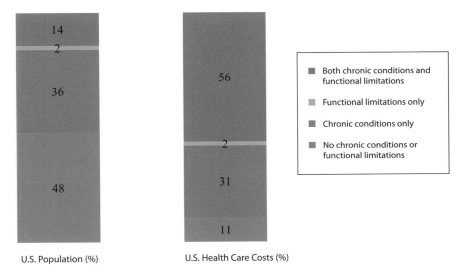

FIGURE 1-1 Population and health care costs for people with chronic conditions and functional limitations, 2010-2011.
SOURCE: Appendix E, Table E-1.

Meanwhile, a large number of Americans have chronic conditions or functional limitations—or both—which are associated with higher needs and, as a result, health care costs (see Figure 1-1). The important message of this figure is that the nearly one-half of Americans (48 percent) who have no chronic condition or functional limitation account for only 14 percent of U.S. health care costs, whereas the 14 percent of Americans who have both chronic conditions and functional limitations account for 56 percent of these costs. Two-thirds of the population with the highest health care costs (top 5 percent spenders) are under age 65 and therefore not part of the Medicare population; further, according to an analysis commissioned for this study (see Appendix E, Figure E-12), the proportion of Medicare spending in the year prior to death remained stable from 1978 to 2006 (most recent comparable data) despite rapidly rising health care costs overall.

Physicians might be assumed to be in a better position than the average nonclinician to judge the likely value of services provided near the end of life.[1] It is therefore telling that when it comes to their own care, many

---

[1] "Value should always be defined around the customer, and in a well-functioning health care system, the creation of value for patients should determine the rewards for all other actors in the system. Since value depends on results, not inputs, value in health care is measured by the outcomes achieved, not the volume of services delivered" (Porter, 2010, p. 2477).

physicians choose much less aggressive treatments than they offer their patients. A 1997 study comparing 78 primary care faculty and residents with 831 of their patients found that the physicians were much less likely than the patients to want five of six specific treatments if they were terminally ill (Gramelspacher et al., 1997). Fifty-nine percent of the physicians had "least aggressive" treatment preferences, while 31 percent had "moderate" treatment preferences.

Although few scientific studies have addressed the subject, a personal essay by Kenneth Murray, M.D., suggests that doctors "don't die like the rest of us. What's unusual about them is not how much treatment they get compared to most Americans, but how little"[2] (Murray, 2011). In a survey of some 765 physicians, most (more than 80 percent) wanted pain medications, one-quarter to one-third wanted antibiotics or intravenous (IV) hydration, and fewer than 10 percent wanted cardiopulmonary resuscitation or mechanical ventilation (Gallo et al., 2003). Likewise, a 2011 survey of some 500 board-certified U.S. physicians found that 96 percent believed "it is more important to enhance the quality of life for seriously ill patients, even if it means a shorter life," while only 4 percent believed it is more important to extend life "through every medical intervention possible" (Regence Foundation and National Journal, 2011, p. 2).

Because people understand the world largely in terms of personal experience, families that have suffered the painful loss of a loved one tend to attribute any aspects of care that went wrong or needed improvement to factors of which they have direct knowledge—the drastic turn of the illness, the conflicting requirements of various care settings, confusion about what clinicians were telling them, the decisions they made when events felt out of control. People in these situations may not recognize that their difficulties resulted largely from systemic problems in need of fundamental solutions. Addressing such systemic factors is the aim of this report.

WHY THIS STUDY IS IMPORTANT NOW

In contemplating an addition to the considerable body of existing work on this topic, the IOM took note of a number of contextual factors that make this new study particularly timely:

---

[2]Dr. Murray is a retired clinical assistant professor of family medicine at the University of Southern California. His essay, first published in *Zócalo Public Square* (Murray, 2011), has been republished in *The Best American Essays 2012* and widely excerpted and republished in the popular media.

- the increasing number of elderly Americans, including those with some combination of frailty, significant physical and cognitive disabilities, multiple chronic illnesses, and functional limitations;
- growing cultural diversity of the U.S. population, which makes it ever more important for clinicians to approach all patients as individuals, without assumptions about the care choices they might make;
- structural barriers in access to care that disadvantage certain population groups;
- a mismatch between the services patients and families need most and the services they can readily obtain;
- palliative care services that do not keep pace with the growing demand;
- wasteful and costly systemic problems, including perverse financial incentives, a fragmented care delivery system, time pressures that limit communication, and a lack of service coordination across programs; and
- the resulting unsustainable growth in costs of the current system over the past several decades.

STUDY CHARGE AND APPROACH

To conduct this study, the IOM assembled a 21-member committee comprising experts in clinical care, aging and geriatrics, hospice and palliative care, pediatrics, consumer advocacy, spirituality, ethics, communications, clinical decision making, health care financing, law, and public policy (see Appendix G for biographical sketches of the committee members). Co-chairs of the committee were Philip A. Pizzo, M.D., former dean of the Stanford University School of Medicine, and David M. Walker, former U.S. comptroller general. The charge to the committee is presented in Box 1-1.

This study was supported by a donor that wishes to remain anonymous and whose identity was unknown to the committee. The sponsor played no role in the selection of the co-chairs or members of the committee or in the committee's work.

The committee's recommendations are based on both scientific evidence and expert judgment. In preparing its recommendations, the committee reviewed the most recent, powerful, and salient evidence that should reshape the U.S. approach to care near the end of life. Because so many aspects of the nation's health care system are undergoing often dramatic changes, in part as a result of the Patient Protection and Affordable Care Act of 2010, the committee had to rely in some cases on preliminary evidence rather than definitive reports. The committee also sought to achieve a deeper understanding of the evidence through the voices and stories of people willing

---

BOX 1-1
Study Charge

The Institute of Medicine (IOM) will conduct a consensus study that will produce a comprehensive report on the current state of medical care for persons of all ages with a serious illness or medical condition who may be approaching death and who require coordinated care, appropriate personal communication (or communication with parents or guardians for children), and individual and family support. The committee will assess the delivery of medical care, social, and other supports to both the person approaching death and the family; person-family-provider communication of values, preferences, and beliefs; advance care planning; health care costs, financing, and reimbursement; and education of health professionals, patients, families, employers, and the public at large. The study will also explore approaches to advance the field. Specifically, the committee will:

1. Review progress since the 1997 IOM report *Approaching Death: Improving Care at the End of Life* and the 2003 IOM report *When Children Die: Improving Palliative and End-of-Life Care for Children and Their Families.* The committee will assess major subsequent events and recommendations that have been implemented as well as those that were not implemented along with remaining challenges and opportunities.
2. Evaluate strategies to integrate care of those with serious illness or medical condition who may be approaching death into a person- and family-centered, team-based framework. Demographic shifts, cultural changes, fiscal realities, and the needs of vulnerable populations will be considered as will advances in technology that affect the provision of care in different settings, most notably in the home. Families are a vital component of the health care team, and the financial and other ramifications for families and society will be considered.
3. Develop recommendations for changes in policy, financing mechanisms and payment practices, workforce development, research and measurement, and clinical and supportive care. These recommendations will align care with individual values, preferences, and beliefs and promote high-quality, cost-effective care for persons with serious illness or medical condition who may be approaching death, as well as with their families.
4. Develop a dissemination and communication strategy to promote public engagement understanding, and action. This strategy will need to consider the fears and anxieties surrounding care for patients who may be approaching death as well as functional dependency, aging and death, and cultural diversity in values, preferences and beliefs.

---

to share their current, direct experiences. Thus, in addition to holding six meetings among its members, the committee received input from patients, family members, clinicians, and advocates through public workshops and additional activities and through an active Web portal to which 578 comments were submitted (see Appendix A).

In conducting this study, the committee used the definitions for *basic palliative care*, *end-of-life care*, *hospice*, *palliative care*, and *specialty palliative care* shown in Box 1-2. Additional definitions relevant to this study are provided in the glossary following Chapter 6. This study also was guided by the principles listed in Box 1-3.

The findings and recommendations presented in this report are intended first and foremost to address the needs of patients and families. They should also assist policy makers, clinicians in various disciplines and their educational and credentialing bodies, leaders of health care delivery and financing organizations, researchers, public and private funders, religious and community leaders, advocates for better care, journalists, and members

---

BOX 1-2
Key Definitions

- **Basic palliative care:** Palliative care that is delivered by health care professionals who are *not* palliative care specialists, such as primary care clinicians; physicians who are disease-oriented specialists (such as oncologists and cardiologists); and nurses, social workers, pharmacists, chaplains, and others who care for this population but are not certified in palliative care.
- **End-of-life care:** Refers generally to the processes of addressing the medical, social, emotional, and spiritual needs of people who are nearing the end of life. It may include a range of medical and social services, including disease-specific interventions as well as palliative and hospice care for those with advanced serious conditions who are near the end of life.
- **Hospice:** "A service delivery system that provides palliative care for patients who have a limited life expectancy and require comprehensive biomedical, psychosocial, and spiritual support as they enter the terminal stage of an illness or condition. It also supports family members coping with the complex consequences of illness, disability, and aging as death nears" (NQF, 2006, p. 3).
- **Palliative care:** Care that provides relief from pain and other symptoms, supports quality of life, and is focused on patients with serious advanced illness and their families. Palliative care may begin early in the course of treatment for a serious illness and may be delivered in a number of ways across the continuum of health care settings, including in the home, nursing homes, long-term acute care facilities, acute care hospitals, and outpatient clinics. Palliative care encompasses hospice and specialty palliative care, as well as basic palliative care.
- **Specialty palliative care:** Palliative care that is delivered by health care professionals who *are* palliative care specialists, such as physicians who are board certified in this specialty; palliative-certified nurses; and palliative care–certified social workers, pharmacists, and chaplains.

BOX 1-3
Guiding Principles for This Study

- All people with advanced illness who may be approaching the end of life are entitled to access to high-quality, compassionate, evidence-based care, consistent with their wishes, that can reasonably be expected to protect or improve the quality and length of their life. Ensuring that access and delivering that care humanely and respectfully is a central clinical and ethical obligation of health care professionals and systems.
- "All people with advanced illness" encompasses all age groups—from neonates, to children, to adolescents, to adults, to the elderly.
- "Patient-centered" and "family-oriented" care is designed to meet physical, cognitive, social, emotional, and spiritual needs, regardless of a patient's age or infirmity; it takes into account culture, traditions, values, beliefs, and language; and it evolves with patient and family needs.
- In this report, "family" means not only people related by blood or marriage but also close friends, partners, companions, and others whom patients would want as part of their care team. As palliative care leader Ira Byock expresses it, family includes all those "for whom it matters."*
- This report's use of the term "vulnerable populations" goes beyond the conventional usage, which applies to people from ethnic, cultural, and racial minorities; people with low educational attainment or low health literacy; and those in prisons or having limited access to care for geographic or financial reasons. Here it includes people with serious illnesses, multiple chronic diseases, and disabilities (physical, mental, or cognitive); the frail elderly; and those without access to needed health services. In this latter sense, almost all people nearing the end of life can rightly be considered a "vulnerable population."
- Near the end of life, clinical care is not a person's sole priority. Patients and families may be deeply concerned with existential or spiritual issues, including bereavement, and with practical matters of coping. Appropriate support in these areas is an essential component of good care.
- The knowledge and skills that enable effective care and communication with patients and families are needed across many different health professions, among generalists as well as specialists. Honest and transparent communication about death and dying—between loved ones, between patients and clinicians, and between policy makers/media and the public—is essential to creating a truly compassionate context for high-quality end-of-life care.
- Measurement of the quality of care for the sickest and most vulnerable patients and their families is necessary to ensure access to and receipt of the highest-quality care, especially given current intense pressures to contain costs. Measurement systems should be transparent and foster accountability of services and programs.
- Innovative, well-designed biomedical, clinical, behavioral, organizational, and health policy research is needed to further improve patient-centered outcomes and ensure system sustainability.

*See http://www.dyingwell.org/springer.htm (accessed December 16, 2014).

of the interested public in learning more about what constitutes good care for people nearing the end of life and the steps necessary to achieve such care for more patients and families.

In taking on this issue at this time, the committee follows in the path of many compassionate and thoughtful people, including the members of past IOM committees whose work resulted in the following reports:

- *Approaching Death: Improving Care at the End of Life* (IOM, 1997);
- *Ensuring Quality Cancer Care* (IOM, 1999);
- *Improving Palliative Care for Cancer* (IOM, 2001b);
- *When Children Die: Improving Palliative and End-of-Life Care for Children and Their Families* (IOM, 2003);
- *Relieving Pain in America: A Blueprint for Transforming Prevention, Care, Education, and Research* (IOM, 2011); and
- *Delivering High-Quality Cancer Care: Charting a New Course for a System in Crisis* (IOM, 2013).

In addition, the IOM's series of reports on improving the quality of care (especially *Crossing the Quality Chasm* [IOM, 2001a] and the work of the Roundtable on Value & Science-Driven Health Care) provide guidance and inspiration for working toward a system that provides the right care—as determined by patients and families together with their health care team—when and where it is needed at a price that is affordable and sustainable. This committee's aim was to build on this past work and to bring compassionate and pragmatic new thinking to bear on the persistent problems affecting care for Americans living with advanced illnesses and nearing the end of life.

STUDY SCOPE

This committee's charge (see Box 1-1) was to examine "medical care for persons of all ages with a serious illness or medical condition who may be approaching death." While this may appear to be a clearly defined assignment, establishing parameters for the study was actually rather complicated. On the one hand, it was obviously infeasible for the committee to examine the entire spectrum of care for chronic illnesses from their earliest stages and manifestations or the full dimensions of frailty. This constraint imposed one limitation on the scope of the study, even though subsets of individuals with progressive chronic and debilitating conditions are highly relevant to the consideration of care in the final phase of life. On the other hand, the committee did not want to define the population of interest too narrowly or arbitrarily and thereby exclude people—or their families or clinicians—who do not consider themselves to be "approaching death." Further, overly narrow definitions of "who is dying" fail any pragmatic test, as the uncertainties of making prognoses amply attest.

In 1982, the Medicare Hospice Benefit set an eligibility criterion of a 6-month prognosis if the disease runs its normal course. The legislation never defined whether this meant median life expectancy or that all persons must be dead within 6 months. Given the inherent limitations of prognostication, health care providers are hard pressed to say which individual patients will live 6 months or less. If the policy that all persons who enter hospice must have illnesses that are certain to be fatal within 6 months is strictly enforced, access to hospice will be extremely limited. On the other hand, expanding hospice services to include persons who would live for years would have important financial implications. Thirty years ago, the 6-month limit might have had some, although weak, medical justification because hospices served primarily people with cancer whose disease progression could be projected fairly accurately. Today hospices serve people with many different diagnoses that follow various and often unpredictable trajectories. With good care, even people who are very ill may survive for many months or several years. The time frame for illnesses or conditions that ultimately will prove fatal is often considerably longer than 6 months and proceeds at a different pace for different individuals.

Assigning people to an "end-of-life" or "terminally ill" category—especially given prognostic uncertainty—also creates undesirable social and personal challenges. Although patients, families, and clinicians may not consider particular individuals—or themselves—to be "dying" (thus, the often preferred formulation "living with cancer" or "living with heart disease"), they still need the kinds of intense management of pain and other symptoms, psychological support, ancillary services, and family supports provided by hospice and palliative care programs. The committee believes the timing of death is a much less important consideration than whether the person is living with a set of conditions that are now causing distress or disability and thus needs services that address those problems, as determined in the context of need and not prognosis. The real challenge is to design models of quality and affordable care that fit the variable trajectories and needs of seriously ill people who are nearing the end of life and their family caregivers.

The same definitional quandary faced the authors of the 1997 IOM study *Approaching Death*, among many others (Hui et al., 2012). That committee, like this one, recognized that its recommendations applied to people "for whom death is imminent and those with serious, eventually fatal illnesses who may live for some time" (IOM, 1997, p. 7). That committee's sense however, was that "those referred to as dying are often thought to be likely to die within a few days to several months," and it generally focused its attention on that group, rather than on people with "an incurable, terminal or fatal illness . . . whose deaths are less predictable and might not come for years" (IOM, 1997, p. 27).

The present committee's resolution of this definitional dilemma is different in character from that of the practicing clinician, confronted with an increasing number of patients with not one but several serious and debilitating conditions that have uncertain prognoses and trajectories. For clinicians, the principle of patient-centeredness must remain paramount. Even though clinicians may be unable to predict the precise course of an individual patient's illnesses,[3] they can nevertheless demonstrate "qualities of compassion, empathy, and responsiveness to the needs, values, and expressed preferences" of the individuals and families in their care (IOM, 2001a, p. 48).

This report similarly concentrates on the population whose medical condition puts them at risk of death in some loosely defined "near future." The committee recognizes that many of the actions and systemic changes that would improve care for people nearing the end of life would be of broad benefit to many other patient groups, especially those with advanced illnesses and the functional limitations that accompany frailty, helping them retain the highest possible degree of functioning and quality of life in their remaining lifetimes, however long they may be. Examples of the improvements the committee recommends that would affect large numbers of patients are those supporting evidence-based services, strengthened patient-clinician relationships, coordination of services, patient-centered and family-oriented care, and the free flow of information, as well as other system features considered hallmarks of high-quality care (IOM, 2001a). However, the charge to the committee did not encompass this broader patient population.

Finally, although the constellation of health challenges leading to death commonly confront people of advancing age, the committee understood the problem of end-of-life care to be relevant throughout the life cycle: infants die, most often of heritable or congenital disorders or sudden infant death syndrome; injuries are the leading cause of death for children; by adolescence and young adulthood, accidents and violence cause more than 70 percent of deaths; by age 45, cancers are the leading cause of death; and by age 65, heart disease is the leading killer (Heron, 2013). No age group is immune from death. The improvements in care and communication that would help population groups most commonly facing the end of life must, therefore, be extended to those of all ages.

---

[3] A recent review of the supportive and palliative care oncology literature found 386 articles (from either 2004 or 2009) that used the term "end of life," but not one provided a definition (Hui et al., 2012).

17 YEARS OF PROGRESS

While much more progress is needed to achieve the vision of an end-of-life care system characterized by high-quality care, compassion, economic value, sustainability, and affordability, the committee wishes to acknowledge and even celebrate the progress made over the past decade and a half. When the *Approaching Death* and *When Children Die* reports were published in 1997 and 2003, respectively, they contained a total of 19 recommendations. These recommendations are summarized in Appendix B, along with information on subsequent progress and remaining gaps.

A great many improvements in end-of-life care resulted from aggressive public- and private-sector efforts. Notable among these was the work of two large foundations—the Robert Wood Johnson Foundation (RWJF)[4] and the Soros Foundation through its Project on Death in America (PDIA)[5]—which together provided millions of dollars to support professional education; research on health services delivery; the creation of models of care and their diffusion; and public engagement, media, and policy initiatives. Dozens of national and regional foundations made important contributions as well. The results of the Study to Understand Prognoses and Preferences for Outcomes and Risks of Treatments (SUPPORT) galvanized many of these efforts (Connors et al., 1995). In brief, this large and rigorous multiyear project demonstrated unequivocally that the "solutions" to the problem of end-of-life care that had been promoted for years would not change clinical practice or the experiences of dying people, in part because of the powerful incentives aligned against them. New approaches were needed.

Major professional and provider organizations, advocacy organizations, and local coalitions have actively supported care improvements and public awareness. For example, in a policy statement released in November 2013, the American Public Health Association (APHA) addressed care for people near the end of life from a public health perspective, calling the burden experienced by those with advanced life-limiting conditions a "public health problem" (APHA, 2013). APHA recommended that the needs of these individuals be addressed through improvements in pain management, advance care planning, use of hospice and palliative

---

[4]RWJF's 10-year, $170 million investment in improving end-of-life care relied on a three-part strategy: improving clinicians' knowledge of and skills in care for the dying, encouraging institutional and policy changes that would facilitate the provision of good end-of-life care, and engaging a broad range of social institutions and leaders in creating a supportive environment for change (http://www.rwjf.org/content/dam/farm/reports/reports/2011/rwjf69582 [accessed December 16, 2014]).

[5]"The mission of PDIA is to understand and transform the culture and experience of dying through initiatives in research and scholarship, the arts and humanities, through innovations in provision of care, through public and professional education and through public policy" (http://www.ncbi.nlm.nih.gov/pmc/articles/PMC1282198 [accessed December 16, 2014]).

care, care coordination, health professional education and training (at both the generalist and specialty levels), and improvements to hospice and palliative care financing and policy. As another example, RWJF's Last Acts campaign involved more than 800 partner organizations, from individual religious congregations and hospices, to the National Association for the Advancement of Colored People (NAACP), to the American Medical Association (De Milto, 2002). Thousands of individual clinicians, researchers, and community leaders worked to move the field forward. State government offices and agencies, many of them participants in the RWJF-funded Community-State Partnerships to Improve End-of-Life Care, achieved various policy advances, as did the federal government, especially through the Health Care Financing Administration (now the Centers for Medicare & Medicaid Services [CMS]), the Agency for Healthcare Research and Quality, and the National Institute of Nursing Research within the National Institutes of Health (NIH).

DYING IN AMERICA: 2014

Several key aspects of dying in America today should be noted as context for this study.

Site of Death

"Death is not what it used to be," the *Approaching Death* report observed in 1997. "In the United States, death at home in the care of family has been widely superseded by an institutional, professional, and technological process of dying" (IOM, 1997, p. 33). Although the proportion of people who die in hospitals has declined in recent years, the last few months of life are characterized by frequent hospital and intensive care stays; as noted, enrollment in hospice often occupies just the last few days of life. Among Medicare fee-for-service beneficiaries, the percentage who died in acute care hospitals declined from 33 percent in 2000 to 25 percent in 2009 (Goodman et al., 2013; Teno et al., 2013). Also in 2009, one-third of Medicare deaths occurred in private residences, 28 percent in nursing homes, and approximately 14 percent elsewhere (Teno et al., 2013).

These percentages vary from one locale to another, depending on local conditions and the availability of nonhospital services, such as nursing homes (Gruneir et al., 2007). The growing number of deaths in nursing homes—approaching 40 percent in Minnesota and Rhode Island as of 2007—is difficult to track, because many studies omit these residents. Nevertheless, the pattern of institution-based death appears to have changed to a considerable extent, in part because of the increased availability of hospice services, which help families provide appropriate care at home near the end of life. Dying at home remains a consistent preference in population surveys and patient interviews (Teno et al., 2013).

Epidemiologic Patterns

Two and a half million Americans died in 2011, according to the most recent data from the Centers for Disease Control and Prevention (Hoyert and Xu, 2012). The nation continues to make progress on key mortality figures since the 1997 *Approaching Death* report was released (see Table 1-1). In general, the dramatic gains in life expectancy that began around 1900 have continued. Life expectancy was 4.8 years longer for women than for men in 2011, although the gap between the sexes has been shrinking (Hoyert and Xu, 2012). Life expectancy for whites (non-Hispanic) was 2.4 years less than that for Hispanics and 3.7 years more than that for blacks.

Table 1-2 presents information about deaths among U.S. children. Infant mortality remains a serious national public health concern: 54 of the world's 224 countries have lower estimated 2013 infant mortality rates than the rate in the United States (CIA, 2014). Still, the U.S. rate fell 12 percent between 2005 and 2011, partly because of a decline in premature births (MacDorman et al., 2013). In general, the number of pediatric deaths due to trauma and other acute causes has declined, while the number attributable to complex chronic conditions has risen. One-third of pediatric deaths are among children with one or more complex chronic conditions. Overall, children and adolescents "live with and die from a wide array of often-rare diseases that require specialized care"; as noted earlier, many of these conditions are different from those that affect adults (see Appendix F).

The 10 leading causes of deaths in the United States are shown in Table 1-3. Heart disease and cancer together account for approximately half of the total. The leading causes vary among different population groups defined by age, race/ethnicity, and other factors.

At least seven of the causes of death listed in Table 1-3 are chronic conditions, the exceptions being unintentional injuries, influenza and pneumonia, and suicide. Nonetheless, taking into account that influenza and

TABLE 1-1 Improvements in U.S. Life Expectancy, 1995-2011

Indicator	1995	2011	Overall Improvement (%)
Average life expectancy at birth	75.8 years	78.7 years	3.8

SOURCES: For 1995: IOM, 1997, citing Anderson et al., 1997; for 2011: Hoyert and Xu, 2012.

TABLE 1-2 Deaths Among U.S. Infants and Children, Rates and Causes, 2009-2010

Indicator	Infants	Ages 1-4	Ages 5-9	Ages 10-14
Number of deaths	24,586	4,316	2,330	2,949
Crude death rate	614.7 per 100,000 live births	26.5 per 100,000	11.5 per 100,000	14.3 per 100,000
Leading causes of death	Prematurity and low birthweight, congenital problems, pregnancy complications, sudden infant death syndrome	Accidents (unintentional injuries), congenital problems, homicide	Accidents (unintentional injuries), cancer, congenital problems, homicide	Accidents (unintentional injuries), cancer, suicide, homicide

SOURCE: Heron, 2013.

pneumonia are most deadly among people whose health is already compromised in some way, as well as the contribution of alcohol use, depression, and other such factors to suicide and unintentional injuries (e.g., fires, falls, drownings, vehicle and pedestrian accidents), all 10 causes are linked in some way to chronic health problems.

The Changing U.S. Population

Dying in America today reflects the overall aging and growing diversity of the U.S. population, as well as the particular vulnerability of certain individuals.

Aging

An increase in the number and proportion of Americans aged 65 and older has been a dominant demographic trend since long before Medicare came into being. Three times the percentage of Americans pass their 65th birthday today as was the case in 1900, and the proportion of the population reaching age 85 is 48 times larger than a century ago (AoA, 2012). Indeed, the percentage of Americans over age 65 is on an upward trajectory from 9 percent in 1960 to a projected 20 percent in 2050 (see Table 1-4).

Greater longevity comes at a cost. With increases in life expectancy, the

TABLE 1-3 Leading Causes of Death, United States, 2010

Cause	Percentage of Deaths
Heart disease	24.2
Cancer (malignant neoplasms)	23.3
Chronic lower respiratory diseases	5.6
Cerebrovascular diseases (e.g., stroke)	5.2
Unintentional injuries	4.9
Alzheimer's disease	3.4
Diabetes mellitus	2.8
Influenza and pneumonia	2.0
Kidney diseases (e.g., nephritis)	2.0
Suicide	1.6

SOURCE: Heron, 2013.

burden of serious illnesses among the nation's Medicare-eligible (65 and older) and old-old (85 and older) populations has risen markedly. Two-thirds of people aged 65 and older suffer from serious, multiple chronic conditions (CDC, 2013). By contrast, 31 percent of those aged 45 to 64 and only 6 percent of those aged 18 to 44 were treated for two or more chronic conditions in 2009 (Machlin and Soni, 2013).

Table 1-5 shows the impact of having multiple chronic conditions on health care costs. In general, Medicare spending rises dramatically with increases in the number of chronic conditions. Beneficiaries with five or more such conditions accounted for nearly two-thirds of Medicare dollars spent in 2007 (Anderson, 2010).

In the future, the aging U.S. population is likely to experience large increases in certain diseases that are costly to treat. Without more effective methods for prevention and early treatment, conditions such as cardio-

TABLE 1-4 Growth in the U.S. Elderly Population, 1960-2050 (projection)

Age Group	1960	2000	2010	2050 (est.)
65+: number	16.6 million	35 million	40.3 million	88.5 million
(% of total population)	(9.2)	(12.4)	(13.0)	(19.8)
85+: number	929,000	4.2 million	5.5 million	19 million
(% of total population)	(0.5)	(1.5)	(1.7)	(4.2)

SOURCES: For 1960 and 2000: He et al., 2005; for 2010: Bureau of the Census, 2010; for 2050: Bureau of the Census, 2008.

TABLE 1-5 Average Medicare Expenditures per Fee-for-Service Beneficiary, by Number of Chronic Conditions, 2010

Number of Chronic Conditions	Average Expenditure ($)
0-1	2,025
2-3	5,698
4-5	12,174
6 or more	32,658

NOTE: The 15 chronic conditions included in this analysis are high blood pressure, high cholesterol, ischemic heart disease, arthritis, diabetes, heart failure, chronic kidney disease, depression, chronic obstructive pulmonary disease, Alzheimer's disease, atrial fibrillation, cancer, osteoporosis, asthma, and stroke.
SOURCE: CMS, 2012.

vascular disease (Pandya et al., 2013) and cancer are likely to consume an increasingly large share of health care resources because even with stable or slightly falling *rates* of illness, the growing number of people in the higher-risk age groups means the *number* of cases will grow. Thus, the number of new cases of cancer is expected to increase by 45 percent between 2010 and 2030 (IOM, 2013).

The number of Americans with Alzheimer's disease and related dementias also is rising rapidly, expected to grow from 5.5 million in 2010 to 8.7 million in 2030 (HHS, 2013), and the prevalence of Parkinson's disease is expected to double in the next 30 years. In 2010, the annual costs of caring for Americans with dementia, including both medical and nursing home care and unpaid care (mostly by family members), were estimated at $157-$215 billion, depending on how informal care was valued (Hurd et al., 2013); for Parkinson's disease, the estimated direct and indirect costs totaled almost $21 billion (Kowal et al., 2013). These high costs can accumulate over a number of years of declining health, despite the tendency for the intensity of medical care to decrease among the oldest members of the population in the last year of life (see Appendix E).

Functional limitations and disabilities likewise increase with age and as death approaches (Chaudhry et al., 2013; Smith et al., 2013). One result is a growing need for nursing home and other long-term care placements. The number of Americans needing long-term care is expected to more than double, reaching 27 million, by 2050 (Senate Commission on Long-Term Care, 2013).

Living for extended periods with serious disease and disability need not be inevitable features of aging, however. Data from the National Long-Term Care Survey show that disability rates can be decreased (NIA, 2010), while data from the Survey of Income and Program Participation show these rates stabilizing since 2000 (Kaye, 2013). In addition, evidence from the Health and Retirement Study indicate that the probability of being cognitively impaired declined from the mid-1990s up until at least 2004, and there is reason for cautious optimism that better control of stroke and heart disease will contribute to reductions in new cases of dementia as well (Rocca et al., 2011). Factors behind these improvements include not only better clinical treatment but also behavioral changes, assistive technologies, and improvements in socioeconomic status that suggest a need for a broad array of interventions—beyond health care—to reduce the burden of disability on older Americans. These improvements are masked, however, by the rapidly increasing number of older adults, which will result in increased need for services despite stable or lower disability rates.

Growing Diversity

The ethnic and cultural composition of the U.S. population is changing. Much has been said about the rapidity with which some U.S. cities and states are becoming "majority minority" places. Many clinicians today and certainly those of the future will care for people of differing ethnic, cultural, religious, and language backgrounds and literacy/health literacy levels; differing traditions and rituals around dying; differing levels of comfort with making critical decisions; differing expectations of the health care system; and differing family compositions, roles, and responsibilities. The strengths, weaknesses, and resilience of families are especially important factors, given the long-term trend to move ever more complex care to the home. Such factors can increase particular risks—in the present context, the risk of poor-quality, high-cost care in the final phase of life—for population groups, or even particular individuals.

Vulnerable Individuals

Many people are among those at heightened risk of poor-quality, high-cost end-of-life care. Beyond the demographic factors discussed above, the following individuals are particularly vulnerable:

- infants and children with congenital disorders, genetic diseases, or cancer;
- people of any age with complex chronic conditions;
- the elderly who have multiple chronic conditions, functional limitations, and frailty;
- people who have mental disorders or cognitive impairments, such as stroke, Alzheimer's disease, or other dementias; and

- people with inadequate access to health services because of geography, immigration status, low income and lack of health insurance, incarceration, and structural features of the health care system.

RESEARCH NEEDS

Areas in which additional research is needed are cited in Chapters 2, 3, and 5. In 2013, the National Institute of Nursing Research—the lead institute within NIH for research on end-of-life care—published a summary of research trends and funding in end-of-life and palliative care for the years 1997-2010 (NINR, 2013). This summary was based on published research supported by both public and private entities. While the report notes that the scientific literature in this area has tripled since 1997 and totaled more than 3,000 publications as of 2010, it cites gaps as well.

In 1997, most research in end-of-life and palliative care was privately funded. While the amount of federal funding for such research has increased dramatically since 1997—from $4.2 million to $61.55 million in 2010—it still represents a very small proportion of the nation's annual investment in biomedical research. Researchers who want to study end-of-life and palliative care topics face an ongoing difficulty in obtaining NIH funding. To evaluate the significance of these proposals adequately, the various NIH institutes would need approval bodies (study sections) devoted to end-of-life questions or larger numbers of people with end-of-life and palliative care expertise serving on existing study sections.

SUMMARY

Despite considerable progress, significant problems remain in providing end-of-life care for Americans that is high quality and compassionate and preserves their choice while being affordable and sustainable. Many of these same challenges apply generally to individuals with chronic and complex medical and mental disorders and reflect the current fragmentation and limitations of the U.S. health care system—a system currently undergoing profound change.

Significant opportunities exist to improve and align financial and programmatic incentives across health and social services programs, develop incentives to implement program models that have demonstrated how to achieve better care at lower cost, better target complex care interventions and tailor resources to individual needs, and use social services to ease the burden on families and enhance quality of life. In some cases, additional research is needed, especially toward improving clinicians' ability to identify individuals at risk of a "bad death." In addition, greater oversight is needed to ensure quality care, control costs, increase transparency, and ensure accountability.

A national strategy for accomplishing the needed changes in the current health care delivery system would necessarily be broad-based, taking into account features of the health care system as it is currently evolving, the way care is provided and the improvements needed, the way health care providers are trained and what they are taught to do, and the awareness and knowledge that would cause the public at large to support and advocate for these changes. Fundamental to this strategy is the need for—and difficult work of—breaking down a range of silos, for example, between "curative" and palliative care, between professional groups so as to foster interdisciplinary practice, and between traditional medical and social services. Development of a specific strategy, therefore, would require the broad engagement of multiple actors in the health care field and social and supporting services sector, as well as the organizations and institutions on which Americans rely for practical assistance, spiritual support, information, and advice as caregivers and as people with life-limiting illnesses. Designing such a complex, multipart strategy involving so many essential participants is beyond the scope of this study, particularly given that the U.S. health system is undergoing so many changes. However, the insights offered in this report regarding problems, challenges, and strengths of the system may be a foundation on which many other efforts can build. These challenges and opportunities are discussed in detail in the following chapters.

ORGANIZATION OF THE REPORT

This report provides a detailed description of important aspects of the current U.S. health care system as they affect Americans nearing the end of life. As noted, the system is changing substantially at present, meaning that the following chapters, which rely heavily on published evidence and analysis, are to some extent a snapshot taken yesterday. An accurate picture of U.S. health care today has not yet developed, and what the system will be tomorrow is not clearly in focus. Nevertheless, much has been learned to date that should enable the implementation of high-quality, cost-effective care that patients and families find compassionate and supportive of their values, goals, and preferences at the end of life.

Chapter 2 describes end-of-life services as they are currently delivered, focusing especially on the role of palliative care. The importance of comprehensive advance care planning and improvements in traditional advance directives is discussed in Chapter 3. Chapter 4 examines the workforce and educational needs of health professionals who care for people nearing the end of life. Chapter 5 reviews the policies and payment systems, particularly those of Medicare and Medicaid, that shape current patterns of care. Finally, public attitudes and beliefs about topics in end-of-life care and elements of potential public education programs are reviewed in Chapter 6.

REFERENCES

Anderson, G. 2010. *Chronic care: Making the case for ongoing care.* Princeton, NJ: Robert Wood Johnson Foundation. http://www.rwjf.org/content/dam/farm/reports/reports/2010/rwjf54583 (accessed July 3, 2013).

Anderson, R. N., K. D. Kochanek, and S. L. Murphy. 1997. Report of final mortality statistics, 1995. *Monthly Vital Statistics Reports* 45(11):1-80.

AoA (Administration on Aging). 2012. *A profile of older Americans: 2012.* http://www.aoa.gov/AoAroot/Aging_Statistics/Profile/index.aspx (accessed January 4, 2014).

APHA (American Public Health Association). 2013. *APHA policy #20134—Supporting public health's role in addressing unmet needs in serious illness and at the end of life.* Washington, DC: APHA. http://www.apha.org/advocacy/policy/policysearch/default.htm?id=1450 (accessed August 5, 2014).

Bureau of the Census. 2008. *Projections of the population by age and sex for the United States: 2010 to 2050.* NP2008-T12. Washington, DC: Bureau of the Census.

Bureau of the Census. 2010. *The older population: 2010. 2010 Census briefs.* http://www.census.gov/prod/cen2010/briefs/c2010br-09.pdf (accessed July 30, 2013).

CDC (Centers for Disease Control and Prevention). 2013. *The state of aging and health in America—2013.* http://www.cdc.gov/aging/pdf/state-aging-health-in-america-2013.pdf (accessed November 12, 2013).

Chaudhry, S. I., T. E. Murphy, E. Gahbauer, L. S. Sussman, H. G. Allore, and T. M. Gill. 2013. Restricting symptoms in the last year of life: A prospective cohort study. *JAMA Internal Medicine* 173(16):1534-1540.

CIA (Central Intelligence Agency). 2014. Country comparison: Infant mortality rate. *The World Factbook.* https://www.cia.gov/library/publications/the-world-factbook/rankorder/2091rank.html (accessed February 6, 2014).

CMS (Centers for Medicare & Medicaid Services). 2012. *Chronic conditions among Medicare beneficiaries.* Baltimore, MD: CMS.

Connors, A. F., N. V. Dawson, N. A. Desbiens, W. J. Fulkerson, L. Goldman, W. A. Knaus, J. Lynn, and D. Ransohoff. 1995. A controlled trial to improve care for seriously ill hospitalized patients: The Study to Understand Prognoses and Preferences for Outcomes and Risks of Treatments (SUPPORT). *Journal of the American Medical Association* 274(20):1591-1598.

Dartmouth Institute for Health Policy and Clinical Practice. undated. *Inpatient days per decedent during the last six months of life, by gender and level of care intensity, 2007.* http://www.dartmouthatlas.org/data/topic/topic.aspx?cat=18 (accessed July 16, 2013).

De Milto, L. 2002. *Assessment of Last Acts program provides recommendations for future direction: Assessing progress and opportunities for the Last Acts initiative.* http://www.rwjf.org/content/dam/farm/reports/program_results_reports/2002/rwjf65521 (accessed June 23, 2014).

Gallo, J. J., J. B. Straton, M. J. Klag, L. A. Meoni, D. P. Sulmasy, N. Wang, and D. E. Ford. 2003. Life-sustaining treatments: What do physicians want and do they express their wishes to others? *Journal of the American Geriatrics Society* 51(7):961-969.

Goodman, D. C., E. S. Fisher, J. E. Wennberg, J. S. Skinner, S. Chasan-Taber, and K. K. Bonner. 2013. *Tracking improvement in the care of chronically ill patients: A Dartmouth Atlas brief on Medicare beneficiaries near the end of life.* http://www.dartmouthatlas.org/downloads/reports/EOL_brief_061213.pdf (accessed March 10, 2014).

Gramelspacher, G. P., X.-H. Zhou, M. P. Hanna, and W. M. Tierney. 1997. Preferences of physicians and their patients for end-of-life care. *Journal of General Internal Medicine* 12(6):346-351.

Gruneir, A., V. Mor, S. Weitzen, R. Truchil, J. Teno, and J. Roy. 2007. Where people die: A multilevel approach to understanding influences on site of death in America. *Medical Care Research and Review* 64(4):351-378.

He, W., M. Sengupta, V. A. Velkoff, and K. A. DeBarros. 2005. *65+ in the United States.* http://www.census.gov/prod/2006pubs/p23-209.pdf (accessed July 30, 2013).

Heron, M. 2013. Deaths: Leading causes for 2010. *National Vital Statistics Reports* 62(6):1-97. http://www.cdc.gov/nchs/data/nvsr/nvsr62/nvsr62_06.pdf (accessed February 5, 2014).

HHS (U.S. Department of Health and Human Services). 2013. *National plan to address Alzheimer's Disease—2013 update.* http://aspe.hhs.gov/daltcp/napa/NatlPlan2013.shtml#intro (accessed November 12, 2013).

Hoyert, D. L., and J. Xu. 2012. Deaths: Preliminary data for 2011. *National Vital Statistics Reports* 61(6):1-52.

Hui, D., M. Mori, H. A. Parsons, S. H. Kim, Z. Li, S. Damani, and E. Bruera. 2012. The lack of standard definitions in the supportive and palliative oncology literature. *Journal of Pain and Symptom Management* 43(3):582-592.

Hurd, M. D., P. Martorell, A. Delavande, K. J. Mullen, and K. M. Langa. 2013. Monetary costs of dementia in the United States. *New England Journal of Medicine* 368(14):1326-1334.

IOM (Institute of Medicine). 1997. *Approaching death: Improving care at the end of life.* Washington, DC: National Academy Press.

IOM. 1999. *Ensuring quality cancer care.* Washington, DC: National Academy Press.

IOM. 2001a. *Crossing the quality chasm: A new health system for the 21st century.* Washington, DC: National Academy Press.

IOM. 2001b. *Improving palliative care for cancer.* Washington, DC: National Academy Press.

IOM. 2003. *When children die: Improving palliative and end-of-life care for children and their families.* Washington, DC: The National Academies Press.

IOM. 2011. *Relieving pain in America: A blueprint for transforming prevention, care, education, and research.* Washington, DC: The National Academies Press.

IOM. 2013. *Delivering high-quality cancer care: Charting a new course for a system in crisis.* Washington, DC: The National Academies Press.

Kaye, H. S. 2013. Disability rates for working-age adults and for the elderly have stabilized, but trends for each mean different results for costs. *Health Affairs* 32(1):127-134.

Kowal, S. L., T. M. Dall, R. Chakrabarti, M. V. Storm, and A. Jain. 2013. The current and projected economic burden of Parkinson's disease in the United States. *Movement Disorders* 28(3):311-318.

MacDorman, M. F., D. L. Hoyert, and T. J. Mathews. 2013. Recent declines in infant mortality in the United States, 2005-2011. *NCHS Data Brief* 120. http://www.cdc.gov/nchs/data/databriefs/db120.htm (accessed February 5, 2014).

Machlin, S. R., and A. Soni. 2013. *Health care expenditures for adults with multiple treated chronic conditions: Estimates from the Medicare Expenditure Panel Survey, 2009.* Washington, DC: CDC. http://www.cdc.gov/pcd/issues/2013/12_0172.htm (accessed February 5, 2014).

Murray, K. 2011. How doctors die: It's not like the rest of us, but it should be. *Zocalo Public Square.* http://www.zocalopublicsquare.org/2011/11/30/how-doctors-die/ideas/nexus (accessed March 1, 2014).

Neuberg, G. W. 2009. The cost of end-of-life care: A new efficiency measure falls short of AHA/ACC standards. *Circulation: Cardiovascular Quality and Outcomes* 2:127-133.

NIA (National Institute on Aging). 2010. *Disability in older adults.* Fact sheet. http://report.nih.gov/nihfactsheets/Pdfs/DisabilityinOlderAdults%28NIA%29.pdf (accessed January 4, 2014).

NINR (National Institute of Nursing Research). 2013. *Building momentum: The science of end-of-life and palliative care. A review of research trends and funding, 1997-2010.* http://www.ninr.nih.gov/sites/www.ninr.nih.gov/files/NINR-Building-Momentum-508.pdf (accessed March 12, 2014).

NQF (National Quality Forum). 2006. *A national framework and preferred practices for palliative and hospice care quality: A consensus report.* Washington, DC: NQF.

Pandya, A., T. A. Gaziano, M. C. Weinstein, and D. Cutler. 2013. More Americans living longer with cardiovascular disease will increase costs while lowering quality of life. *Health Affairs* 32(10):1706-1714.

Porter, M. E. 2010. What is value in health care? Perspective. *New England Journal of Medicine* 363(26):2477-2481.

Regence Foundation and National Journal. 2011. *Living well at the end of life: A national conversation.* http://syndication.nationaljournal.com/communications/NationalJournal RegenceDoctorsToplines.pdf (accessed June 23, 2014).

Rocca, W. A., R. C. Petersen, D. S. Knopman, L. E. Hebert, D. A. Evans, K. S. Hall, S. Gao, F. W. Unverzagt, K. M. Langa, E. B. Larson, and L. R. White. 2011. Trends in the incidence and prevalence of Alzheimer's disease, dementia, and cognitive impairment in the United States. *Alzheimer's & Dementia* 7(1):80-93.

Senate Commission on Long-Term Care. 2013. *Report to the Congress.* http://www.chhs.ca.gov/OLMDOC/Agenda%20Item%206-%20Commission%20on%20Long-Term%20Care-%20Final%20Report%209-26-13.pdf (accessed December 2, 2013).

Smith, A. K., L. C. Walter, Y. Miao, W. J. Boscardin, and K. E. Covinsky. 2013. Disability during the last two years of life. *JAMA Internal Medicine* 173(16):1506-1513.

Teno, J. M., P. L. Gozalo, J. P. Bynum, N. E. Leland, S. C. Miller, N. E. Morden, T. Scupp, D. C. Goodman, and V. Mor. 2013. Change in end-of-life care for Medicare beneficiaries: Site of death, place of care, and health care transitions in 2000, 2005, and 2009. *Journal of the American Medical Association* 309(5):470-477.

2

The Delivery of Person-Centered, Family-Oriented End-of-Life Care

For most people, death does not come suddenly. Instead, dying is an inevitable result of one or more diseases that must be managed carefully and compassionately over weeks, months, or even years, through many ups and downs. This chapter examines the ways in which health care providers manage that process. Evidence shows that—regardless of whether curative treatments are also undertaken—a palliative approach often offers the best chance of maintaining the highest possible quality of life for the longest possible time for those living with advanced serious illness.

Death is not a strictly medical event. Ideally, health care harmonizes with social, psychological, and spiritual supports. Health care makes important contributions as patients near the end of life: it relieves pain, discomfort, and other symptoms and effects of disease; it can facilitate achieving maximum possible functioning; it can help alleviate depression and anxiety; it can ease the burden on loved ones and facilitate constructive family dynamics; and sometimes it can extend life for a period of time. It can achieve all these things by combining science with compassion; by adjusting treatments to the unique needs of the individual patient; and by taking into account the patient's and family's spiritual and cultural context, interests, roles, and strengths. The committee believes, therefore, that care of people nearing the end of life should be preeminently patient-centered and family-oriented.

The importance of family is emphasized throughout this chapter. As articulated in the guiding principles presented in Chapter 1 (see Box 1-3), the committee construes the term "family" broadly to encompass spouses, blood relatives, in-laws, step-relatives, fiancés, significant others, friends, caring neighbors, colleagues, fellow parishioners or congregants, and other people with a personal attachment to the person with advanced serious illness—in other words, the people "for whom it matters."

Also emphasized throughout this chapter—as throughout this report— is the importance of providing the services needed by people with advanced serious illnesses in a *coordinated* way. This coordination can be accomplished through many different types of structures and arrangements, depending on available resources, payment schemes, and cultural and social preferences. No one service delivery pattern fits all.

This chapter begins by reviewing the current situation with respect to end of life: the trajectories and symptoms of death; and salient features of current end-of life care delivery, including the providers of care, the importance of primary care, the problem of burdensome transitions across care settings, and the challenge of unwanted and uncoordinated care. Next is an examination of palliative care, including hospice, as an established approach to providing the best possible quality of life for people of all ages who have an advanced serious illness or are likely approaching death. The chapter then looks at efforts to measure and report on the quality of care near the end of life, and suggests a set of core quality components. This is followed by a discussion of the problem of prognosis alluded to in Chapter 1. The chapter then focuses on family caregivers, who constitute a generally invisible, undertrained, financially and emotionally stressed, and growing workforce. After outlining research needs related to the delivery of patient-centered, family-oriented end-of-life care, the chapter ends with the committee's findings, conclusions, and recommendation for broad-scale improvement in this area.

REVIEW OF THE CURRENT SITUATION

Trajectories and Symptoms Near the End of Life

The Institute of Medicine (IOM) report *Approaching Death: Improving Care at the End of Life* (IOM, 1997) depicts three prototypical trajectories near the end of life:

- a sudden death from an unexpected cause (such as a motor vehicle accident, myocardial infarction, or stroke);
- a steady decline from a progressive disease with a terminal phase (such as cancer); and
- an advanced illness marked by a slow decline with periodic crises and eventual sudden death (such as chronic lung disease or congestive heart failure).

For children (as described in Appendix F), the three most common trajectories near the end of life are sudden death (from trauma), fluctuating decline (such as worsening heart failure), and constant medical fragility (as with some neurologic impairments).

To a patient or family, these categories may appear to overlap. A person dying suddenly from an unexpected cause may have had serious underlying health problems; someone experiencing a steady decline may also enjoy many good days; and a person with a generally slow decline may suffer a sudden steep deterioration in health status.

Another way to view trajectories near the end of life is to focus on functional status. In a prospective cohort study that included 491 participants who initially were not disabled, were at least 70 years old at the start of the study, and died during the 13-year course of the study, disabilities (or "restricting symptoms") remained relatively constant from 12 months before death until 5 months before death, when they began to increase rapidly (Chaudhry et al., 2013). Twenty percent of the study population demonstrated disability 1 year before death, 27 percent at 5 months before death, and nearly 60 percent in the month before death. Similarly, in a study of 8,232 decedents enrolled in the Health and Retirement Study between 1995 and 2010, the prevalence of disability increased from 28 percent 2 years before death to 56 percent in the month before death (Smith et al., 2013b).

As is emphasized later in this chapter in the section on prognosis, it is difficult to predict an individual patient's disease or disability trajectory. While the course of a disease varies greatly from one individual to another, and people often have multiple diseases and debilitating conditions near the end of life, it may be possible to identify likely patient needs based on patient and disease characteristics, informing service delivery needs. At the individual level, the committee believes health care providers are best advised to develop, frequently review and revise, and implement care plans tailored to individual circumstances.

Individual circumstances that influence personalized care plans include the disease process; the patient's physical, social, spiritual, and cultural environments and supports (e.g., difficulties in obtaining culturally and linguistically appropriate care); and the patient's experience with both physical and psychological symptoms. Some of the major physical and psychological symptoms people face toward the end of life are identified in *Approaching Death* in a list that remains relevant today (IOM, 1997, pp. 76-78):

- pain;
- diminished appetite and wasting (anorexia-cachexia syndrome);
- weakness and fatigue (asthenia);

- shortness of breath (dyspnea) and cough;
- nausea and vomiting;
- difficulty swallowing (dysphagia);
- bowel problems (constipation, diarrhea);
- mouth problems (dry mouth, sores, dental problems, infections);
- skin problems (itching, dryness, chapping, acne, sweating, sensitivity to touch, pressure sores, dark spots);
- tissue swelling (lymphedema);
- accumulation of liquid in the abdomen (ascites);
- confusion;
- dementia;
- anxiety; and
- depression.

Other problems experienced by many patients nearing the end of life are not necessarily disease related but common to the experience of aging. Examples include incontinence, falls and mobility problems, delirium, depression, and abuse and neglect.

Children nearing the end of life face symptoms similar to those of adults. Studies of children with cancer have found the patient symptoms most frequently reported by parents to be pain, fatigue, dyspnea, change in behavior, and loss of appetite (Pritchard et al., 2010; Wolfe et al., 2000).

The varied trajectories and symptoms experienced by people with advanced serious illnesses pose special challenges for health care providers, especially if the patient has multiple coexisting conditions. A drug or treatment prescribed for one condition may be contraindicated for another; unexpected interactions among drugs may occur. Moreover, the availability of personal, physical, social, and other resources influences how care needs related to decreases in functional status are addressed. Box 2-1 highlights another important challenge noted also in Chapter 1: many elderly people with advanced serious illnesses have dementia or cognitive impairments.

Providers of Care Near the End of Life

The health care institutions most involved in care near the end of life are hospitals, nursing homes, long-term acute care facilities, home health agencies, and hospices, as well as outpatient clinical settings. The health professions most involved are physicians, nurses, and social workers. Besides specialists trained and certified in hospice and palliative medicine, the involved physicians include primary care clinicians, hospitalists, and specialists in treating advanced serious diseases, such as cancer and heart disease. Nursing personnel involved in end-of-life care include advanced

---

BOX 2-1
Dementia as an Example of the Challenges in End-of-Life Care

Many elderly people in their final months or years have combinations of chronic diseases that include dementia. People with dementia cannot consistently communicate effectively with health care workers or participate actively and routinely in their care. A study of 163 elderly, non-critically ill patients in the emergency department of an academic medical center found that 37 percent had cognitive dysfunction (Carpenter et al., 2011). Such impairments hamper clinicians' efforts to obtain accurate medical histories, make timely and accurate medical diagnoses, and initiate proper treatment (Han et al., 2011). Such impairments can also prevent patients from adhering to discharge instructions designed to prevent future problems and emergencies (Hustey et al., 2003).

Dementia may add another layer of complexity to disparities in medical decision making among racial and ethnic minority groups. A systematic review of 20 articles on end-of-life care among African Americans, Hispanics, Asian Americans, and Caucasians with dementia found treatment differences at the end of life that may be due to "the double disadvantage of dementia and ethnic minority status" (Connolly et al., 2012, p. 359). The study found that Asian Americans and African Americans with dementia were more likely than others to initiate artificial nutrition, and African Americans were more likely to receive blood transfusions, mechanical ventilation, and intensive care unit care, and less likely to have treatment withheld or to complete advance directives.

---

practice nurses, other registered nurses, practical nurses, and nursing assistants, with specialty certifications available at all these levels. Social workers, chaplains, pharmacists, rehabilitation therapists, direct care workers (such as home health aides), family caregivers, and hospice volunteers also participate in end-of-life care in large numbers. Family caregivers are discussed later in this chapter, while other personnel are discussed in Chapter 4.

The Importance of Primary Care

Primary care[1] plays a crucial role for many people with advanced serious illnesses because primary care clinicians often are best positioned to coordinate the patient's health services across multiple specialties, ensure continuity of care across the patient's life span, and understand the capabili-

---

[1] An IOM report defines primary care as "the provision of integrated, accessible health care services by clinicians who are accountable for addressing a large majority of personal health care needs, developing a sustained partnership with patients, and practicing in the context of family and community" (IOM, 1996, p. 31).

As my 88-year-old father-in-law was in decline with eight different chronic conditions, he had more specialists than we could keep track of, and nobody was steering the ship. Most of all, his pain was poorly managed, but finding an outpatient palliative care physician was impossible, even in a city like Los Angeles. He resisted hospice mainly because he thought that meant he was giving up, so he continued to suffer and experience recurring runs to the emergency room. When he finally agreed to home hospice, his care and condition improved dramatically, and during the final month he lived under hospice he was comfortable, he had heartfelt conversations with all 11 of his children, and he died in peace and dignity in his home. It was a good death, but the period of serious, progressive illness before hospice was a nightmare, because hospice-type care is kept out of reach until the last moments of life. *

*Quotation from a response submitted through the online public testimony questionnaire for this study. See Appendix C.

ties of family members. Primary care clinicians include family physicians, general internists, general pediatricians, and geriatricians; primary care nurse practitioners; and some physician assistants. These clinicians often treat patients who are nearing the end of life and require identification and treatment of multiple physical symptoms, as well as psychosocial support. In addition to treatment of one or more advanced serious illnesses and their comorbidities, their patients variously may need assistance in advance care planning and health care decision making, counseling, referrals to hospice and specialty palliative care, referrals to other relevant specialists and to social service and home health agencies, and coordination of care.

Care coordination, including communication among all providers and between providers and the patient and family, is especially crucial because care near the end of life can involve many health professionals, multiple chronic conditions, and rapidly emerging complex problems with medical and social dimensions. Primary care often is expected to carry out this care coordination function. However, the high use of specialty care by elderly people with multiple chronic conditions makes coordination difficult. This difficulty is illustrated by a cross-sectional study in Washington State of 2,000 Group Health plan members who had chronic conditions and were eligible to enroll in a Medicare Advantage Special Needs Plan. In that study, continuity of primary care was associated with more coordinated care for patients who were low users of specialty care, but not for patients who were high specialty care users[2] (Liss et al., 2011).

A literature review of coordination in end-of-life cancer care between primary care physicians and oncologists found "preliminary evidence that the continued involvement of primary care physicians in cancer care is valued by patients, may influence care experiences and outcomes, and serves identifiable functions," such as "meeting patients' needs for communication and emotional support" (Han and Rayson, 2010, p. 33). The authors of this literature review further noted, "Data are particularly lacking on the nature and outcomes of care coordination occurring specifically between primary care physicians and oncologists" (Han and Rayson, 2010, p. 34). For example, one study using the Surveillance, Epidemiology, and End Results (SEER)-Medicare database[3] for 1992-2002 found that advanced lung cancer patients who were seen by their usual primary care provider during their final hospitalization had 25 percent reduced odds of admission to critical care units (Sharma et al., 2009).

Current trends support the development of "medical homes," which are distinguished by seven essential features: a personal physician, physician-directed medical practice, a whole-person orientation, coordination (or at least integration) of care, quality and safety as hallmarks, enhanced access to care, and appropriate payment mechanisms (American Academy of Family Physicians et al., 2007). One of the "joint principles" of medical homes adopted by the American Academy of Family Physicians, American Academy of Pediatrics, American College of Physicians, and American Osteopathic Association describes a whole-person orientation:

> The personal physician is responsible for providing for all the patient's health care needs or taking responsibility for appropriately arranging care with other qualified professionals. This includes care for all stages of life: acute care, chronic care, preventive services, and *end of life care*. (American Academy of Family Physicians et al., 2007, p. 1, emphasis added)

Attention to the spectrum of needs of persons near the end of life and their families thus is highly consistent with the goals of the medical home approach.

Medical homes are commonly used in the care of children. Pediatricians in medical homes provide end-of-life care "by proactively coordinating care; facilitating consistent communication for better decision-making; providing

---

[2]In this study, coordination was defined based partly on the coordination measure from the short form of the Ambulatory Care Experiences Survey, continuity of care was based on a formula that involved the number of primary care clinicians seen by a patient during 1 year and the number of visits to each primary care clinician, and high use of specialty care was defined as 10 or more specialty care visits in 1 year.

[3]The SEER-Medicare database comprises Medicare beneficiaries diagnosed with cancer.

anticipatory guidance; and helping to manage symptoms and social distress; and helping with medical decision-making" (Tripathi et al., 2012, p. 113). These activities are seen as consistent with palliative care, as described later in this chapter, and should be offered from the time of diagnosis onward, according to the American Academy of Pediatrics (AAP, 2013).

Strongly related to the primary care needs of many older people with advanced serious illnesses are their needs for geriatric care. Geriatricians routinely provide care for vulnerable older adults with complex conditions (Warshaw et al., 2008). Providing appropriate palliative care is a core value of this subspecialty of both internal medicine and family medicine (Besdine et al., 2005). Many of the needs of older people can also be met by geron-tological advanced practice nurses (Hendrix and Wojciechowski, 2005).

Addressing the palliative needs of people near the end of life and their families is consistent with the expertise, approach, and values of primary care across the life span.

The Problem of Burdensome Transitions

Patients often experience multiple transitions near the end of life, and they suffer the consequences of the resultant discontinuities in care. Medication errors, disruptions in care planning, and failures to coordinate care all are implicated in poorly managed transitions between care settings, including between hospitals and nursing homes or private homes. Following discharge from hospital to home, the lack of a single point of contact and of nurse involvement in follow-up care can be unsettling to patients and families (Swan, 2012). Transitions characterized by these deficits or those that are simply difficult for sick, confused patients and their families to manage are considered "burdensome." Transitions between care settings can be confusing and overwhelming to patients, especially seriously ill patients, and their families and can result in preventable readmissions or emergency department visits. Often, appropriate follow-up referrals are not made, follow-up with relevant health care professionals is not sufficiently timely, psychological and social needs are not addressed, and potentially useful personnel such as social workers, pharmacists, health educators, and rehabilitation therapists are not engaged (Abrashkin et al., 2012; Feigenbaum et al., 2012).

Preventable hospital readmissions are frequently a consequence of poorly managed transitions. As many as one-fifth of Medicare fee-for-service beneficiaries discharged from the hospital to the community in 2003-2004 were readmitted within 30 days, and one-half of them did not see their physician in the interim (Jencks et al., 2009). Between 2000 and 2009, the rate of health care transitions—both in the last 90 days and in the last 3 days of life—among fee-for-service Medicare beneficiaries increased

(Teno et al., 2013). Among transitions in the last 3 days of life, more than 20 percent were to an acute care hospital.

In what may be the start of a favorable trend, the Medicare readmission rate did fall slightly in 2012, to 18.4 percent (Gerhardt et al., 2013). This decline was perhaps related to recent initiatives aimed at reducing readmissions. For example, Aetna Medicare Advantage members in the mid-Atlantic region who received care under what was called the Transitional Care Model had a 29 percent 3-month readmission rate, compared with a 39 percent rate among matched nonparticipants; they also experienced far fewer hospital days on average during the 3 months postdischarge (Naylor et al., 2013). The Transitional Care Model entailed assignment of a transitional care nurse at the time of admission to assess needs and develop and implement the discharge plan. Similarly, an intervention designed to encourage patients and family caregivers to play a more active role in care transitions led to lower readmission rates at both 30 and 90 days in a large integrated care delivery system in Colorado (Coleman et al., 2006). This intervention included guidance from a "transitions coach," as well as encouragement and tools to improve communication across settings. Another intervention, in an academic medical center, led to lower hospital utilization within 30 days of discharge by using a "nurse discharge advocate" to conduct patient education, arrange follow-up appointments, and assist with reconciliation of medications (Jack et al., 2009). More recently, the Centers for Medicare & Medicaid Services' (CMS's) Quality Improvement Organization Program, Community-based Care Transitions Program, and Hospital Readmissions Reductions Program introduced a penalty that reduces payments to hospitals with a disproportionate readmission rate for particular conditions beginning in 2012. This initiative, which incorporates aspects of several of these other programs, has demonstrated success in reducing hospital readmission rates (Brock et al., 2013; CMS, 2013a, 2014a,b; James, 2013).

To reduce readmission rates and improve primary care, the U.S. Department of Veterans Affairs (VA) has used Patient Aligned Care Teams (PACTs) with nurse case managers. In Madison, Wisconsin, a VA program called Coordinated-Transitional Care (C-TraC) used experienced nurses as case managers to consult with patients by telephone, rather than in home visits (Kind et al., 2012). These nurses followed protocols intended to educate and empower the patient and caregiver in medication management, ensure medical follow-up, educate the patient and caregiver to respond to "red flags" indicating a worsening medical condition, and ensure that the patient and caregiver knew whom to contact. Readmission rates were 23 percent among C-TraC patients in 2010-2012, compared with 34 percent at baseline. The 23 percent rate is still higher than the 18.4 percent national average for 2012 noted above, but this difference may reflect differences in patient characteristics.

According to a meta-review of 57 meta-analyses of randomized clinical trials, community-based disease management programs[4] have been shown to reduce hospital readmission rates for patients with heart failure, coronary heart disease, and asthma (Benbassat and Taragin, 2013). On the other hand, disease management programs for several other types of patients and inpatient-based programs generally have been less successful. A systematic review of 21 randomized clinical trials involving transitions of patients from the hospital to another setting found that 9 of the interventions resulted in a statistically significant positive effect on readmission (Naylor et al., 2011); all 9 interventions involved nurses, and 6 of these involved home visits.

Transfers to and from nursing homes are also important to end-of-life care in at least two ways. First, as noted in Chapter 1, the percentage of deaths occurring in nursing homes has been greater recently than it was in the years prior to the publication of *Approaching Death* (IOM, 1997). As end-of-life care moves away from hospitals and toward nursing homes and individual homes, the quality of care near the end of life in nonhospital settings becomes more important (Flory et al., 2004). Second, many nursing home residents with dementia, in particular, face burdensome transitions and may experience interventions that cause discomfort and produce little if any gain:

> The late stages of dementia are characterized by major challenges to quality of life, including inability to communicate, initiate movement, or walk; difficulty eating and swallowing; agitation; incontinence; and a high risk of infection and pressure ulcers. The sources of suffering for individuals with dementia go beyond fear, depression, and confusion and include significant physical symptoms, including pain, coughing, choking, dyspnea, agitation, and weakness. . . . Nearly all family members of nursing home residents with advanced dementia report that comfort is the primary goal for their care. Nonetheless, a minority of Medicare decedents with dementia are referred to hospice before death, and repeated burdensome transitions between hospitals and nursing homes and feeding tube placement commonly occur, despite lack of evidence of quality of life or survival benefit. (Unroe and Meier, 2013, p. 1212)

In one sense, nursing homes face a dilemma in providing care near the end of life. Although nursing homes typically are a frail elderly person's final residence, federal and state agencies and national accreditation entities hold them to standards that can be more suitable to life-prolonging

---

[4]Disease management programs coordinate services, over time and across settings, for patients with multiple serious conditions (Ellrodt et al., 1997).

care than to addressing quality of life and comfort near the end of life. As a result, "evidence indicates that nursing homes undertreat pain, especially in cognitively impaired and minority residents" (IOM, 2011, p. 141).

Unwanted Care and Lack of Coordination and Continuity: An Illustration

Box 2-2 presents a family narrative illustrating several dimensions of care near the end of life that is neither needed nor desired, neither coordinated nor continuous. Those dimensions include a failure to implement advance directives, an excessive number of burdensome transitions, repeated miscommunications with the family, inadequate pain management and apparent overuse of sedation, insensitive communication with the patient, and an inordinate delay in referral to hospice. Chapter 3 examines in detail the importance of communication about patients' values, goals, and informed preferences. Such communication can help patients avoid unwanted care and ensure that they receive care that is consistent with their personal goals and values.

How frequently does this scenario occur? The incident recounted in Box 2-2 took place despite the active involvement of at least one clearly articulate family advocate; many people near the end of life lack this advantage. Other accounts of unwanted treatment that fails to accord with patient preferences are reported in generalist publications (Butler, 2013; Krieger, 2012; Rauch, 2013), in comments submitted to the committee online by members of the public, and in subsequent chapters of this report.

The IOM Committee on Improving the Quality of Cancer Care recently underscored the importance of patient preferences, saying, "In the setting of advanced cancer, the cancer care team should provide patients with end-of-life care consistent with their needs, values, and preferences" (IOM, 2013, p. 138). Current conditions appear to fall far short of this goal. The same IOM report notes that according to recent studies, clinicians ask for patient preferences in medical decisions only about half the time. (See also Chapter 3.)

THE PALLIATIVE APPROACH

Palliative care can be considered an umbrella term that encompasses a spectrum of approaches to delivering care for people with serious advanced illness. Various organizations have put forward conceptual or functional definitions of palliative care, suggesting that it

- "seeks to prevent, relieve, reduce, or soothe the symptoms of disease or disorder without effecting a cure" (IOM, 1997, p. 31).

BOX 2-2
The Impact of Unwanted, Uncoordinated Treatment:
A Family Narrative

The subject of this narrative is a New England man who died at age 98, several years after telling his family and signing directives to exclude "heroic" measures at the end of his life. His daughter recounts his experience:

In 2010, he had been suffering from a form of senile dementia progressively for at least 10 years, though his physical health was excellent. The death of his wife, however, in May of that year, caused him greater confusion and anxiety than he had ever experienced. . . .

Early in the morning on December 7, 2010, the staff at the assisted living facility, where he lived in Maine, found him on the floor. They phoned an ambulance and he was taken to a nearby hospital, where a left hip fracture was diagnosed. . . .

The surgery was "successful" and my father "recovered" post-operatively very well. However, his agitation—presumably prompted by pain, unfamiliar surroundings, lack of comprehension of the circumstances—increased daily. . . .

In the 4 weeks prior to his death, my father lived under the care of five different institutions in two states. Only the last place, the hospice, appeared willing or able to provide care and comfort to a man who was obviously at the end of his life.

After he had been in the hospital in Maine for 12 days, a social worker phoned one morning to say an ambulance was on its way to take him to a hospital in Haverhill, Massachusetts, where his medications would be "adjusted." . . . The transfer was already in progress; we, the family, were merely being notified.

When we arrived at the hospital in Maine, distraught at the short notice, we asked to see the doctor who was discharging my father. A psychiatrist, he explained the reasons for my father's abrupt discharge. According to medical practice, it was well known (from patients who could give a reliable history) that post-op pain is gone after 3 days. Given the state my father was in—he was groaning in evident agony—I began to suspect that the situation was purposely misunderstood by the professionals in charge of his care.

It was clear that there was no good future for my father: I knew his comprehension could not be improved medically; only his physical activity and his mental agitation could be subdued by drugs. Distressed myself, I pleaded with this psychiatrist that all my father needed was "care and comfort," a phrase my own doctor had assured me was the medically acceptable option. At this, the psychiatrist looked me straight in the eye and said, "I'm sorry, but because of my own personal and religious beliefs, I am not able to discuss that with you."

When we arrived at the Haverhill facility—which we only then discovered was a mental hospital—my father was already admitted to a ward of mostly elderly patients who, we had been told, were being treated for medical as well as psychiatric problems. However, it was there that an aide, trying to help my father to the toilet, recoiled in horror when he saw the staples still holding the incision site together, asking, "How do we get him to the toilet with a broken hip?"

A staff social worker . . . seemed surprised that this new patient had come from Maine, but then remembered that their marketing person had just visited the Maine hospital. My father's transfer was apparently the first success of their new marketing campaign.

She told us that on Monday morning we would be called for a family meeting to consider my father's care. . . . His distress and confusion steadily increased. By Sunday, he was hostile, even to us (we had never seen that before) and obviously paranoid. . . .

Monday morning came, and no one contacted us. I phoned both the social worker and the nurses' station on the floor, but no one was available to talk to me about my father. Fifteen minutes after my last phone call, my sister received a call from the Haverhill hospital to inform her that they were transferring my father to a nearby regional hospital emergency room. Why? Because he was dehydrated and had an elevated white cell count.

When we got to the emergency department and saw my father, he was heavily sedated. . . . We were later told that my father was not dehydrated and that actually his white cell count was only slightly elevated. The Haverhill mental hospital had kept him the three nights required for reimbursement by Medicare and then got rid of him.

The staff at the regional hospital were terrific. . . . We agreed to have him admitted to their "Adult Behavior Unit." . . . Despite his dementia, my father had somehow retained the old-fashioned courtesy and personal decorum of a by-gone era—being addressed by well-meaning young staff members as "Sweetie" added to his bewilderment. He hated being there. . . . A few days after Christmas, when it was evident that my father wasn't going to improve and neither could he stay there, a thoughtful and efficient social worker suggested a hospice center also in Haverhill.

The hospice staff was uniformly kind, supportive, unhurried, and caring; they provided a wonderfully peaceful place to live while dying. He died 4 days later, and we still regret that he didn't get there sooner.

[He] died on January 2, 2011, 65 years to the day that he was discharged from the Army after serving in the Pacific during World War II.

SOURCE: Stephens, 2011. Reprinted with permission from WBUR and Sarah Stephens.

- "is a broader term that includes hospice care as well as other care that emphasizes symptom control, but does not necessarily require the presence of an imminently terminal condition or a time-limited prognosis. Palliative care may include a balance of comfort measures and curative interventions that varies across a wide spectrum" (VA, 2008, p. 2).
- is "specialized medical care for people with serious illnesses. It is focused on providing patients with relief from the symptoms, pain, and stress of a serious illness—whatever the diagnosis. The goal is to improve quality of life for both the patient and the family" (CAPC, 2013).
- is "an approach that improves the quality of life of patients and their families facing the problem associated with life-threatening illnesses, through the prevention and relief of suffering by means of early identification and impeccable assessment and treatment of pain and other problems, physical, psychological, and spiritual" (WHO, 2002, p. 84).
- "focuses on achieving the best possible quality of life for patients and their family caregivers, based on patient and family needs and goals and independent of prognosis. Interdisciplinary palliative care teams assess and treat symptoms, support decision-making and help match treatments to informed patient and family goals, mobilize practical aid for patients and their family caregivers, identify community resources to ensure a safe and secure living environment, and promote collaborative and seamless models of care across a range of care settings (i.e., hospital, home, and nursing home)" (Meier, 2011, p. 344).
- "provides relief from pain and other distressing symptoms; affirms life and regards dying as a normal process; intends neither to hasten or postpone death; integrates the psychological and spiritual aspects of patient care; offers a support system to help patients live as actively as possible until death; offers a support system to help the family cope during the patient's illness and in their own bereavement; uses a team approach to address the needs of patients and their families, including bereavement counseling, if indicated; will enhance quality of life, and may also positively influence the course of illness; is applicable early in the course of illness, in conjunction with other therapies that are intended to prolong life, such as chemotherapy or radiation therapy, and includes those investigations needed to better understand and manage distressing clinical complications" (WHO, 2013).[5]

---

[5]A separate World Health Organization definition of palliative care for children is cited later in this chapter.

- "means patient and family-centered care that optimizes quality of life by anticipating, preventing, and treating suffering. Palliative care throughout the continuum of illness involves addressing physical, intellectual, emotional, social, and spiritual needs and to facilitate patient autonomy, access to information, and choice" (Dahlin, 2013; HHS, 2008).

A content analysis of these seven definitions was developed for this report. That analysis revealed four essential attributes of palliative care, used in constructing the definition of palliative care used in this report:

Palliative care provides relief from pain and other symptoms, supports quality of life, and is focused on patients with serious advanced illness and their families.

Palliative care may begin early in the course of treatment for a serious illness and may be delivered in a number of ways and across the continuum of health care settings, including the home, assisted living facilities, nursing homes, long-term acute care facilities, acute care hospitals, and outpatient clinics. It encompasses

- *hospice care,* usually including services required under the Medicare Hospice Benefit (described in more detail in Chapter 5);
- *basic (or, as it is sometimes called in the literature, "primary") palliative care,* delivered by health care professionals who are *not* palliative care specialists, such as primary care clinicians, physicians who are disease-oriented specialists (such as oncologists and cardiologists), and others (such as nurses, social workers, pharmacists, and chaplains) who care for this population but are not certified in palliative care; and
- *specialty palliative care,* delivered by health care professionals who *are* palliative care specialists, such as physicians who are board certified in this specialty, palliative-certified nurses,[6] and palliative care-certified social workers, pharmacists, and chaplains.

Specialty palliative care currently is most commonly hospital based and offered as a consultative service, although growth recently has been seen in specialty palliative care services in outpatient settings, at home, in nursing homes, and in long-term acute care facilities (CAPC, 2011; NHPCO,

---

[6]Palliative nurses are certified in one of seven certification programs, such as programs for advanced certified hospice and palliative nurse and certified hospice and palliative nursing assistant (NBCHPN®, 2013). Chapter 4 reviews these programs.

2012a, 2013). A survey of 20 outpatient palliative care practices revealed that almost all anticipate substantial growth (Smith et al., 2013a).

The delivery of palliative care has been studied in racially and ethnically diverse patients. In a review of care provided to 1,999 seriously ill African American and Hispanic patients at a safety net hospital, 65 percent of African Americans and 70 percent of Hispanics elected do-not-resuscitate (DNR) orders following palliative care consultation (Sacco et al., 2013). On admission, by comparison, 80 percent of African American patients and 71 percent of Hispanic patients had unknown DNR status, and 20 percent and 29 percent, respectively, had elected no DNR status; 29 percent of all patients were referred to hospice. These findings suggest that palliative care consultations can help overcome gaps in information that lead to unwanted, intensive interventions near the end of life. Language barriers may also hamper palliative care consultations for some populations. Elderly people who communicate in Asian languages, for example, have been found to have difficulty finding nursing homes where they can communicate with staff members (Vega, 2014).

Growth in Hospice Use

Hospice is an essential approach to addressing the palliative care needs of patients with limited life expectancy and their families. In 1995, 17 percent of all U.S. deaths—some 390,000 decedents—were users of hospice (IOM, 1997); by 2011, this figure had risen to 45 percent of U.S. deaths, or more than 1 million decedents (NHPCO, 2012a).

Hospice emerged as a modern concept in the United Kingdom in the mid-20th century as a result of the pioneering work of Dame Cicely Saunders, a physician, nurse, and social worker. The approach and concept were popularized in the United States partly through the writing of Elisabeth Kubler-Ross (NHPCO, undated). For people with a terminal illness or at high risk of dying in the near future, hospice is a comprehensive, socially supportive, pain-reducing, and comforting alternative to technologically elaborate, medically centered interventions. It therefore has many features in common with palliative care, and indeed in this report is considered a subset of palliative care. Various definitions of hospice exist that reiterate these points:

- The IOM report *Approaching Death* offers three definitions: a discrete site of care; an organization that provides and/or arranges for services to patients in homes or other settings; and "an approach to care for dying patients based on clinical, social, and metaphysical or spiritual principles" (IOM, 1997, p. 31).

- The VA defines hospice as "a mode of palliative care, often associated with specific characteristics of the individual receiving the care, diagnosed with a known terminal condition with a prognosis less than 6 months, and desiring therapies with a palliative intent for the terminal condition" (VA, 2008, p. 2).
- The National Quality Forum (NQF), in *A National Framework and Preferred Practices for Palliative and Hospice Care Quality*, defines hospice as "a service delivery system that provides palliative care for patients who have a limited life expectancy and require comprehensive biomedical, psychosocial, and spiritual support as they enter the terminal stage of an illness or condition. It also supports family members coping with the complex consequences of illness, disability, and aging as death nears" (NQF, 2006, p. 3).

With the understanding that in discussing particular studies, the terms employed by their authors are used, this report uses the NQF definition of hospice.

As noted in Chapter 1, whereas hospice programs originally were designed primarily to serve people with cancer, hospices now also serve large numbers of people with heart problems, Alzheimer's disease, kidney disease, and other conditions, including (especially before improvements in drug treatments) HIV/AIDS. As one clinician told the committee in open testimony, "Hospices are known and trusted in their communities" (Harrold, 2013), and hospice use has attained mainstream status.

By 2012 there were 5,500 hospice programs in the United States, reflecting a steady increase since the first such program opened in 1974 (NHPCO, 2013). (Note that one commercial or nonprofit entity may operate multiple hospice programs, each at a different site.) Nearly three in five of these programs were free-standing or independent, while the rest were part of a hospital system, home health agency, or nursing home. In 2012, more than three-fourths of the programs admitted fewer than 500 patients, and the (mean) average daily census of the programs was 149 patients. New hospice programs opening in 2008-2009 were more likely to be for-profit than those that began operation in earlier years. There also is a trend toward larger hospices (Thompson et al., 2012). The VA has shown a commitment to providing veterans with high-quality hospice and specialty palliative care (Daratsos and Howe, 2007; Edes et al., 2007). Hospice and palliative care is part of the VA's standard medical benefits package, and palliative care consultation teams are available at all VA hospitals in the United States.

Hospice services are available to many children with serious chronic diseases, as described in Appendix F. That appendix points to an increasing share of deaths among seriously ill children occurring at home, but with substantial racial differences (such as a smaller proportion of African American children dying at home) nationally and in some states. Still, children appear to have far less access than adults to hospice. Hospices responding to a 2007 survey typically cared for only 1-20 children per year (Friebert, 2009).

Volunteers are an important part of hospice services and, in fact, are required under hospice conditions of participation for Medicare and Medicaid.[7] A 2006 study of volunteer participation in 305 hospice programs found an average of 0.7 volunteer hours per patient per week (Block et al., 2010). The researchers then matched use of volunteers with an associated survey of 57,000 family members of decedents. Hospice programs with the greatest use of volunteers had the highest overall ratings for quality of care. Using volunteers can also increase access to hospice care in some circumstances. For example, prison volunteers have helped make hospice a viable service for fellow inmates who are dying, including elderly prisoners serving long sentences and prisoners with AIDS (Casavecchia, 2011; Mitchell, 2013).

People frequently associate hospice use with earlier death and abandonment of treatment. The reality is very different. Some evidence suggests that on average, hospice patients live longer than similarly ill nonhospice patients. For example, hospice patients outlived nonhospice patients by an average of 29 days in a study of almost 4,500 Medicare beneficiaries in the late 1990s and early 2000s (Connor et al., 2007). In a study of 7,879 Medicare beneficiaries who died of advanced non-small-cell lung cancer between 1991 and 1999, 26 percent of hospice patients and 21 percent of nonhospice patients survived 1 year from diagnosis, and 6.9 percent of hospice patients and 5.5 percent of nonhospice patients survived 2 years (Saito et al., 2011).

As the discussion of the evidence for the effectiveness of palliative care later in this chapter further shows, addressing the physical, emotional, and support needs of patients through a palliative approach may actually extend life expectancy, in addition to improving the quality of life and increasing patient and family satisfaction. Box 2-3, for example, describes a case in which hospice tailored services to meet the needs of a seriously ill elderly woman who was contemplating suicide.

Growing Support for Palliative Care

First hospice and later a broader palliative care approach arose during the latter part of the 20th century. Palliative care is consistent with the biopsychosocial model of care, prominent in the mental health field for the

---

[7]42 CFR § 418.78 Conditions of Participation: Volunteers.

BOX 2-3
Hospice Responds to a Patient's Unique Needs

In an interview with a hospice and palliative medicine specialist, an introspective 86-year-old woman with progressive congestive heart failure and multiple comorbidities, including depression, was contemplating suicide. The physician suggested she consider hospice to maximize her quality of life, prevent her from feeling like a burden to her family, and help her and the family make medical and social decisions concordant with her goals (Kutner, 2010). At the beginning of her ensuing hospice stay, the woman was "upset about hospice in general, specific caregivers, and medical decisions" (Triveldi and Delbanco, 2011, p. 645). But discussions with family members and health professionals, including assurances that she could disenroll from hospice, proved reassuring (Kutner, 2010). Members of her health care team later reported: "In the end, she and the hospice caregivers developed a style that suited all concerned, enabled her to stay in her home, relieved her discomfort, and facilitated her death at home. With hospice's assistance, she was able to die as she wished—in her home with dignity, control, and comfort" (Triveldi and Delbanco, 2011, p. 645). Death came 22 months after the initial interview with the physician.

---

past three decades, which views patients in a broader context than their disease state and attends to relationships between physical and mental health (Curlin, 2013; Engel, 1980). In the United States, higher percentages of dying patients—and far more patients with noncancer diagnoses—receive hospice or palliative care services compared with other countries, such as Canada, England, and Germany (Klinger et al., 2013).

Much of the appeal of palliative care flows from its dual emphasis on (1) providing support that enables patients to remain for as long as possible at home or in the least restrictive and least intensive setting of care and (2) ensuring that patients receive care consistent with their values, goals, and informed preferences, including avoiding the discomfort of unwanted tests and procedures that may not be necessary or beneficial. With palliative care,

> [p]atients are able to remain in their homes as a consequence of better family support, care coordination, and home care and hospice referrals; more hospital admissions go directly to the palliative care service or hospice program instead of a high-cost intensive care unit (ICU) bed; patients not benefiting from an ICU setting are transferred to more supportive settings; and non-beneficial or harmful imaging, laboratory, specialty consultation, and procedures are avoided. (Meier, 2011, p. 350)

Over the past two decades, hospital-based palliative care programs have grown from very small numbers to, by 2011, a presence in 67 percent of U.S. hospitals with at least 50 beds (CAPC, 2013), 85 percent of U.S. hospitals with more than 300 beds, 54 percent of public hospitals, and 26 percent of for-profit hospitals (CAPC, 2011). Such programs are especially common in large hospitals and those affiliated with medical schools (CAPC, 2013). In seven states and the District of Columbia, 80 percent of all hospitals had these services in 2011, while six states had such services in fewer than 40 percent of hospitals (CAPC, 2011). In addition, almost 70 percent of children's hospitals had a palliative care program in 2012 (Feudtner et al., 2013). Access to inpatient palliative care varies by geography and type of hospital, with hospitals in the south, for-profit and public hospitals, and those that are sole community providers less likely to offer it (Goldsmith et al., 2008).

Several factors have contributed to the rise of palliative care since the release of *Approaching Death* (IOM, 1997):

- increases in the numbers and needs of elderly Americans,
- recognition of the numbers and needs of family caregivers,
- greater prevalence of chronic diseases, and
- public attention to controversies and legal cases regarding the right to die and assisted suicide (Meier, 2010).

In addition, a growing body of research and data has emerged to support the use of palliative care, as discussed in the evidence review below.

Successful clinical experiences and the support of consumer groups, influenced by high rates of patient and family satisfaction, have also contributed to broader use of palliative care. For example, the cancer advocacy group C-Change strongly supports "increasing the use of palliative care throughout treatment" (Santiago, 2013, p. 5).

Other specialty societies and authorities are beginning to recommend integration of palliative care into disease-specific treatment and care. Beyond the field of cancer, palliative care is supported by groups advocating improved care in renal disease (Molony, 2013) and neurology (Shaw, 2010). Authorities also recommend integrating evidence-based specialty medical care and palliative care for patients with heart failure (Goodlin, 2009).

In general, however, acceptance of recommendations to counsel patients about palliative care appears to be slow. In a national survey of cardiologists, for example, less than one-half of respondents said they would discuss palliative care in the case of two hypothetical elderly patients with late-stage heart failure, as recommended by clinical guidelines (Matlock et al., 2010). This departure from cardiology guidelines was especially pronounced in regions with high use of health care services in the last 6 months of life.

My long-time best friend just died of a slowly progressive brain tumor. Over the 5 years since his diagnosis, he slowly lost ability to use his left side, his vision, and finally his speech. However, thanks to the diligence of family and hospice, friends, and a few respectful caregivers, he spent the last few weeks of his life comfortably at home, almost constantly in the presence of family, friends, and his most diligent wife. He spent these days listening to his favorite music, reading poetry, discussing new ideas and old ones, holding hands, and giving hugs. His final weeks were the most peaceful imaginable! Such a profoundly meaningful exit is indeed rare.

The "medicalization" of the end of life which is pervasive in America creates many obstacles to the experience of my friend. The relatively "new" (but very old) palliative care movement in this country cannot come to fruition soon enough!*

---

*Quotation from a response submitted through the online public testimony questionnaire for this study. See Appendix C.

Illustrative Palliative Care Processes

The MD Anderson Cancer Center's Supportive and Palliative Care Service illustrates how palliative care can function in hospital and outpatient settings. A palliative care consultant meets with patients and families, and together they develop treatment goals and identify problems. Early introduction of palliative care helps ensure a greater level of comfort for patients during the entire course of treatment (Bruera and Hui, 2010).

The clinical process begins with an assessment, using one of several validated assessment instruments (Hui, 2008).[8] To meet palliative care needs throughout an illness, regular palliative care assessment is then incorporated into patient care. Box 2-4 summarizes recent efforts to improve and standardize the assessment process.

Using initial assessment results, palliative care consultants can help direct relevant assistance, in conformance with patient and family treatment goals. For example, one problem common among cancer patients but difficult to identify is depression. As appropriate, the palliative care team

---

[8]Examples include the Edmonton Symptom Assessment System; the Memorial Delirium Assessment Scale; and instruments used to assess the patient's performance status, which helps determine eligibility for certain cancer therapies and is believed to help predict survival, quality of life, and functioning (Hui, 2008).

BOX 2-4
Palliative Care Screening in the Hospital

Hospital palliative care is most commonly provided by a consultation service based in the hospital. A key question is which inpatients could benefit from a palliative care consultation, and when. The Center to Advance Palliative Care convened a consensus panel to develop checklists for identifying these patients.

The panel determined that every hospital, including specialty hospitals, should identify patients at high risk for unmet palliative care needs using a screening process on admission that looks for

- a potentially life-limiting or life-threatening condition; and
- five primary criteria of (1) whether the attending physician would not be surprised if the patient died within 12 months or before adulthood; (2) frequent hospital admissions; (3) admissions prompted by physical or psychological symptoms that are difficult to control; (4) complex care requirements; and (5) a decline in function, feeding intolerance, or unintended decline in weight; and when possible to identify, also looks for
- secondary criteria, including, for example, admission from a nursing home or similar facility, hip fracture, and lack of advance care planning.

The panel also proposed a similar but separate checklist for assessing patients daily during their hospital stay, as appropriate. This checklist looks for

- a potentially life-limiting or life-threatening condition; and
- five primary criteria of (1) whether the attending physician would not be surprised if the patient died within 12 months or before adulthood; (2) physical or psychological symptoms that are difficult to control; (3) intensive care unit (ICU) stay of 7 or more days; (4) lack of documentation of or clarity about goals of care; (5) disagreements or uncertainty among patient, family, and/or staff about medical decisions and treatment preferences; and when possible to identify, also looks for
- secondary criteria, including, for example, emotional distress of the patient or family, medical team considering patient as a candidate for feeding tube placement, tracheostomy, ethics consults, or other similar procedures or services.

The main components of palliative care assessment include pain and other symptoms, social and spiritual factors, patient's understanding of the illness and prognosis and treatment options, development of patient-centered goals of care, and discharge planning.

SOURCE: Weissman and Meier, 2011.

helps minimize medications that may contribute to depression, rules out comorbidities that may contribute to depression, provides or arranges for counseling or psychotherapy, and prescribes antidepressant medications as needed (Dev and Sivesind, 2008).

Other palliative care processes focus on spiritual and cultural aspects of care. For example, chaplaincy services, the most visible mode of spiritual services, are described in Chapter 4. The importance of spiritual services is underscored by the spiritual distress experienced by many patients near the end of life (Hui et al., 2011).

Palliative Care for Children

The World Health Organization (WHO) has developed a definition of palliative care specifically for children, which states in part: "Palliative care for children is the active total care of the child's body, mind and spirit, and also involves giving support to the family" (WHO, 2013).[9] Palliative care for children differs from adult palliative care based on the stage of child development, which affects communication and the patient's understanding of illness and death; differences between children's diseases and causes of death and those of adults; greater involvement of family members as direct caregivers and decision makers; and the emotional impact of the child's illness on parents and siblings (Zhukovsky, 2008).

One important development since the IOM report *When Children Die* (IOM, 2003) was issued is the emergence of several sets of guidelines for pediatric palliative care. These include guidelines of the National Hospice and Palliative Care Organization (NHPCO, 2009) and the Children's Oncology Group and Association of Pediatric Hematology and Oncology Nurses (Ethier et al., 2010), and the National Cancer Institute's "PDQ" for health professionals on pediatric supportive care, including care at the end of life (NCI, 2014).

Assessment scales that are age- and developmentally appropriate are used in evaluating pediatric patients. For pain, for example, behavioral observation scales often are used for children under 4 years of age, while faces, photographic or drawing scales, color-analog scales, body maps, and other

---

[9]The WHO definition includes the following additional characteristics of pediatric palliative care, which WHO states should apply to other pediatric chronic disorders, not just life-threatening illnesses: "It begins when illness is diagnosed, and continues regardless of whether or not a child receives treatment directed at the disease. Health providers must evaluate and alleviate a child's physical, psychological, and social distress. Effective palliative care requires a broad multidisciplinary approach that includes the family and makes use of available community resources; it can be successfully implemented even if resources are limited. It can be provided in tertiary care facilities, in community health centres and even in children's homes" (WHO, 2013).

tools may be appropriate for children ages 3-7 (Zhukovsky, 2008). Adult visual analog scales and verbal rating scales are often used for children over age 8. Likewise, diverse interventions are used to manage pain, including the cognitive-behavioral strategies of distraction, imagery, thought stopping, exercise, relaxation, modeling, desensitization, art therapy, music therapy, and play therapy.

As noted in Appendix F, most pediatric deaths take place in hospitals, and the majority of these deaths occur in critical care units, often with an escalating array of procedures, such as mechanical ventilation. Since 2005, children's hospitals, in particular, have developed pediatric palliative care teams for children with long-term advanced serious illness and/or a broad array of symptoms. The pediatric palliative care approach combines the continuity of care and patient-centeredness usually associated with primary care with highly specialized clinical services. It complements, rather than replaces, curative and related life-extending specialty services.

Since 1997, for example, a palliative care program at Children's Hospital Boston and Dana-Farber Cancer Institute has coordinated care, helped families make difficult treatment decisions, focused on easing the child's pain and suffering, and provided extensive bereavement services (Groopman, 2014). A longitudinal cohort study of 515 patients receiving care from six hospital-based pediatric palliative care programs found that 70 percent of the patients survived at least 1 year after receiving their first palliative care consultation (Feudtner et al., 2011).

States implementing pediatric palliative care programs through Medicaid include California, Colorado, Florida, New York, North Carolina, North Dakota, and Washington (NHPCO, 2012b). Massachusetts has independently funded and implemented a pediatric palliative care program (Bona et al., 2011). Excellus BlueCross BlueShield, serving Upstate New York, developed CompassionNet, a pediatric palliative care program in 2001, serving more than 1,000 families of children with life-threatening illnesses (Excellus BlueCross BlueShield, 2011). The program enhances regular health insurance coverage with social and support services, many of which are not traditionally covered by health insurance, to improve quality of life for both child and family. Services are carefully tailored to each family's unique needs.

Support for family members is an essential part of pediatric palliative care, beginning in the first days of life. Today, babies born even 16 weeks prematurely often survive, but their survival may require painful and uncomfortable interventions and may result in serious, lifelong disabilities, which places a significant burden on parents who must make fateful decisions. As a result, it has been suggested that the same attention given to end-of-life decisions for adults be given to end-of-life decisions for children (Dworetz, 2013).

BOX 2-5
Lessons from Pediatric Care

Pediatrics has long been associated with an emphasis on the importance of the family. The benefits of this family focus remain applicable as patients grow older. Pediatric patient- and family-centered care reflects six core values: listening to and respecting each child and family; flexibility in policies, procedures, and practices; sharing information with patients and families; providing and ensuring formal and informal support; collaborating with patients and families at all levels of health care; and empowering children and families (Committee on Hospital Care and Institute for Patient- and Family-Centered Care, 2012).

In addition, as described in the text, pediatrics assesses a child's behavioral readiness to determine his or her role in making medical decisions, rather than relying on a vague, subjective opinion. End-of-life pediatric care also includes a strong component of bereavement services and consideration of family survivorship.

Moreover, in light of today's changing population demographics (see Chapter 1), pediatrics offers a perspective on how to deal with new family structures—single parents, smaller families and households, and blended families—and the care needs of people of diverse ethnic, cultural, and racial backgrounds.

Finally, although adult and pediatric palliative care differ in important ways, lessons from such care for children can be applied by policy makers and clinicians to improve the care provided to adults, as described in Box 2-5.

Palliative Care in Nonhospital Settings

Although most palliative care programs are hospital based, the palliative approach ideally is available as well wherever patients with serious advanced illness are, including in long-term care facilities, in outpatient clinical settings, and at home. A literature review focused on four "sentinel articles" found that palliative care outside inpatient settings can enhance patient satisfaction; improve symptom control and quality of life; reduce health care utilization; and, in a population of lung cancer patients, lengthen survival (Rabow et al., 2013).

Some nursing homes provide residents with access to palliative care through palliative care consultants, services provided by hospice staff to residents not enrolled in hospice, or enhanced training of nursing home staff (CAPC, 2008; Meier, 2010). Training in some instances has focused on pain management and quality improvement (Robert Wood Johnson Foundation, 2004). Community-based palliative care programs, other than those provided by hospices, are also beginning to appear, although these programs are developing unsystematically, and so at present lack standardization with respect to management processes, services, and methods of integration with other health services (Kamal et al., 2013). Home health agencies, too, are beginning to offer palliative care services (Labson et al., 2013). Advances in communication technology, such as remote monitoring systems that can alert off-site health professionals to changes in a patient's vital signs or medical status, may spur additional growth in such programs.[10]

In New Mexico, a Hospital at Home® project, conducted by Presbyterian Healthcare Services and inspired by developmental work at Johns Hopkins University, assisted patients with congestive heart failure, chronic obstructive pulmonary disease (COPD), and other serious conditions that put them at risk of repeated hospital admissions (Cryer et al., 2012). Services included diagnostic services, arrangements for medical supplies and equipment, transportation, daily physician house calls, and home visits from a nurse once or twice per day. The project succeeded in meeting Presbyterian's core quality metrics 100 percent of the time for 323 patients and achieved higher patient satisfaction ratings than usual care. Other examples appear in Chapter 5.

Palliative care does not always have to be provided by specialist clinicians. In fact, to meet the palliative care needs of all people with advanced serious illness who are likely approaching death, palliative care precepts must be integrated across the continuum of care and generally embraced by clinicians who care for this population. For example, an article by oncology palliative care specialists describes the important role of basic, or "primary," palliative care as "delivered every day in the oncology office" (Cheng et al., 2013, p. 84). These authors stress the importance of several actions by the office-based oncologist: a "repeating conversation" on coping with cancer, use of a symptom assessment scale, a spiritual assessment, and referral to a hospice information visit for patients with a prognosis of 3-6 months. Delivery of basic palliative care by primary care and regular specialist physicians would help meet a rising demand that exceeds the supply of palliative care specialists, simplify demands on patients and families, and reinforce existing relationships (Quill and Abernethy, 2013).

---

[10]Monitoring technologies in development in 2013 included a sensor mat that is placed under the mattress to monitor a patient's sleep patterns, heart rate, and breathing rate; a videoconferencing "robot" to help physicians conduct real-time virtual consultations; cloud-based applications to help patients track vital signs and access their plan of care; and remote monitoring sensors that can be placed throughout the home to detect falls and missed medications. Several of these products have already been approved by the U.S. Food and Drug Administration (InformationWeek, 2013).

Interdisciplinary Team Approach

The interdisciplinary team approach that typically distinguishes palliative care contributes to the development and implementation of comprehensive plans of care, helps ensure coordination of care, enhances the anticipation and remediation of problems that arise during transitions and crises, facilitates quality improvement, and contributes to good pain management (Meier, 2011). According to Mitchell and colleagues (2012, p. 3), "The high-performing team is now widely recognized as an essential tool for constructing a more patient-centered, coordinated, and effective health care delivery system," with the patient and family at the team's center.

Since the publication of *Approaching Death* in 1997, hospice and palliative medicine has become a defined physician specialty, and palliative care has also become a specialty area in the professions of nursing, social work, and chaplaincy (as described in more detail in Chapter 4) (ABMS, 2013; American Osteopathic Association, 2013; APC, 2013; NASW, 2013; NBCHPN®, 2013). In addition to palliative medicine specialists, palliative nurses, social workers, and chaplains, team members may include, for example, pharmacists, dietitians or nutritionists, physical therapists, occupational therapists, psychotherapists, speech-language pathologists, and others such as art or music therapists and child life specialists (Adams et al., 2011; American Occupational Therapy Association, 2011; American Society of Health System Pharmacists, 2002; Cruz, 2013; Hebert et al., 2011; NASW, 2013, 2014; Pollens, 2004; Puchalski et al., 2009; Vitello, 2008). A team with such broad composition is most likely to have the competence and time to meet patients' needs involving medication management, loss of appetite, functional limitations, depression, difficulties in swallowing and communicating, spiritual guidance, and other problems arising, perhaps for the patient's first time, during an advanced stage of illness (NQF, 2006).[11]

The interdisciplinary approach should begin with the initial patient assessment. For example, a nurse may perform the initial assessment, which leads to the involvement of other professional team members as appropriate. The composition of the team depends, to a large extent, on resource availability. In a smaller hospital, in rural settings, and under conditions of

---

[11]To give one example of team composition, Kaiser Permanente's TriCentral Palliative Care program, a model that serves patients at home instead of only in the hospital, has estimated the following full-time equivalent staff complement for a census of 30 palliative care patients: 0.4 physician, 2.2 registered nurses, 1.2 social workers, 1.2 certified home health aides, 0.3 intake and liaison registered nurse, 0.6 clinical nurse specialist supervisor, 0.2 chaplain, 0.3 program director, and 1.0 clerk, for a total staff-to-patient ratio of 1:4, plus volunteers. The program includes patient care conferences every 1-2 weeks (Brumley and Hillary, 2002, p. 26). In pediatric palliative care, as noted in Appendix F, staffing patterns are "remarkably diverse."

a shortage of specialized personnel, teams may be more rudimentary than is the case in large, well-staffed academic medical centers. Identification of which interdisciplinary team members are necessary in any particular situation is part of the assessment process.

Evidence for the Effectiveness of Palliative Care

As noted, a growing evidence base supports the effectiveness of palliative care for those nearing the end of life. A study of 524 dying patients at five VA medical centers and affiliated nursing homes and clinics in 2006-2007 showed that those who received inpatient palliative care consultations had significantly better outcomes in five of six domains studied: information and communication, access to home care services, emotional and spiritual support, well-being and dignity, and care around the time of death (Casarett et al., 2008). A trend toward higher scores for the sixth domain, bereavement services, was not statistically significant. The VA's well-established, highly rated Home Based Primary Care Program for patients with complex chronic disabling diseases includes palliative care services (Beales and Edes, 2009). This program has been in place for four decades, and provides comprehensive longitudinal primary care and palliative care delivered by an interdisciplinary team in the homes of veterans with serious chronic disabling conditions. The program is associated with a 24 percent lower total cost of VA care per patient per year.

A landmark study of palliative care published in 2010 found that it can lead to improved quality of life and greater longevity when provided concurrently with disease-focused care (Temel et al., 2010). In this 3-year study, 151 patients with metastatic non-small-cell lung cancer at Massachusetts General Hospital were randomly assigned at the time of diagnosis to either palliative care or no palliative care, and all patients also received standard oncology treatment. Quality-of-life scores were an average of 6.5 points higher for the palliative care group on the 136-point Functional Assessment of Cancer Therapy-Lung (FACT-L) scale. Symptoms of depression were nearly 2.5 times more common in the non–palliative care group (38 percent versus 16 percent). Moreover, median survival was 30 percent longer for the palliative care group (11.6 months versus 8.9 months), even though fewer patients in that group received aggressive care near the end of life (defined in the study as receipt of chemotherapy within 2 weeks of death, admission to hospice 3 days or less before death, or no admission to hospice care) (33 percent versus 54 percent). The authors conclude that palliative care, begun early in the course of treatment, led to significant improvements in quality of life and mood and was associated with longer survival in this population.[12] Illustrating this study's importance, the American Society of Clinical Oncology cited it as a "strong evidence base" in formulating a provisional clinical opinion (now also adopted in guidelines of the National Comprehensive Cancer Network) advising oncologists to offer palliative care concurrently with standard specialty care, beginning at the time of diagnosis (NCCN, 2013; Simone and Jones, 2013; Smith et al., 2012).

Other studies tend to confirm that palliative care benefits patients. A systematic review of 23 studies conducted in Australia, Canada, Italy, Norway, Spain, Sweden, the United Kingdom, and the United States found that use of expert home palliative care teams more than doubled the odds of dying at home (Gomes et al., 2013). This review further found that home palliative care reduced the symptom burden for patients, while usual care increased it.

In a randomized controlled trial of 512 patients hospitalized with life-limiting diseases in Denver, Portland (Oregon), and San Francisco in 2002-2003, palliative care patients, compared with "usual care" patients, had greater satisfaction with communication and the care experience and fewer critical care unit admissions. No differences in survival or symptom control were found (Gade et al., 2008).

A randomized controlled trial of 322 patients with advanced cancer in New Hampshire and Vermont in 2003-2008 found that a specific psycho-educational palliative care intervention led to higher scores on quality of life and mood (Bakitas et al., 2009). No differences were found in symptom intensity, hospital days, critical care unit admissions, or emergency department visits. The intervention (Educate, Nurture, Advise Before Life Ends, or ENABLE) consisted of four weekly education sessions, with monthly follow-up sessions conducted by an advanced practice nurse.

---

[12]A follow-up analysis of this study explored whether the increased survival rates of the palliative care patients resulted from improvements (that is, reductions) in depression alone. The analysts found that "the data do not support the hypothesis that treatment of depression mediated the observed survival benefit from [early palliative care]" (Pirl et al., 2012, p. 1310). The effect of palliative care on patient longevity is of considerable interest. However, the effects of palliative care on life span—and the factors that may account for those effects—remain unclear. According to Meier (2011, p. 349), "Conjectures accounting for the possibility that palliative care and hospice may prolong life include reduction in depression, which is an independent predictor of mortality in multiple disease types; avoidance of the hazards of hospitalization and high-risk medical interventions; reduction in symptom burden; and improved support for family caregivers that permits patients to remain safely at home." The association between palliative care and increased life span is a promising target for further research.

A number of studies suggest that specialty palliative care has the capacity to

- improve information and communication, access to home care services, emotional and spiritual support, well-being and dignity, and care around the time of death (Casarett et al., 2008);
- reduce depression, enhance quality of life, and increase survival (Temel et al., 2010);
- reduce critical care unit mortality (Elsayem et al., 2006); and
- prevent emergency department visits, hospitalizations, and deaths away from home (Brumley et al., 2007).

The case for greater use of and support for specialty palliative care can be made based on clinical, economic, and ethical considerations: "Early provision of specialty palliative care improves quality of life, lowers spending, and helps clarify treatment preferences and goals of care" (Parikh et al., 2013, p. 2350).

With respect to hospice, high quality of care in hospice overall has been well established in the literature for three decades. As early as 1984, hospice was associated with greater patient satisfaction when compared with conventional care for patients with serious illness nearing the end of life (Kane et al., 1984). As noted earlier, there is suggestive evidence that hospice use may be associated with longer survival (Connor et al., 2007; Saito et al., 2011). Hospice was also found to improve care for people with the difficult diagnosis of dementia in a survey of 538 bereaved family members in Alabama, Florida, Massachusetts, Minnesota, and Texas (Teno et al., 2011). In that study, the family members of patients who received hospice services "at the right time" reported fewer unmet needs, fewer concerns about quality of care, higher quality of care, and better quality of dying. In a survey of 292 family members of deceased nursing home residents enrolled in hospice, 64 percent rated the quality of care rendered before hospice care began as good or excellent for both physical and emotional symptoms (Baer and Hanson, 2000). For quality of care after hospice care began, ratings increased to 93 percent for physical symptoms and 90 percent for emotional symptoms. And in a 10-item family satisfaction survey involving bereaved family members of nearly 1,600 people who died of chronic diseases in 2000, overall satisfaction was found to be better in home hospices than in hospitals, nursing homes, and home health agencies (Teno et al., 2004) (see Table 2-1).

THE PURSUIT OF QUALITY IN CARE NEAR THE END OF LIFE

Two aspects of the quality of palliative care are especially important for establishing accountability: first, which components of palliative care

TABLE 2-1 Family Satisfaction with Alternative Models for End-of-Life Care by Last Site of Care, 2000

Indicator of Family Satisfaction	Hospital (%)	Nursing Home (%)	Home Health Services (%)	Home Hospice (%)
Patient did not receive enough help with pain	19	32	43	18
Patient did not receive enough help with shortness of breath	19	24	38	26
Patient did not receive enough emotional support	52	56	70	35
Physician did not satisfy family desire for contact	52	31	23	14
Family had enough contact with physician but had concerns about physician communication	27	18	27	18
Patient was not always treated with respect	20	32	16	4
Family had concerns about own emotional support	38	36	46	21
Family had concerns about having enough information about what to expect while patient was dying	50	44	32	29
Staff did not know enough about patient's medical history	15	20	8	8
Overall quality of care was excellent	47	42	47	71

SOURCE: Teno et al., 2004.

contribute most to better patient care outcomes, and second, which metrics are most useful for evaluating the quality of care delivered by individual providers. Current efforts to measure and report on these aspects of care are described below. Opportunities to overcome limitations of these efforts are then reviewed, followed by the committee's proposed core components of quality care near the end of life.

Approaches to Improving Quality of Care Near the End of Life

Care of patients with serious advanced illness near the end of life is complex. Various interventions have been implemented and evaluated to identify aspects of quality care near the end of life that lead to positive outcomes and patient and family satisfaction. A systematic review of 23 studies of interventions to improve continuity of care, care coordination, or transitions between settings of care for people with serious illness found the best, yet moderate, evidence for improvement in patient or family satisfaction; evidence generally was weak for other outcomes, including patient or family quality of life, caregiver burden, and utilization of health care resources (Dy et al., 2013). The greatest success in improving satisfaction was achieved through interventions that combined components of a coordinator of care, patient and/or family involvement through health education or another form of assistance, and/or additional patient assessment. Other interventions studied incorporated care plans and use of a palliative care specialist. Quantifying the impact of these components on outcomes was not possible because of the heterogeneity of the studies included in the review. The reviewers also found that "many studies were limited by numerous methodological issues such as insufficient power for reported outcomes (primarily utilization), measuring outcomes not specifically targeted by the intervention, and using measurement tools (especially for quality of life outcomes) not specific for populations with advanced disease" (p. 443).

A broader systematic review, conducted by essentially the same team, found similar methodological deficiencies in many of the 90 studies included in the analysis (AHRQ, 2012). Still, the authors found moderate evidence for improvements in satisfaction with interventions targeting continuity, coordination, and transitions between care settings. Those interventions that incorporated patient-centered quality improvement components, such as patient, family, or caregiver education and self-management, showed the strongest evidence of effectiveness. Evidence was moderate for improvements in health care utilization outcomes among interventions that targeted communication and decision making, but specific quality improvement methods were not assessed for these types of interventions.

Methodological challenges relating to individual interventions (e.g., insufficient statistical power) and larger-scale reviews of interventions (e.g., lack of meta-analysis) make it difficult to quantify the impact of specific components on quality of care and quality of life. Still, information can be gleaned from these studies and reviews, which show that moderate evidence exists to support the impact of some quality improvement interventions on outcomes including satisfaction with care among patients nearing the end of life and their families.

Use of end-of-life care pathways has also been the subject of a systematic review; in this case, researchers found no clinical trials meeting their criteria for high-quality research design that evaluated the benefits of end-of-life care pathways for quality of care and quality of life (Chan and Webster, 2013). The researchers suggest that this gap in the literature reflects a clear need to investigate the effectiveness of pathways and other guidelines for end-of-life care.

Current Quality Measurement and Reporting Efforts

In the mid-2000s, a group building on efforts of the Robert Wood Johnson Foundation's Critical Care End-of-Life Peer Workgroup used a consensus process to develop 18 proposed measures for assessing the quality of palliative care (Mularski et al., 2006). Of these, 14 address processes of care at the patient level, while 4 address structural aspects of critical care delivery. The proposed set of measures was designed to stimulate further work on measurement and enhancement of the quality of palliative care.

NQF (2012) has endorsed 14 evidence-based quality measures for palliative and end-of-life care. (NQF calls these items "measures," but because they are broad categories, they might better be termed "criteria" or "domains.") The NQF measures are as follows:

- pain screening, for hospice and palliative care (NQF #1634);
- pain assessment, for hospice and palliative care (NQF #1637);
- patients treated with an opioid who are given a bowel regimen (NQF #1617);
- patients with advanced cancer assessed for pain at outpatient visits (NQF #1628);
- dyspnea treatment, for hospice and palliative care (NQF #1638);
- dyspnea screening, for hospice and palliative care (NQF #1639);
- patients admitted to an intensive care unit who have care preferences documented (NQF #1626);
- treatment preferences, for hospice and palliative care (NQF #1641);
- percentage of hospice patients with documentation in the clinical record of a discussion of spiritual/religious concerns or documentation that the patient/caregiver did not want to discuss such concerns (NQF #1647);

- comfortable dying (NQF #0209);
- hospitalized patients who die an expected death with an implant-able cardioverter defibrillator (ICD) that has been deactivated (NQF #1625);
- family evaluation of hospice care (NQF #0208);
- Consumer Assessments and Reports of End of Life (NQF #1632); and
- bereaved family survey (NQF #1623).

In 2013 the National Consensus Project for Quality Palliative Care (NCP) released a new set of Clinical Practice Guidelines, rooted, as the name suggests, more in consensus than in evidence for effectiveness (Dahlin, 2013). The NCP is a collaborative effort of the American Academy of Hospice and Palliative Medicine, Center to Advance Palliative Care, Hospice and Palliative Nurses Association, National Association of Social Workers, National Hospice and Palliative Care Organization (NHPCO), and National Palliative Care Research Center. The Clinical Practice Guidelines are divided into eight domains:

- structure and processes of care;
- physical aspects of care;
- psychological and psychiatric aspects of care;
- social aspects of care;
- spiritual, religious, and existential aspects of care;
- cultural aspects of care;
- care of the patient at the end of life; and
- ethical and legal aspects of care.[13]

To illustrate the complexity of these domains, the domain "care of the patient at the end of life" emphasizes multiple preferred practices, including assessment and management of symptoms; documentation and communication with patient, family, and all health care providers about signs and symptoms of the dying process; family guidance; and bereavement support both before and after death, all the while keeping social, spiritual, and cultural concerns in mind. The same domain includes four guidelines, with a list of associated criteria. The guidelines center on (1) identification, communication, and management of signs and symptoms; (2) care planning;

---

[13]The NCP domains are generally consistent with the quality domains suggested by the American Geriatrics Society and emphasized in the *Approaching Death* report (IOM, 1997): physical and emotional symptoms; support of function and autonomy; advance care planning; aggressive care near death—site of death, cardiopulmonary resuscitation (CPR), and hospitalization; patient and family satisfaction; global quality of life; family burden; survival time; provider continuity and skill; and bereavement.

(3) postdeath care; and (4) bereavement support. An interdisciplinary team approach is considered essential.

A large set of quality indicators was developed through a RAND Corporation effort called Assessing Care of Vulnerable Elders (ACOVE) (Wenger et al., 2007). While these indicators cover numerous conditions and care processes and the entire continuum of care, from screening and prevention to diagnosis, treatment, and follow-up, end of life is considered a particular condition within ACOVE. Illustrating how these measures can be used, researchers applied 16 ACOVE indicators for end-of-life care and pain management to the care of almost 500 patients who died at the University of California, Los Angeles, Medical Center between April 2005 and April 2006 (Walling et al., 2010). These indicators, which could be measured using information found in patient medical records, fit into three domains: eliciting goals of care, pain assessment and management, and dyspnea assessment and management. Of note, these domains have content overlap with NQF-endorsed measures. The researchers found that physician-patient/family communication was "the most striking area in need of quality improvement" (p. 1061). Deficits were also found in assessing breathing difficulties, documenting deactivation of ICDs, and establishing bowel regimens for patients taking opioids. The study found further that critical care units addressed goals of care only about half the time. High scores were obtained for pain assessments, pain treatment, and treatment for breathing difficulties (dyspnea).

In conjunction with the effort of CMS to establish quality measures for evaluating hospices, the Carolinas Center for Medical Excellence (the Quality Improvement Organization in North and South Carolina), in conducting the PEACE (Prepare, Embrace, Attend, Communicate, Empower) Project, initially identified 174 measures in the literature, from governmental agencies including the Agency for Healthcare Research and Quality (AHRQ) and CMS and from previous quality measurement efforts by NQF and the RAND Corporation. Of these 174 measures, 88 were submitted to a technical expert panel for review (Schenck et al., 2010). The panel gave high ratings to 34 measures, falling within all eight domains of the NCP's Clinical Practice Guidelines, but most heavily in the domain of physical aspects of care. In a related exercise, 39 instruments measuring mainly physical, psychological, or social aspects of palliative care, identified through a literature review, received high psychometric ratings (Hanson et al., 2010).

Specific new quality indicators have been advocated. One opinion, for example, is that quality standards should prohibit placing feeding tubes in people with advanced dementia, in line with recommendations of leading professional groups (Fischberg et al., 2013; Unroe and Meier, 2013).

Limitations of Current Quality Measurement and Reporting Efforts

There are important opportunities to improve existing quality measures for care near the end of life. The NQF-endorsed measures listed above reflect substantive limitations. Of these 14 items, 4 involve pain, 3 patient preferences, 3 bereaved family or close friend perceptions of the quality of care, 2 dyspnea, 1 ICD, and 1 "comfortable dying" (NQF, 2012). While NQF's Consumer Assessments and Reports of End of Life (CARE) survey assesses decision making using a postdeath survey of the bereaved family, there is no NQF-endorsed measure of shared decision making that asks the seriously ill person about his/her perceptions of the quality of care and the quality of shared decision making. Current NQF-endorsed measures also do not adequately measure the experience of caregiving, advance care planning, concordance with patient preferences, burdensome transitions, or the timeliness of referral to palliative care services. Presumably, these omissions result from a lack of evidence validating specific measures in any of these areas.

Patient and family satisfaction has been used as a relatively common indicator of the quality of end-of-life care. But the measurement of family satisfaction is subject to methodological inconsistencies—for example, the use of qualitative versus quantitative methods or direct versus indirect questions to ascertain satisfaction (Aspinal et al., 2003). Indirect methods may illuminate specific components of care that affect satisfaction and perceived quality of care. An examination of 117,000 surveys from 819 hospices in 2005, for instance, found that family members were more likely to rate hospice services as excellent if they, as family members, were regularly informed about the patient's condition and treatment, if they could identify a single nurse as being in charge of the patient's care, and if they believed the hospice was providing them with the right amount of emotional support (Rhodes et al., 2008). Still, the measurement of satisfaction may be influenced by factors other than quality per se, such as sociodemographic factors or fulfilment of expectations (Aspinal et al., 2003).

Efforts to establish criteria for evaluating the quality of care near the end of life are ongoing. As previously mentioned, a preliminary set of 18 quality measures or criteria was developed through a consensus process in the mid-2000s (Mularski et al., 2006). However, a systematic review of 16 publications on quality indicators for palliative care led researchers to conclude that, while a number of quality indicators have been identified, few development processes for these indicators have been described in detail, and additional specification of methodological characteristics is needed (Pasman et al., 2009). An update to that review identified an additional 13 publications containing 17 sets of quality indicators (including 9 new sets and 8 sets also identified in the previous review) and again determined that further development of indicators is needed (De Roo et al., 2013).

In nursing homes, place of death (in the nursing home or in the hospital) and hospice enrollment were identified as important quality measures for end-of-life care, ones that could be measured using existing administrative data, such as the Minimum Data Set, Medicare enrollment files, and Medicare claims data (Mukamel et al., 2012). Both of these measures were found to be more effective in identifying low-quality than high-quality outliers. Illustrating how these two measures can be used, a study of decedents nationwide between 2003 and 2007 found that within nursing homes, residents with dementia were more likely than other residents to use hospice and to avoid transfer to a hospital as the place of death (Li et al., 2013). Residents of nursing homes with a high prevalence of dementia were also more likely than residents of other nursing homes to use hospice.

Measurement of care components agreed upon as constituting quality care may identify systematic variation in care quality. For example, smaller or independent hospices may be less likely than larger or chain-affiliated programs to achieve comprehensive implementation of preferred practices identified by NQF (Carlson et al., 2011).[14] A similar issue arises regarding place of death—namely, the probability that a person will die in a critical care unit, in another type of hospital unit, or in a more comfortable setting. On this measure, geography appears to be a significant factor, at least for people with cancer. Nationwide, from 2003 to 2007, about 29 percent of Medicare decedents with advanced cancer died in a hospital, but rates ranged from 7 percent in Mason City, Iowa, to 47 percent in Manhattan (Goodman et al., 2010).

Coordination of care is a linchpin of high-quality end-of-life and palliative care and is particularly difficult to measure. An examination of 111 root-cause analysis reports submitted by outpatient departments to the VA's National Center for Patient Safety in 2005-2012 showed that most delays in diagnosis and treatment involved poor communication and coordination among health professionals, other staff, and patients. "Failures in the process of follow-up and tracking of patients were especially prominent, mentioned in more than half of the reports" (Giardina et al., 2013, p. 1371).

At times, quality scores turn out to be unrelated to quality of care, or facilities meeting standards have widely varying performance on recognized quality measures. For example, the Health Resources and Services

---

[14]Similarly, an American Society of Clinical Oncology initiative to measure office-based practices' adherence to cancer care guidelines found that showing physicians how well their practice performed failed to lead to measurable improvements in performance. The authors speculate that this failure may relate to small practices' lack of financial resources to institute formal quality improvement efforts (Blayney et al., 2012).

Administration and the Center for Medicare & Medicaid Innovation use an assessment developed by the National Committee for Quality Assurance (NCQA) to certify community health centers as patient-centered medical homes. One study found that while all 30 of the surveyed centers met criteria for becoming an NCQA-recognized patient-centered medical home, no association was found between performance on the NCQA assessment that determines this recognition and the quality of patient care (Clarke et al., 2012). In what may be of particular interest to advocates of improved end-of-life care, the authors note that the NCQA assessment does not include measures reflecting the provision of social or "enabling" services, such as assistance in obtaining government benefits, transportation, and community outreach. Experience suggests the great difficulty of devising standards that take into account factors as diverse as staff composition, clinical performance, provision of ancillary and supporting services, and quality improvement efforts. Overall, any effort to recognize high-quality care near the end of life faces formidable methodological challenges.

Opportunities for Enhancing Measurement and Reporting

According to the IOM (2013, p. 301), "Cancer care quality measures provide a standardized and objective means for assessing the quality of cancer care delivered," and objective measures can serve the same function for end-of-life care. That report's recommendation on quality measurement (Recommendation 8) entails developing "a national quality reporting program for cancer care as part of a learning health care system" (p. 301). To this end, the report says, "the Department of Health and Human Services should work with professional societies to:

- Create and implement a formal long-term strategy for publicly reporting quality measures for cancer care that leverages existing efforts.
- Prioritize, fund, and direct the development of meaningful quality measures for cancer care with a focus on outcome measures and with performance targets for use in publicly reporting the performance of institutions, practices, and individual clinicians.
- Implement a coordinated, transparent reporting infrastructure that meets the needs of all stakeholders, including patients, and is integrated into a learning health care system" (IOM, 2013, pp. 301-302).

In any setting and at any stage of life, high-quality health care is "safe, effective, patient-centered, timely, efficient, and equitable" (IOM, 2001, p. 40). The third of these characteristics, patient-centeredness, is especially important for patients near the end of life. Care marked by preset protocols and impersonal treatment can deprive patients of their essential dignity, autonomy, and comfort. The committee believes it is essential for end-of-life care to reflect awareness of the individual's personal history and unique physical, emotional, intellectual, cultural, spiritual/religious, financial, and social situation, as well as the roles of family members and other key individuals in the person's life. High-quality patient-centered care at the end of life should also, to the extent possible, reflect patients' values, goals, and informed preferences (see Chapter 3); maintain quality of life under the constraints of advancing disease; and support family and other caregivers.

Health policy makers recently have been focusing on identifying high-quality providers as a means of improving the overall quality of health care, and end-of-life care is no exception. Hospices face a financial penalty (a 2 percentage point reduction in the market basket percentage increase for a particular fiscal year) under the Affordable Care Act (ACA) for failure to report on quality measures endorsed by a "consensus-based entity"[15] (CMS, 2013b; see also Meier, 2011, p. 353). Initial implementation of this Hospice Quality Reporting Program (HQRP) by CMS called for hospices to report on only two measures: the NQF #0209 pain measure ("the number of patients who report being uncomfortable because of pain at the initial assessment who report that pain was brought to a comfortable level within 48 hours") and a structural measure addressing the organization's Quality Assessment and Performance Improvement Plan. Beginning in 2014, however, these previously used measures will be discontinued, and hospices will be required under the HQRP to complete and submit to CMS the Hospice Item Set, which collects data on seven NQF-endorsed measures:

- patients treated with opioid who are given a bowel regimen (NQF #1617),
- pain screening (NQF #1634),
- pain assessment (NQF #1637),
- dyspnea treatment (NQF #1638),
- dyspnea screening (NQF #1639),
- treatment preferences (NQF #1641), and
- beliefs/values addressed (if desired by the patient) (modified from NQF #1647).

Starting in 2015, in addition to the Hospice Item Set quality reporting requirements, CMS will require that hospices complete the Hospice Experience of Care Survey, which will gather information from caregivers of

---

[15]Patient Protection and Affordable Care Act of 2010, Public Law 111-148, 111th Cong., 2d Sess. (January 5, 2010), § 3004(c).

deceased hospice patients about patient and family experiences with hospice care (CMS, undated; HHS, 2013).

Palliative care programs, by contrast, are not required to report on the quality of the care they provide, nor are accountable care organizations or large systems. The result is a lack of transparency and accountability. There is no consensus on quality measures to use for this purpose or a general approach for determining the locus of accountability for the quality of end-of-life care—the palliative care program or the physician, the hospital where the program is based, or the entire hospital or other integrated system?

A voluntary advanced certification program for palliative care programs has been created by the Joint Commission, which accredits hospitals and other providers of care. Advanced certification is accorded to "hospital inpatient programs that demonstrate exceptional patient and family-centered care and optimize the quality of life for patients (both adult and pediatric) with serious illness" (Joint Commission, 2014a). Certification criteria include whether the program employs an organized interdisciplinary approach, uses practice guidelines, directs the clinical management of patients and coordinates care, offers round-the-clock availability of the full range of palliative care services, and includes a measurement-based quality improvement component (Joint Commission, 2014b). While programs are required to collect data on at least four performance measures, including two clinical measures, the Joint Commission does not specify which measures must be implemented; each program may choose the performance measures that are most important and relevant and thus necessitate review and analysis. As of May 2014, 66 programs had received certification under this program (Joint Commission, 2014c).[16]

In addition, a task force of the American Academy of Hospice and Palliative Medicine and an advisory group of the Hospice and Palliative Nurses Association have begun collaborating to identify a core set of evidence-based performance measures that would apply to all hospice and palliative care programs across care settings. This effort, called "Measuring What Matters," has the aim of developing a list of basic, advanced, and "aspirational" measures that build on the work on the NCP domains and guidelines and the NQF measures, as well as other previously developed measures (American Academy of Hospice and Palliative Medicine, undated-a). A technical advisory panel referred 34 measures to a clinical user panel, which narrowed the list down to 12 existing measures from

---

[16]The first five programs accorded certification, in 2012, were those based at Regions Hospital, St. Paul, Minnesota; Strong Memorial Hospital, Rochester, New York; Mount Sinai Medical Center, New York, New York; St. Joseph Mercy Oakland, Pontiac, Michigan; and The Connecticut Hospice, Inc., Branford, Connecticut (HealthPartners, 2012).

the PEACE Project, NQF, ACOVE, NHPCO, and NCQA/the American Medical Association-Physician Consortium for Performance Improvement (PCPI) that fall within six of the eight NCP domains (American Academy of Hospice and Palliative Medicine, undated-a,b). The list will be culled further. The broad applicability of the selected measures and the development of a common denominator, a task that is planned for the next phase of this effort, will allow for benchmarking and comparison across programs and settings (American Academy of Hospice and Palliative Medicine, undated-c).

Proposed Core Components of Quality End-of-Life Care

Many stakeholders—patients, caregivers, families, the public, health professionals, health care administrators, payers, and policy makers—would benefit from an authoritative, validated list of the core components of quality end-of-life care. Core components would apply to care near the end of life of every type, provided in every setting. They would include not only hospice and palliative care but also the usual care received by people with advanced serious illness who likely are approaching death, which may be provided by primary care physicians, physician specialists, nurses, and other personnel in hospitals, nursing homes, assisted living facilities, outpatient clinics, private homes, and other settings.

Unfortunately, the evidence base falls short of supporting the establishment of such a validated list. Nonetheless, the committee proposes a list of components, based on existing quality indicators, the existing literature, the committee members' expert judgment, and their varied and extensive experience. This list, shown in Table 2-2, is advanced to suggest an agenda for research and policy development, because each item included should be tested to determine whether it is supported by clinical findings across a wide range of patients and by the opinions of patients, families, and clinicians involved in care near the end of life. In addition, the most valid way to measure each of the proposed components of quality end-of-life care will need to be identified.

Key to all 12 of these core components is flexibility and individual tailoring over time, reflecting patient and family priorities and preferences. Those involved in a patient's care must be nimble in responding to individual needs and evolving circumstances. Regular meetings between the care team and the patient and family may facilitate achieving these components of quality end-of-life care as the patient's and family's needs evolve over time.

TABLE 2-2 Proposed Core Components of Quality End-of-Life Care

Component	Rationale
Frequent assessment of patient's physical, emotional, social, and spiritual well-being	Interventions and assistance must be based on accurately identified needs.
Management of emotional distress	All clinicians should be able to identify distress and direct its initial and basic management. This is part of the definition of palliative care, a basic component of hospice, and clearly of fundamental importance.
Offer referral to expert-level palliative care	People with palliative needs beyond those that can be provided by non-specialist-level clinicians deserve access to appropriate expert-level care.
Offer referral to hospice if the patient has a prognosis of 6 months or less	People who meet the hospice eligibility criteria deserve access to services designed to meet their end-of-life needs.
Management of care and direct contact with patient and family for complex situations by a specialist-level palliative care physician	Care of people with serious illness may require specialist-level palliative care physician management, and effective physician management requires direct examination, contact, and communication.
Round-the-clock access to coordinated care and services	Patients in advanced stages of serious illness often require assistance, such as with activities of daily living, medication management, wound care, physical comfort, and psychosocial needs. Round-the-clock access to a consistent point of contact that can coordinate care obviates the need to dial 911 and engage emergency medical services.
Management of pain and other symptoms	All clinicians should be able to identify and direct the initial and basic management of pain and other symptoms. This is part of the definition of palliative care, a basic component of hospice, and clearly of fundamental importance.
Counseling of patient and family	Even patients who are not emotionally distressed face problems in such areas as loss of functioning, prognosis, coping with diverse symptoms, finances, and family dynamics, and family members experience these problems as well, both directly and indirectly.
Family caregiver support	A focus on the family is part of the definition of palliative care; family members and caregivers both participate in the patient's care and require assistance themselves.

TABLE 2-2 Continued

Component	Rationale
Attention to the patient's social context and social needs	Person-centered care requires awareness of patients' perspectives on their social environment and of their needs for social support, including at the time of death. Companionship at the bedside at time of death may be an important part of the psychological, social, and spiritual aspects of end-of-life care for some individuals.
Attention to the patient's spiritual and religious needs	The final phase of life often has a spiritual and religious component, and research shows that spiritual assistance is associated with quality of care.
Regular personalized revision of the care plan and access to services based on the changing needs of the patient and family	Care must be person-centered and fit current circumstances, which may mean that not all the above components will be important or desirable in all cases.

NOTE: The proposed core components of quality end-of-life care listed in this table were developed by the committee. Most of the components relate to one of the domains in the Clinical Practice Guidelines for Quality Palliative Care set forth by the National Consensus Project for Quality Palliative Care (Dahlin, 2013).

THE PROBLEM OF PROGNOSIS

The problem of prognosis—establishing the life expectancy of a patient with an advanced serious illness or medical condition who is likely approaching death—is important for several reasons. A patient's prognosis

- has important personal implications, affecting the patient's state of mind and decisions about how to spend the next several weeks or months and the family's support for the patient;
- has financial implications that may affect the patient's and family's decisions about earning and spending;
- has family caregiver implications, affecting family caregivers' understanding of what will be expected of them and for how long;
- has clinical implications, affecting decisions about treatment of the illness and of comorbid conditions, and referrals to hospice and social services;

BOX 2-6
Prognosis and the Medicare Hospice Benefit

Under the Medicare Hospice Benefit, the patient's prognosis may have negative practical consequences. As discussed in Chapter 5, one of the eligibility requirements for the Medicare Hospice Benefit is an expected prognosis of 6 months or less if the disease runs the expected course. According to the former medical director of a home hospice, for example, when a patient's pulmonologist determined that her chronic obstructive pulmonary disease (COPD) prognosis was more than 6 months, the pulmonologist effectively discharged her from hospice against her will. She thereby lost access to regular nursing care and other supportive services and died less than 2 months later. The writer offers the opinion that patients' eligibility for hospice should be based on "their demonstrated need for supportive care services—in other words, based on the weight of their symptoms, their level of functional impairment, or the burden their illness imposes on caregivers" (Groninger, 2012, p. 455).

- may have legal implications, affecting the preparation and implementation of advance directives[17]; and
- affects eligibility for hospice care under the Medicare Hospice Benefit (see Box 2-6).

Prognostic Uncertainties

Predicting prognosis is easier for certain diseases, such as solid-tumor metastatic cancers, than for many other common and serious conditions, such as stroke, heart failure, COPD, end-stage renal disease, frailty, dementia, and Parkinson's disease. Among elderly people especially, assessing the overall prognosis may be difficult because these patients frequently suffer from two or more such conditions. Predicting the time course and prognosis of disabling genetic or congenital disorders that affect children is similarly problematic.

Although most people have high levels of disability by the last few months of life, the trajectory of disability, like life expectancy, is difficult to

---

[17]For example, the New Jersey Supreme Court's holding that prognosis, broadly defined, affects the legality of decisions to withhold or withdraw life-sustaining treatment in accordance with patients' determined preferences: *In re Quinlan*, 70 N.J. 10, 355 A2d 647 (1976); *Matter of Jobes*, 108 N.J. 335, 529 A2d 434 (1987); and *Matter of Peter by Johanning*, 108 N.J. 365, 529 A2d 419 (1987).

predict, even when people with the same medical condition are compared. Variation in disability trajectories "poses challenges for the proper allocation of resources to care for older persons at the end of life" (Gill et al., 2010, p. 1180). Nevertheless, an increasing level of disability, combined with frailty and accumulating symptoms, may be the most useful signal of the need for palliative care assessment and subsequent provision of palliative services.

Predictive Models

Expected longevity is typically the major focus of prognosis. An appendix to *Approaching Death* (IOM, 1997, Appendix D) describes efforts to develop clinical forecasting models, especially for acute myocardial infarction, coma, pediatric intensive care, and critical care. The discussion emphasizes several limitations of such models, some of which are technical: statistical limitations, inherent imperfections, and inadequate accounting for disease specificity and the effects of interventions. However, other limitations may be inherent in the predictive process: death is not the only outcome of interest; critical illness is a dynamic process; the models' complexity impedes their usefulness; and the perspective of the model differs from the perspective of the patient or family.

Since the release of that report, new forecasting models have emerged. Table 2-3 lists components of these models, and as this table reveals, there

TABLE 2-3 Factors Used to Predict Mortality in Five Illustrative Prognostic Models

Factors	PIPS*	PaP	CARING	HRS	Cheng
Cancer or metastatic disease (any site)	X		X	X	
Malignant effusion					X
Liver metastases	X				
Lung disease				X	
Heart failure				X	
Diabetes				X	
Anorexia or loss of weight	X	X			X
Dyspnea		X			
Age (with more points for each older age category; applies to adults only)				X	

continued

TABLE 2-3 Continued

Factors	PIPS*	PaP	CARING	HRS	Cheng
Sex				X	
General health status	X				
Mental test score	X				
Performance status	X	X			X
Critical care unit admission with multiorgan failure			X		
Hospital admissions (two or more)			X		
Nursing home residence			X		
Applicability of two or more noncancer hospice guidelines			X		
Current tobacco use				X	
Body mass index				X	
Pulse rate	X				
White blood count	X	X			
Platelet count	X				
Lymphocyte count or lymphopenia		X			
Hypercalcemia					X
C-reactive protein	X				
Urea	X				
Bathing				X	
Walking several blocks				X	
Pushing/pulling large objects				X	
Managing money				X	
Physician's survival prediction (in weeks)		X			

NOTES: CARING = Cancer, Admissions ≥2, Residence in a nursing home, Intensive care unit admit with multiorgan failure, ≥2 Noncancer hospice Guidelines; HRS = Health and Retirement Study; PaP = Palliative Prognostic; PIPS = Prognosis in Palliative Care Study.

*These factors were found in the PIPS study to predict survival at both 2 weeks and 2 months. Factors found to predict survival at 2 weeks only were dyspnea, dysphagia, bone metastases, and alanine transaminase. Factors found to predict survival at 2 months only were primary breast cancer, male genital cancer, tiredness, loss of weight, lymphocyte count, neutrophil count, alkaline phosphatase, and albumin.

SOURCES: PIPS: Gwilliam et al., 2011; PaP: Pirovano et al., 1999; CARING: Fischer et al., 2006; HRS: Lee et al., 2006; Cheng: Cheng et al., 2013.

is little overlap. (A forecasting model for pediatric mortality is mentioned in Appendix F.)

A systematic review determined that the most accurate of 13 models for predicting life expectancy in patients with advanced, incurable cancer is the Palliative Prognostic (PaP) score, along with a PaP variant that includes dementia (D-PaP) (Krishnan et al., 2013). PaP scores estimate survival at 1 month, and the PaP model has been externally validated (Maltoni et al., 1999; Pirovano et al., 1999). The authors of the systematic review note the need for further research to establish reliable prognoses across a broader spectrum of time and to determine the effect of the use of prognostic tools on the quality of end-of-life care.

With regard to non-disease-specific models, a systematic review of 16 indices predicting mortality risk in people over age 60 in community, hospital, or nursing home settings "identified several high-quality prognostic indices." However, the authors found that "there is insufficient evidence at this time to recommend the widespread use of prognostic indices in clinical practice" (Yourman et al., 2012, p. 190). According to the authors, limitations of the models include potential bias and failure to predict either very low or very high risk of mortality—precisely the information most likely to be useful to clinicians. The conclusion that these limitations may impede a clinician's ability to apply prognostic models in a clinical setting appears to bear out the skepticism expressed in *Approaching Death* (IOM, 1997, Appendix D).

The following are examples of the many studies presenting prognostic models:

- A British prospective cohort study based at multiple palliative care centers—the Prognosis in Palliative Care Study (PIPS)—produced a composite model for predicting survival of cancer patients at 2 weeks and 2 months (Gwilliam et al., 2011). This model has not been externally validated (Krishnan et al., 2013).
- Another study identified criteria for determining the likelihood of dying within 1 year. According to the study authors, these "CARING" criteria can be used at the time of hospital admission to determine whether the patient is ready for palliative care (Fischer et al., 2006). This model has been validated (Youngwerth et al., 2013).
- Still another study used 1998 Health and Retirement Study data for people over age 50 living in the community to identify 12 independent predictors of mortality within 4 years (Lee et al., 2006). According to the systematic review of non-disease-specific indices cited above, this model "was well calibrated and showed very good discrimination," although it was not externally validated

(Yourman et al., 2012, p. 186). While this model shows promise, its relevance to the population that is near the end of life has not yet been demonstrated given that it is currently validated only for mortality within 4 years.

Acute Physiology and Chronic Health Evaluation (APACHE) and ePrognosis are two tools that can be used to assess prognosis in clinical settings. APACHE is a scoring system that uses predictor variables and measures collected shortly after a patient's admission to the intensive care unit to determine severity of disease and likelihood of in-hospital mortality (Knaus et al., 1985, 1991; Wong and Knaus, 1991). ePrognosis is a website and software application that aggregates prognostic indices to provide clinicians with information about patients' possible mortality outcomes based on answers to questions about certain predictor variables (such as those listed in Table 2-3) (ePrognosis, 2014).

There are also informal methods for developing prognoses, with less proven reliability. A group of palliative care specialists in oncology, for example, concluded that "it is relatively easy to predict which patients have less than six months to live" (Cheng et al., 2013, p. 85). According to these authors, four factors ("Cheng" factors shown in Table 2-3) "should all trigger discussion about hospice" (p. 85).

Another informal tool that has been used to identify patients for whom palliative care may be appropriate is the "surprise" question: "Would I be surprised if this patient died in the next 12 months?" (Moss et al., 2008, 2010). While not perfect, the "surprise" question can be applied simply and effectively by health care professionals as a way to identify patients with a poor prognosis.

It should be cautioned, however, that "there will always be some uncertainty in prognosis" (Smith et al., 2013c, p. 2448). For example, if a physician knows a patient belongs to a group with a 25 percent risk of dying within 6 months, the physician still does not know whether this particular patient is in the 25 percent subset or the 75 percent subset. Smith and colleagues (2013c) recommend that physicians be honest with patients about the boundaries of predictive knowledge, address patients' and families' emotions about uncertainty, and help them live in the present despite an uncertain prognosis (see also Chapter 3).

FAMILY CAREGIVERS

Family caregivers (with family defined broadly; see the guiding principles in Box 1-3 in Chapter 1) provide many types of assistance to people with a chronic disease or disabling condition. An estimated 66 million Americans, or 29 percent of the adult population, are caregivers; nearly two-thirds are women (National Alliance for Caregiving, 2009). They provide an average of 20 hours of services per week and are heavily involved in assisting with instrumental activities of daily living. Information about the number and responsibilities of family caregivers is not available specifically for the population nearing the end of life. This report uses the term "family caregivers" to describe people in this role; other terms used include "informal caregivers," "carers," "primary caregivers," and "volunteer caregivers." Whatever the term, these individuals often exhibit extraordinary commitment, provide incalculable value, and face significant burdens in carrying out the caregiver role.

While many family members readily assume this responsibility—and may not consider it a "burden" at all—it takes a largely unrecognized toll. The toll increases when family caregivers must administer medications (including opioid pain relievers); maintain complex equipment; and perform the physical labor of feeding (and possibly preparing special diets), bathing, toileting, changing and cleaning, dressing, turning, and transporting a family member (National Alliance for Caregiving, 2009; Reinhard et al., 2012). Caregiving takes a psychological toll when family members worry about performing all those tasks safely and well, when caregiving keeps them from meeting responsibilities to other family members, when their loved one is frightened or in pain, when they receive little training or guidance, and when they do not receive help in managing their own fears (National Alliance for Caregiving, 2009). When the patient is a child, the family caregiver role is made more difficult by the relative youth and inexperience of the parents, the frequent need to travel long distances to obtain subspecialty pediatric care, deep strains on the parents' relationship with each other, and the vulnerability of siblings to profound emotional stress (Sourkes, 2013).

I belong to a caregivers group which is supportive. People who are not caregivers don't understand the continuous burden of the role and seem to think it can be walked away from or put aside forever or for a while. Not so. The stress feels as if I'm constantly holding my breath. That combined with dealing with financial concerns, the medical and insurance communities is just too much. . . . Transportation is also a barrier; just getting the sick person to appointments is physically demanding, and visiting in the hospital is wearying. Parking is a big expense. Pushing a wheelchair is physically demanding.*

---

*Quotation from a response submitted through the online public testimony questionnaire for this study. See Appendix C.

Caregiving also takes a financial toll when families face high out-of-pocket costs for services and equipment or when family income decreases because family caregivers must reduce their work hours or leave their jobs altogether (Evercare and National Alliance for Caregiving, 2007; Feinberg et al., 2011; National Alliance for Caregiving, 2009). Employer support may therefore be crucial for employed family caregivers. Aware of caregiver absenteeism and lost productivity, some employers offer greater flexibility in working hours and location or other special assistance (Coalition to Transform Advanced Care, 2013).

Given an explicit choice, most people would prefer to spend their last weeks and days in their own home, free of pain, clean and comfortable, and in control—not in emergency departments, hospitals, and critical care units away from family and familiar surroundings (see Chapter 3). As discussed earlier in this chapter, new models of home and community health care delivery and improved communication technologies are making that choice increasingly possible; however, adequate support for family caregivers remains an unmet need.

It took all of our savings to keep my husband at home. And it took five of us to give him the round-the-clock care he needed. *

---

*Quotation from a response submitted through the online public testimony questionnaire for this study. See Appendix C.

In previous generations, caregiving was a widely expected role of women in families, and caregiving responsibilities often lasted only briefly, as people died at younger ages or sooner after the onset of a serious illness. Today's families are smaller, and many women work outside the home. Moreover, not only may caregiving be needed for lengthy periods, but also it is becoming more complex, requiring management of medical equipment and medication regimens, wound care, nutrition, mental health care, use of community resources, and so on—for the most part with no formal training (Feinberg, 2013; Reinhard et al., 2012). Some key information about family caregivers appears in Table 2-4.

Meanwhile, the demand for family caregiving is growing with the rising prevalence of chronic diseases (Feinberg, 2013), as well as the long-term care trends that encourage more care at home and fewer nursing home placements (see Chapter 5). And the ratio of potential caregivers (people aged 45 to 64) to people 80 and older is expected to fall from 7:1 in 2010 to 4:1 by 2030 (Redfoot et al., 2013).

TABLE 2-4 Some Key Facts About U.S. Family Caregivers

Subject	Figure	Descriptor
Supply of family caregivers	4:1	Projected ratio of potential caregivers (aged 45-64) to people potentially in need (over 80) in 2030 (Redfoot et al., 2013)
Medication management	78%	Of caregivers that perform medical/nursing tasks, the proportion regularly administering drugs (average 5-9 medications per day) (Reinhard et al., 2012)
No home visits	69%	Proportion of caregivers not assisted with home visits by a health professional (Reinhard et al., 2012)
Caregivers who are employed	73%	Proportion of caregivers employed at some time while caregiving (National Alliance for Caregiving, 2009)
Caregiving for parents	72%	Proportion of employed workers serving as caregivers who care for a parent or parent-in-law (Mendes, 2011)
Caregiving for elderly people	67%	Proportion of employed workers serving as caregivers who care for someone over age 75 (Mendes, 2011)
Duration of caregiving	55%	Proportion of employed workers serving as caregivers who have been doing so for 3 years or longer (Mendes, 2011)
Worker absenteeism	6.6 days	Employed family caregivers' average annual number of days of employed work lost as a result of caregiving (Witters, 2011)
Lost productivity	$25.2 billion	Annual cost of lost productivity due to absenteeism caused by family caregiving (Witters, 2011)
Economic impact	$450 billion	Value of family caregiving services in 2009 (Feinberg et al., 2011)

In theory, family caregivers should be in an ideal position to foster patient-centered care, starting with an understanding of the patient's health status, helping to identify care goals, and participating in the development of the plan of care (Gillick, 2013). But such participation requires support from the health care team. Although palliative care tends to provide such support, even families involved in palliative care often feel unprepared to perform the caregiving role (Abernethy et al., 2008; Kilbourn et al., 2011; Payne et al., 1999). And patients and families not receiving palliative care may lack any systematic caregiver support.

We share the care of my mother-in-law with worsening dementia. The fragmentation of care is challenging, even for professional health care providers. Home support is almost non-existent, and we tremble regarding the limited options when/if her needs exceed what we can provide in our homes.*

---

*Quotation from a response submitted through the online public testimony questionnaire for this study. See Appendix C.

Personal attributes that help in the caregiver role include adaptability and resilience, and caregivers benefit from the constructive involvement of other family members. But they are at risk of loss of control, loss of identity, and loss of relationships, as well as exhaustion and eventual bereavement (Sourkes, 2013). In addition,

> Caregivers are at increased risk of disease because of the burden and difficulties associated with caregiving. A lot don't sleep or eat right. They neglect themselves, so they're at higher risk of depression and anxiety, coronary types of problems and are more prone to getting sick. (Vuong, 2013, quoting Dr. Linda Ercoli, Assistant Professor of Psychiatry, University of California, Los Angeles)

Results of a systematic review of 19 studies from six countries (Canada, Israel, Norway, Saudi Arabia, the United Kingdom, and the United States) were inconclusive as to whether gender, age, and relationship to the patient affect caregiver stress. In 8 of the studies, however, stress was found to increase as the patient's condition worsened and death approached (Williams and McCorkle, 2011).

Family caregivers receive services as well as provide them. Those services may include respite care (temporary custodial care of the patient) and bereavement services—counseling, assistance with arrangements, and other supports for as long as 1 year after a death—which are a component of quality palliative care. Both respite and bereavement services are covered under the Medicare Hospice Benefit (CMS, 2012).

AARP, the National Alliance for Caregiving, and other groups have helped call attention to the extent of and challenges entailed in family caregiving. However, research on family caregivers' roles, needs, behavior, health risks, success in performance, interaction with professional members of the health care team, and use of respite care and other support services is not highly developed. Research on family caregiving remains sparse, perhaps reflecting its lack of visibility as compared with the services offered by health care professionals.

Family caregivers have received some protections from the federal government. The Family and Medical Leave Act of 1993 guarantees up to 12 weeks of job-protected unpaid leave for attending to the care needs of a spouse, child, or parent, but not other family members (DOL, 2013). The National Family Caregiver Support Program, established by the Older Americans Act, as amended in 2000, has helped increase awareness of the importance of family caregivers by establishing the caregiver as a client and providing family counseling, support groups, training, and respite care (AoA, 2012; Feinberg, 2013). The ACA includes multiple references to caregivers and may help them by promoting models of care that prevent or facilitate transitions between care settings (Feinberg, 2013). Medicaid's Cash & Counseling program, available in about 15 states, permits beneficiaries to pay family members modest sums for home care services in some cases (National Resource Center for Participant-Directed Services, 2013). And family caregivers of seriously injured veterans (who served after September 11, 2001) may receive a stipend, comprehensive training, medical services, and other services under the VA Program of Comprehensive Assistance to Family Caregivers (VA, 2013).

An IOM committee investigating health care workforce needs for an aging America took note of the importance of integrating family caregivers into health care teams and providing them with better training. One recommendation of that committee reads: "Public, private, and community organizations should provide funding and ensure that adequate training opportunities are available in the community for informal caregivers" (IOM, 2008, p. 255).

RESEARCH NEEDS

A comprehensive review of studies on end-of-life care (NINR, 2013) undertaken since the publication of *Approaching Death* (IOM, 1997) identifies a shortage of research on the changing demographic characteristics of populations experiencing serious advanced illnesses or multiple chronic conditions, especially kidney and liver conditions and HIV/AIDS. According to the National Institute of Nursing Research (NINR) report, "Issues related to economics, ethics, and access must be integrated into new research paradigms[,] and attention to culture, ethnicity, and minorities must be made to produce a measurable shift in the focus of research grants, the sources of funding dollars, and the dissemination of meaningful results to inform and educate the public" (NINR, 2013, pp. xi-xii). The report suggests that public-private partnerships could help fill these research gaps and improve the delivery of hospice and palliative care.

This chapter has identified numerous important areas for further research, including

- the prevalence and nature of care that is neither beneficial nor wanted, and practical ways to avoid it;
- the effect of palliative care on longevity;
- the elements of palliative care likely to offer the greatest improvements in quality of life;
- evidence-based measures of quality end-of-life care, beyond those identified to date by NQF and including aspects of the proposed core components listed in Table 2-2;
- family caregivers' roles, needs, behavior, health risks, success in performance, interaction with other members of the health care team, and use of respite care and other support services;
- reliable approaches to prognosis that start earlier in the disease trajectory, and assessment of whether more accurate prognoses lead to improvements in quality of life and other outcomes of care; and
- the effects and value of specific types of clinical innovations in delivering end-of-life care.

Pediatric-related research needs may be especially pressing. Appendix F suggests the need for research in the following areas for children near the end of life:

- comparative effectiveness studies of different approaches to symptom management and bereavement support;
- analyses of care received in emergency departments, outpatient settings, and hospices and through home health agencies;
- cohort studies examining the effect of palliative care on outcomes and on the patient experience; and
- studies of how best to staff, manage, and finance hospital-based pediatric palliative and community-based pediatric hospice services.

A general lack of investment in research on palliative care is identified in a review of the palliative care landscape referenced earlier in this chapter (Meier, 2011). That review suggests that the National Institutes of Health (NIH), in particular, can make important contributions in this field. In 2006-2010, NIH funded 240 percent more palliative care projects than it did in 2001-2005, but palliative care still accounted for only a fraction of 1 percent of all NIH grants (Gelfman et al., 2010).

Given that palliative care is inherently patient-centered, the Patient-Centered Outcomes Research Institute (PCORI) may be a potential funding source for research in this field going forward. PCORI was established under the ACA, and its research "is intended to give patients a better understanding of the prevention, treatment, and care options available, and the science that supports those options"[18] (PCORI, 2014). In developing its research priorities, PCORI reviewed previous comparative effectiveness prioritization efforts and found 10 common priority areas for such research; palliative care was one of these areas (PCORI, 2012). While its own national priorities and research agenda do not specifically call for research on palliative care, many of the topics highlighted are relevant to this field, including prognostication, shared decision making, health care teams, and differences in patient preferences.

Besides concerns about the *quantity* of research on topics related to end-of-life care, there are concerns about the *quality* of such research. One concern is that an emphasis on developing quantifiable results through such traditional methods as randomized controlled trials tends to omit key questions, such as why a treatment was effective, how patients viewed their experience, and what mechanisms caused the outcomes observed (Fleurence et al., 2013; Steinhauser and Barroso, 2009; see also IOM, 2009, p. 31).[19] Efforts to broaden the types of investigations used in comparative effectiveness research and involve consumers in the design and execution of studies may help address this concern (Fleurence et al., 2013).

One potentially rich area of research involves linking major academic medical centers to community-based settings, using treatment results experienced by large numbers of patients to show which treatments work best for whom, and then disseminating that information back to clinicians and patients in useful ways (Westfall et al., 2007). This approach, typical of a "learning health care system," would transform the nation's clinical trials enterprise (IOM, 2012, especially p. 15, Table 2-1) and is endorsed in the recent IOM report on cancer care (IOM, 2013).

Practice-based research networks (PBRNs) are one practical way to conduct "practice-relevant" research in community-based settings. For example, PBRNs that are supported by AHRQ link primary care practices in research relevant to community-based health care (AHRQ, 2013). Each PBRN includes at least five primary care practices; most of the research conducted by the current 131 networks has focused on underserved, low-income, and minority populations (Peterson et al., 2012). PBRNs are even collaborating to create consortia of research networks (Calmbach et al., 2012; Peterson et al., 2012).

---

[18]Patient Protection and Affordable Care Act of 2010, Public Law 111-148, 111th Cong., 2d Sess. (January 5, 2010), § 6301.

[19]Randomized controlled trials may also exclude patients with multiple chronic conditions or chronic conditions combined with disabilities (Fleurence et al., 2013). This exclusion can leave out many people nearing the end of life. Trials also typically ignore family-related factors, including the role of family caregivers. In general, moreover, clinical trials assess only the efficacy of an intervention under carefully controlled conditions, not its effectiveness in the real world.

Significant resources to facilitate the conduct of high-quality palliative care and end-of-life research have emerged since *Approaching Death* (IOM, 1997) was published. The National Palliative Care Research Center, acting in partnership with the Center to Advance Palliative Care, provides a mechanism for establishing research priorities, preparing a new generation of researchers, and coordinating and supporting studies aimed at improving care (NPCRC, 2013). The Palliative Care Research Cooperative Group, established in 2010, offers a mechanism for connecting researchers and clinicians across varied clinical settings and facilitating timely completion of complex studies, including randomized controlled trials, by pooling resources and expertise across sites (Abernethy et al., 2010).

FINDINGS, CONCLUSIONS, AND RECOMMENDATION

Findings

This study yielded the following findings on the delivery of person-centered, family-oriented end-of-life care.

Burdensome Transitions

People nearing the end of life often experience multiple transitions between health care settings, including high rates of apparently preventable hospitalizations. These transitions can fragment the delivery of care and create burdens for patients and families (Coleman et al., 2006; Jencks et al., 2009; Naylor et al., 2013; Teno et al., 2013).

Growth of Hospice

The role of hospice in end-of-life care has been increasing in the past two decades. Hospice grew from being the locus of 17 percent of all U.S. deaths in 1995 to 45 percent in 2011 (IOM, 1997, p. 40; NHPCO, 2012a).

Growth of Specialty Palliative Care

The years since *Approaching Death* (IOM, 1997) was published also have seen the emergence and growth of specialty palliative care. By 2011, fully 85 percent of all hospitals with 300 or more beds reported having palliative care services (CAPC, 2011, 2013; see also Chapter 4 for information about the number of board-certified hospice and palliative physicians and certified nurses).

Provision of Palliative Care

The guidelines and expert advice of professional associations encourage oncologists, cardiologists, and other disease-oriented specialists to counsel patients about palliative care. Nevertheless, widespread adoption of the practice of timely referral to palliative care appears to be slow, despite support for integrating and improving the basic level of knowledge of palliative care among all clinicians who treat patients with serious advanced illness (Cheng et al., 2013; Goodlin, 2009; IOM, 2013; Matlock et al., 2010; Molony, 2013; Quill and Abernethy, 2013; Shaw, 2010; Smith et al., 2012).

Interdisciplinary Teams for Palliative Care

Besides physician specialists in hospice and palliative medicine, members of palliative care interdisciplinary teams often include specialty advanced practice nurses and registered nurses, social workers, chaplains, pharmacists, rehabilitation therapists, direct care workers, and family members (Adams et al., 2011; American Occupational Therapy Association, 2011; American Society of Health System Pharmacists, 2002; Brumley and Hillary, 2002; Cruz, 2013; Hebert et al., 2011; Meier, 2011; NASW, 2013, 2014; NQF, 2006; Pollens, 2004; Puchalski et al., 2009; Vitello, 2008).

Impact of Hospice and Palliative Care on Longevity

Some evidence suggests that on average, palliative care patients (including hospice patients) may live longer than similarly ill patients receiving usual care (Connor et al., 2007; Saito et al., 2011; Temel et al., 2010).

Impact of Palliative Care on Quality of Life

Palliative care has been associated with a higher quality of life, as measured by indicators that include information and communication, access to home care, emotional and spiritual support, well-being and dignity, care at time of death, and a lighter symptom burden (Casarett et al., 2008; Gomes et al., 2013; Rabow et al., 2013; Temel et al., 2010).

Prognosis

Since *Approaching Death* was published in 1997, new predictive models have emerged that enhance clinicians' ability to make valid and reliable medical prognoses. Lack of adequate prognostication may prevent some patients from receiving appropriate hospice care because of the 6-month prognosis rule in the Medicare Hospice Benefit (described in Chapter 5) (Fischer et al., 2006; Gwilliam et al., 2011; Krishnan et al., 2013; Pirovano et al., 1999; Tax Equity and Fiscal Responsibility Act of 1982[20]; IOM, 1997, Appendix D; for commentary on the 6-month rule, see, e.g., Groninger, 2012).

Family Caregiving

With an aging population, demand for family caregiving is increasing. At the same time, the types of tasks being performed by family caregivers are expanding from personal care and household tasks to include medical/ nursing tasks, such as medication management and other services for those near the end of life. Three in 10 U.S. adults are family caregivers (National Alliance for Caregiving, 2009; Redfoot et al., 2013; Reinhard et al., 2012). Information about the number and responsibilities of caregivers specifically for those nearing the end of life is not available.

Conclusions

Care near the end of life can be complex. People with serious advanced illness and their families could benefit from all clinicians having a basic level of competence in addressing the palliative care needs of this population. Such patients and their families may further require the involvement of interdisciplinary teams of professionals specifically trained in palliative care. Such care teams—whether available in hospitals, long term acute care facilities, nursing homes, hospices, clinics, or patients' homes—combine services and expertise to meet the broad needs of patients and families. However, palliative care currently is unavailable in many geographic areas and in many settings where people with advanced serious illness receive care. Transformational change is required, building on evidence about high-quality, compassionate, and cost-effective care that is person-centered and family-oriented and available wherever patients nearing the end of life may be. A further need is to continue to build and strengthen that evidence base while responding to challenges posed by new communication and biomedical technologies, growing demands on caregivers, and demographic change.

Approaching Death (IOM, 1997) was published 17 years ago. Then, hospice was well on its way to achieving mainstream status, and palliative care was in the early stages of development. Now, hospice is in the mainstream, and palliative care is well established in hospitals and in the

---

[20]Tax Equity and Fiscal Responsibility Act of 1982 (TEFRA), Public Law 97-248, section 122.

professions of medicine, nursing, social work, and chaplaincy. Yet many clinicians and families still appear to not regard palliative care as an essential component of high-quality care. The needed shift among the public and health care providers toward recognizing all that hospice and palliative care can achieve remains incomplete.

Recommendation 1. Government health insurers and care delivery programs as well as private health insurers should cover the provision of comprehensive care for individuals with advanced serious illness who are nearing the end of life.

Comprehensive care should

- be seamless, high-quality, integrated, patient-centered, family-oriented, and consistently accessible around the clock;
- consider the evolving physical, emotional, social, and spiritual needs of individuals approaching the end of life, as well as those of their family and/or caregivers;
- be competently delivered by professionals with appropriate expertise and training;
- include coordinated, efficient, and interoperable information transfer across all providers and all settings; and
- be consistent with individuals' values, goals, and informed preferences.

Health care delivery organizations should take the following steps to provide comprehensive care:

- All people with advanced serious illness should have access to skilled palliative care or, when appropriate, hospice care in all settings where they receive care (including health care facilities, the home, and the community).
- Palliative care should encompass access to an interdisciplinary palliative care team, including board-certified hospice and palliative medicine physicians, nurses, social workers, and chaplains, together with other health professionals as needed (including geriatricians). Depending on local resources, access to this team may be on site, via virtual consultation, or by transfer to a setting with these resources and this expertise.
- The full range of care that is delivered should be characterized by transparency and accountability through public reporting of aggregate quality and cost measures for all aspects of the health

care system related to end-of-life care. The committee believes that informed individual choices should be honored, including the right to decline medical or social services.

REFERENCES

AAP (American Academy of Pediatrics). 2013. Pediatric palliative care and hospice care commitments, guidelines, and recommendations. *Pediatrics* 132(5):966-972.

Abernethy, A. P., D. C. Currow, B. S. Fazekas, M. A. Luszcz, J. L. Wheeler, and M. Kuchibhatla. 2008. Specialized palliative care services are associated with improved short- and long-term caregiver outcomes. *Support Care Cancer* 16:585-597.

Abernethy, A. P., N. M. Aziz, E. Basch, J. Bull, C. S. Cleeland, D. C. Currow, D. Fairclough, L. Hanson, J. Hauser, D. Ko, L. Lloyd, R. S. Morrison, S. Otis-Green, S. Pantilat, R. K. Portenoy, C. Ritchie, G. Rocker, J. L. Wheeler, S. Y. Zafar, and J. S. Kutner. 2010. A strategy to advance the evidence base in palliative medicine: Formation of a palliative care research cooperative group. *Journal of Palliative Medicine* 13(12):407-413. http://www.ncbi.nlm.nih.gov/pubmed/21105763 (accessed September 20, 2013).

ABMS (American Board of Medical Specialties). 2013. *2012 ABMS certificate statistics.* Chicago, IL: ABMS.

Abrashkin, K. A., H. J. Cho, S. Torgalkar, and B. Markoff. 2012. Improving transitions of care from hospital to home: What works? *Mount Sinai Journal of Medicine* 79(5):535-544.

Adams, J. A., D. E. Bailey, Jr., R. A. Anderson, and S. L. Docherty. 2011. Nursing roles and strategies in end-of-life decision making in acute care: A systematic review of the literature. *Nursing Research and Practice* 2011:527834.

AHRQ (Agency for Healthcare Research and Quality). 2012. *Improving healthcare and palliative care for advanced and serious illness: Closing the quality gap—revisiting the state of the science.* Rockville, MD: AHRQ.

AHRQ. 2013. *Practice-Based Research Networks (PBRNs).* http://pbrn.ahrq.gov (accessed September 9, 2013).

American Academy of Family Physicians, AAP, American College of Physicians, and American Osteopathic Association. 2007. *Joint principles of the patient-centered medical home.* Shawnee Mission, KS: American Academy of Family Physicians. http://www.aap.org/en-us/professional-resources/practice-support/quality-improvement/Documents/Joint-Principles-Patient-Centered-Medical-Home.pdf (accessed August 9, 2013).

American Academy of Hospice and Palliative Medicine. undated-a. *Measuring What Matters.* http://aahpm.org/quality/measuring-what-matters (accessed March 4, 2014).

American Academy of Hospice and Palliative Medicine. undated-b. *Top twelve measures—background information, evidence, and Clinical User Panel (CUP) comments.* http://aahpm.org/uploads/education/MWM%20Top%2012%20Measure%20Information%20and%20Comments.pdf (accessed July 23, 2014).

American Academy of Hospice and Palliative Medicine. undated-c. *Frequently asked questions (FAQs) about Measuring What Matters.* http://aahpm.org/uploads/education/MWM%20FAQ%20List.pdf (accessed July 23, 2014).

American Occupational Therapy Association. 2011. *The role of occupational therapy in palliative care.* Bethesda, MD: American Occupational Therapy Association. http://www.aota.org/~/media/Corporate/Files/AboutOT/Professionals/WhatIsOT/PA/Facts/FactSheet_PalliativeCare.ashx (accessed August 24, 2013).

American Osteopathic Association. 2013. *Specialties and subspecialties.* Chicago, IL: American Osteopathic Association. http://www.osteopathic.org/inside-aoa/development/aoa-board-certification/Pages/specialty-subspecialty-certification.aspx (accessed September 21, 2013).

American Society of Health System Pharmacists. 2002. ASHP statement on the pharmacist's role in hospice and palliative care. *American Journal of Health System Pharmacy* 59(18):1770-1773.

AoA (Administration on Aging). 2012. *National Family Caregiver Support Program (OAA Title IIIE).* http://aoa.gov/aoa_programs/hcltc/caregiver (accessed August 27, 2013).

APC (Association of Professional Chaplains). 2013. *The Association of Professional Chaplains introduces palliative care specialty certification.* News release. May 1. Schaumburg, IL: APC.

Aspinal, F., J. Addington-Hall, R. Hughes, and I. J. Higginson. 2003. Using satisfaction to measure the quality of palliative care: A review of the literature. *Journal of Advanced Nursing* 42(4):324-339.

Baer, W. M., and L. C. Hanson. 2000. Families' perceptions of the added value of hospice in the nursing home. *Journal of the American Geriatrics Society* 48(8):879-882.

Bakitas, M., K. D. Lyons, M. T. Hegel, S. Balan, F. C. Brokaw, J. Seville, J. G. Hull, Z. Li, T. D. Tosteson, I. R. Byock, and T. A. Ahles. 2009. Effects of a palliative care intervention on clinical outcomes in patients with advanced cancer: The Project ENABLE II randomized controlled trial. *Journal of the American Medical Association* 302(7):741-749.

Beales, J. L., and T. Edes. 2009. Veteran's Affairs home based primary care. *Clinics in Geriatric Medicine* 25(1):149-154.

Benbassat, J., and M. I. Taragin. 2013. The effect of clinical interventions on hospital readmissions: A meta-review of published meta-analyses. *Israel Journal of Health Policy Research* 2:1.

Besdine, R., C. Boult, S. Brangman, E. A. Coleman, L. P. Fried, M. Gerety, J. C. Johnson, P. R. Katz, J. F. Potter, D. B. Reuben, P. D. Sloane, S. Studenski, G. Warshaw, and American Geriatrics Society Task Force on the Future of Geriatric Medicine. 2005. Caring for older Americans: The future of geriatric medicine. *Journal of the American Geriatrics Society* 53(Suppl. 6):S245-S256.

Blayney, D. W., J. Severson, C. J. Martin, P. Kadlubek, T. Ruane, and K. Harrison. 2012. Michigan oncology practices showed varying adherence rates to practice guidelines, but quality interventions improved care. *Health Affairs* 31(4):718-727.

Block, E. M., D. J. Casarett, C. Spence, P. Gozalo, S. R. Connor, and J. M. Teno. 2010. Got volunteers? Association of hospice use of volunteers with bereaved family members' overall rating of the quality of end-of-life care. *Journal of Pain and Symptom Management* 39(3):502-506.

Bona, K., J. Bates, and J. Wolfe. 2011. Massachusetts' Pediatric Palliative Care Network: Successful implementation of a novel state-funded pediatric palliative care program. *Journal of Palliative Medicine* 14(11):1217-1223.

Brock, J., J. Mitchell, K. Irby, B. Stevens, T. Archibald, A. Goroski, J. Lynn, and Care Transitions Project Team. 2013. Association between quality improvement for care transitions in communities and rehospitalizations among Medicare beneficiaries. *Journal of the American Medical Association* 309(4):381-391.

Bruera, E., and D. Hui. 2010. Integrating supportive and palliative care in the trajectory of cancer: Establishing goals and models of care. *Journal of Clinical Oncology* 28(25):4013-4017. http://jco.ascopubs.org/content/28/25/4013.short (accessed September 20, 2013).

Brumley, R. D., and K. Hillary. 2002. *The TriCentral Palliative Care Program toolkit.* Oakland, CA: Kaiser Permanente.

Brumley, R. D., S. Enquidanos, P. Jamison, R. Seitz, N. Morgenstern, S. Saito, J. McIlwane, K. Hillary, and J. Gonzales. 2007. Increased satisfaction with care and lower costs: Results of a randomized trial of in-home palliative care. *Journal of the American Geriatric Society* 55(7):993-1000.

Butler, K. 2013. *Knocking on heaven's door.* New York: Scribner.

Calmbach, W. L., J. G. Ryan, L.-M. Baldwin, and L. Knox. 2012. Practice-Based Research Networks (PBRNs): Meeting the challenges of the future. *Journal of the American Board of Family Medicine* 25(5):572-576.

CAPC (Center to Advance Palliative Care). 2008. *Improving palliative care in nursing homes.* http://www.capc.org/support-from-capc/capc_publications/nursing_home_report.pdf (accessed March 24, 2014).

CAPC. 2011. *A state-by-state report card on access to palliative care in our nation's hospitals.* New York: CAPC. http://www.capc.org/reportcard (accessed September 19, 2013).

CAPC. 2013. *Defining palliative care.* New York: CAPC. http://www.capc.org/building-a-hospital-based-palliative-care-program/case/definingpc (accessed August 15, 2013).

Carlson, M. D., C. Barry, M. Schlesinger, R. McCorkle, R. S. Morrison, E. Cherlin, J. Herrin, J. Thompson, M. L. Twaddle, and E. H. Bradley. 2011. Quality of palliative care at U.S. hospices: Results of a national survey. *Medical Care* 49(9):803-809.

Carpenter, C. R., E. R. Bassett, G. M. Fischer, J. Shirshekan, J. E. Galvin, and J. C. Morris. 2011. Four sensitive screening tools to detect cognitive dysfunction in geriatric emergency department patients: Brief Alzheimer's Screen, Short Blessed Test, Ottawa 3DY, and the caregiver-completed AD8. *Academic Emergency Medicine* 18(4):374-384.

Casarett, D., A. Pickard, F. A. Bailey, C. Ritchie, C. Furman, K. Rosenfeld, K. Shreve, Z. Chen, and J. A. Shea. 2008. Do palliative consultations improve patient outcomes? *Journal of the American Geriatric Society* 56(4):593-599.

Casavecchia, K. 2011. *Inside view.* http://npha.org/2011/11/29/inside-view (accessed March 11, 2014).

Chan, R., and J. Webster. 2013. End-of-life care pathways for improving outcomes in caring for the dying. *Cochrane Database of Systematic Reviews* 1:CD008006.

Chaudhry, S. I., T. E. Murphy, E. Gahbauer, L. S. Sussman, H. G. Allore, and T. M. Gill. 2013. Restricting symptoms in the last year of life: A prospective cohort study. *JAMA Internal Medicine* 173(16):1534-1540.

Cheng, M. J., L. M. King, E. R. Alesi, and T. J. Smith. 2013. Doing palliative care in the oncology office. *Journal of Oncology Practice* 9(2):84-88.

Clarke, R. M. A., C. Tseng, R. H. Brook, and A. F. Brown. 2012. Tool used to assess how well community health centers function as medical homes may be flawed. *Health Affairs* 31(3):627-634.

CMS (Centers for Medicare & Medicaid Services). 2012. *Medicare benefit policy manual: Chapter 9—coverage of hospice services under hospital insurance.* http://www.cms.gov/Regulations-and-Guidance/Guidance/Manuals/Downloads/bp102c09.pdf (accessed April 18, 2014).

CMS. 2013a. *Quality improvement organizations.* http://www.cms.gov/Medicare/Quality-Initiatives-Patient-Assessment-Instruments/QualityImprovementOrgs/index.html?redirect=/qualityimprovementorgs (accessed June 18, 2014).

CMS. 2013b. *Hospice quality reporting.* http://www.cms.gov/Medicare/Quality-Initiatives-Patient-Assessment-Instruments/Hospice-Quality-Reporting/index.html?utm_medium=email&utm_source=govdelivery (accessed February 6, 2014).

CMS. 2014a. *Community-based care transitions program.* http://innovation.cms.gov/initiatives/CCTP (accessed June 18, 2014).

CMS. 2014b. *Readmissions reduction program.* http://www.cms.gov/Medicare/Medicare-Fee-for-Service-Payment/AcuteInpatientPPS/Readmissions-Reduction-Program.html (accessed June 18, 2014).

CMS. undated. *User guide for hospice quality reporting data collection.* http://www.cms.gov/Medicare/Quality-Initiatives-Patient-Assessment-Instruments/Hospice-Quality-Reporting/Downloads/UserGuideforDataCollection-.pdf (accessed June 18, 2014).

Coalition to Transform Advanced Care. 2013. *Summary Report of National Summit on Advanced Illness Care.* http://advancedcarecoalition.org/wp-content/uploads/2012/11/2013-Summit-Summary-.pdf (accessed January 14, 2014).

Coleman, E. A., C. Parry, S. Chalmers, and S. J. Min. 2006. The care transitions intervention: Results of a randomized controlled trial. *Archives of Internal Medicine* 166(17): 1822-1828.

Committee on Hospital Care and Institute for Patient- and Family-Centered Care. 2012. Patient- and family-centered care and the pediatrician's role. *Pediatrics* 129(2):394-404.

Connolly, A., E. L. Sampson, and N. Purandare. 2012. End-of-life care for people with dementia from ethnic minority groups: A systematic review. *Journal of the American Geriatrics Society* 60(2):351-360.

Connor, S. R., B. Pyenson, K. Fitch, C. Spence, and K. Iwasaki. 2007. Comparing hospice and nonhospice patient survival among patients who die within a three-year window. *Journal of Pain and Symptom Management* 33(3):238-246.

Cruz, M. L. 2013. *Patient-centered care: How physical therapy can help patients who need palliative care.* http://physical-therapy.advanceweb.com/Features/Articles/Patient-Centered-Care.aspx (accessed August 24, 2013).

Cryer, L., S. B. Shannon, M. Van Amsterdam, and B. Leff. 2012. Costs for "hospital at home" patients were 19 percent lower, with equal or better outcomes compared to similar inpatients. *Health Affairs* 31(6):1237-1242.

Curlin, F. 2013. *Addressing spiritual concerns in care of patients at the end of life.* Presentation at Meeting of the IOM Committee on Approaching Death: Addressing Key End-of-Life Issues, Houston, TX, July 22.

Dahlin, C., ed. 2013. *Clinical practice guidelines for quality palliative care.* 3rd ed. Pittsburgh, PA: National Consensus Project for Quality Palliative Care. http://www.hpna.org/multimedia/NCP_Clinical_Practice_Guidelines_3rd_Edition.pdf (accessed August 20, 2013).

Daratsos, L., and J. L. Howe. 2007. The development of palliative care programs in the Veterans Administration: Zelda Foster's legacy. *Journal of Social Work in End-of-Life & Palliative Care* 3(1):29-39.

De Roo, M. L., K. Leemans, S. J. Claessen, J. Cohen, H. R. Pasman, L. Deliens, A. L. Francke, and EURO IMPACT. 2013. Quality indicators for palliative care: Update of a systematic review. *Journal of Pain and Symptom Management* 46(4):556-572.

Dev, R., and D. Sivesind. 2008. Depression, Chapter 14. In *The MD Anderson supportive and palliative care handbook*, 4th ed., edited by E. Bruera and A. Elsayem. Houston, TX: The University of Texas MD Anderson Cancer Center.

DOL (U.S. Department of Labor). 2013. *Wage and hour division: Family and Medical Leave Act.* http://www.dol.gov/whd/fmla (accessed August 27, 2013).

Dworetz, A. 2013. End of life, at birth. *New York Times,* August 4.

Dy, S. M., C. Apostol, K. A. Martinez, and R. A. Asiakson. 2013. Continuity, coordination, and transitions of care for patients with serious and advanced illness: A systematic review of interventions. *Journal of Palliative Medicine* 16(4):436-445.

Edes, T., S. Shreve, and D. Casarett. 2007. Increasing access and quality in Department of Veterans Affairs care at the end of life: A lesson in change. *Journal of the American Geriatrics Society* 55(10):1645-1649.

Ellrodt, G., D. J. Cook, J. Lee, M. Cho, D. Hunt, and S. Weingarten. 1997. Evidence-based disease management. *Journal of the American Medical Association* 278(20):1687-1692.

Elsayem, A., M. L. Smith, L. Parmley, J. L. Palmer, R. Jenkins, S. Reddy, and E. Bruera. 2006. Impact of a palliative care service on in-hospital mortality in a comprehensive cancer center. *Journal of Palliative Medicine* 9(4):894-902.

Engel, G. L. 1980. The clinical application of the biopsychosocial model. *American Journal of Psychiatry* 137(5):535-544.

ePrognosis. 2014. *ePrognosis: How to use.* http://eprognosis.ucsf.edu/case-examples.php (accessed June 24, 2014).

Ethier, A. M., J. Rollins, and J. Stewart. 2010. *Pediatric oncology palliative and end-of-life care resource.* Chicago, IL: Association of Pediatric Hematology/Oncology Nurses.

Evercare and National Alliance of Caregiving. 2007. *Evercare study of family caregivers: What they spend, what they sacrifice. The personal financial toll of caring for a loved one.* http://www.caregiving.org/data/Evercare_NAC_CaregiverCostStudyFINAL20111907. pdf (accessed April 17, 2014).

Excellus BlueCross BlueShield. 2011. *CompassionNet: Surrounding families with support.* https:// www.excellusbcbs.com/wps/wcm/connect/230a33e7-7d80-49b5-ada9-dee141b62c0b/ WEBCompassionNet10thAnniversary.pdf?MOD=AJPERES&CACHEID=230a33e7-7d80-49b5-ada9-dee141b62c0b (accessed May 28, 2014).

Feigenbaum, P., E. Neuwirth, L. Trowbridge, S. Teplitsky, C. A. Barnes, E. Fireman, J. Dorman, and J. Bellows. 2012. Factors contributing to all-cause 30-day readmissions: A structured case series across 18 hospitals. *Medical Care* 50(7):599-605.

Feinberg, L. 2013. *Policies and Family Caregiving.* Presentation at Meeting of the IOM Committee on Approaching Death: Addressing Key End-of-Life Issues, Menlo Park, CA, May 29.

Feinberg, L., S. C. Reinhard, A. Houser, and R. Choula. 2011. *Valuing the invaluable: 2011 update—The growing contribution and costs of family caregiving.* Washington, DC: AARP, Public Policy Institute. http://assets.aarp.org/rgcenter/ppi/ltc/i51-caregiving.pdf (accessed August 27, 2013).

Feudtner, C., T. I. Kang, K. R. Hexem, S. J. Friedrichsdorf, K. Osenga, H. Siden, S. E. Friebert, R. M. Hays, V. Dussel, and J. Wolfe. 2011. Pediatric palliative care patients: A prospective multicenter cohort study. *Pediatrics* 127(6):1094-1101.

Feudtner, C., J. Womer, R. Augustin, S. Remke, J. Wolfe, S. Friebert, and D. Weissman. 2013. Pediatric palliative care programs in children's hospitals: A cross-sectional national survey. *Pediatrics* 132(6):1063-1070.

Fischberg, D., J. Bull, D. Casarett, L. C. Hanson, S. M. Klein, J. Rotella, T. Smith, C. P. Storey, J. M. Teno, E. Widera, and HPM Choosing Wisely Task Force. 2013. Five things physicians and patients should question in hospice and palliative medicine. *Journal of Pain and Symptom Management* 45(3):595-605.

Fischer, S. M., W. Gozansky, A. Sauaia, S. J. Min, J. S. Kutner, and A. Kramer. 2006. A practical tool to identify patients who may benefit from a palliative approach: The CARING criteria. *Journal of Pain and Symptom Management* 31(4):285-292.

Fleurence, R., J. V. Selby, K. Odom-Walker, G. Hunt, D. Meltzer, J. R. Slutsky, and C. Yancy. 2013. How the Patient-Centered Outcomes Research Institute is engaging patients and others in shaping its research agenda. *Health Affairs* 32(2):393-400.

Flory, J., Y. Young-Xu, I. Gurol, N. Levinsky, A. Ash, and E. Emanuel. 2004. Place of death: U.S. trends since 1980. *Health Affairs* 23(3):194-200.

Friebert, S. 2009. *NHPCO facts and figures: Pediatric palliative and hospice care in America.* Alexandria, VA: NHPCO. http://www.nhpco.org/sites/default/files/public/quality/ Pediatric_Facts-Figures.pdf (accessed March 5, 2014).

Gade, G., I. Venohr, D. Conner, K. McGrady, J. Beane, R. H. Richardson, M. P. Williams, M. Liberson, M. Blum, and R. Della Penna. 2008. Impact of an inpatient palliative care team: A randomized controlled trial. *Journal of Palliative Medicine* 11(2):180-190.

Gelfman, L. P., Q. Du, and R. S. Morrison. 2010. An update: NIH research funding for palliative medicine 2006-2010. *Journal of Palliative Medicine* 16(2):125-129.

Gerhardt, G., A. Yemane, P. Hickman, A. Oelschlaeger, E. Rollins, and N. Brennan. 2013. Medicare readmission rates showed meaningful decline in 2012. *Medicare & Medicaid Research Review*. http://www.cms.gov/mmrr/Briefs/B2013/mmrr-2013-003-02-b01.html (accessed January 5, 2014).

Giardina, T .D., B. J. King, A. P. Ignaczak, D. E. Paull, L. Hoeksema, P. D. Mills, J. Neily, R. R. Hemphill, and H. Singh. 2013. Root cause analysis reports help identify common factors in delayed diagnosis and treatment of outpatients. *Health Affairs* 32(8):1368-1375.

Gill, T. M., E. A. Gahbauer, L. Han, and H. G. Allore. 2010. Trajectories of disability in the last year of life. *New England Journal of Medicine* 362:1173-1180.

Gillick, M. R. 2013. The critical role of caregivers in achieving patient-centered care. *Journal of American Medical Association* 310(6):575-576.

Goldsmith, B., J. Dietrich, Q. Du, and R. S. Morrison. 2008. Variability in access to hospital palliative care in the United States. *Journal of Palliative Medicine* 11(8):1094-1102.

Gomes, B., N. Calanzani, V. Curiale, P. McCrone, and I. J. Higginson. 2013. Effectiveness and cost-effectiveness of home palliative care services for adults with advanced illness and their caregivers. *Cochrane Database of Systematic Reviews* 6:CD007760.

Goodlin, S. J. 2009. Palliative care in congestive heart failure. *Journal of the American College of Cardiology* 54(5):386-396.

Goodman, D. C., E. S. Fisher, C.-H. Chang, N. E. Morden, J. O. Jacobson, K. Murray, and S. Miesfeldt. 2010. Quality of end-of-life cancer care for Medicare beneficiaries: Regional and hospital-specific analyses. *Dartmouth Atlas*. Lebanon, NH: Dartmouth College.

Groninger, H. 2012. A gravely ill patient faces the grim results of outliving her eligibility for hospice benefits. *Health Affairs* 31(2):452-455.

Groopman, J. 2014. Lives less ordinary: Chronically ill children are living longer than ever. How should we care for them? *The New Yorker*, January 20.

Gwilliam, B., V. Keeley, C. Todd, M. Gittins, C. Roberts, L. Kelly, S. Barclay, and P. C. Stone. 2011. Development of Prognosis in Palliative Care Study (PIPS) predictor models to improve prognostication in advanced cancer: Prospective cohort study. *British Medical Journal* 343:d4920.

Han, J. H., S. N. Bryce, E. W. Ely, S. Kripalani, A. Morandi, A. Shintani, J. C. Jackson, A. B. Storrow, R. S. Dittus, and J. Schnelle. 2011. The effect of cognitive impairment on the accuracy of the presenting complaint and discharge instruction comprehension in older emergency department patients. *Annals of Emergency Medicine* 57(6):662-667.

Han, P. K., and D. Rayson. 2010. The coordination of primary and oncology specialty care at the end of life. *Journal of the National Cancer Institute Monographs* 40:31-37.

Hanson, L. C., L. P. Scheunemann, S. Zimmerman, F. S. Rokoske, and A. P. Schenck. 2010. The PEACE project review of clinical instruments for hospice and palliative care. *Journal of Palliative Medicine* 13(10):1253-1260.

Harrold, J. 2013. Testimony presented to inform the IOM Committee on Approaching Death: Addressing Key End-of-Life Issues, Washington, DC, February 20.

HealthPartners. 2012. *The Joint Commission awards first advanced certifications for palliative care*. News release. February 27. https://www.healthpartners.com/public/newsroom/newsroom-article-list/02-27-12.html (accessed August 21, 2013).

Hebert, K., H. Moore, and J. Rooney. 2011. The nurse advocate in end-of-life care. *Ochsner Journal* 11(4):325-329.

Hendrix, C. C., and C. W. Wojciechowski. 2005. Chronic care management for the elderly: An opportunity for gerontological nurse practitioners. *Journal of the American Academy of Nurse Practitioners* 17(7):263-267.

HHS (U.S. Department of Health and Human Services). 2008. Medicare and Medicaid programs: Hospice conditions of participation, final rule. *Federal Register* 73(109):32088-32220. http://www.gpo.gov/fdsys/pkg/FR-2008-06-05/pdf/08-1305.pdf (accessed June 10, 2014).

HHS. 2013. Medicare program; FY2014 hospice wage index and payment rate update; hospice quality reporting requirements; and updates on payment reform. *Federal Register* 78(152):48234-48281. http://www.gpo.gov/fdsys/pkg/FR-2013-08-07/pdf/2013-18838.pdf (accessed June 18, 2014).

Hui, D. 2008. Comprehensive palliative care assessments. Chapter 3. In *The MD Anderson Supportive and Palliative Care Handbook,* 4th ed., edited by E. Bruera and A. Elsayem. Houston: The University of Texas MD Anderson Cancer Center.

Hui, D., M. de la Cruz, S. Thorney, H. A. Parsons, M. Delgado-Guay, and E. Bruera. 2011. The frequency and correlates of spiritual distress among patients with advanced cancer admitted to an acute palliative care unit. *American Journal of Hospice and Palliative Medicine* 28(4):264-270.

Hustey, F. M., S. W. Meldon, M. D. Smith, and C. K. Lex. 2003. The effect of mental status screening on the care of elderly emergency department patients. *Annals of Emergency Medicine* 41(5):678-684.

InformationWeek. 2013. *Remote patient monitoring: 9 promising technologies.* July 30. http://www.informationweek.com/mobile/remote-patient-monitoring-9-promising-technologies/d/d-id/1110968?page_number=1 (accessed January 10, 2014).

IOM (Institute of Medicine). 1996. *Primary care: America's health in a new era.* Washington, DC: National Academy Press.

IOM. 1997. *Approaching death: Improving care at the end of life.* Washington, DC: National Academy Press.

IOM. 2001. *Crossing the quality chasm: A new health system for the 21st century.* Washington, DC: National Academy Press.

IOM. 2003. *When children die: Improving palliative and end-of-life care for children and their families.* Washington, DC: The National Academies Press.

IOM. 2008. *Retooling for an aging America: Building the health care workforce.* Washington, DC: The National Academies Press.

IOM. 2009. *Initial national priorities for comparative effectiveness research.* Washington, DC: The National Academies Press.

IOM. 2011. *Relieving pain in America: A blueprint for transforming prevention, care, education, and research.* Washington, DC: The National Academies Press.

IOM. 2012. *Envisioning a transformed clinical trials enterprise in the United States: Establishing an agenda for 2020: Workshop summary.* Washington, DC: The National Academies Press.

IOM. 2013. *Delivering high-quality cancer care: Charting a new course for a system in crisis.* Washington, DC: The National Academies Press.

Jack, B. W., V. K. Chetty, D. Anthony, J. L. Greenwald, G. M. Sanchez, A. E. Johnson, S. R. Forsythe, J. K. O'Donnell, M. K. Paasche-Orlow, C. Manasseh, S. Martin, and L. Culpepper. 2009. A reengineered hospital discharge program to decrease rehospitalization: A randomized trial. *Annals of Internal Medicine* 150(3):178-187.

James, J. 2013. Medicare Hospital Readmissions Reduction Program: To improve care and lower costs, Medicare imposes a financial penalty on hospitals with excess readmission. *Health Affairs Health Policy Brief.* http://healthaffairs.org/healthpolicybriefs/brief_pdfs/healthpolicybrief_102.pdf (accessed June 18, 2014).

Jencks, S. F., M. V. Williams, and E. A. Coleman. 2009. Rehospitalizations among patients in the Medicare fee-for-service program. *New England Journal of Medicine* 360(14): 1418-1428.

Joint Commission. 2014a. *Facts about the advanced certification program for palliative care.* http://www.jointcommission.org/certification/palliative_care.aspx (accessed June 2, 2014).

Joint Commission. 2014b. *Eligibility for advanced certification for palliative care.* http://www.jointcommission.org/certification/eligiblity_palliative_care.aspx (accessed June 2, 2014).

Joint Commission. 2014c. *Certification programs.* http://www.qualitycheck.org/Certification List.aspx (accessed June 2, 2014).

Kamal, A. H., D. C. Currow, C. S. Ritchie, J. Bull, and A. P. Abernethy. 2013. Community-based palliative care: The natural evolution for palliative care delivery in the U.S. *Journal of Pain and Symptom Management* 46(2):254-264.

Kane, R. L., J. Wales, L. Bernstein, A. Leibowitz, and S. Kaplan. 1984. A randomized controlled trial of hospice care. *Lancet* 1984(2):890-892.

Kilbourn, K., A. Costenaro, S. Madore, K. DeRoche, D. Anderson, T. Keech, and J. S. Kutner. 2011. Feasibility of a telephone-based counseling program for informal caregivers of hospice patients. *Journal of Palliative Medicine* 14(11):1200-1205.

Kind, A. J. H., L. Jensen, S. Barczi, A. Bridges, R. Kordahl, M. A. Smith, and S. Asthana. 2012. Low-cost transitional care with nurse managers making mostly phone contact with patients cut rehospitalization at a VA hospital. *Health Affairs* 31(12):2659-2667.

Klinger, C. A., D. Howell, D. Zakus, and R. B. Deber. 2013. Barriers and facilitators to care for the terminally ill: A cross-country case comparison study of Canada, England, Germany, and the United States. *Palliative Medicine* 28(2):111-120.

Knaus, W. A., E. A. Draper, D. P. Wagner, and J. E. Zimmerman. 1985. APACHE II: A severity of disease classification system. *Critical Care Medicine* 13(10):818-829.

Knaus, W. A., D. P. Wagner, E. A. Draper, J. E. Zimmerman, M. Bergner, P. G. Bastos, C. A. Sirio, D. J. Murphy, T. Lotring, and A. Damiano. 1991. The APACHE III prognostic system: Risk prediction of hospital mortality for critically ill hospitalized adults. *Chest* 100(6):1619-1636.

Krieger, L. M. 2012. The cost of dying: It's hard to reject care even as costs soar. *Mercury News,* February 5. http://www.mercurynews.com/cost-of-dying/ci_19898736 (accessed June 28, 2013).

Krishnan, M., J. S. Temel, A. A. Wright, R. Bernacki, K. Selvaggi, and T. Balboni. 2013. Predicting life expectancy in patients with advanced incurable cancer: A review. *Journal of Supportive Oncology* 11(2):68-74.

Kutner, J. S. 2010. An 86-year-old woman with cardiac cachexia contemplating the end of her life: Review of hospice care. *Journal of the American Medical Association* 303(4): 349-356.

Labson, M. C., M. M. Sacco, D. E. Weissman, and B. Gornet. 2013. Innovative models of home-based palliative care. *Cleveland Clinic Journal of Medicine* 80(Suppl. 1):e530-e535.

Lee, S. J., K. Lindquist, M. R. Segal, and K. E. Covinsky. 2006. Development and validation of a prognostic index for 4-year mortality in older adults. *Journal of the American Medical Association* 295(7):801-808.

Li, Q., N. T. Zheng, and H. Temkin-Greener. 2013. Quality of end-of-life care of long-term nursing home residents with and without dementia. *Journal of the American Geriatrics Society* 61(7):1066-1073.

Liss, D. T., J. Chubak, M. L. Anderson, K. W. Saunders, L. Tuzzio, and R. J. Reid. 2011. Patient-reported care coordination: Associations with primary care continuity and specialty care use. *Annals of Family Medicine* 9(4):323-329.

Maltoni, M., O. Nanni, M. Pirovano, E. Scarpi, M. Indelli, C. Martini, M. Monti, E. Arnoldi, L. Piva, A. Ravaioli, G. Cruciani, R. Labianca, and D. Amadori. 1999. Successful validation of the palliative prognostic score in terminally ill cancer patients. Italian Multicenter Study on Palliative Care. *Journal of Pain and Symptom Management* 17(4):240-247.

Matlock, D. D., P. N. Peterson, B. E. Sirovich, D. E. Wennberg, P. M. Gallagher, and F. L. Lucas. 2010. Regional variations in palliative care: Do cardiologists follow guidelines? *Journal of Palliative Medicine* 13(11):1315-1319.

Meier, D. E. 2010. The development, status, and future of palliative care. In *Palliative care: Transforming the care of serious illness,* edited by D. E. Meier, S. L. Isaacs, and R. G. Hughes. Hoboken, NJ: Jossey-Bass.

Meier, D. E. 2011. Increased access to palliative care and hospice services: Opportunities to improve value in health care. *Milbank Quarterly* 89(3):343-380.

Mendes, E. 2011. Most caregivers look after elderly parent; invest a lot of time. *Gallup Well-Being,* July 28. http://www.gallup.com/poll/148682/caregivers-look-elderly-parent-invest-lot-time.aspx (accessed August 25, 2013).

Mitchell, K. 2013. Colorado prison hospice program helps inmates die with dignity. *Denver Post,* February 17. http://www.denverpost.com/ci_22607208/colorado-prison-hospice-program-helps-inmates-die-dignity (accessed March 10, 2014).

Mitchell, P., M. Wynia, R. Golden, B. McNellis, S. Okun, C.E. Webb, V. Rohrbach, and I. Von Kohorn. 2012. *Core principles and values of effective team-based health care.* Discussion paper. Washington, DC: The National Academies Press.

Molony, D. 2013. Testimony presented to inform the IOM Committee on Approaching Death: Addressing Key End-of-Life Issues, Houston, TX, July 23.

Moss, A. H., J. Ganjoo, S. Sharma, J. Gansor, S. Senft, B. Weaner, C. Dalton, K. MacKay, B. Pellegrino, P. Anantharaman, and R. Schmidt. 2008. Utility of the "surprise" question to identify dialysis patients with high mortality. *Clinical Journal of the American Society of Nephrology* 3(5):1379-1384.

Moss, A. H., J. R. Lunney, S. Culp, M. Auber, S. Kurian, J. Rogers, J. Dower, and J. Abraham. 2010. Prognostic significance of the "surprise" question in cancer patients. *Journal of Palliative Medicine* 13(7):837-840.

Mukamel, D. B., T. Caprio, R. Ahn, N. T. Zheng, S. Norton, T. Quill, and H. Temkin-Greener. 2012. End-of-life quality of care measures for nursing homes: Place of death and hospice. *Journal of Palliative Medicine* 15(4):438-446.

Mularski, R. A., J. R. Curtis, J. A. Billings, R. Burt, I. Byock, C. Fuhrman, A. C. Mosenthal, J. Medina, D. E. Ray, G. D. Rubenfeld, L. J. Schneiderman, P. D. Treece, R. D. Truog, and M. M. Levy. 2006. Proposed quality measures for palliative care in the critically ill: A consensus from the Robert Wood Johnson Foundation Critical Care Workgroup. *Critical Care Medicine* 34(Suppl. 11):S404-S411.

NASW (National Association of Social Workers). 2013. *NASW standards for practice in palliative and end-of-life care.* Washington, DC: NASW.

NASW. 2014. *NASW professional social work credentials and advanced practice specialty credentials.* Washington, DC: NASW. https://www.socialworkers.org/credentials/list.asp (accessed January 8, 2014).

National Alliance for Caregiving. 2009. *Caregiving in the U.S.* Bethesda, MD: National Alliance for Caregiving. http://www.caregiving.org/data/Caregiving_in_the_US_2009_full_report.pdf (accessed March 11, 2014).

National Resource Center for Participant-Directed Services. 2013. *Cash & Counseling.* Chestnut Hill, MA: Boston College. http://www.bc.edu/schools/gssw/nrcpds/cash_and_counseling.html (accessed January 15, 2014).

Naylor, M. D., L. H. Aiken, E. T. Kurtzman, D. M. Olds, and K. B. Hirschman. 2011. The importance of transitional care in achieving health reform. *Health Affairs* 30(4):746-754.

Naylor, M. D., K. H. Bowles, K. M. McCauley, M. C. Maccoy, G. Maislin, M. V. Pauly, and R. Krakauer. 2013. High-value transitional care: Translation of research into practice. *Journal of Evaluation in Clinical Practice* 19(5):727-733.

NBCHPN® (National Board for Certification of Hospice and Palliative Nurses). 2013. *Pittsburgh, PA: National Board for Certification of Hospice and Palliative Nurses.* http://www.nbchpn.org (accessed September 20, 2013).

NCCN (National Comprehensive Cancer Network). 2013. *Clinical practice guidelines in oncology—palliative care.* Version 2.2013. Fort Washington, PA: NCCN.

NCI (National Cancer Institute). 2014. *Pediatric supportive care (PDQ®).* http://www.cancer. gov/cancertopics/pdq/supportivecare/pediatric/Patient/page1 (accessed March 12, 2014).

NHPCO (National Hospice and Palliative Care Organization). 2009. *Standards of practice for pediatric palliative care and hospice.* Alexandria, VA: NHPCO.

NHPCO. 2012a. *NHPCO facts and figures: Hospice care in America.* Alexandria, VA: NHPCO. http://www.nhpco.org/sites/default/files/public/Statistics_Research/2012_Facts_ Figures.pdf (accessed July 7, 2013).

NHPCO. 2012b. *Pediatric concurrent care. Alexandria,* VA: NHPCO. http://www.nhpco. org/sites/default/files/public/ChiPPS/Continuum_Briefing.pdf (accessed May 25, 2014).

NHPCO. 2013. *NHPCO's facts and figures: Hospice care in America.* Alexandria, VA: NHPCO. http://www.nhpco.org/sites/default/files/public/Statistics_Research/2013_Facts_ Figures.pdf (accessed January 7, 2014).

NHPCO. undated. *History of hospice care.* Alexandria, VA: NHPCO. http://www.nhpco.org/ history-hospice-care (accessed February 5, 2014).

NINR (National Institute of Nursing Research). 2013. *Building momentum: The science of end-of-life and palliative care—a review of research trends and funding, 1997-2010.* http://www.ninr.nih.gov/sites/www.ninr.nih.gov/files/NINR-Building-Momentum-508.pdf (accessed July 26, 2013).

NPCRC (National Palliative Care Research Center). 2013. *Mission.* New York: Icahn School of Medicine. http://npcrc.org/content/37/mission.aspx (accessed September 20, 2013).

NQF (National Quality Forum). 2006. *A national framework and preferred practices for palliative and hospice care quality: A consensus report.* Washington, DC: NQF.

NQF. 2012. *Palliative care and end-of-life care: A consensus report.* Washington, DC: NQF. http://www.qualityforum.org/Publications/2012/04/Palliative_Care_and_End-of-Life_ Care%E2%80%94A_Consensus_Report.aspx (accessed February 7, 2014).

Parikh, R. B., R. A. Kirch, T. J. Smith, and J. S. Temel. 2013. Early specialty palliative care—translating data in oncology into practice. *New England Journal of Medicine* 369(24):2347-2351.

Pasman, H. R., H. E. Brandt, L. Deliens, and A. L. Francke. 2009. Quality indicators for palliative care: A systematic review. *Journal of Pain and Symptom Management* 38(1):145-156.

Payne, S., P. Smith, and S. Dean. 1999. Identifying the concerns of informal carers in palliative care. *Palliative Medicine* 13:37-44.

PCORI (Patient-Centered Outcomes Research Institute). 2012. *National priorities for research and research agenda.* Washington, DC: PCORI. http://www.pcori.org/assets/PCORI-National-Priorities-and-Research-Agenda-2012-05-21-FINAL1.pdf (accessed July 24, 2014).

PCORI. 2014. *About us.* http://www.pcori.org/about-us/landing (accessed July 24, 2014).

Peterson, K. A., P. Darby Lipman, C. J. Lange, R. A. Cohen, and S. Durako. 2012. Supporting better science in primary care: A description of Practice-Based Research Networks (PBRNs) in 2011. *Journal of the American Board of Family Medicine* 25(5):565-571.

Pirl, W. F., J. A. Greer, L. Traeger, V. Jackson, I. T. Lennes, E. R. Gallagher, P. Perez-Cruz, R. S. Heist, and J. S. Temel. 2012. Depression and survival in metastatic non-small-cell lung cancer: Effects of early palliative care. *Journal of Clinical Oncology* 30(12):1310-1315.

Pirovano, M., M. Maltoni, O. Nanni, M. Marinari, M. Indelli, G. Zaninetta, V. Petrella, S. Barni, E. Zecca, E. Scarpi, R. Labianca, D. Arnadori, and G. Luporini. 1999. A new palliative prognostic score: A first step for the staging of terminally ill cancer patients. *Journal of Pain and Symptom Management* 17(4):231-239.

Pollens, R. 2004. Role of the speech-language pathologist in palliative hospice care. *Journal of Palliative Medicine* 7(5):694-702.

Pritchard, M., E. A. Burghen, J. S. Gattuso, N. K. West, P. Gajjar, D. K. Srivastava, S. L. Spunt, J. N. Baker, J. R. Kane, W. L. Furman, and P. S. Hinds. 2010. Factors that distinguish symptoms of most concern to parents from other symptoms of dying children. *Journal of Pain and Symptom Management* 39(4):627-636.

Puchalski, C., B. Ferrell, R. Virani, S. Otis-Green, P. Baird, J. Bull, H. Chochinov, G. Handzo, H. Nelson-Becker, M. Prince-Paul, K. Pugliese, and D. Sulmasy. 2009. Improving the quality of spiritual care as a dimension of palliative care: The report of the Consensus Conference. *Journal of Palliative Medicine* 12(10):885-904.

Quill, T. E., and A. P. Abernethy. 2013. Generalist plus specialist palliative care: Creating a more sustainable model. *New England Journal of Medicine* 368(13):1173-1175.

Rabow, M. W., E. Kvale, L. Barbour, J. B. Cassel, S. Cohen, V. Jackson, C. Luhrs, V. Nguyen, S. Rinaldi, D. Stevens, L. Spragens, and D. Weissman. 2013. Moving upstream: A review of the evidence of the impact of outpatient palliative care. *Journal of Palliative Medicine* 16(12):1540-1549.

Rauch, J. 2013. How not to die. *The Atlantic.* http://www.theatlantic.com/magazine/archive/2013/05/how-not-to-die/309277 (accessed February 2, 2014).

Redfoot, D., L. Feinberg, and A. Houser. 2013. *The aging of the baby boom and the growing care gap: A look at future declines in the availability of family caregivers.* Washington, DC: AARP, Public Policy Institute. http://www.aarp.org/content/dam/aarp/research/public_policy_institute/ltc/2013/baby-boom-and-the-growing-care-gap-insight-AARP-ppi-ltc.pdf (accessed August 26, 2013).

Reinhard, S. C., C. Levine, and S. Samis. 2012. *Home alone: Family caregivers providing complex chronic care.* Washington, DC: AARP, Public Policy Institute.

Rhodes, R. L., S. L. Mitchell, S. C. Miller, S. R. Connor, and J. M. Teno. 2008. Bereaved family members' evaluation of hospice care: What factors influence overall satisfaction with services? *Journal of Pain and Symptom Management* 35(4):365-371.

Robert Wood Johnson Foundation. 2004. *Community-state partnerships to improve end-of-life care: An RWJF national program.* Princeton, NJ: Robert Wood Johnson Foundation.

Sacco, J., D. R. Deravin Carr, and D. Viola. 2013. The effects of the palliative medicine consultation on the DNR status of African Americans in a safety net hospital. *American Journal of Hospice and Palliative Care* 30(4):363-369.

Saito, A. M., M. B. Landrum, B. A. Neville, J. Z. Avanian, J. C. Weeks, and C. C. Earle. 2011. Hospice care and survival among elderly patients with lung cancer. *Journal of Palliative Medicine* 14(8):929-939.

Santiago, K. C. 2013. Testimony presented to inform the IOM Committee on Approaching Death: Addressing Key End-of-Life Issues, Washington, DC, February 20.

Schenck, A. P., F. S. Rokoske, D. D. Durham, J. G. Cagle, and L. C. Hanson, 2010. The PEACE project: Identification of quality measures for hospice and palliative care. *Journal of Palliative Medicine* 13(12):1451-1459.

Sharma, G., J. Freeman, D. Zhang, and J. S. Goodwin. 2009. Continuity of care and ICU utilization during end of life. *Archives of Internal Medicine* 169(1):81-86.

Shaw, G. 2010. Special report: Bringing palliative care to neurology. *Neurology Today* 10(19):16-17. http://journals.lww.com/neurotodayonline/Fulltext/2010/10070/Special_Report__Bringing_Palliative_Care_to.5.aspx (accessed September 19, 2013).

Simone, C. B. II, and J. A. Jones, 2013. Palliative care for patients with locally advanced and metastatic non-small cell lung cancer. *Annals of Palliative Medicine* 2(4):178-188.

Smith, A. K., J. N. Thai, M. A. Bakitas, D. E. Meier, L. H. Spragens, J. S. Temel, D. E. Weissman, and M. W. Rabow. 2013a. The diverse landscape of palliative care clinics. *Journal of Palliative Medicine* 16(6):661-668. http://www.ncbi.nlm.nih.gov/pubmed/23662953 (accessed September 19, 2013).

Smith, A. K., L. C. Walter, Y. Miao, W. J. Boscardin, and K. E. Covinsky. 2013b. Disability during the last two years of life. *JAMA Internal Medicine* 173(16):1506-1513.

Smith, A. K., D. B. White, and R. M. Arnold. 2013c. Uncertainty: The other side of prognosis. *New England Journal of Medicine* 368(26):2448-2450.

Smith, T. J., S. Temin, E. R. Alesi, A. P. Abernethy, T. A. Balboni, E. M. Basch, B. R. Ferrell, M. Loscalzo, D. E. Meier, J. A. Paice, J. M. Peppercorn, M. Somerfield, E. Stovall, and J. H. Van Roenn. 2012. American Society of Clinical Oncology provisional clinical opinion: The integration of palliative care into standard oncology care. *Journal of Clinical Oncology* 30(8):880-887.

Sourkes, B. 2013. *Transforming end-of-life care, panel: Family caregivers.* Presentation at Meeting of the IOM Committee on Approaching Death: Addressing Key End-of-Life Issues, Menlo Park, CA, May 29.

Steinhauser, K. E., and J. Barroso. 2009. Using qualitative methods to explore key questions in palliative care. *Journal of Palliative Medicine* 12(8):725-729.

Stephens, S. A. 2011. *My father's end-of-life treatment: Not what he had in mind.* http://commonhealth.wbur.org/2011/10/my-fathers-end-of-life-treatment-not-what-he-had-in-mind (accessed August 11, 2013).

Swan, B. A. 2012. A nurse learns firsthand that you may fend for yourself after a hospital stay. *Health Affairs* 31(11):2579-2582.

Temel, J. S., J. A. Greer, A. Muzikansky, E. R. Gallagher, S. Admane, V. A. Jackson, C. M. Dahlin, C. D. Binderman, J. Jacobsen, W. F. Pirl, J. A. Billings, and T. J. Lynch. 2010. Early palliative care for patients with metastatic non-small-cell lung cancer. *New England Journal of Medicine* 363(8):733-742.

Teno, J. M., B. R. Claridge, V. Casey, L. C. Welch, T. Wetle, R. Shield, and V. Mor. 2004. Family perspectives on end-of-life care at the last place of care. *Journal of the American Medical Association* 291(1):88-93.

Teno, J. M., P. L. Gozalo, I. C. Lee, S. Kuo, C. Spence, S. R. Connor, and D. J. Casarett. 2011. Does hospice improve quality of care for persons dying from dementia? *Journal of the American Geriatrics Society* 59(8):1531-1536.

Teno, J. M., P. L. Gozalo, J. P. Bynum, N. E. Leland, S. C. Miller, N. E. Morden, T. Scupp, D. C. Goodman, and V. Mor. 2013. Change in end-of-life care for Medicare beneficiaries: Site of death, place of care, and health care transitions in 2000, 2005, and 2009. *Journal of the American Medical Association* 309(5):470-477.

Thompson, J. W., M. D. A. Carlson, and E. H. Bradley. 2012. U.S. hospice industry experienced considerable turbulence from changes in ownership, growth, and shift to for-profit status. *Health Affairs* 31(6):1286-1293.

Tripathi, S. S., G. P. Cantwell, A. Ofir, D. Serrecchia, and S. Peck. 2012. Pediatric palliative care in the medical home. *Pediatric Annals* 41(3):112-116.

Triveldi, N. S., and T. Delbanco. 2011. Update: An 86-year-old woman with cardiac cachexia contemplating the end of her life: Review of hospice care. *Journal of the American Medical Association* 306(6):645.

Unroe, K. T., and D. E . Meier. 2013. Quality of hospice care for individuals with dementia. *Journal of the American Geriatric Society* 61(7):1212-1214.

VA (U.S. Department of Veterans Affairs). 2008. *Palliative Care Consult Teams (PCCT).* VHA directive 2008-006. http://www.va.gov/vhapublications/ViewPublication.asp?pub_ID=1784 (accessed June 18, 2014).

VA. 2013. *Services of family caregivers of post-9/11 veterans.* http://www.caregiver.va.gov/
support/support_benefits.asp (accessed August 27, 2013).

Vega, T. 2014. As parents age, Asian-Americans struggle to obey a cultural code. *New York
Times*, January 14. http://www.nytimes.com/2014/01/15/us/as-asian-americans-age-their-
children-face-cultural-hurdles.html?hp&_r=0 (accessed January 17, 2014).

Vitello, P. 2008. Hospice chaplains take up bedside counseling. *New York Times,* October 28.
http://www.nytimes.com/2008/10/29/nyregion/29hospice.html?pagewanted=all&_r=0
(accessed September 20, 2013).

Vuong, Z. 2013. Alzheimer's disease takes its toll on families, caregivers. *San Gabriel Valley
Tribune News,* May 3. http://www.sgvtribune.com/general-news/20130504/alzheimers-
disease-takes-its-toll-on-families-caregivers (accessed August 27, 2013).

Walling, A., S. M. Asch, K. Lorenz, C. P. Roth, T. Barry, K. L. Kahn, and N. S. Wenger. 2010.
The quality of care provided to hospitalized patients at the end of life. *Archives of Internal Medicine* 170(12):1057-1063.

Warshaw, G. A., E. J. Bragg, L. P. Fried, and W. J. Hall. 2008. Which patients benefit the most
from a geriatrician's care? Consensus among directors of geriatrics academic programs.
Journal of the American Geriatrics Society 56(10):1796-1801.

Weissman, D. E., and D. E. Meier. 2011. Identifying patients in need of a palliative care assessment in the hospital setting: A consensus report from the Center to Advance Palliative
Care. *Journal of Palliative Medicine* 14(1):1-6.

Wenger, N. S., C. P. Roth, P. Shekelle, and the ACOVE Investigators. 2007. Introduction to
the Assessing Care of Vulnerable Elders-3 quality indicator measurement set. *Journal of
the American Geriatrics Society* 55:S247-S252.

Westfall, J. M., J. Mold, and L. Fagnan. 2007. Practice-based research: "Blue highways" on
the NIH roadmap. *Journal of the American Medical Association* 297(4):403-406.

WHO (World Health Organization). 2002. *National cancer control programmes: Policies and
managerial guidelines.* 2nd ed. Geneva, Switzerland: WHO.

WHO. 2013. *Cancer: WHO definition of palliative care.* Geneva, Switzerland: WHO. http://
www.who.int/cancer/palliative/definition/en/# (accessed August 17, 2013).

Williams, A.-L., and R. McCorkle. 2011. Cancer family caregivers during the palliative,
hospice, and bereavement phases: A review of the descriptive psychosocial literature.
Palliative and Supportive Care 9(3):315-325.

Witters, D. 2011. Caregiving costs U.S. economy $25.2 billion in lost productivity. *Gal-
lup Well-Being,* July 27. http://www.gallup.com/poll/148670/caregiving-costs-economy-
billion-lost-productivity.aspx (accessed August 26, 2013).

Wolfe, J., H. E. Grier, N. Klar, S. B. Levin, J. M. Ellenbogen, S. Salem-Schatz, E. J. Emanuel,
and J. C. Weeks. 2000. Symptoms and suffering at the end of life in children with cancer.
New England Journal of Medicine 342(5):326-333.

Wong, D. T., and W. A. Knaus. 1991. Predicting outcome in critical care: The current status of
the APACHE prognostic scoring system. *Canadian Journal of Anaesthesia* 38(3):374-383.

Youngwerth, J., S. J. Min, B. Statland, R. Allyn, and S. Fischer. 2013. Caring about prognosis:
A validation study of the CARING criteria to identify hospitalized patients at high risk
for death at 1 year. *Journal of Hospital Medicine* 8(12):696-701.

Yourman, L. C., S. J. Lee, M. A. Schonberg, E. W. Widera, and A. K. Smith. 2012. Prognostic
indices for older adults: A systematic review. *Journal of the American Medical Association* 307(2):182-192.

Zhukovsky, D. S. 2008. Palliative care in pediatrics. Chapter 16. In *The MD Anderson supportive and palliative care handbook,* 4th ed., edited by E. Bruera and A. Elsayem.
Houston: The University of Texas MD Anderson Cancer Center.

3

Clinician-Patient Communication and Advance Care Planning

There are many barriers to clear communication on people's preferences for end-of-life care. Albeit well intentioned, past efforts to ensure that patients' wishes are known and followed have fallen short, even when codified into legislation and regulation, as a result of multiple factors:

- the natural reluctance of patients, families, and clinicians to explore death and dying;
- a fragmented health care system that can make the discussion of end-of-life preferences "someone else's problem";
- poor-quality communication in the conversations that are held, often in hurried or crisis situations; and
- inadequate structural supports for advance care planning, including clinician training, payment, and record keeping.

The "living will"—conceived as a document designed to protect people's legal right to have the amount and kinds of medical treatment they want even if they can no longer express that choice themselves—was perceived as the solution for Americans' concerns about being "hooked up to machines" for long periods or, conversely, being protected against premature "pulling of the plug." Nonetheless, this legal approach has been disappointingly ineffective in improving the care people nearing the end of life receive and in ensuring that this care accords with their informed preferences.

This chapter describes some of the reasons for that failure and the evolution of new and potentially more effective approaches to advance care planning. These approaches share the following features:

- They do not consider advance care planning a one-time activity, but instead emphasize discussion of goals, values, and care preferences among individuals, family, health care agents, and care providers over the life span. Ideally, these discussions would start early in adulthood, addressing global values and the identification of potential surrogate decision makers, and focusing on more specific treatment preferences for older persons and those facing serious illness. With changes in health status, they would take on increasing specificity. "Putting it in writing" remains important but does not substitute for the discussion.
- They emphasize appointment of a health care agent[1]; encourage adequate preparation of that agent for future decision making; and support discussions of care choices among individuals, the agent, and the primary clinician.
- They respect and accommodate the different cultural, ethnic, and spiritual values of the diverse U.S. population.

A measure of control over the final phase of life appears achievable in most situations today if patients, families, and clinicians have these essential conversations. The best experiences occur when there are reliable systems for eliciting, recording, and using information about patients' preferences; when clinicians are trained to carry out these tasks effectively and are properly compensated for doing so; and when, regardless of care setting—home, nursing home, hospital, intensive care, rehabilitation facility, or under hospice care—patients' wishes are known and respected to the extent possible. Instead, however, there are strong professional, cultural, and financial incentives for continuing treatment beyond the point where it benefits patients.

This chapter examines the current state of advance care planning—who participates and the ways in which it affects clinical care, patient and caregiver outcomes, and the costs of care. It then describes the way age, disability, and personal background may affect attitudes about and experiences with advance care planning. Next, fundamental to the advance care planning process is clear empathetic communication between clinicians and patients, which can lead to shared decision making. Accordingly, the chapter explores the elements of good communication in this process. This is followed by discussion of several model advance care planning programs

---

[1]These individuals are variously called surrogates, proxies, or agents. A health care agent is an individual designated in an advance directive, while a health care proxy is any designated substitute decision maker, including a guardian or conservator. A surrogate is a person who, by default, becomes the decision maker for an individual who has no appointed proxy (HHS, 2008). In this report, the term "health care agent" is generally used. The form that names the agent is often called a durable power of attorney for health care.

and the committee's proposed life cycle model for advance care planning. The chapter ends by outlining research needs and presenting the committee's findings, conclusions, and recommendations on alignment of care with patient preferences.

BACKGROUND

Americans express strong views when asked about the kinds of care they want when they are seriously ill and approaching death. As noted in earlier chapters, in general they prefer to die at home, and they want to remain in charge of decisions about their care (CHCF, 2012; Fischer et al., 2013; Gruneir et al., 2007; Tang, 2003). However, evidence suggests these wishes are not likely to be fulfilled:

- In 2009, one in four adults aged 65 and older died in an acute care hospital, 28 percent died in a nursing home, and one in three died at home (Teno et al., 2013). Among all decedents, 30 percent were in an intensive care unit (ICU) in the month preceding death.
- An estimated 40 percent of all adult medical inpatients are incapable of making their own treatment decisions because of unconsciousness, cognitive impairment, or inability to express a choice (Raymont et al., 2004).
- Among nursing home residents, 44-69 percent cannot make their own medical decisions (Kim et al., 2002).
- Fully 70 percent of decedents participating in the Health and Retirement Study who were aged 60 and older at death and who faced treatment decisions in the final days of their lives were incapable of participating in these decisions (Silveira et al., 2010).
- The vast majority of critically ill patients cannot participate directly in decision making (Nelson et al., 2006), nor are they likely even to have met the intensivist physicians caring for them (Gay et al., 2009).

The Institute of Medicine (IOM) report *Approaching Death* (IOM, 1997) reviews many of the then-recognized shortcomings of the advance directive approach:

- patients' and families' lack of awareness of or interest in completing forms;
- clinicians' unwillingness to adhere to patients' wishes;
- difficulties in having meaningful family conversations about patients' wishes and in making choices in the face of prognostic uncertainty;

- lack of institutional support and processes for completing advance directives; and
- cultural and legal factors, including resistance within the medical culture as well as differences in families' cultural traditions.

A study of public views conducted around the same time that report was published reinforced these concerns (American Health Decisions, 1997). Respondents noted that there are many reasons why they or their loved ones avoid talking about death, including that it is upsetting or depressing or is an issue to be addressed in the future. They also felt that the medical system's emphasis on achieving cure and sustaining life "even when death is inevitable—can ironically result in treatments that prolong life 'unnaturally' and cause unnecessary suffering."

Some of the problems identified 17 years ago have since diminished or been remedied, while others have become more acutely apparent. The mischaracterization of advance care planning as "death panels" during debates about the Affordable Care Act (see Chapter 6) suggests that misunderstandings about the process have persisted and, indeed, intensified.

The remainder of this section reviews the four-decade history of advance directives/advance care planning. Before proceeding, however, a note about these two terms is in order. *Approaching Death* draws a useful distinction between advance directives (documents written or completed by patients) and the broader concept of advance care planning. As Box 3-1 describes, advance care planning is a process for setting goals and plans with respect to medical treatments and other clinical considerations. It brings together patients, families, and clinicians "to develop a coherent care plan that meets the patients' goals, values, and preferences" (Walling et al., 2008, p. 3896). It can begin at any point in a person's life, regardless of his or her current health state; is revisited periodically; and becomes more specific as changing health status warrants.

As anticipated in *Approaching Death*, the current emphasis has evolved considerably from a debate about specific legal forms and living wills to acceptance of the more general concept of advance care planning (Sabatino, 2010). Because much of the large body of research in this area focuses on advance directives (a tangible product) rather than the broader and more difficult to document topic of advance care planning, this chapter likewise talks about directives. It should be noted, however, that while the committee consistently found shortcomings in advance directives, it is more optimistic about the potential benefits of advance care planning.

The following historical review draws on a report prepared by the U.S. Department of Health and Human Services (HHS, 2008) titled *Advance Directives and Advance Care Planning*. That report resulted from a request by Congress in 2006 that HHS conduct a study of advance directives and how to promote their use.

For decades, people with advanced serious illnesses relied almost unquestioningly on their physicians' judgment regarding treatment matters, trusting that physicians would act in their patients' best interests as a matter of professional and personal ethics. As technology and medicine advanced, increasingly intensive interventions could keep people alive with breathing tubes and feeding tubes and high doses of powerful drugs. In many cases, people recovered and resumed their former lives, but in other cases, the lives these technologies sustained were not optimal.

Around the time public awareness of the darker potential of "heroic measures" was growing, so was the consumer rights movement. In that context, Americans sought to assert their right to control whether life-sustaining treatments were used in their care, especially when the outcome was doubtful. Among the earliest attempts to codify this new right was the California Natural Death Act of 1976[2] (Towers, 1978), which made the written advance directives of terminally ill patients binding on their physicians. The California law was quickly followed by similar actions in other states and upheld in state and federal courts. In 1990, Congress passed the Patient Self-Determination Act,[3] which required all health care facilities receiving reimbursement from Medicare or Medicaid "to ask patients whether they have advance directives, to provide information about advance directives, and to incorporate advance directives into the medical record" (HHS, 2008, p. x), setting the stage for subsequent emphasis on this type of form.

Public concern about advance directives increased in the wake of several well-publicized legal cases that centered on the right to withdraw treatment from people lacking decision-making capacity. At the same time, new state laws outlined do-not-resuscitate protocols—medical orders signed by a clinician—for use outside as well as within the hospital. Building on this concept of having medical orders in place to guide treatment, a new model was pioneered in Oregon for recording a broader range of preferences. These Physician Orders for Life-Sustaining Treatment (POLST), now being approved in an increasing number of states (see Box 3-1 and Annex 3-2) and described later in this chapter, are actionable in and out of the hospital, even in emergency situations.

Regional and national efforts to encourage advance care planning have

---

[2]Natural Death Act, Ch. 1439, 1976 Cal. Stat. 6478 (enacting Cal. Health & Safety Code § 7188 (repealed 2000)).

[3]The Patient Self-Determination Act, Omnibus Budget Reconciliation Act of 1990, Public Law 101-508 §§ 4206 and 4751, 104 Stat. 1388-155 and 1388-204 (1991).

BOX 3-1
Terms Related to Advance Care Planning

Advance care planning entails a number of different kinds of instruments. In this report, the committee has tried to maintain the distinctions among them, but the medical literature reviewed does not always do so, and there is confusion even in the field. Terms appearing in this report with respect to advance care planning are defined as follows, with the understanding that in discussing particular studies, the committee uses the terms employed by their authors.

Advance care planning refers to the whole process of discussion of end-of-life care, clarification of related values and goals, and embodiment of preferences through written documents and medical orders. This process can start at any time and be revisited periodically, but it becomes more focused as health status changes. Ideally, these conversations (1) occur with a person's health care agent and primary clinician, along with other members of the clinical team; (2) are recorded and updated as needed; and (3) allow for flexible decision making in the context of the patient's current medical situation.

Advance directive refers to several types of patient-initiated documents, especially living wills and documents that name a health care agent. People can complete these forms at any time and in any state of health that allows them to do so.

- *Living will*—a written (or video) statement about the kinds of medical care a person does or does not want under certain specific conditions (often "terminal illness") if no longer able to express those wishes.
- *Durable power of attorney for health care*—identifies the person (the health care agent) who should make medical decisions in case of the patient's incapacity.

Medical orders are created with and signed by a health professional, usually a physician (in some states, a nurse practitioner or physician assistant), for someone who is seriously ill. Because they are actual doctor's orders, other health professionals, including emergency personnel, are required to follow them.

---

evolved. Community Conversations on Compassionate Care (CCCC),[4] operating in Upstate New York, was launched with a press conference of spiritual leaders in Rochester, New York, in 2002 to encourage everyone aged 18 and older to start early advance care planning discussions. The Center for Practical Bioethics works extensively in the Midwest and throughout the

---

[4]See https://www.compassionandsupport.org/index.php/for_patients_families/advance_care_planning/community_conversations (accessed December 16, 2014).

- *Physician Orders for Life-Sustaining Treatment (POLST)[a]*—physician orders covering a range of topics likely to emerge in care of a patient near the end of life, an innovation that began in Oregon in the early 1990s, gradually spread to a few states, and is increasingly being adopted nationwide. The orders cross care settings and are honored in the community in an emergency. As of December 2013, the POLST Paradigm Task Force had endorsed the POLST programs of 16 states,[b] and another 12 states were developing POLST implementation plans (National POLST, 2012f).
- *Do-not-resuscitate,[c] do-not-intubate, do-not-hospitalize orders*—medical orders covering specific treatments that are written in a health care facility, but do not cross care settings and are not necessarily honored in the community. An out-of-hospital do-not-resuscitate is a do-not-resuscitate medical order that pertains when a patient is outside of a health care facility setting (for example, a hospital or nursing home), and is intended to ensure that a patient will not be resuscitated against his or her wishes by emergency medical personnel.

---

[a]The names of similar forms in different states vary. They include MOLST (Medical Orders for Life-Sustaining Treatment), MOST (Medical Orders for Scope of Treatment), POST (Physician Orders for Scope of Treatment), COLST (Clinical Orders for Life-Sustaining Treatment), SMOST or SPOST (Summary of Physician Orders for Scope of Treatment), and TPOPP (Transportable Physician Order for Patient Preference). The approach is referred to as the POLST paradigm, and the state organizations or coalitions that oversee the implementation of these medical order programs are referred to as POLST paradigm programs. Program names vary among the states overseeing these forms as well. This chapter uses POLST to apply to all these variations unless the text is referring to a specific program with a different name. See also http://www.polst.org.

[b]California, Colorado, Georgia, Hawaii, Idaho, Louisiana, Montana, New York, North Carolina, Oregon, Pennsylvania, Tennessee, Utah, Washington, West Virginia, and Wisconsin (Wisconsin has been endorsed only regionally).

[c]Because of the high likelihood that resuscitation near death will be unsuccessful and will only cause injury and distress, the term "do not *attempt* resuscitation" is also used. It has been suggested that "allow natural death" may be a less threatening term than "do-not-resuscitate" (Venneman et al., 2008).

United States to effectively engage various population groups through religious, veterans, and other organizations with which they are connected and makes advance directives and related resources available through its Caring Conversations® initiative.[5] Nationally, the American Bar Association Commission on Law and Aging[6] has produced a comprehensive "Consumer's

---

[5]See https://www.practicalbioethics.org/resources/caring-conversations (accessed December 16, 2014).

[6]See http://www.americanbar.org/groups/law_aging.html (accessed December 16, 2014).

Toolkit for Health Care Advance Planning" covering important issues such as selecting a health care agent and weighing odds of survival, as well as state-specific advance care planning information (American Bar Association, 2005). National Healthcare Decisions Day[7] has been held on or near April 16 since 2008. This 50-state public awareness campaign is designed to motivate people to select a health care agent and prepare a living will, to advise them where to obtain these documents, and to link them to resources that can help in having difficult conversations. More recently, The Conversation Project[8] was launched by author Ellen Goodman in 2010 as a grassroots public campaign designed to change and increase the conversation around end-of-life care long before a medical crisis occurs (see Chapter 6 for more detail on these and other initiatives).

Medicare covers a one-time initial preventive physical examination (the Welcome to Medicare Preventive Visit) that includes end-of-life planning as a required service for Medicare beneficiaries who desire it (CMS, 2012a). Although this is a one-time service for which the physician is paid, it is seldom used. Of the millions of beneficiaries newly enrolled in 2011, Medicare paid for preventive visits for only approximately 240,000 (CMS, 2012b); the number who chose to receive the advance care planning information is unknown, but was undoubtedly smaller.

At present, all 50 U.S. states and the District of Columbia have laws supporting advance directives and the appointment of a health care agent (through what is often called a durable power of attorney for health care; see Box 3-1) (Gillick, 2010). An examination of policies regarding advance directives in a dozen large nations around the world[9] found that "the U.S. stands alone in terms of attention paid to advance directives, perhaps due to the emphasis on individual rights and [a] highly litigant system" (Blank, 2011, p. 210). This chapter examines what the U.S. effort in this area over the past 40 years has accomplished. (For a discussion of the 2009 controversy over death panels, see Chapter 6.)

THE CURRENT STATE OF ADVANCE CARE PLANNING AND WHAT IT ACHIEVES

The ethical principle of autonomy underlies much of the thinking about advance care planning in the United States. But the principle of autonomy—particularly with a growing segment of the population that highly values

---

[7]See http://www.nhdd.org/public-resources (accessed December 16, 2014).

[8]See http://theconversationproject.org (accessed December 16, 2014).

[9]The other countries in this review were Brazil, China, Germany, India, Israel, Japan, Kenya, Netherlands, Taiwan, Turkey, and the United Kingdom. Usage of advance directives is low in other countries, even in those whose legal systems allow them (Blank, 2011).

other principles, such as family cohesion—is showing signs of stress. Trying to determine in advance how one might want to be treated in some hypothetical future state is highly problematic (Loewenstein, 2005). Moreover, according to the President's Council on Bioethics (2005, p. xix), the process gives "major ethical weight to personal autonomy and choice and personal pride in self-sufficiency. But in so doing, it deliberately ignores the truth of human interdependence and of our unavoidable need for human presence and care." And human presence and care are exactly what is needed by the overwhelming proportion of people unable to make their own decisions near the end of life.

Who Have Made Their Wishes Clear?

It's always too early, until it's too late.
—The Conversation Project, 2013

Most people have no documentation of their wishes regarding end-of-life care, and few have talked with either their family or physician about the subject (Clements, 2009). (See also the subsequent discussion of specific population groups.) A 2013 national survey of nearly 2,100 Americans aged 18 and older found that, while 90 percent believe having family conversations about wishes at the end of life is important, fewer than 30 percent have done so (The Conversation Project, 2013).

---

*I have served as a clinical chaplain in home health hospices and as an independent health care ethics consultant and educator for community-based organizations over the past 10 years. I have learned over this time that it is extremely difficult for patients and their families and caregivers to address end-of-life decisions. Changes in the patient's physical, mental, and spiritual states, the news of the diagnosis, the impact on family, friends, caregivers, and even the community at large, all contribute to the emotional stress of decision making at this point in a person's life.**

---

*Quotation from a response submitted through the online public testimony questionnaire for this study. See Appendix C.

According to results of a 2012 survey (CHCF, 2012), the demographic groups most likely to have had a discussion about end-of-life issues with a loved one were those aged 65 and older, whites, people with higher education and income, and those with one or more chronic conditions (see the next section for discussion of differences among population groups). And while 42 percent of respondents reported having such a discussion, only 23 percent had put their wishes in writing. More than three-quarters of respondents said they would "definitely" or "probably" want to talk with their doctor about their wishes for medical treatment toward the end of life if they were seriously ill (47 and 32 percent, respectively); however, more than 90 percent said a doctor had never asked them about those issues. Among respondents aged 65 or older—the prime age group for having chronic illnesses—84 percent had not been asked.

The older people are, the more likely they are to have participated in some kind of advance care planning activity, as shown in Table 3-1. Other factors that increase the likelihood of having an advance directive include more education, having a close family member or confidant, recent hospital admission, and having a close family member who died with pain or suffering (Carr and Khodyakof, 2007). Although marital status and number of children did not affect the likelihood of having an advance directive in the study by Carr and Khodyakof (2007), those with dependent children were significantly less likely than those without dependent children to have any advance care planning documents in place (Nilsson et al., 2009).

According to the HHS (2008) review, advance care planning is least likely to take place in hospitals and intensive care settings, perhaps because of patients' physical, mental, or cognitive state or because the overriding impulse is to provide what the authors call aggressive treatment. By contrast, nursing home residents are more likely than individuals in other care settings to complete advance directives.

Why People Do Not Participate in Advance Care Planning

Many factors contribute to whether people complete some sort of advance directive form. For example, people who believe doctors, not patients, should make decisions about health care and those who have a greater fear of death are significantly less likely to complete a form (Carr and Khodyakov, 2007). However, when people reluctant to complete advance directives hear the personal stories of others who have had to make end-of-life decisions for a loved one without any guidance, the desire to save their family from these painful experiences can become a prime motivator for putting their own wishes in writing (Halpern, 2012a; Steinhauser et al., 2000a).

The many and varied requirements embedded in state laws covering advance directives also discourage their completion. Problems include poor readability and lack of clarity in some state-mandated forms; restrictions on who can serve as health care agents and limitations on their authority; procedural requirements, including the need for witness signatures or no-

TABLE 3-1 Participation in Advance Care Planning Activities, U.S. Adults

	Associated Press-National Opinion Research Center (AP-NORC),[a] 2013 (people 40+) (%)	National Council on Aging (NCOA)-United Healthcare-USA Today,[b] 2013 (people 60+) (%)	California HealthCare Foundation (CHCF),[c] 2012 (all ages) (%)	Excellus BlueCross BlueShield Upstate New York,[d] 2013 (working-age population) (%)
Have an advance directive	47	54	23	
Discussed care preferences with a loved one	41	62	42 (higher among those 65 and older)	
Designated a health care power of attorney (or equivalent)		49	—	58

SOURCES:

[a]Tompson et al., 2013: telephone survey conducted by the AP-NORC Center for Public Affairs Research from February 21 through March 27, 2013, among a nationally representative sample of 1,019 American adults aged 40 and older.

[b]NCOA et al., 2013: telephone survey conducted by Penn Schoen Berland from April 4 through May 3, 2013, among a national sample of adults, including 1,007 respondents aged 60 or older, and an oversample of low-income adults aged 60 and older, including those with three or more chronic health conditions and those living in Birmingham (Alabama), Indianapolis (Indiana), Los Angeles (California), Orlando (Florida), and San Antonio (Texas).

[c]CHCF, 2012: statewide survey conducted by Lake Research Partners from October 26 through November 3, 2011, among a representative sample of 1,669 Californians aged 18 and older, including 393 respondents who had lost a loved one in the previous 12 months.

[d]Personal communication, P. Bomba, Community Conversations on Compassionate Care and employer groups, March 1, 2014. Upstate New York data were collected as part of a serial data collection on advance care planning among ~6,000 employees of Excellus BlueCross BlueShield and other subsidiaries in Upstate New York since 2002. Results reflect a 2013 data update. (http://www.compassionandsupport.org/pdfs/research/2006_Employee_Health_Care_Decisions_Survey_Results_Report.pb.092406.FINAL.pdf [accessed December 16, 2014]).

tarization; inadequate reciprocity across states; and inadequate reflection of different religious, cultural, and social characteristics of individuals and families (Castillo et al., 2011).

According to Fried and colleagues (2010, p. 2329), advance care planning "may best be understood as a health behavior, for which individuals have highly varied motivation, barriers and facilitators, and self-efficacy regarding their participation." It may be efficacious to tailor information to the readiness of individuals to participate in specific advance care planning activities, an approach similar to how the stages of change model has been used to help people adopt health-promoting behaviors, such as smoking cessation (Orleans and Cassidy, 2011).[10] A stages of change strategy for advance care planning would approach people differently depending on whether they needed help in completing an advance directive, naming a health care agent, or communicating their preferences to their physician or family members (Fried et al., 2010). Individuals vary greatly in their readiness to participate in each of these activities.

A 2012 California survey (CHCF, 2012) asked adults (all ages) whether they had spoken with a loved one about their wishes for end-of-life medical treatment. Among those who had not, the most important reasons given were

- too many other things to worry about right now (41 percent);
- don't want to think about death or dying (26 percent), cited by 38 percent of Latinos and 26 percent of Asians and Pacific Islanders, but only 15 percent of African Americans and of non-Latino whites; and
- family member did not want to discuss it (13 percent).

Another reported reason patients (versus the public) do not participate in advance care planning is that they "would rather concentrate on staying alive than talk about death" (Ganti et al., 2007; Knauft et al., 2005, p. 2190).

Reluctance to engage in advance care planning sometimes originates in patients' sense that the initiative to do so should come from clinicians—hence "the importance of clinicians bringing up advance care planning with their patients who may be fearful of discussing the topic with family or be waiting for some one else to initiate discussion" (Phipps et al., 2003,

---

[10]In the Orleans and Cassidy (2011) review, the stages of change are specified as precontemplation (not thinking about participating in the activity yet), contemplation (thinking about participating in the next 6 months), preparation (planning to complete the activity in the next 30 days), action (participated in the activity within the past 6 months), and maintenance (participated in the activity more than 6 months ago).

p. 553). Finally, people often do not realize they have a terminal disease, what that disease is, or that they are dying (Gardiner et al., 2009).

My mother died in January 2012. She was in a nursing home for the last 7 weeks of her life and in a hospital for 2 weeks prior to that. At no time did a doctor or nurse say to me, "I'm sorry, but there is nothing we can do for your mother—let's plan for her to have an easy death. *

*Quotation from a response submitted through the online public testimony questionnaire for this study. See Appendix C.

The Choice of a Health Care Agent

With respect to the choice of a health care agent, the following general points apply:

- Married people overwhelmingly choose their spouse (Carr and Khodyakov, 2007). Spousal proxies have been found to be more accurate than adult children in their assessment of an elder's wishes (Parks et al., 2011; but see the quote below for a counterexample), with wives being more accurate than husbands (Zettel-Watson et al., 2008).
- Unmarried and widowed parents choose a child and rarely some other relative, friend, or professional, although in families with only one or two children, a child is less likely to be selected (Carr and Khodyakov, 2007).
- People without a spouse or children choose another relative, such as a sister or a brother or perhaps a friend or a colleague (Carr and Khodyakov, 2007).

The above pattern is not universal, however, and "individuals will innovate to meet their own needs and the presumed needs of their loved ones" (Carr and Khodyakov, 2007, p. 188)—for example, when they believe decision making would be too stressful. Being a health care agent is a difficult job and an extra burden on an already stressed spouse, partner, parent, or child. Close family members may be unable to separate their feelings from the needs of the situation, be unwilling to face the prognosis or talk through the patient's wishes, or be unable to handle conflicts that arise among family members or with clinical staff. Family members who can answer yes to the following questions are less likely to struggle with the agent role: Do

My mother was 99 when she fell, fractured her hip, had a mild heart attack, and became unconscious. EMTs [emergency medical technicians] took her to the hospital. The surgeon there said she needed a hip operation to relieve the pain. I knew Mom would not want that. For several years, she had told me and my stepfather that she "was ready to go" and didn't care about living to 100. Her quality of life had clearly deteriorated.

When I saw Mom in the ICU, she was surrounded by beeping monitors and tubes, with nurses running in and out. Her head thrashed from side to side, and she couldn't recognize anyone. She kept repeating, "I already died once, why am I still here?" and "Let me go, let me go." It was heartbreaking.

Some years earlier, Mom told me she had assigned me her health care durable power of attorney. I never asked to see the documents, because I thought it would be "impolite." The day of Mom's crisis, I found out that my stepfather, who was devastated and grieving, had health care power of attorney for Mom, and I was merely the backup. Shockingly, he agreed to the operation, which was scheduled to begin in 3 hours, and I had no legal power to stop it.

I had a hard talk with my stepfather and reminded him of Mom's wishes. An hour before the operation, he agreed to talk to a hospice representative, who said Mom was eligible for hospice at their facility. Three hours later, Mom was in a quiet, machine-free hospice room, on increased pain medication, looking much more tranquil, with calm, relaxed breathing. She died 10 hours later, in that peaceful state. I know we did what she wanted. *

---

*Quotation from a response submitted through the online public testimony questionnaire for this study. See Appendix C.

you have prior experience as someone's health care agent, and have you had prior conversations with the patient about treatment preferences? (Majesko et al., 2012). Box 3-2 lists some of the key considerations in an individual's choice of a health care agent.

An obvious and important consideration is the availability of the agent. In a survey of almost 300 physicians regarding their recent experiences with

---

BOX 3-2
What to Keep in Mind When Choosing a Health Care Agent

The person you select as an agent must:

- Meet legal criteria (for example, be a competent adult and at least age 18 years)
- Be willing to speak on your behalf
- Be willing to act on your wishes
- Be able to separate his/her own feelings from yours
- Live close by or be willing to come
- Know you well
- Understand what is important to you
- Be willing to talk with you now about sensitive wishes
- Be willing to listen to your wishes
- Be able to work with those providing your care to carry out your wishes
- Be available in the future
- Be able to handle potential conflicts between your family, close friends

SOURCE: Compassion and Support, 2010, p. 7.

---

patient decision making, most (73 percent) reported having to make major decisions for patients, for various reasons. One in five reported difficulty contacting agents, and one in four reported never having talked to agents personally (Torke et al., 2009).

Most states have established default systems for authorizing surrogates. Thus, even if a proxy form is not signed or if the chosen health care agent is not reasonably available, a priority list of people who can make decisions if the patient cannot is generally in place. State laws vary, but such lists generally start with the immediate family. In some states, lists include domestic partners or close friends or senior officials in religious organizations, and in some, they include physicians, often in consultation with an ethics committee or other physician (in other states, physicians cannot take on this role). To the extent possible, default surrogates are charged with making decisions (substituted judgment) reflecting to the extent possible the patient's likely decisions, best interests, instructions if any, or personal values (American Bar Association, 2009; Kohn and Blumenthal, 2008).[11] If patients have not thoroughly discussed their wishes, however, it is unlikely that surrogates,

---

[11]Ostensibly, these laws provide the maximum feasible protection of the wishes of the incapacitated person and "the fundamental right to make health care decisions for oneself" (Kohn and Blumenthal, 2008, p. 9) (as expressed in the laws of Illinois, Louisiana, and Utah, for example).

even family members, can accurately gauge what those preferences would be despite believing to the contrary (Kohn and Blumenthal, 2008).

Although surrogacy laws meet most situations, they fall short, for example, in serving families in which intergenerational and group decision making are highly valued or cultural groups more likely to select a non-family member as health care agent (Kohn and Blumenthal, 2008). Further, the underlying presumption of health care proxy statutes is that people will have a spouse, child, sibling, or close friend whom they can name as their agent. Many people, especially among the elderly, have no such person. While data on the number of such people are lacking, they may represent 3 to 4 percent of the nursing home population alone (Karp and Wood, 2003). In many states, should they become unable to make or communicate their own health care decisions, no one has the authority to make those decisions unless a court deems them legally incompetent and appoints a guardian. Because such guardians may be strangers with little or no evidence of the patient's prior wishes, there is no assurance their decisions will be what the patient would have chosen. In the absence of clear guidance from the patient and in light of the consequent uncertainty, the default decision often is to treat the patient's various conditions regardless of likely benefit.

Do Clinicians Follow Patients' Previously Expressed Wishes?

Data on the impact of advance directives on the treatment received by patients suggest that directives are not always followed. In one large study, for example, 92 percent of people had recorded a preference for what the authors call comfort-focused care in their living will, but this desire was "poorly correlated with treatment delivered" (Kelley et al., 2011, p. 240). In a study of advanced cancer patients, 13 percent received life-extending treatment in the last week of life despite a stated preference for treatment focused on relieving pain and discomfort (Mack et al., 2010b).

While the predominant conversation about advance care planning focuses on people who want to avoid intensive and nonbeneficial medical interventions, the recent controversy over "death panels" (see Chapter 6) makes clear that many Americans worry about being denied care, and some clinicians believe patients may fear they will give up on care too soon (Gutierrez, 2012). Yet while some people, at least in the abstract, do want every treatment the health system can offer (Pew Research Center, 2013; Veysman, 2010), a study of people aged 60 and older at the time of death revealed that fewer than 2 percent (10 subjects) of those with a living will wanted "all care possible" (Silveira et al., 2010). In another study, involving people with advanced cancer who were aware they were terminally ill, just 17 percent wanted supposed life-extending treatment (Mack et al., 2010b).

If patients with serious advanced illness receive less intensive treatment than desired, the difference may reflect a lack of treatment options. For example, one study found more frequent mismatches between desire for intensive treatment and services received for patients with cancer than for those with congestive heart failure or chronic obstructive pulmonary disease. The authors conclude that "it is probable that many [cancer] patients reached a point in the course of their illness where treatment options were limited regardless of the patient's preferences" (Cosgriff et al., 2007, p. 1570).

Physician Concerns

Several studies have explored the extent to which physicians comply with directives such as living wills and what factors may influence their actions in this regard. One such study found that most primary care physicians would honor a patient's advance directive even if it were 5 years old (80 percent) or even if the patient's spouse requested continued resuscitative care (74 percent).[12] Fear of legal liability was a concern, including for one-third and one-half of respondents in these situations, respectively (Burkle et al., 2012), and for a large percentage of emergency physicians (58 percent) (Marco et al., 2009). In general, physicians believe their liability risk is greater if they, mistakenly, do not attempt resuscitation than if they provide it against patient wishes (Burkle et al., 2012). As in so many other instances, the default is to treat.

Burkle and colleagues (2012) found that almost 60 percent of the physicians in their study were not likely to honor the wishes of patients whose advance directives indicated they wanted to "pass away in peace" if such patients were in a sudden acute situation (ventricular fibrillation) and likely to be treated successfully (including 45 percent who considered it unlikely that they would honor the advance directive and 14 percent who were unsure). The fact that the remainder would honor patients' directives in such a situation suggests that, despite several decades of experience, some 40 percent of physicians remain confused about the purpose and interpretation of advance directives. This is true even among emergency medical personnel and hospital residents likely to be called upon under urgent circumstances. Several small studies have shown that some clinicians assume a living will's instructions apply even if the patient does not have the requisite terminal condition or persistent unconsciousness (Mirarchi et al., 2008, 2009, 2012).

---

[12]By contrast, a survey involving more than 10,000 physicians found that more than half (55 percent) would not consider halting life-sustaining therapy because the family demanded it; for 29 percent, that decision would depend on circumstances (Kane, 2010).

System/Logistical Challenges

Patients' advance care preferences cannot be followed if the record of those preferences cannot be found and/or is not up to date. People's preferences change over time and with hospitalization (Chochinov et al., 1999; Ditto et al., 2006; Fried et al., 2007), which may partially explain why the actual preferences of patients differ from what is documented in their medical record (Volandes et al., 2012a,b). Yung and colleagues (2010) found that advance directives for 53 percent of patients (aged 75 and older and in fragile health) who said they gave them to their health care provider were not in their medical record, nor was there any indication of their existence. This percentage was much higher—83 percent—for a separate cohort of patients aged 65 and older and also in fragile health. For patients who said they had not provided an advance directive to their provider but had communicated information about their health care agent, that person's name and contact information was in the medical record zero percent of the time for patients under age 75 and 16 percent of the time for those aged 75 and older.

Even if the clinician remembers the conversation and the patient's wishes, recording those preferences is critical "in a health-care system that relies on teams of providers in different settings" (Yung et al., 2010, p. 866) and in which frequent care transitions occur near the end of life (Lakin et al., 2013). Researchers attempting to track the continuity of advance care planning documentation across care settings found that when patients transitioned from provider office to hospital or emergency department, the likelihood that advance care planning documentation would be available and/or in concordance "was no greater than chance" (Yung et al., 2010, p. 865). As discussed in detail in the section on electronic health records later in this chapter, data standards for electronic health records that help promote document portability, availability, and agreement do not require robust documentation of advance care planning.

The implementation of advance directives for pediatric patients entails several particular barriers. For example, emergency department personnel are uncomfortable honoring them, schools may not accept them, and parents seeking to honor their children's wishes encounter negative reactions from others (Lotz et al., 2013).

Conflicting Views

There are two schools of thought regarding how binding advance directive instructions should be: one is that they should be followed strictly, and the other holds that "it is simply not possible for people to anticipate [their future] decisions about life-preserving treatment with any degree of accuracy" (Bomba et al., 2012; Sahm et al., 2005, p. 297). Further, prior instructions may not fit the current situation or reflect advances in treatment options. These problems, it is said, are compounded by the lack of clarity in the wording of many advance planning documents. The question is not just what they mean in some abstract sense but what they meant to the person who completed them, who now can no longer amplify or explain and whose mind may have changed with time and altered circumstances.

A German study found that nonclinicians had a much more flexible approach than clinical personnel to interpreting advance directives (Sahm et al., 2005). The authors conclude that the uncertainties around decision making are a strong argument for employing sound clinical judgment in the final phases of a patient's life. They suggest that a preferable alternative to rigid advance directives is comprehensive advance care planning, which can take into account a broader array of issues and social relationships and can include spiritual and cultural matters, as well as practical concerns.

Taking this argument a step further are those who recommend that advance care planning's main objective should not be to make advance treatment decisions, but "to prepare patients and surrogates to work with their clinicians to make the best possible in-the-moment medical decisions" (Sudore and Fried, 2010, p. 259). It is suggested that health care agents need this flexibility because they will have to live with the decisions they make (Vig et al., 2006). In one study, the majority of patients (55 percent) gave their surrogates leeway to consider the benefits and burdens of treatment and "specify processes rather than outcomes in their preferences for end-of-life care" (Shapiro, 2012, p. 226).

Conflicts in the implementation of advance directives occur in certain typical situations: when the directive requests a type or intensity of care that, at the time of the event, is judged by clinicians or family not to be in the patient's best interest, and when the health care agent disagrees with the patient's request. State laws differ regarding the circumstances under which families can override advance directives. In addition, many hospitals have nonbeneficial care policies and/or refer such cases to the ethics committee for resolution.

Does Advance Care Planning Affect Patient and Caregiver Outcomes?

Advance care planning influences the quality of care and patient and family satisfaction in several ways:

- People who participate in advance care planning generally but not always choose treatment focused on relieving pain and discomfort over life-extending treatments and enroll in hospice earlier, thereby avoiding many physical and psychological stresses (Mack et al., 2010b; Wright et al., 2008).

- Advance care planning gives patients and families the opportunity to start preparing mentally and emotionally for death (Martin et al., 1999; Steinhauser et al., 2000a).
- Advance care planning supports several of the primary concerns of people with life-limiting illnesses: involvement, clear communication, shared decision making (Steinhauser et al., 2000b), and a sense of control (Edwards et al., 2010; Martin et al., 1999).
- By stating the kind of care they want in advance, patients may alleviate the burden of decision making on family members (Billings, 2012; Detering et al., 2010).
- Among children and youth, participation in systematic advance care planning programs may enhance positive emotions and facilitate communication, lead to treatment modifications (for example, withdrawal of ventilator support and addition of opioid analgesia), and support having death occur at home (Lotz et al., 2013).

Comparing the survival of patients with and without advance care planning[13] before stem cell transplant therapy revealed that those without such documents were significantly more likely to die within 1 year of transplant than those who had them (Ganti et al., 2007). This finding led researchers to conclude that the discussions were not deleterious to patients and that those "who did not engage in [advance care planning] were the most likely to face a situation in which [it] might have helped" (p. 5647). Another study found that discussions of do-not-resuscitate orders did not result in worse psychosocial functioning, including greater anxiety or depression, among either patients or caregivers (Stein et al., 2013).

The impact of advance care planning for the elderly has been studied, and the results parallel those found in other population groups. Elders do engage in such discussions, most often with family present, if given an opportunity to reflect on their goals, values, and beliefs; to articulate and document their treatment preferences; and to choose a health care agent. Those who have these discussions are almost three times as likely to have their end-of-life wishes both known and followed, and their family members suffer significantly less stress, anxiety, and depression after their loved one's death (Detering et al., 2010).[14]

---

[13]Advance care planning is defined in this study as having one or more of the following: a living will, a power of attorney for health care, or life support instructions (Ganti et al., 2007). No distinction is drawn between completion of such a document with and without comprehensive discussion with the physician.

[14]Of those receiving the advance care planning intervention, 10 percent of patients' wishes were unknown; 3 percent of patients' wishes were known but not followed.

Research related specifically to advance care planning among people with heart failure, chronic obstructive pulmonary disease, cancer, and dementia, discussed in Annex 3-1 at the end of this chapter, provides many insights into the role of advance care planning in several of the most common causes of death in the United States. It reveals that for each of these conditions, high-quality palliative care, which includes the goal-setting activities of advance care planning, would be an important parallel focus of treatment, but in each case is not the current standard of care.

What Are the Effects of Advance Care Planning on Health Care Agents and Families?

Health care agents and surrogates (including those who are family members) are critically important for the 44 to 69 percent of nursing home residents with decisional impairment (Kim et al., 2002). Agents may also make decisions for large numbers of geriatric patients who retain decision-making capacity yet defer decisions to family members (Vig et al., 2007).

Even when patients' preferences are clear to health care agents—which too often they are not (Fried and O'Leary, 2008)—the decisions these agents must make do not come without difficulty (Schenker et al., 2012). Moreover, "surrogates are not perfect ambassadors of patient preferences" (Vig et al., 2006, p. 1688). Often, caregivers (usually family members) want life-sustaining measures used even when patients do not (Phipps et al., 2003). At times, health care agents may be required to make a decision at odds with patients' expressed wishes (to die at home, for example) when clinical circumstances evolve differently than anticipated.

Health care agents' decisions inevitably are colored by their own wishes and care preferences, feelings of overwhelming responsibility, religious beliefs, and the desire for family consensus (Fritch et al., 2013; Schenker et al., 2012). Interviews with health care agents have revealed the broad range of bases on which they make their decisions: conversations with patients, the agents' own beliefs and preferences, input from others close to the family, shared values and life experiences, and written documents (Vig et al., 2006).

When health care agents cannot meet patients' requests, they feel regret or guilt that may lead to complicated grief and bereavement (Fried and O'Leary, 2008; Topf et al., 2013).[15] Family decision making can have a significant and sometimes long-term negative psychological impact, including stress, guilt, doubt, grief, and even increased thoughts of suicide, especially among spouses (Abbott et al., 2013; Wendler and Rid, 2011). Wendler and

---

[15]Complicated grief is long-lasting and shares elements of both depression and posttraumatic stress disorder. For a full description, see http://www.health.harvard.edu/fhg/updates/Complicated-grief.shtml (accessed December 16, 2014).

TABLE 3-2 Stresses on Health Care Agents and Examples of Potential Remedies

Stressor	Potential Remedy
Uncertainty about patient preferences	More thorough advance care planning
Uncertainty about prognosis	Conversation about key decision points
Discomfort with the hospital environment	Familiarizing family members with the hospital; explaining why certain procedures are followed, who directs various aspects of care, and whom to ask for what
Discomfort with the logistics of making decisions	Ensuring that information is conveyed in a thorough and unhurried manner; use of a shared decision-making model
Poor communication by clinicians	Targeted communication training for clinical staff; limiting the number of clinicians with whom the health care agent must deal
Uncertainty and guilt	Providing support and positive reinforcement for health care agent decisions and adequate subsequent counseling

SOURCES: Majesko et al., 2012; Vig et al., 2007; Wendler and Rid, 2011.

Rid (2011) reviewed the literature on health care agent stressors and identified a number of problems commonly reported by agents, some of which appear to be at least partly remediable (see Table 3-2).

Risk factors for complicated grief among bereaved caregivers include fewer years of education, younger age of the deceased, and lower satisfaction with social support (Allen et al., 2013). The care provided by hospices may lead to positive health outcomes, including survival, among the bereaved and may help some people avoid long-term depression and other consequences of complicated grief (Christakis and Iwashyna, 2003). A hospital-based family support specialist who maintains connections with health care agents can provide emotional, communication, decision, and anticipatory grief support (White et al., 2012).

Negative mental health effects among family members of ICU patients in one study were markedly higher (reaching 82 percent) if family members believed the information received from the staff to be too rushed, unclear, or incomplete or if they shared in end-of-life decision making (Azoulay et al., 2005). Having an advance directive reduces bereaved family members' concerns about physician communication or lack of information (Teno et al., 2007). Health care agents may also be helped by previous decision-making experiences; effective coping strategies; supportive life circumstances; a belief that their decisions will result in a "good" outcome; and having a clinician who is available and who provides frank information, recommendations, and respect (Back et al., 2010; Vig et al., 2007).

An approach to working with families that supports both emotional reasoning and medical requirements has been suggested, allowing patients, families, and physicians to "expand their medical focus to include disease-modifying and symptomatic treatments and attend to underlying psychological, spiritual, and existential issues" (Back et al., 2003, p. 439). Health care agents who have been well prepared, who have the support of other family members and the clinical team, and who have been given some reasonable leeway in carrying out their role will be able to do so with fewer long-lasting negative effects. Effective preparation has been shown to be best achieved when the patient-agent discussion is guided by a trained facilitator (or other knowledgeable person), when there is an opportunity to discuss concerns, and when patient misconceptions regarding the likely outcomes of treatment are corrected (Fried et al., 2002; Jezewski et al., 2007; Kirchhoff et al., 2010). Grief and bereavement are a natural corollary to losing a loved one; unrelieved stress-related problems are not.

Does Advance Care Planning Affect Health Care Costs?

The purpose of comprehensive advance care planning is to ensure that people receive the care they desire and minimize the burden on their families. In doing so, an additional benefit may be lower health care costs. This is useful to know given that proposals to expand and improve advance care planning programs will almost certainly be met with the argument that they are "too expensive." The evidence presented in this section suggests just the contrary.

Several large studies have attempted to assess the impact of advance care planning on health care costs. One found no association between advance care planning (either reported completion of an advance directive or discussion of care preferences) and Medicare expenditures in the last 6 months of life (Kelley et al., 2011). Another study compared costs for people who had "treatment-limiting advance directives" and those who did not (Nicholas et al., 2011). People with such directives had lower rates of life-sustaining treatment (34 percent versus 39 percent), were less likely to die in the hospital (37 percent versus 43 percent), and were more likely to use hospice (40 percent versus 26 percent). All these care differences were statistically significant. But again, median fee-for-service Medicare spending in the last 6 months of life was not significantly different for the two groups ($21,008 for the treatment-limiting group versus $21,614 for the group without a treatment-limiting advance directive).

Another analysis of this study compares spending for decedents in low-spending regions of the country (who were significantly more likely to have a treatment-limiting advance directive) with spending for decedents in higher-spending regions (Nicholas et al., 2011). Although the two groups had similar cause-of-death and comorbidity patterns, the costs of care in the last 6 months were substantially different. The largest differential was between spending for people with a treatment-limiting advance directive in low-spending regions ($14,153) and spending for those without a directive in high-spending regions ($26,616). These data further suggest that having an advance directive made no statistically significant difference in predicted spending in the low- and medium-spending regions; in the high-spending regions, however, a treatment-limiting advance directive might save $5,585 per death, primarily as a result of lower hospital utilization rates. Thus, this study demonstrates "a statistically and economically significant relationship between advance directives and regional practice patterns" (Nicholas et al., 2011, p. 1452).

A large portion of hospital costs at the end of life is associated with ICU care. One study found that among Americans who died, the cost of a terminal hospitalization with an ICU stay was an estimated $38,000, compared with $13,000 if ICU care was not included (both of these figures are in 2010 dollars) (Zilberberg and Shorr, 2012).

Assessing patients' end-of-life preferences and providing care congruent with their values, along with coordinating the care provided by different clinicians and institutions, produces important improvements in clinical care. In one such model program, the Sutter Health Advanced Illness Management program, this combination of approaches appeared to save about $2,000 per month per patient in direct care costs (Meyer, 2011).

Lower rates of hospital deaths and higher rates of hospice enrollment occur when the care team pays attention to more than patients' physical condition—specifically, to their religious and spiritual concerns (Flannelly et al., 2012). Such whole-person care "may assist patients in recognizing less aggressive [end-of-life] care options that remain consistent with their religious/spiritual beliefs" (Balboni et al., 2011, p. 5389). In this study, the estimated care costs in the last week of life for cancer patients who reported high spiritual support were $2,441 less than costs for those who reported less spiritual support.[16]

Finally, in a cohort of 603 advanced cancer patients, 188 reported discussing their end-of-life care preferences with their physicians (Zhang et al., 2009). Costs of care in the last week of life were 36 percent lower among

---

[16]These findings were adjusted to take into account potential confounders such as advance directives and advance care planning.

patients who had the care discussion, amounting to savings of $1,041 per patient in 2008 dollars.

ADVANCE CARE PLANNING AND TREATMENT PREFERENCES AMONG SPECIFIC POPULATION GROUPS

This section describes what is known about advance care planning and treatment preferences among people in specific groups described by age, disability state, religious affiliation, ethnicity, and literacy level. An important caveat is that all of these groups include individuals with a full range of attitudes and preferences, and the generalities that may be derived from population studies may not apply at all to a specific patient and family. Chapter 1 of this report notes the importance of patient-centered care for people nearing the end of life; the wide variation in preferences that exists in any group reinforces the need for end-of-life care that approaches each individual and family as unique.

Children and the Elderly

Children

The typical barriers to conducting advance care planning in adult populations—reluctance to discuss dying, cultural norms that support family-level decisions, clinician time constraints, unpredictable disease trajectories, and insufficient clinician preparation to conduct such discussions—also are present when the patient is a child.[17] In addition, the process is made more difficult by concerns regarding the child's cognitive and emotional development and both the child's and parents' readiness to participate in such conversations; the emotional burden on parents and caregivers; differences in understanding of prognosis between clinician and child/parent; unrealistic expectations among parents; and the need for a three-way conversation and communication among parents, children, and clinicians (Durall et al., 2012).

Nonetheless, advance care planning models suitable for children and adolescents have been developed. Even suitable adult advance directives have been used successfully with younger people. When combined with in-depth counseling (such as Gundersen Health System's Respecting Choices model, discussed later in this chapter), they have greatly increased the proportion of adolescent patients who give their families the leeway to "do what is best at the time," increased information available to the patient and family and improved patient understanding about end-of-life decisions, and

---

[17]The term "child" here encompasses adolescents.

I am a pediatrician, specializing in care of children living with HIV. Discussions regarding end-of-life care of children are always difficult. Many family members (and health professionals) shy away from the issue. Speaking directly with the child or adolescent is both extremely important and extremely difficult. Spiritual care is often neglected, as it is kept separate from medical discussions.

There is great need to treat the child as a child—a complex, multi-faceted individual—and not as an impersonal medical case. Children have much greater insight into their own conditions and realities than they are given credit. The death of a child is and should be heart-breaking. However, end-of-life care should not be treated as a taboo subject, especially when speaking directly with the child/adolescent. Successes in end-of-life care for children come from strong, supportive relationships with health care providers, counselors, spiritual leaders, and family members. *

---

*Quotation from a response submitted through the online public testimony questionnaire for this study. See Appendix C.

---

increased patient and family agreement about decisions to limit treatment (Lyon et al., 2009, 2013).

Five Wishes,[18] an advance directive written in nontechnical language, includes identification of a health care agent, as well as choices about medical and nonmedical treatment and comfort. Wish 5—"what I want my loved ones to know"—lets patients describe how they want to be remembered and in a group of adolescents and young adults, was deemed the most helpful part of the document (Wiener et al., 2008). *Five Wishes* is available in child and adolescent/young adult versions (Wiener et al., 2012).

Available guidelines for making end-of-life treatment decisions for pediatric patients tend to be broad, and research has yet to fully establish their usefulness in clinical settings (Hinds et al., 2010). Making decisions that will not forestall the death of a terminally ill child and involving the child in the decision that will end his or her life "are startling concepts," say Hinds and colleagues (2010, p. 1049). From these authors' vantage point of working in pediatric oncology, enabling a peaceful death is part of providing care of the highest quality. The way these decisions are made and a respectful reaction to parents' decisions "can color all of their pre-

---

[18]See http://www.agingwithdignity.org/five-wishes.php (accessed December 16, 2014).

ceding treatment-related interactions, and may influence how well parents emotionally survive the dying and death of their child" (Hinds et al., 2010, p. 1049).

The capacity or incapacity of children to participate in end-of-life decision making cannot be assumed and must be individually determined at each decision point (Hinds et al., 2010). This capacity begins at least by age 10 and in some cases by age 6, and depends in part on children's own appraisal of their health and well-being. Because of their experiences, many children are perceptive judges of the balance between the burdens and benefits of treatment. Even children aged 5-6 can be capable of remarkably insightful abstract leaps and often express their views in drawings and stories, for example.

Few studies of pediatric advance care planning have been conducted, and those generally have involved small numbers of patients and families. A recent review found three reports of systematic advance care planning programs specifically for children, all in the United States (Lotz et al., 2013).[19] Although the three program models had similar overall designs, they differed in care setting, target population, participants, and advance directive used. These programs increased completion of advance directives and parents' initiation of discussions about treatment, and both patients and physicians made increasing use of the programs over time.

The importance of involving children in these discussions is illustrated by research among 24 pairs of adolescents with AIDS and their family decision makers, which found that family members did not recognize when their child wanted to have an end-of-life conversation (Garvie et al., 2012). The great majority of the adolescents (90 percent) wanted to talk about end-of-life issues before entering the dying phase, including 48 percent who thought the best timing for end-of-life decisions was before getting sick and another 24 percent who wanted to have conversations throughout the illness trajectory: before getting sick, when first diagnosed, when first sick, and when dying. While parents may be reluctant to have end-of-life discussions when their child's health is relatively stable (Edwards et al., 2012), most clinicians (71 percent in the Durall et al. [2012] study) believe advance care planning discussions often happen too late in the course of disease. Anticipatory guidance and reflection on the goals of care during times of both stability and worsening illness are useful (Edwards et al., 2012). Families are more likely to take advantage of palliative care options when they and the care team recognize earlier in the clinical course that a cure is unrealistic and focus instead on reducing suffering (Wolfe et al., 2000).

From the sparse research available, it is clear that parents of children

---

[19]They are the FACE Intervention (Lyon et al., 2009), the Footprints Model (Toce and Collins, 2003), and Respecting Choices (Hammes et al., 2005).

who will not survive need time for making decisions and preparing for their child's death. Understanding parents' end-of-life decision making for their children necessitates consideration of the reason, understanding, and emotion they bring to their responsibilities and their roles as parents and as decision makers (Bluebond-Langner et al., 2007). Factors that help parents improve their decision-making capability are opportunities to make decisions that accord with the family's traditions and values, clear and complete understanding of the child's condition, and opportunities within each clinical encounter to build trust and reinforce parents' competence (Hinds et al., 2010; Lannen et al., 2010). In sum, believing "they have acted as 'good parents' in such a situation is likely to be very important to their emotional recovery from the dying and death of their child" (Hinds et al., 2010, p. 1058).

The Elderly

Older Americans are more likely than those who are younger to have thought about their end-of-life preferences or completed an advance directive (CHCF, 2012; Pew Research Center, 2013; Tompson et al., 2013). The higher rate of any kind of consideration of end-of-life care reflects age-related increases in the prevalence of chronic illnesses, dementia, other cognitive impairments, frailty, and disability. In one large study,[20] the proportion of people with one or more disabilities increased from 28 percent 2 years before death to more than half (56 percent) in the last month of life (Smith et al., 2013a).

In one study of more than 5,000 65-year-old individuals, most were able to articulate their preferences for end-of-life care, and most said they would reject life-extending treatment if they had a terminal illness involving either cognitive impairment or severe physical pain (Carr and Moorman, 2009). That these survey respondents were more likely to avoid life-sustaining treatments in the case of cognitive impairment than in the case of physical pain may indicate the relative importance of these experiences. A separate study, however, found that while pain control was ranked as the most important attribute among both patients and physicians, mental awareness was ranked lower in importance among physicians than among patients (Steinhauser et al., 2000a). "This discrepancy between what patients value and what physicians rate as important could lead physicians to advocate for (or encourage the patient's family to select)

---

[20]In this study of 8,232 people over age 50 who died while enrolled in the Health and Retirement Study between 1995 and 2010, disability was defined as needing help with at least one of the following activities of daily living: dressing, bathing, eating, getting in or out of bed, walking across the room, and using the toilet.

treatments that do not mesh with the patient's preferences" (Carr and Moorman, 2009, p. 769).

Infrequently considered is that an older person's net financial worth is positively associated with participating in any type of advance care planning, regardless of demographic, health, and psychological characteristics. People with higher incomes are more likely to engage in estate and financial planning,[21] an activity that frequently includes or otherwise may trigger some aspects of health-related planning, such as establishing a durable power of attorney for health care (Carr, 2012b).

Differences Across Disability Groups

People with Cognitive Impairments

Determining whether an individual patient has the cognitive capacity to participate meaningfully in decisions about end-of-life treatments is a challenge to clinicians, and "physicians regularly fail to recognize incapacity" (Sessums et al., 2011, p. 420). Such a determination is especially challenging when it involves people who live in community group homes and other community settings (rather than in state institutions), especially if they have no family, guardian, or health care agent. Challenges further emerge because of a "lack of clear standards and regulatory guidelines protecting these individuals when institutionalized that do not transfer to the more independent, 'least-restrictive' environments of privatized group homes" (Artnak, 2008, p. 240).

Determining capacity generally requires tests of whether patients can understand, retain, and use information about proposed treatment in the decision-making process; appreciate the significance of the decision and use reason in making it; and communicate their choice (Raymont et al., 2004; Sessums et al., 2011). Capacity is task specific. People who lack the decision-making capacity to make certain medical decisions—especially high-risk or exceedingly complex ones—may nevertheless retain the capacity to make simpler decisions and even to choose a health care agent they trust. However, determinations of capacity are not standardized, and although many different instruments for assessing capacity exist, their precision and suitability for different clinical settings vary considerably.[22]

---

[21] An intriguing recent report found in four analyses that saving money, in itself, is a buffer against anxiety about death by providing a sense of control over one's fate and protecting people from existential fears (Zaleskiewicz et al., 2013).

[22] Sessums and colleagues (2011) recommend three capacity-assessing instruments suitable for use in a physician office visit: the Aid to Capacity Evaluation (ACE), the Hopkins Competency Assessment Test (HCAT), and Understanding Treatment Disclosure (UTD). These instruments have robust likelihood ratios (sensitivity/specificity) and moderate to strong levels of evidence.

In some situations, physicians may rely heavily on the views of family members as well as their own knowledge of the fragile health of their patients with intellectual disabilities (Wagemans et al., 2013). Clear communication—verbal and nonverbal—and efforts to avoid possible misunderstandings by using language free of jargon are vital for clinicians serving such patients (Tuffrey-Wijne and McEnhill, 2008).

A study of factors influencing parents' resuscitation decisions for their institutionalized children with severe developmental disabilities found that a concerted effort to explain treatment options and end-of-life issues resulted in some families' making a change from full-resuscitation to do-not-resuscitate status (Friedman and Gilmore, 2007). Family members, religious leaders, and discussions with physicians had the greatest influence on those who chose full resuscitation. Families' perceptions of the child's quality of life or discomfort did not appear to affect the decision.

Homeless or "Unbefriended" Patients

"Unbefriended" patients who have neither decision-making capacity nor a surrogate decision maker are at particular risk of not having their wishes known or followed. Physicians and institutions need clear guidance on how to handle the care of such patients, with the Veterans Health Administration's "detailed and transparent process . . . [being] a model for other institutions" (Berlinger et al., 2013, p. 51). That policy describes a collaborative approach that involves the hospital's senior leadership and guides professionals on how to collaborate with legal counsel if a court-appointed guardian is needed.

Homeless people might be assumed to be a quintessential "unbefriended" population, with high rates of cognitive challenges due in part to underlying mental health problems, substance abuse, and isolation (Karp and Wood, 2003). A test of whether homeless people can and will complete a counseling session on advance care planning and an advance directive was conducted in Minneapolis (Song et al., 2010). More than one-quarter of the subjects completed an advance directive, with a higher rate of completion (38 percent) being seen among those who received guidance from a counselor. About one-third of the group had someone (often a family member) whom they wanted to make decisions about their care in specific clinical situations.

Having a single health professional make unilateral decisions for an unbefriended patient is ethically unsatisfactory in terms of protecting patient autonomy and establishing transparency. Equally troublesome is "waiting until the patient's medical condition worsens into an emergency so that consent to treat is implied" (Berlinger et al., 2013, p. 51), which compromises patient care and prevents any thorough and thoughtful consideration of patient preferences or best interests.

People with Physical Disabilities

People are not well able to foresee their own (or others') capacity to adapt to a disability (Stein, 2003), which means that others' assessments of quality of life, a fundamentally subjective judgment, are not necessarily in accord with those of people with disabilities. The "paradox" of high perceived quality of life despite serious and persistent disabilities has been acknowledged for some time (Albrecht and Devlieger, 1999; King et al., 2012).

People with severe neuromuscular diseases, such as Duchenne's muscular dystrophy or amyotrophic lateral sclerosis, are not necessarily well served by advance directive language that refers to "extreme disability" as a reason to withhold or withdraw treatment because of the lack of context provided (Stein, 2003). The core definition of quality of life for many people with disabilities is "living well," and the underlying factors contributing to living well are consistent across disabilities: health status, social connectedness, being oneself (that is, able to continue doing things important to the person), and financial security (Murphy et al., 2009). The possibility of quality of life for people with disabilities nearing the end of life often is ignored (Gill, 2010). Even health care providers familiar with people with disabilities and their lives may hold negative views about their quality of life. According to disability rights advocate Diane Coleman in testimony provided to the committee, "Unfortunately, the disability community . . . has a lot of experience with devaluation by physicians and other health care providers, devaluation that leads to pressure to forego life-sustaining treatment" (Coleman, 2013).

One approach suggested to improve the relevance and suitability of advance care planning to people with disabilities is to reconsider including disabling conditions as a reason for limiting treatment in living wills and make greater efforts to help health care agents understand the complex choices involved when a medical condition or injury might lead to substantial disability (Stein, 2003).

Differences Among Religious Groups

The majority of patients at the end of their lives find religion to be important; however, these needs are supported only minimally or not at all by the current health care system (Balboni et al., 2007). Research has documented a strong role of religious affiliation, although not necessarily denominational affiliation, in both advance care planning and the nature of treatment preferences at the end of life. In a large survey of mostly white, non-Hispanic individuals aged 64-65, those from tradition-ally defined religious groups (categorized as conservative, moderate, or liberal Protestant; Catholic; other; and no religion) had similar treatment preferences given two end-of-life scenarios, and the majority of people in all religious subcategories "would reject life-sustaining treatments if faced with an incurable terminal illness" (Sharp et al., 2012, p. 288). However, people holding fundamentalist views,[23] regardless of denomination, were significantly more likely to want life-sustaining treatments than their non-fundamentalist counterparts, even after controlling for sociodemographic factors and health status. Two specific attitudes accounted for this differ-ence: fundamentalists were less likely to believe that quality of life is more important than just staying alive and more likely to say that their religious or spiritual beliefs would guide their medical decisions. Similarly, in another study, conservative Protestants and those attributing great importance to religion/spirituality had a lower likelihood of engaging in advance care planning (Garrido et al., 2013). Beliefs about God's control of life's length and adherence to values supporting the use of all available treatments were the main factors accounting for the relationships between religiosity and advance care planning.

Additional spiritual beliefs that influence both treatment choices and how those choices are made relate to the origin of illness and well-rooted confidence that miracle cures can occur or that "those who believe in God do not have to plan for end-of-life care" (Balboni et al., 2013; Johnson et al., 2008, p. 1956). For instance, in a prospective, multicenter cohort study, researchers found that positive religious coping (constructive reliance on faith, e.g., through seeking God's love and care) was associated with receipt of intensive life-prolonging medical care near the end of life (Phelps et al., 2009). Positive religious coping among patients remained a strong predictor of intensive life-prolonging care despite statistically accounting for known demographic (age and race) and psychosocial confounders, including patients' acknowledgment of terminal illness and completion of advance directives. Thus, the choice of life-prolonging therapies near the end of life among "religious copers" may be driven by their belief in God's divine healing or hope for a miraculous cure through intensive medical care.

The research literature also identifies a strong interaction between religiosity/spirituality and certain racial/ethnic group membership (Buck and Meghani, 2012; Johnson et al., 2005; Winter et al., 2007). Recent data from the Pew Research Religion and Public Life Project (reported in

---

[23]Defined as "agreeing or agreeing strongly with both of the two statements: (1) the Bible is God's word and everything happened or will happen exactly as it says and (2) the Bible is the answer to all important human problems" (Sharp et al., 2012, p. 283).

more detail in Chapter 6) reveal that most white mainline Protestants (72 percent), white Catholics (65 percent), and white evangelical Protestants (62 percent) would stop medical treatment if they had an incurable disease and were suffering a great deal of pain. Most black Protestants (61 percent) and Hispanic Catholics (57 percent), by contrast, would tell their physician to "do everything possible to save their lives" (Pew Research Center, 2013, p. 16).

Despite this well-documented relationship between race/ethnicity and preference for intensive life-sustaining treatment at the end of life, mechanisms explaining this relationship are not fully understood. In a large, single-site study with a predominantly African American sample, those who were highly religious and/or spiritual were more likely to have a designated decision maker for end-of-life decisions (Karches et al., 2012). In this study, religious characteristics were not significantly associated with the likelihood of having an advance directive or do-not-resuscitate order. In another study, the effect of race on end-of-life decisions was only partially mediated by a measure of guidance by God's will (Winter et al., 2007). The authors conclude that other dimensions of spirituality or unique constructs not pertaining to spirituality and religiosity may operate simultaneously in explaining end-of-life preferences among racial subgroups. Thus, pathways to the use of intensive measures to extend life are multifactorial and may go beyond religious beliefs (see the following subsection).

Differences Across Racial, Ethnic, and Cultural Groups[24]

Patients' backgrounds, culture, ethnicity, and race influence their perceptions about life, illness, suffering, dying, and death and the meaning they ascribe to these events. These perceptions in turn affect preferences for the kinds of care people want, how much they want to know about their situation and choices, whether and how they want to make treatment choices, whom they want to make those choices if they cannot, and the role of the family in the entire process (Blank, 2011; Kagawa-Singer and Blackhall, 2001).

In the coming years, rapid growth in the proportion of U.S. elderly that are members of racial/ethnic minority groups will challenge clinicians to communicate more effectively with people of many cultural traditions. Between 2010 and 2030, the U.S. white, non-Hispanic population aged 65 and older is expected to increase by 59 percent, whereas the minority population of the same age group will increase by 160 percent (Greenberg, 2011). It is vital, therefore, that clinicians be aware of common differences

---

[24]The terms used to describe population groups in this section vary and are generally those used by the authors cited.

in perception among racial, ethnic, and cultural groups so that at the very least, they can ask the right probing questions and have a firmer basis for individualized understanding of patients and their families.

As noted above, although there are many differences among individual perspectives and actions within groups, the *general* pattern in minority populations is one of a lack of advance care planning and a preference for more intensive treatments; poorer communication with clinicians is part of this pattern. Although patients and families may not follow clinicians' advice and recommendations, "avoiding such communication increases the likelihood of poor end-of-life decision making" (Curtis and Engelberg, 2011, p. 283).

In many cultures, collective family decision making—and even sometimes the paternalistic decisions of the family patriarch—is considered as important or more so than patient autonomy (Blank, 2011). Having made reference to the collective wisdom of the family in every other aspect of their lives to that point, dying individuals cannot realistically be expected to make decisions completely on their own or to name a single health care agent. In a presentation to the committee, Rebecca Dresser, a member of the President's Council on Bioethics (2002-2009), suggested that bioethics has had an unintended and at times negative consequence by focusing on autonomy and ignoring guidance and support (Dresser, 2013).

The fact that racial and ethnic minority individuals are less likely to use advance directives or choose hospice care has been noted in numerous studies in different population groups (Johnson et al., 2008; Ko and Berkman, 2010; Ko and Lee, 2013; Muni et al., 2011; Phipps et al., 2003; Waite et al., 2013; Zaide et al., 2013). At the same time, many authors have found associations between minority race or ethnicity and the receipt of more intensive end-of-life care (see, for example, Barnato et al., 2007; Mitchell and Mitchell, 2009; Muni et al., 2011). This pattern may result from a lack of information about advance planning documents and hospice (Wicher and Meeker, 2012) or from lower levels of general or health literacy (Volandes et al., 2008b). However, Volandes and colleagues (2008a) warn that "while attention to patients' culture is important, it is also important to avoid ascribing choices to culture that may actually reflect inadequate comprehension" (p. 700). Despite the often high-pressure, complex situations in which end-of-life decisions must be made, clinicians cannot make assumptions about preferences or take communication shortcuts without jeopardizing the quality of care.

The available body of evidence suggests that multiple factors are at work in forming patient and family preferences and in translating those preferences into care (see Table 3-3). As Ko and Lee (2013, p. 6) state, "Taken together, race/ethnicity can be thought of as a proxy for personal, cultural, and social contexts, so that an individual's values, beliefs, and per-

TABLE 3-3 Summary of Patient and Family Factors in End-of-Life Decision Making Among Individuals of Different Races, Ethnicities, and Cultures

Factor	Selected Source(s)
A combination of beliefs, preferences, and values	Johnson et al., 2008
Spiritual beliefs	Wicher and Meeker, 2012
Knowledge about advance directives	Wicher and Meeker, 2012
Historical mistrust of the health care system	Kagawa-Singer and Blackhall, 2001; Wicher and Meeker, 2012
Cultural beliefs about family involvement	Blank, 2011; Kagawa-Singer and Blackhall, 2001; Ko and Berkman, 2010; Yennurajalingam et al., 2013a,b
Desire to avoid emotional distress for self or family by discussing death, fear, denial	West and Hollis, 2012
"Don't want to think about dying" or family already aware of care preferences	Carr, 2012a
Disagreement between patient and family preferences for treatment	Muni et al., 2011; Phipps et al., 2003
Patients and physicians each waiting for the other to initiate the discussion	Phipps et al., 2003
Extent to which family engages in estate planning	Carr, 2011, 2012b
Literacy level	Waite et al., 2013
Socioeconomic status*	Carr, 2012b

*Although racial/ethnic differences in ICU care were found after controlling for socioeconomic status, once a patient is in the ICU, socioeconomic status may not make a difference (Muni et al., 2011).

sonal circumstances are necessary for [understanding] his or her [advance care planning]."

A relative lack of advance care planning is seen among black, Hispanic, and Asian patients across socioeconomic groups. It is seen as well across care settings, including hospitals and nursing homes and even in intensive care, where patients are least likely to be able to make their own decisions and the need for such planning is greatest (Frahm et al., 2012; Muni et al., 2011; Reynolds et al., 2008). "Advance directives, which are generally accepted in western civilization, hold little or no relevance within the [black and minority ethnic] population" (Cox et al., 2006, p. 20), including Asian cultures, in which family decision making predominates (Blank, 2011), and American Indian cultures, which hold different views from those typical of the white, non-Hispanic population regarding autonomy and informed consent (Colclough and Brown, 2013).

Asians

Whereas one U.S. study of patients with head and neck cancers found that more than 81 percent did not want anyone else present at the time of diagnosis (Kim and Alvi, 1999), patients from family-centered cultures such as the Japanese are more likely to want a relative present for such difficult conversations (Fujimori and Uchitomi, 2009). A review of the literature indicates that Asian patients in general may be less likely than patients of other cultural backgrounds to want an estimate of life expectancy and more likely to have family present when receiving bad news (Fujimori and Uchitomi, 2009). In a separate study of more than 500 Japanese cancer patients, Fujimori and colleagues (2007) found that married patients, those with less helplessness/hopelessness, and those with more formal education preferred to discuss life expectancy. Still, the majority of these patients preferred to have their physician explain the status of their illness, break bad news honestly and in a way that is easy to understand, and explain the treatment plan.

African Americans

As noted, African Americans are less likely than white non-Hispanics to express any treatment wishes or to have written advance care planning documents. Compared with whites, they also are more likely to report inadequate or problematic communication with physicians (Trice and Prigerson, 2009), to have greater concerns about staying informed about the illness, and to give the care their family member received a lower rating (Welch et al., 2005). In response, some efforts have been made to carefully tailor the messages regarding advance care planning to African American (as well as other cultural) communities. One example is the comprehensive approach of Gloria Anderson called "What Y'all Gon' Do With Me?: The African-American Spiritual and Ethical Guide to End of Life Care" (Anderson, 2006).

A study involving New York State nursing homes found lower rates of hospice use and higher rates of in-hospital deaths among blacks than whites: 40 percent of black patients and 24 percent of white patients died in hospitals, a differential accounted for largely by a higher use of feeding tubes and a lower use of do-not-resuscitate and do-not-hospitalize orders among black patients (Zheng et al., 2011). Overall, according to the authors (p. 996), "Other conditions being equal, residents from facilities with higher concentrations of blacks have higher risk of in-hospital death and lower probability of using hospice." Further examination is needed of why differentials in use occur by diagnosis and type of nursing home, and especially how these differentials may affect quality of care and outcomes.

Some evidence suggests that the gap between African American and white patients in the use of hospice has been shrinking. Between 1992 and 2000, the hospice use rate for whites doubled and for African Americans increased almost four-fold (Han et al., 2006). Differences by race and ethnicity still are seen, however (see Table 3-4). Blacks are underrepresented in the proportion of deaths that occur in hospice, which has been attributed, at least in part, to the Medicare Hospice Benefit's requirement that enrollees give up curative efforts (Wicher and Meeker, 2012).

The well-documented historical abuse of African Americans in medical research, dating back more than 150 years, continues to ripple throughout the health care enterprise in many parts of the United States. The author of the award-winning book *Medical Apartheid* says people tried to discourage her from writing the book, claiming that "any acknowledgment of abuse will drive African Americans from sorely needed medical care. However, a steady course of lies and exploitation has already done this" (Washington, 2006, pp. 386-387). This history and profound lack of trust may be one

TABLE 3-4 Race and Ethnicity of U.S. Decedents, and Hospice Patients, 2011

	White, non-Hispanic (%)	African American, non-Hispanic (%)	Hispanic (%)	Multiracial (%)	Asian, Hawaiian, Other Pacific Islander (%)
Race and ethnicity of U.S. decedents aged 35 and over (2011, preliminary)[a]	80.9	10.9	5.5	N/A	2.1
Race and ethnicity of U.S. hospice patients (2011)	82.8	8.5	6.2[b]	6.1	2.4

[a]Fully 99 percent of hospice patients were aged 35 and older in 2011.
[b]The National Hospice and Palliative Care Organization (NHPCO) reports Hispanic ethnicity separately from race.
SOURCES: Hoyert and Xu, 2012; NHPCO, 2013.

reason why African Americans may prefer intensive life-sustaining treatment near the end of life and believe that advance care planning and hospice may deny them wanted services (Johnson et al., 2008, 2011; Lepore et al., 2011; West and Hollis, 2012).

Some believe that poor physician communication skills contribute to this lack of trust (Gordon et al., 2006). In a study of physician-patient relationships, however, the issue on which African American and white respondents were in closest agreement was whether they had complete trust in their physician; African American respondents rated all other measures of relationship quality significantly lower compared with white respondents (Smith et al., 2007).

Hispanics/Latinos

Compared with other minority populations, less research has been done among Hispanics/Latinos on end-of-life preferences and decision making. The available studies suggest, however, that they follow the general pattern seen among cultural and ethnic minority populations as previously described (Carr, 2012a). Extent of knowledge about and attitudes toward advance directives are strong predictors of whether such directives are completed among both Hispanics and whites, and disparities in rates of completion may be due to differences in these factors (Ko and Lee, 2013). Greater acculturation was found to increase the likelihood of having an advance directive among older Latinos (Kelley et al., 2010).

Interviews with 147 Latinos aged 60 and older from Los Angeles–area senior centers found that most (84 percent) would prefer care focused on relieving pain and discomfort if they became seriously ill, yet nearly half (47 percent) had never discussed these preferences with either their family or their physicians (Kelley et al., 2010). Interviewees expressed a strong preference for family involvement in decision making about end-of-life care, whether or not they were incapacitated. In another study, 71 percent of hospitalized Latinos had not had a discussion about advance directives with clinical personnel (Fischer et al., 2012). Latinos who had had such a discussion were just as likely as any other population group members to have an advance directive on file, suggesting that the primary barrier to overcome is the low rate of such discussions.

System Factors in Decision Making

Mack and colleagues (2010a, p. 1537) conclude that "wider issues within the health care system . . . could explain the major disparity we identified. . . . White patients may have greater continuity of providers and sites of care, with the confirmation of [do-not-resuscitate] orders and documentation of preferences, for example, at every encounter. Alternatively, racial bias on the part of health care providers about patient preferences could have a role."

Several potential system barriers to advance care planning and completion of advance directives have been identified. For example, doctors' belief that African American patients "are more likely to prefer intensive, life-sustaining treatment" (Barnato et al., 2011, p. 1663) may lead to an overestimation of an African American individual's preference for such treatment. This may be one reason black patients tend to receive life-extending measures even when they have stated a preference for symptom-directed care (Mack et al., 2010a) and why the hospital care they receive is more likely to involve intensive services (Barnato et al., 2006, 2007).

Some patients may simply need more information about advance directives, the advance care planning process, and hospice and palliative care options (Johnson et al., 2008; Wicher and Meeker, 2012; Zaide et al., 2013). As a practical matter, health care providers need to be sure that the relevant discussions with all patients, regardless of race, ethnicity, language, and health literacy level, are unhurried, culturally appropriate, free of confusing medical terms and concepts, and adequately understood by the patient and family. Physicians can be part of that discussion, but may not in all cases be the most appropriate person to lead a lengthy conversation; bicultural and bilingual patient navigators or other trained laypersons may be helpful in talking to patients and their families about advance care planning. Materials in languages other than English and designed for low-literacy populations may also improve knowledge, understanding, and rates of advance care planning (Fischer et al., 2012).

Differences Across Literacy Levels

Levels of both general literacy and health literacy—defined as "the degree to which individuals have the capacity to obtain, process, and understand basic health information and services needed to make appropriate health decisions" (Ratzan and Parker, 2000, p. vi)—affect engagement in advance care planning and the preparation of advance directives.

General Literacy

Most advance directives (which often contain complex legal constructions and descriptions of medical technologies and procedures) require at least a 12th-grade reading level (Castillo et al., 2011). The 2003 National Assessment of Adult Literacy found that 14 percent of the total U.S. population aged 16 and older have below-basic prose literacy, and adults 65 and older account for more than one-quarter of these individuals (Baer et al.,

2009). And while adults with income below 125 percent of the poverty level accounted for 24 percent of the adult population in 2003, they represented 56 percent of those with below-basic prose literacy.

Predictions are that the general English literacy of the U.S. population will decline as a result of several factors, including continued low high school graduation rates; continued low reading and math performance among U.S. schoolchildren, particularly blacks and Hispanics; and the increasing number of immigrants (Kirsch et al., 2007; Parker et al., 2008). In 2011, almost 61 million U.S. residents aged 5 and older spoke a language other than English at home, and 7 percent of those residents—4.3 million people—spoke English "not at all." For 38 million Americans, the language spoken at home is Spanish, and for 23 million more, it is something else—with Chinese, French, German, Korean, Tagalog, and Vietnamese each being spoken by more than 1 million people (Ryan, 2013).

Health Literacy

According to an IOM (2004) report, approximately 90 million people have low health literacy. As a result, they would be likely to have significant difficulty navigating the health care system and/or completing a range of tasks key to self-managing complex chronic conditions successfully. In general, people with low health literacy experience more hospitalizations, use more emergency care, and are less able to interpret medication labels and health messages appropriately than those with higher health literacy (Berkman et al., 2011). Low-literacy seniors have poorer health status than their more health-literate counterparts. Such difficulties are likely to escalate near the end of life.

Health literacy "is not simply the ability to read. It requires a complex group of reading, listening, analytical, and decision-making skills, and the ability to apply these skills to health situations" (NNLM, 2013). Frequently measured and highly correlated health literacy components are "the ability to interpret documents, read and write prose (print literacy), use quantitative information (numeracy), and speak and listen effectively (oral literacy)" (Berkman et al., 2011, p. ES-1), with oral literacy being less frequently assessed. Numeracy skills are especially important in understanding prognoses, risks of treatment, and the expression of clinical uncertainty.

The 2003 National Assessment of Adult Literacy assessed the health literacy of U.S. adults using multiple measures. The test content encompassed clinical and prevention topics, as well as navigation of the health care system (Kutner et al., 2006). Key results (all statistically significant at the 0.05 level) mirror those for general literacy:

- The health literacy of 36 percent of U.S. adults was basic or below and was "proficient" for only 12 percent.
- White (non-Hispanic) and Asian/Pacific Islander adults had higher average health literacy than other groups.
- Those aged 65 and older had lower average health literacy than younger adults, and 29 percent of adults aged 65 and older had below-basic health literacy.

Low health literacy affects certain population subgroups disproportionately: people of lower socioeconomic status, racial and ethnic minorities, people with disabilities, those with psychiatric and other cognitive disorders, and the elderly. Nevertheless, "people of all ages, races, incomes, and education levels—not just people with limited reading skills or people for whom English is a second language—are affected by limited health literacy" (ODPHP, 2010, p. 4).

Multiple studies have shown that health literacy affects health care utilization, outcomes, and costs (Berkman et al., 2011). Individuals with low health literacy whose difficulties are compounded by the emotional stress and debilitation of an advanced disease may have difficulty reading, comprehending, and/or signing insurance forms or complicated advance directive documents. In one study of almost 800 patients aged 55 to 74, almost one-half of those with adequate literacy, just more than one-quarter of those with marginal literacy, and only one-eighth of those with low literacy reported having an advance directive (Waite et al., 2013). Uncertainties about care preferences among less health-literate groups suggest a need for culturally sensitive decision-making tools that take literacy into account (Sudore et al., 2010).

ELEMENTS OF GOOD COMMUNICATION IN ADVANCE CARE PLANNING

Elements of good communication in advance care planning include open, clear, and respectful communication between clinician and patient; good communication with families and health care agents; and shared decision making and patient-centered care.

Clinician-Patient Communication

Open, clear, and respectful communication between health care professional and patient is a precondition for effective advance care planning. It also is critical to developing a therapeutic relationship and negotiating and carrying out a treatment plan. Moreover, it is professionally rewarding and personally satisfying for clinicians, and reduces anxiety and uncertainty for patients (Dias et al., 2003).

A National Cancer Institute (NCI) monograph on improving patient-centered communication is organized around six major goals:

- fostering healing relationships,
- exchanging information,
- responding to emotions,
- managing uncertainty,
- making decisions, and
- enabling patient self-management (Epstein and Street, 2007).

Several of these goals are major topics in this report and in this chapter in particular. Authors of the NCI monograph point out the interrelationships among these goals and the variability in information about each of them.

After-death interviews with 205 families of adult decedents included several questions related to advance care planning. Although total "quality of dying and death scores" were not influenced by whether the patient had an advance directive, "higher scores were associated with communication about treatment preferences, compliance with treatment preferences, and family satisfaction regarding communication with the health care team" (Curtis et al., 2002, p. 17). Specific components of communication associated with a better-quality dying experience included how well the health care team listened to the family[25] and explained the patient's condition "in language they can understand and in terms that are meaningful in their lives" (Curtis et al., 2002, p. 27).

While in-the-moment decision making may provide the most accurate reflection of patients' wishes at the time a decision is needed, this approach entails numerous barriers. For example, considering all the implications of a decision—medical, psychological, logistical, financial, caregiving—may be nearly impossible for patients and health care agents under such circumstances; many of them may not want to think about these issues and the current trajectory of a serious advanced illness, and clinicians may not have the time to discuss them. Nevertheless, clinicians—especially those who do not have a lengthy previous relationship with the patient—need this input.

According to Sudore and Fried (2010, p. 257), what matters most to patients "is the potential outcomes of treatment." Asking patients about the outcomes they most hope for or fear is a way to identify values and prefer-

---

[25]Previous research indicated that when physicians talked to patients about advance directives, they spent two-thirds of the time talking; discussed attitudes toward uncertainty only 55 percent of the time; and asked about patients' values, goals, and reasons for treatment preferences 34 percent of the time (Tulsky et al., 1998).

ences in a way that may be more actionable than asking whether they want or do not want specific interventions. And because opinions change over time, discussions of this type need to be repeated. Good questions include "What information would you like to know?," "Who else should be given the information and be involved in decision making?," and "How should that information be presented?" (Russell and Ward, 2011). A review of the international literature[26] suggests that cancer patients' information preferences are affected by four factors: setting, manner of communicating bad news, what and how much information is provided, and emotional support (Fujimori and Uchitomi, 2009).

Despite the importance of good clinician-patient communication, many impediments to such communication exist. Some are inherent in the previously discussed issues concerning specific populations. Others relate to physicians themselves, including a lack of training, insufficient time, competing needs, and personal discomfort in discussing terminal prognoses and death. Walling and colleagues (2008) identify the following reasons for a lack of the effective clinician-patient communication needed for advance care planning:

- reluctance to give patients bad news, with doctors' physiological responses to breaking bad news showing that it is stressful for them to do so;
- physicians' avoidance of discussions of negative prognoses because of some combination of uncertainty and not wanting to engender hopelessness;
- lack of evidence about the best timing for discussions of future treatment options and the above-noted changing concerns of patients over the course of illness that may warrant repeat discussions;
- reluctance on the part of patients to discuss these matters; and
- time constraints and distractions (pagers, for example).

"There is too little time during our appointments to discuss everything we should" was the most common barrier to advance care planning mentioned by almost two-thirds of 56 physicians responding to one survey, with wanting to maintain patients' hope being the next most frequently cited (by 23 percent) (Knauft et al., 2005).

Lack of time to identify patients' preferences can contribute to misunderstandings if doctors rely instead on their own instincts and experience. Two studies found that even specially trained palliative care physicians who

---

[26]This systematic review of English-language research papers was conducted by investigators in Japan, but they note that most of the research they found reported on experiences in Western countries.

had had lengthy initial consultations with their patients most commonly assessed the patients' medical decision-making preferences (how actively they wanted to participate in making treatment decisions) incorrectly (Bruera et al., 2001, 2002).

The following sections look at four topics that exemplify the challenges of end-of-life communications: discussing prognosis, handling emotional encounters, nurturing patients' hope, and addressing spirituality and religion.

Discussing Prognosis

Shortcomings in existing prognostic tools and methods contribute to a lack of clarity about disease prognosis that weighs on physicians and clouds communication (Smith et al., 2013b; see also Chapter 2). Population-based estimates of the course of disease do not exclude the possibility that an individual patient will be an exception at the short or long tail of longevity. Not only is estimating prognosis difficult, but so, too, as noted above, is the process of communicating it to patients and families (Lamont and Christakis, 2003). Numerous studies have shown that to compensate, physicians tend to provide prognosis estimates infrequently or to give overly optimistic estimates of survival. The more long-standing the physician-patient relationship, the more likely it is that the physician will make an inaccurate, overpessimistic prediction of prognosis (Christakis and Lamont, 2000). It is not surprising, then, that interviews with terminally ill patients and their caregivers reveal considerable uncertainty about life expectancy among both groups, even within a few weeks of death (Fried et al., 2006).

A study involving palliative care specialists found that almost all of their consultations (93 percent) included some prognostic information and more pessimistic than optimistic cues, gave greater emphasis to quality of life than to length of survival, focused on the situation of the particular patient rather than population-based estimates as the patient neared death, and tended to provide more pessimistic views when talking to family members without the patient present (perhaps because the patient was too ill to participate) (Gramling et al., 2013).

Often family members and health care agents do not understand, have not been made aware of, or cannot accept their loved one's serious prognosis (see also the discussion of good communication with families and health care agents below). Both patients and family members frequently "don't hear" negative messages about prognosis (Fried et al., 2003) and tend to interpret even negative information optimistically—not because physicians are unclear or families do not understand numerical risk information, but because of psychological factors and belief in the power of positive thinking (Wachterman et al., 2013; Zier et al., 2012). On the other hand, even a single pessimistic statement from an oncologist can reduce patients' unchecked optimism (Robinson et al., 2008).

Bringing physician and patient views into greater alignment is necessary to give patients the best opportunity to make realistic and informed choices about their care. One strategy is to make clear that the plan of treatment may go well, but that it may not effect a cure of the underlying disease. Oncologists make such statements in less than half of patient visits (46 percent) (Robinson et al., 2008), and even so, patients often do not understand them (Weeks et al., 2012).

Handling Emotional Encounters

Patients living with advanced serious illnesses experience significant distress, and their need to make difficult decisions about treatment contributes to this suffering. These treatment decisions can be fraught with uncertainty and are often clouded by a fear of death. Such distress is known to be highly prevalent among cancer patients in particular, with up to 60 percent of selected populations acknowledging emotional difficulties (Carlson et al., 2010, 2012; Gao et al., 2010; Zabora et al., 2001). Many factors contribute to this distress, including managing physical symptoms, adjusting to changes in social or occupational roles, and navigating the emotional ups and downs of cancer remission and progression (Anderson et al., 2008). In addition, most patients face multiple decisions about treatment throughout the course of their illness. These decisions vary from discrete choices about surgery to more general decisions about philosophies of treatment and balances between risk and reward.

Much of the research on clinician management of emotional encounters comes from studies of cancer patients, and it has found that clinicians do not consistently handle patients' and families' expressions of emotions well (Loewenstein, 2005; Pollak et al., 2007). In fact, research suggests that empathetic responses by physicians to patients' expressed emotions are relatively rare, despite physicians' high confidence in being able to address patients' concerns and the frequency with which such concerns are expressed. Analysis of audiotapes from almost 400 conversations between oncologists and 270 patients with advanced cancer[27] revealed that opportunities for the oncologists to show empathy arose in patients' remarks some 292 times in 398 conversations (Pollak et al., 2007). Some 68 percent of these remarks were direct (e.g., "I have been really depressed lately"), and one-third were indirect (e.g., "Oh, no. What do we do now?").

Emotions can arise in patients in response to several broad categories of issues: symptoms, diagnosis, and treatment; social issues; the health care

---

[27]Most of these 270 patients had at least a 6-month relationship with their oncologist.

system, and death and dying (Anderson et al., 2008). Common words used to express such emotion are "concern," "scared," "worried," "depressed," and "nervous," which would appear to be patently emotion laden. Yet "when clinicians repeatedly miss patients' expressions of emotion, patients eventually cease to express emotion," and an important opportunity to relieve patient distress is foregone (Anderson et al., 2008, p. 808).

In these situations, clinicians can respond with statements or questions that are "continuers" (those that name the patient's emotion, express understanding, show respect or support, or seek to explore the emotion further) or with "terminators" (statements that seek to cut off the discussion). Pollak and colleagues (2007) found that oncologists responded with terminators 73 percent of the time. Patients learn not to raise these issues when met with such responses (see also Butow et al., 2002).

Gender is a predictor of the use of more empathetic language, with women using more such language. In addition, the extent to which oncologists self-identified as more socioemotional than technical-scientific in their orientation also predicted the use of empathetic language (Pollak et al., 2007). In this connection, a survey of oncologists (48), oncology physician assistants (26), and oncology nurses (22) found that most of the physicians (70 percent) described themselves as "technological and scientific," while substantial majorities of the nurses (82 percent) and physician assistants (68 percent) described themselves as "social and emotional" (Morgan et al., 2010). Because the nurses and physician assistants also reported more comfort with psychosocial talk, the authors of this study suggest that the differences across professions in responding to patient emotion "could have important implications for the design of future oncology care teams" (p. 16), as well as for health professions education.

Dealing with patients' emotions is one of the more challenging tasks of the already difficult job of caring for people likely to die. Care and support for the clinicians who do this work may reduce clinician stress and burnout and make an important contribution to improving the care they provide (Mack and Smith, 2012).

Nurturing Patients' Hope

As suggested above, a primary reason physicians are not more candid about discussing prognosis is that they believe "discussing end-of-life care will take away the patient's hope," which might affect treatment outcomes (Ganti et al., 2007, p. 5647). However, research suggests that honest conversations do not rob patients and families of hope or lead to depression, and that being truthful does not hasten death (Shockney and Back, 2013). By adopting a communication approach that simultaneously emphasizes "hoping for the best and preparing for the worst," doctors allow for important opportunities to learn from patients and families what they need, what they fear, and what is possible (Back et al., 2003, p. 439).

Ways to encourage hope in a context of greater candor do exist. Certainly, clinicians can emphasize what can be done (managing pain and symptoms, providing emotional support and care, maintaining dignity, and providing practical assistance); explore realistic goals of care; and discuss the priorities for day-to-day living (Clayton et al., 2005). The importance of the latter topic is suggested by research showing that patients and caregivers are sometimes reluctant to discuss the future because they are so focused on the here and now (Knauft et al., 2005).

Addressing Spirituality and Religion

Attention to patients' spiritual needs can improve the quality of communication among clinicians, patients, and families and reduce the gap between the health care patients want and expect and what they receive (Edwards et al., 2010). Findings from numerous studies indicate that some patients feel that a lack of spiritual support is an important communication gap (e.g., Curtis et al., 2004; Peteet and Balboni, 2013). Many clinicians, too, believe that spiritual support is an important aspect of care (Puchalski and Ferrell, 2010). These findings parallel the goals of palliative care, with its attention to body, mind, and spirit, and of patient-centeredness, which encompasses "compassion, empathy, and responsiveness to the needs, values, and expressed preferences of the individual patient" (IOM, 2001, p. 48). As physician and ethicist Daniel Sulmasy (2009, p. 1635) puts it:

> if physicians and other healthcare professionals have sworn to treat patients to the best of their ability and judgment, and the best care treats patients as whole persons, then to treat patients in a way that ignores the fundamental meaning that the patient sees in suffering, healing, life, and death is to treat patients superficially and to fall short of the best ability and judgment.

A final general consideration is that, although spirituality and religion may be powerful forces for relief of suffering for certain individuals, this does not mean physicians should encourage patients toward religious practices "as something 'medically indicated' for health" (Sulmasy, 2009, p. 1636). The healing benefits of spiritual practice may not be achievable through external exhortation in any case, and may be possible only when they form part of a person's intrinsic belief system.

Good Communication with Families and Health Care Agents

Family involvement is an essential feature of advance care planning, and the family's understanding of the illness and its treatment and likely course can help reinforce—or undermine—the work of the care team. In unexpected situations, when a sudden devastating illness or injury occurs, the same need for careful communication and family involvement occurs. These situations are made more difficult by the likelihood that no prior relationships exist among patient, family, and clinicians and when the patient's condition requires redirecting efforts from resuscitative treatment to palliative care (Limehouse et al., 2012a,b). When there is conflict within the family, moreover, a health care agent is less likely to make decisions in agreement with the patient's wishes (Parks et al., 2011).

Much experience with communication in family meetings has been gained in the long-term care setting. There, individuals may experience significant mental as well as physical declines during their residence, and family meetings are an important component of care. Family meetings have been found to be most successful when they occur at times other than crises and are used to share information, manage emotions, establish goals, and support decision making (Ceronsky and Weissman, 2011). Well-established guidelines exist for conducting such meetings effectively, and opportunities for improving family meetings through cross-learning across care settings may be useful (Hudson et al., 2008; McCusker et al., 2013). In the intensive care setting, conferences in which family members are given opportunities to speak and share their concerns reduce conflict with the doctor over care decisions and family dissatisfaction with the process of making those decisions (McDonagh et al., 2004).[28]

Physicians have avoided such conversations for various reasons—perhaps an unwillingness to reveal the limits of medical knowledge; a desire to avoid causing patients and families undue distress; or, as discussed above, concern about causing a loss of hope. Avoiding these conversations may be misguided, however, because it denies families and health care agents the opportunity to prepare emotionally and logistically for their loved one's death (Apatira et al., 2008; Evans et al., 2009, p. 52).

Families' and health care agents' perceptions of prognosis may be affected by patients' physical appearance, how they have handled previous illnesses, their strengths, and their will to live, as well as by the family members' and agents' own optimism, intuition, and faith. Thus, families attempt to meld and balance these factors with the information provided by the clinician. For example, as Boyd and colleagues (2010, p. 1274) note,

---

[28]In this study, audiotapes of 51 family conferences, involving 214 family members and led by 36 different physicians, were made and analyzed. On average, clinicians spoke more than 70 percent of the time.

"discussing prognosis in terms of outcomes of populations of 'similar' patients may fall short if physicians do not also recognize and appreciate that surrogates also view unique attributes of the patient as relevant."

Interviews with 179 health care agents for ICU patients at an academic medical center revealed that most (87 percent) wanted physicians to discuss an uncertain prognosis, and only 12 percent preferred to avoid such a discussion in case the prognosis was incorrect (Evans et al., 2009). Health care agents wanted to discuss prognosis despite uncertainty because they believed uncertainty is unavoidable. They also felt that discussing uncertainty leaves room for realistic rather than false hope (some noting that they looked for hope elsewhere) and that physicians were the best and only source for this information. Sharing information during such discussions increases trust in the physician. In addition, having this information allows health care agents to better support the patient and other family members, gives them time to prepare to make difficult life support decisions, and allows time to say good-bye and prepare for possible bereavement (Apatira et al., 2008; Evans et al., 2009). Rather than avoiding discussion of the likelihood of death, some health care agents want physicians to practice "complete honesty," although there is a range of receptivity to this information (Evans et al., 2009).

My father had progressive bladder cancer and also was an Alzheimer's patient who lived at home with our mother. As our father's disease progressed, both his physical and mental health deteriorated. Our mother also passed away quite unexpectedly, so his care was completely transferred to my sister and me. We became frustrated by the lack of communication between the doctor's office and us. It did not appear the treatments our father was receiving were working, and he had difficulty understanding why he had to go to the doctor's for a treatment that caused immediate pain and then prolonged discomfort. Phone calls, faxes, and e-mails were not answered. We found the only way we could obtain information or answers to questions was to physically enter the doctor's office and request a face-to-face meeting. Since I lived 5 hours away, it was necessary to schedule the meetings during my half of the week at our father's home. The doctor even scheduled a surgery for our father near the end of his life. *

---

*Quotation from a response submitted through the online public testimony questionnaire for this study. See Appendix C.

Conversations involving withdrawal of life support are inevitably difficult for all parties. Health care agents themselves are divided as to whether they want the physician to make a recommendation in such situations. In one study of 169 agents, 56 percent preferred to receive the physician's recommendation, while 42 preferred not to (2 percent had no preference) (White et al., 2009). This differential was not related to health care agents' demographic characteristics. These findings suggested to the authors that physicians should not routinely provide recommendations about withdrawing life support and instead be flexible in their approach to advising surrogates in such situations, taking into consideration whether such advice is appropriate, desired by the surrogate, and necessary "to ensure that decisions reflect the patient's values and preferences" (White et al., 2009, p. 324).

Shared Decision Making and Patient-Centered Care

Increasingly, informing and involving patients regarding the decisions about their care is recognized as a standard for good care (Fowler et al., 2013). This evolution in thinking has occurred in recent decades with respect to patient-clinician communication around care decisions broadly and is particularly relevant in the context of advance care planning. "Shared decision making emerged as a compromise in the longstanding debate about the relative role of patient autonomy and provider beneficence in medical decision-making" (Stark and Fins, 2013, p. 13).

In May 2013, an editorial in the *British Medical Journal* called for an equal-footing partnership between patients and doctors. The editorial also acknowledged that "achieving such a partnership is a challenge. Years of paternalism have left doctors and patients unprepared for a different type of interaction" (Godlee, 2013, p. 1).[29]

Shared decision making is neither clearly nor consistently defined in the research literature, and more robust research methods are needed to gauge its effects more precisely (Lipkin, 2013). Nonetheless, it clearly shares characteristics and a development path with the notion of patient-centered care. Indeed, shared decision making is one aspect of patient-centeredness, an essential component of quality care. Shared decision making encompasses

- eliciting and understanding the patient's perspective;
- understanding the patient's psychosocial and emotional context;

---

[29]A number of articles on the topic of shared decision making from the *British Medical Journal* have been collected at http://www.bmj.com/specialties/shared-decision-making (accessed December 16, 2014).

- developing a shared understanding of the clinical problem and its appropriate treatment, given the patient's goals, preferences, and values; and
- empowering patients, which is achieved through active involvement of patients in decision making (LeBlanc and Tulsky, in press).

For patients with advanced serious illnesses, shared decision making is intended to create a context in which future decisions can be made that remain true to patients' preferences. This approach eschews the idea of specific, checkbox-style advance directives, and emphasizes participation by patients and, importantly, their families, as well as their health care agents (who may be family members), whose thoughtful selection is strongly endorsed by current practice. According to Gillick (2013, p. 575), "For frail elders and patients with advanced illness, many of whom have multiple chronic diseases, patient-centered care is impossible without caregiver involvement . . . [and] . . . the critical role of caregivers deserves considerably more attention from clinicians."

A narrative synthesis of some 37 articles on shared decision making in palliative care identifies several important themes (Bélanger et al., 2010). Although patients prefer shared decision making (preferred by 40-73 percent of patients surveyed in five studies) and it is important to them, they often are not afforded the chance to participate. In addition, the effects of participation on patient outcomes (anxiety and depression, patient satisfaction, and life expectancy) are not yet clear, and both barriers to and facilitators of shared decision making have been identified. Barriers include patients' and families' unrealistic expectations of treatment; the way options are framed for patients; delaying decisions to follow predetermined patterns of care; and providing information too gradually so that when a decision is needed all the information is not in hand. Facilitators include clinicians providing sufficient, realistic information; presenting choices; and using tools to aid patients in decision making.

How Patients Make Decisions

Advance care planning is founded on the expectation that people, once presented with evidence and facts, will make rational choices based on well-established views and preferences (Swindell et al., 2011). The growing field of behavioral economics is challenging both the notion of "rational choice" and the presence of "well-established views." Clinicians assisting patients benefit from understanding of biases and "rules of thumb" by which patients make decisions (Swindell et al., 2010). Examples of these decision-making methods as they might emerge in end-of-life situations include

- being unduly influenced by a memorable event (such as news reports of the extremely rare cases in which someone in a coma for many years "miraculously" returns to consciousness);
- believing that some exceptional factor will prevent a patient's disease from following its usual course;
- being influenced by unrelated past occurrences (such as a relative's successful recovery from a serious disease or difficult, painful death); and
- preferring inaction to avoid harm (such as declining opioid drugs early in the illness so that "they will work when I need them"), even though this inaction may cause greater harm than action.

Such biases and heuristics can unintentionally thwart what patients themselves see as their best interest and goals (Swindell et al., 2010). Clinicians who understand the ways in which patients' decision making is not always rational can help patients reflect on their biases and to see whether doing so changes their expressed preferences (Halpern, 2012a; Swindell et al., 2011).

Insights into the psychology of human decision making can be used "to develop, test, and implement scalable interventions that improve the quality of the health decisions made by patients, family members, and providers" (Halpern, 2012b, p. 2789). "Choice architecture" takes into account the ways "choices are presented and the environment in which decisions are made," adjusting them so that better decisions result (Halpern, 2012b, p. 2789).

Gaps between people's intentions and their behavior are a prominent theme in the end-of-life field. A prime example is the gap between people believing in the importance of advance directives and discussions about end-of-life wishes and their taking action in accordance with that belief (CHCF, 2012; The Conversation Project, 2013). Certainly patients have been shown to vary a great deal in the extent to which they want to be involved in decisions about their end-of-life care, and it may be possible to encourage and support good decision making without relying on unrealistic expectations about patient engagement.

Choice architecture employs a number of key strategies designed to improve the decision environment, including use of defaults and precommitment (Nease et al., 2013). The precommitment approach takes into account that most people place a higher value on present or imminent events than on events that will occur in the future. Advance care planning is an example of an action that has fairly steep immediate costs (contemplation of one's mortality and the possibility of being unable to make decisions) and benefits that may appear only theoretical. The younger and healthier the person is, the more theoretical those benefits may seem. Default or "opt-out" choices assign patients a provisional decision; if they want to make a different decision, they can, but must actively do so.[30] All default options in the health care system (for example, aggressive care unless stated otherwise) carry biases. Choice architecture seeks to make these biases explicit and, in some cases, encourage changing the default to one that is generally preferred by patients and clinicians. By doing so, biases that currently drive decisions may be undone, and patient choice may be enhanced. According to Halpern and colleagues (2013, p. 412), "A hallmark of defaults is that they lead gently, without restricting any options." A randomized study of patients with incurable lung cancer found that when the patients were presented with an advance directive in which the default was palliative care, they were significantly more likely to elect that option than were patients given a standard advance directive or one that defaulted to life-extending treatment (Halpern, 2012b; Halpern et al., 2013). In studies in which a hypothetical advance directive used forgoing life-sustaining interventions as the default, many more study participants indicated that this was their preference than was the case if they had to actively choose that option (Kressel and Chapman, 2007; Kressel et al., 2007).

The important implication of the research by Kressel and colleagues is that "people might not have well-formulated, strongly held views on what forms of care at the end of life will best promote their values" (Halpern et al., 2013, p. 409). Rather than reflecting deeply ingrained preferences, their responses to advance directive document choices may be constructed at the time they are asked to provide them, similar to what has been observed with respect to other health care choices (Halpern et al., 2007). This hypothesis was tested with 132 patients having incurable lung disease and no prior directive (Halpern et al., 2013). Patients were randomly assigned to be presented with one of three advance directives that differed only in their embedded default options. While most of the patients chose what the authors called comfort-oriented care, the proportion making that choice was much higher in the group receiving the "comfort default" directive. When, subsequently, the study design was explained to patients along with the data showing how defaults had affected the choices of the patient groups, only 2.1 percent of participants reconsidered their selections, and no patients revised their original choices. This result suggests that changes to the way advance directives are structured that make it simple for patients to choose the kind of care most patients prefer (always with the option to

---

[30] An early successful application of "opt-out" decision making was designed to encourage people to participate in an employer-subsidized 401(k) savings plan. Automatically enrolling employees unless they actively opted out "materially increase[d] participation while maintaining a high level of employee satisfaction" (Nease et al., 2013, p. 245).

choose otherwise) might "provide a novel way to improve end-of-life care for large populations of seriously ill patients" (Halpern et al., 2013, p. 414).

Decision Aids

Decision aids have been developed to guide discussion, support patients, and make discussion of difficult issues easier.[31] Recognizing that patients nearing the end of life are likely to be in a state of decline, the designers of these aids generally attempt to make their completion as low burden as possible. Many of these tools have been tested and used in the palliative care setting or with cancer patients, and many of them apply to a single decision, such as whether to place a feeding tube in a cognitively impaired patient.

Even an apparently simple open-ended question such as "What is your understanding of your illness?"—certainly fundamental to a discussion of choices—can have significant clinical utility. A study of patient responses to this question found substantial differences among patient groups: 77 percent of patients with cancer could name or describe their condition, sometimes using precise biomedical terms; 39 percent of patients with congestive heart failure and 41 percent with chronic obstructive pulmonary disease could do so; and some patients (particularly those with limited education) had little knowledge or understanding of their illness (Morris et al., 2012). Patients' responses to this question may, therefore, signal the opportunity for clinicians to provide more information about the illness, discuss how it may affect the patients' lives, and describe its likely course, as well as reveal whether patients have unmet emotional needs.

Decision aids are of three general types: those used in face-to-face encounters; those designed for use outside clinical encounters (take-home materials, for example); and those that use some intervening medium, such as telephone or video (Elwyn et al., 2010). Results of randomized trials of video decision aids, reported in Table 3-5, show that across the board, participants were comfortable with the decision aids and found them useful. According to the authors of one of these studies, "Physicians often underestimate the emotional resilience of patients and their desire to be involved in this decision-making process" (El-Jawahri et al., 2010, p. 309).

A research team at the forefront of developing and evaluating decision aids defines them as follows:

Decision support interventions help people think about choices they face: they describe where and why choice exists; they provide information about

---

[31]For example, the question "Are you at peace?" may be a sufficient screening question to identify patients for whom fuller spiritual assessment or specialized services are needed (Steinhauser et al., 2006).

options, including, where reasonable, the option of taking no action. These interventions help people to deliberate, independently or in collaboration with others, about options, by considering relevant attributes; they support people to forecast how they might feel about short, intermediate and long-term outcomes which have relevant consequences, in ways which help the process of constructing preferences and eventual decision making, appropriate to their individual situation. (Elwyn et al., 2010, p. 705)

Video is not the only effective medium for decision aids. In another recent study involving 120 patients with metastatic cancer who were no longer receiving curative therapy (55 intervention patients, 65 control

TABLE 3-5 Effects of Video Materials on Health Care Decisions Among Selected Audiences

Video Content	Result	Audience
Patient with advanced dementia (Deep et al., 2010)	Proportion choosing comfort care* increased from 50% to 89%	General population over age 40
Goals of care (life-prolonging, basic, or comfort care*) (Volandes et al., 2012a)	80% of viewers chose comfort care,* compared with 57% in control group	Patients in skilled nursing facilities
Goals of care (El-Jawahri et al., 2010)	91% of viewers chose comfort care,* compared with 22% in control group	People with advanced cancer
Cardiopulmonary resuscitation (CPR) (Volandes et al., 2013)	20% of viewers wanted CPR, compared with 48% in control group	People with advanced cancer
CPR (Epstein et al., 2013)	40% of viewers had their advance care plans documented 1 month after the intervention, compared with 15% in control group; viewers' preferences for CPR changed significantly postintervention, with 24% no longer wanting CPR	People with pancreatic or hepatobiliary cancer
Goals of care (Volandes et al., 2012b)	Statistically significant decreases in proportion who wanted CPR or ventilation	People with advanced cancer

*The phrase "comfort care" was used by the authors and described as care that maximizes comfort and alleviates pain or suffering.

patients), the intervention group received a pamphlet ("Living with Advanced Cancer") and a discussion with a psychologist about preferences and values (Stein et al., 2013). Those receiving the intervention had do-not-resuscitate orders placed earlier and were less likely to die in the hospital than patients in the control group. Previous research had indicated that providing the pamphlet alone caused patients distress; with the addition of the discussion with a psychologist, no negative impact on patients or caregivers was found.

The timing of the use of decision aids also is important. By the time a patient is admitted to a hospital palliative care unit, for example, many of the most significant decisions may have been made, or patients may be too sick or preoccupied to participate (Matlock et al., 2011).

MODEL ADVANCE CARE PLANNING INITIATIVES

The National Quality Forum's National Framework and Preferred Practices for Palliative and Hospice Care Quality includes seven preferred practices related to advance care planning (NQF, 2006). They reflect many of the issues raised in this chapter, and many build on positive experiences with model advance care planning initiatives that have improved the effectiveness of the process or its reach in the population. The seven practices are as follows:

- Document the designated surrogate/decision maker in accordance with state law for every patient in primary, acute, and long-term care and in palliative and hospice care.
- Document the patient/surrogate preferences for goals of care, treatment options, and setting of care at first assessment and at frequent intervals as conditions change.
- Convert the patient treatment goals into medical orders, and ensure that the information is transferable and applicable across care settings, including long-term care, emergency medical services [EMS], and hospital care, through a program such as the Physician Orders for Life-Sustaining Treatment (POLST) program.
- Make advance directives and surrogacy designations available across care settings, while protecting patient privacy and adherence to Health Insurance Portability and Accountability Act (HIPAA) of 1996 regulations, for example, by using Internet-based registries or electronic personal health records.
- Develop health care and community collaborations to promote advance care planning and the completion of advance directives

for all individuals, for example, the Respecting Choices and Community Conversations on Compassionate Care programs.

- Establish or have access to ethics committees or ethics consultation across care settings to address ethical conflicts at the end of life.
- For minors with decision-making capacity, document the children's views and preferences for medical care, including assent for treatment, and give them appropriate weight in decision making. Make appropriate professional staff members available to both the child and the adult decision maker for consultation and intervention when the child's wishes differ from those of the adult decision maker (NQF, 2006, pp. 42-45).

These standards reflect several innovations in advance care planning that have occurred since *Approaching Death* (IOM, 1997) was published. These innovations overcome some of the difficulties experienced with conventional advance directives related to timing, relevance, lack of support, and unavailability when needed.

Physician Orders for Life-Sustaining Treatment

The POLST paradigm is an approach to advance care planning designed to ensure that seriously ill or frail patients can choose the treatments they want or do not want and that their wishes are documented and will be honored in an emergency (National POLST, 2012a). POLST is a clinical process designed to facilitate communication between health care professionals and patients, their families, their health care agents, or their designated surrogates. The process encourages shared, informed medical decision making. The result is a set of portable medical orders, POLST forms (see Annex 3-2), that respects the patient's goals for care with regard to the use of cardiopulmonary resuscitation; artificially administered nutrition; and other medical interventions, such as intubation and future hospitalization (Bomba et al., 2012; National POLST, 2012a). Medical intervention options generally are described as "comfort measures only," "limited additional interventions," and "full treatment" and align with the intensity of the desired interventions. "Comfort measures only" indicates that the primary goal for care is maximizing comfort. If comfort needs cannot be met in the patient's location, the patient is transported to a clinical care setting where those needs can be met. "Comfort measures" are medical care and treatment provided with the primary goal of relieving pain and other symptoms and reducing suffering, and may include offering food and fluids by mouth; turning the patient in bed; providing wound care; and providing oxygen, suctioning, and other manual treatment of airway obstruction for comfort. "Limited additional interventions" includes comfort measures plus some medical interventions, such as administration of antibiotics and intravenous fluids. "Full treatment" includes measures provided in the other two categories, as well as use of additional medical interventions, such as intubation or mechanical ventilation.[32]

These medical orders support the person's preferences with respect to treatment, preferred site for receiving care, and death, and can be reviewed and revised as needed (Bomba et al., 2012; National POLST, 2012a). They are intended to stay with patients near the end of life as they are transferred from home to hospital or any other type of care facility and to be in force wherever patients may be. POLST are followed in all care settings and by all health care professionals, including emergency medical services personnel, who in an emergency, cannot interpret a living will or take orders from a health care agent (Bomba et al., 2012; National POLST, 2012b,c).

POLST are not intended for everyone; they are for people with serious illnesses or frailty whose health care professionals would not be surprised if they died within the next year, based on their current health status and prognosis. POLST also are appropriate for patients who reside in a long-term care facility or receive long-term services at home as a result of frailty, and for persons of advanced age who want to avoid or receive any or all life-sustaining treatment. Among vulnerable populations, including persons with disabilities, POLST are intended only for seriously ill or frail patients facing end of life, not the entire population (Bomba et al., 2012; National POLST, 2012a).

The POLST process begins with the clinician's preparing for the discussion by first reviewing the patient's current health status and prognosis to ensure that POLST are appropriate for that patient. The second step entails retrieving and reviewing completed advance directives and prior do-not-resuscitate and/or POLST forms; the third, determining the patient's capacity to make POLST decisions; and the fourth, educating the decision maker about POLST. A conversation or series of conversations between the patient and trained clinicians helps define the patient's values, beliefs, and goals for care that will drive the choice of interventions. The discussion can occur in all clinical care settings, including the physician's office, the long-term care facility, the hospital, or the patient's home. If the patient lacks the capacity to make medical decisions outlined on the POLST form, discussion occurs with the health care agent or the appropriate surrogate, identified under state law. The clinician reviews possible treatment options on the entire POLST form and ensures shared, informed medical decision making. The POLST form is signed by the physician, because it represents

---

[32]Each state POLST paradigm program is responsible for developing that state's POLST form; therefore, the forms vary from state to state. Forms from various states are available at http://www.polst.org/educational-resources/resource-library (accessed December 16, 2014).

a set of medical orders; in some states, nurse practitioners are authorized to sign the form. The conversation should also be documented in the patient's medical record (Bomba et al., 2012).

The POLST form typically is printed in a bright, neon color so it is difficult to overlook on the patient's home refrigerator or in an inches-thick medical chart. It is written in plain language, avoiding both medical and legal jargon, and intended to be based on conversations among the clinician, the patient, and the health care agent (Bomba et al., 2012; National POLST, 2012d).

The physician (or nurse practitioner, if state scope-of-practice regulations allow) should review the POLST form periodically as required by law, and also if

- the patient is transferred from one care setting or care level to another,
- there is a substantial change in the patient's health status (for better or worse), or
- the patient or other decision maker changes his or her mind about treatment.

The advantages of POLST forms are such that their use is supported by the American Hospital Association, AARP, the National Hospice and Palliative Care Organization, and other groups. At the community level, a project sponsored by Excellus BlueCross and BlueShield in Upstate New York has worked to educate the community about that state's POLST program (called Medical Orders for Life-Sustaining Treatment [MOLST]) (Compassion and Support, 2014a). The project has engaged employers, insured members, and clinicians in efforts to increase advance care planning and adherence to patients' informed preferences (see also Chapter 6).

The POLST form is neither an advance directive nor a replacement for advance directives (Bomba et al., 2012; National POLST, 2012e). Both advance directives and the POLST form are helpful advance care planning documents for communicating patient wishes when appropriately used. As discussed in this chapter, one of the principal problems with the "living will" type of advance directive is that it may have been completed when a person was in relatively good health. At that point, it is almost impossible for people to predict the kind of care they would want in some future, more compromised state. Another problem is that clinicians often are unaware of the existence of the advance directive and do not always follow it if they are, if only because they believe patients' former wishes are not relevant in their current situation. Finally, advance directives often do not accompany patients as they transfer between care settings. The POLST form is designed to overcome these limitations. Salient features of the POLST form

TABLE 3-6 Differences Between POLST and Advance Directives

Characteristics	POLST	Advance Directives
Intended for	People who are seriously ill	All adults
Applies to	Current care	Future care
Form completed by	Health care professionals, based on in-depth discussion with their patients	Patients
Resulting form	Medical orders	Advance directive
Health care agent or surrogate role	Can engage in discussion if patient lacks capacity	Cannot complete
Portability	Clinician responsibility	Patient/family responsibility
Periodic review	Clinician responsibility	Patient/family responsibility

SOURCE: Adapted from Bomba et al., 2012.

and the ways in which it differs from advance directives are summarized in Table 3-6.

Like advance directives, POLST forms allow patients to choose a range of intensities of care, from comfort measures only to full treatment, and to indicate whether they want emergency medical services personnel to attempt resuscitation. In one study of more than 700 patients with POLST in place, 42 percent specified comfort measures only, 47 percent specified limited interventions, and 12 percent specified full treatment (Hickman et al., 2010).

Effects of POLST on Patient Care

The developers of the POLST paradigm have conducted a number of studies to document its effects. These studies have yielded the following findings:

- The treatment preferences of nursing home residents without a POLST form were less likely to be reflected in medical orders, and their preferences for treatment other than cardiopulmonary resuscitation were less likely to be recorded (Hickman et al., 2010).
- Nursing home residents with POLST comfort measures only orders were less likely to receive life-prolonging treatments than those with POLST limited treatment or full treatment orders and those with traditional do-not-resuscitate and traditional full-code orders (Hickman et al., 2010).

- Having a POLST form made no difference in the amount of symptom care patients received (Hickman et al., 2010).
- Treatments provided to nursing home residents were highly consistent with POLST orders for resuscitation (98 percent), medical interventions including hospitalization (91 percent), and antibiotic administration (93 percent), but less consistent with orders regarding use of feeding tubes (64 percent) (Hickman et al., 2011).
- Patients whose POLST orders specified higher levels of medical treatment received that treatment (Hammes et al., 2012; Hickman et al., 2011).
- Care diverged from that specified in POLST orders only rarely (Hammes et al., 2012).
- One-half to three-quarters of patients with a POLST form specifying no resuscitation attempt nevertheless had orders for limited additional interventions or full treatment, which can include other medical interventions or life-sustaining treatments (Fromme et al., 2012; Hickman et al., 2009).

New York authorized the statewide use of MOLST in all care settings in 2008 after a successful 3-year community pilot was conducted to ensure that emergency medical services personnel could read and follow do-not-resuscitate and do-not-intubate orders on the MOLST form (Compassion and Support, 2008). Standardized professional training and community education materials, policies and procedures, and a quality assurance program were developed. Community-wide quality and implementation data were collected from emergency medical services, hospitals, nursing homes, hospices, assisted living facilities, enriched housing facilities, and Program of All-inclusive Care for the Elderly (PACE) programs in two Upstate New York counties (Caprio and Gillespie, 2008; Compassion and Support, undated-b).

California authorized the use of POLST in 2009, and efforts have been made to encourage facilities in the state, including nursing homes, to adopt their use. Among 283 respondents to a survey of state nursing homes, 69 percent reported that they had admitted a resident who had a POLST form (Wenger et al., 2012). Overall, 54 percent of nursing home residents had a POLST form. Fewer than 10 percent of nursing homes reported any difficulties in following the POLST orders or having emergency personnel follow them; however, problems that reportedly did arise with more frequency included

- difficulty in retrieving original POLST forms from other facilities (62 percent of respondents),

- difficulty in getting physicians to complete (38 percent) and sign (34 percent) the forms,
- family disagreement with the content of the forms (28 percent), and
- difficulty in interpreting POLST orders to make treatment decisions (21 percent).

Oregon researchers conducted a small survey of emergency medical services personnel to learn the impact of POLST on their work. They found that POLST orders affected both treatment and decisions regarding whether to transport patients to a hospital (Schmidt et al., 2013). Another recent study of 58,000 decedents in Oregon found that nearly 31 percent had POLST forms entered in Oregon's POLST registry. Among those whose completed POLST forms stated a preference for comfort measures only ("Patient prefers no transfer to hospital for life-sustaining treatments. Transfer if comfort needs cannot be met in current location."), that preference was highly likely to be honored (Fromme et al., 2014, p. 2). Only 6.4 percent of these decedents died in a hospital, compared with 34.2 percent of decedents without a POLST form in the registry. This suggests that such forms can be effective in limiting unwanted life-sustaining treatment.

New POLST programs in many states have carried out substantial community engagement efforts with diverse audiences. These efforts are intended to provide education about the program, especially how the POLST form differs from conventional advance directives; to obtain consumer and professional input; and to build momentum for statewide adoption (examples include the efforts of New York, described at http://www.compassion andsupport.org, and those of the Massachusetts Department of Public Health [2011]).

Challenges to POLST

Although many states have or are working to implement POLST, opposition to the paradigm has emerged in some communities, in some cases as a result of confusion between POLST and advance directives. For example, disability rights advocates successfully lobbied against Connecticut's effort to enact POLST legislation in spring 2013 because they felt POLST limited rather than expanded patient options (Hargrave, 2013). Some Catholic theologians and organizations, including the Catholic Medical Association, have also raised objections to POLST (Brugger et al., 2013; Nienstedt et al., 2013), while others have endorsed them when used properly (Catholic Bishops of New York State, 2011). In a letter to the committee, the Catholic Health Association, which takes the view that portable medical documents such as POLST forms can be useful, emphasized the importance of "attending to some of the identified shortcomings and risks of these documents"

(Rodgers and Picchi, 2013, p. 2). Their concerns related to POLST include the following:

- The definition of whom POLST are for—The core idea is that POLST are for people who are seriously ill and near the end of life, but deviations from that notion have been seen.[33]
- Relevant training of health professionals—People who work with POLST, especially emergency personnel and staff of long-term care facilities, need training in the POLST process; effective communications regarding its use; and other skills, such as an understanding of the applicability of a POLST form in a given situation so they do not deny treatment for remediable problems that are not imminently life-threatening.
- Potential lack of meaningful conversation—Clinicians may simply check off the boxes on the POLST form without having the necessary conversations with patients and health care agents. In New York State, an eight-step protocol has been developed to guide clinician-patient/family interactions so as to ensure thoughtful MOLST discussions (Bomba et al., 2012).
- Significance of the clinician's signature—Physicians or other clinicians sign the form, but attest only that the orders are to the best of their knowledge consistent with the patient's current medical condition and preferences, not that they participated in the discussion of the orders. But the POLST form cannot be viewed as "simply another form to be completed by the health care professional, separated from the context of the advance care planning that is essential to the POLST paradigm" (Rodgers and Picchi, 2013, p. 2), because physicians are accountable for the medical orders in the form when they sign it.
- Voluntary nature of POLST—Perhaps especially in long-term care facilities and other institutional settings, the fundamental voluntary nature of POLST, in whole or in part, must be safeguarded, and completion of a POLST form should not be a requirement.

Respecting Choices

One of the best-known advance directive initiatives is Respecting Choices, a community-wide effort begun in 1991 in LaCrosse, Wisconsin.

---

[33]For example, Delaware's Division of Public Health asked medical providers to discontinue using the state's MOLST form until it could be revised because the agency determined it was being used for non–terminally ill patients, which is "beyond the legal parameters set forth in regulation 4304" (Delaware Health and Social Services, 2012).

Initially working with the city's major health systems, the program was aimed not only at encouraging people to complete advance directives, although that is a challenging task in itself, but also at changing the institutional and professional culture and routines to promote and respect advance care planning in a comprehensive way (AHRQ, 2010; Gundersen Health System, 2014a,b). The program produces educational materials for patients; trains facilitators to discuss end-of-life questions with patients and prepare them for the end of life; and ensures that advance directives are available in patients' medical records, now electronically. The project has also adopted the POLST paradigm (Hammes et al., 2012). Each health system promised to

- initiate advance care planning for each patient long before a medical crisis occurs,
- skillfully assist each willing patient with an individualized planning process,
- ensure that any plans created are clear and complete,
- have plans available to the health professionals who may participate in decision making when the patient is incapacitated, and
- follow plans appropriately and respect the values and preferences of the patient as allowed by law and organizational policy (Hammes, 2003, p. 2).

Making such a program work effectively requires embedding advance care planning in the community's larger health system to enable professionals to communicate and collaborate on making improvements, creating ongoing monitoring and feedback loops for quality improvement, and sustaining the effort with ongoing financial support and staff training (Hammes, 2003). Two years after the implementation of the Respecting Choices program, a study found that among 540 decedents, 85 percent had a written advance directive, which in almost all cases (95 percent) was found in the patient's medical record (Hammes and Rooney, 1998). In general, treatment preferences captured in the directives were followed when end-of-life treatment decisions were made. Accomplishing all this requires "nothing less than a cultural shift in the health care sector" (in der Schmitten et al., 2011, p. 8).

An early review of Respecting Choices describes six ways in which this program differs from conventional advance care planning initiatives, which help account for its success in achieving care in greater accord with patient wishes:

- It treats advance care planning as an ongoing process, not as an event designed to produce a product.

- It shifts the focus of end-of-life decision making away from document completion and toward facilitating discussion of values and preferences.
- It shifts the locus of planning from hospitals and physicians to the community and family.
- It does not assume the physician is crucial to the process, but promotes extensive training of nonphysician community volunteers.
- It refocuses discussion of preferences away from autonomy and toward personal relationships, for example, by asking the question, "How can you guide your loved ones to make the best decisions for you?".
- It works with hospitals and area physician offices to ensure that completed advance directives are available in patients' charts (Prendergast, 2001, p. N37).

The LaCrosse initiative has been used as a model for advance care planning programs for specific settings and populations, such as nursing homes (in der Schmitten et al., 2011), and for patients with advanced chronic illnesses, such as heart failure, who may be experiencing disease complications or frequent hospitalizations (Schellinger et al., 2011; see also Annex 3-1). Respecting Choices leader Bernard Hammes (2003) describes several barriers to implementation that must be overcome if the program is to be successfully replicated. First is the need to allow sufficient time to train health professionals and discussion facilitators. At the time Hammes was writing, the program recommended a 14-hour training program for facilitators and had found efforts to shorten this time unsuccessful. Hammes (2003) also cites as barriers the need to make the necessary system changes that establish advance care planning as the routine way to offer care and the need for funding for the costs of the program. Hammes acknowledges as well that transferring this model to more culturally diverse regions of the United States would be a challenge because a highly diverse population makes it more difficult to normalize the advance care planning conversation. In addition, many older people are accustomed to thinking of advance directives as "living wills"—a one-time recording of their wishes intended solely to preserve autonomy. They need to understand the new program's more organic, discussion-based approach that evolves over time with clinical situations and health status.

Electronic Health Records

Electronic storage of advance directives, statements of wishes, health care proxies, or other relevant materials—either in the patient's electronic

---

BOX 3-3
New York State's eMOLST

New York State's eMOLST program is an example of well-coordinated electronic documentation of advance care choices. eMOLST is a secure Web-based application that clinicians can use with patients. The application's standardized clinical process emphasizes shared, informed decision making in completing the eMOLST form. In addition, a Chart Documentation Form provides details about the eMOLST discussion, including information on patients' values, beliefs, and goals for care; capacity determination; and the framework for making MOLST decisions, based on who makes the decision and where it is made, in accordance with New York State's Public Health Law.

eMOLST forms are created as pdf documents, which can be printed out for patients to keep and for insertion in paper-based medical records. The forms can also be stored or linked in electronic health records. Thus, the forms and supporting documentation are accessible regardless of whether an electronic health record is in use.

In addition, the forms become part of the state's eMOLST registry, an electronic database that allows for ready round-the-clock availability of eMOLST forms and the detailed Chart Documentation Form. With this system, health care providers, including emergency personnel, can have access to eMOLST forms and supporting documentation at any time or place.

SOURCES: Compassion and Support, 2013, 2014b, undated-a.

---

health record or an external database—holds promise for solving some current problems with these documents. An example is described in Box 3-3.

A 2013 telephone survey of New York nursing homes found that almost 58 percent had implemented eMOLST, while 61 percent indicated interest in the program. A similar survey of hospices in the state found that 38 percent had implemented eMOLST, while 44 percent were interested. A similar survey of hospitals is under way.[34]

In theory, electronic systems should facilitate finding advance planning documents when critical decisions must be made. If records use a standard template, it may be easier to locate the relevant information to determine whether current care preferences are reflected in the medical record (Yung et al., 2010). According to Wilson and colleagues (2013, p. 1093), "Standardization is a fundamental prerequisite for efficient production and effective delivery of services," and electronic systems can—although they do

---

[34]Personal communication, P. A. Bomba, Community Conversations on Compassionate Care, 2013.

not always—achieve standardization. Another potential advantage of having advance directives in electronic health records is that they can remind clinicians to inquire whether patients' care preferences have changed and whether they wish to update the identity and contact information for their health care agent. For example, Partners Health System has pioneered an innovative and complete electronic health record module that supports appropriate discussion and documentation of end-of-life planning (Block, 2013). The module includes areas for documenting individuals' preferences for receiving information about their illness, their understanding of their illness, and their goals and fears. Some of the other diverse and innovative ways in which clinicians and institutions are using electronic means to support advance care planning are described in Table 3-7.

Currently, however, there are some gaps in practice. Not all advance directive registries are linked to patients' electronic health records. In addition, while electronic health records have increased the documentation of advance directives, they have resulted in "an increase in inaccurate

TABLE 3-7 Selected Examples of the Use of Electronic Health Records and Other Technologies to Support End-of-Life Planning

Example	Outcome
Discharge summary template in the electronic health record to include care wishes expressed and health care agent (Lakin et al., 2013)	Given a modest incentive payment and feedback, clinicians recorded this information for more than 90% of patients discharged, compared with 12% of clinicians not offered these inducements.
Various models providing an electronic registry for 24-hour access to POLST forms and related documents (Zive and Schmidt, 2012)	Some models (such as New York's eMOLST) also enable completion of standardized forms that can be integrated into patients' electronic health records.
Web-based systems for education about end-of-life choices, forms and assistance in their completion, and document storage (Klugman and Usatine, 2012)	A Nevada pilot ended because of low usage and budget cuts; more than 5,000 accounts were created for a Texas repository in its first 3 years, and it was appreciated for its "ease of use."
Interactive computer program that helps users clarify values and goals and record care preferences (Schubart et al., 2012)	In preliminary stages; a pilot shows the computer program had good reliability in representing patients' general wishes and preferences.
Advance directive module in patient portals, alongside modules encouraging personal management of health (Bose-Brill and Pressler, 2012)	In preliminary stages; there is growing interest in and use of portals by patients.

advance directive documentation from labeling errors made in transfer of information to the [electronic health record]," and systems of advance care planning and electronic health records have not yet been well coordinated (Bose-Brill and Pressler, 2012, p. 286). For example, EpicCare is one of the principal electronic health record systems adopted by U.S. health care providers. A study of the availability of advance care planning documents (including living wills, POLST forms, information about health care agents, and do-not-resuscitate orders) was conducted among active patients in EpicCare's ambulatory care electronic health record system (Wilson et al., 2013). The study found that, while 51 percent of those aged 65 and older had such a document, only about one-third of their records included a scanned document—the only type that includes signatures, which are required to make them legally valid. Minority patients were less likely to have a scanned document. Additional problems included a lack of standardization in where in the record advance care planning information is recorded, thwarting easy retrieval, and a time lag between completion of advance care planning documents and their appearance in the electronic record.

Under the Health Information Technology for Economic and Clinical Health (HITECH) Act,[35] Medicare and Medicaid have provided significant financial incentives for hospitals and physicians to engage in "meaningful use" of certified electronic health record technology (CMS, 2014). To receive these payments, physicians and hospitals must show they are "meaningfully using" electronic records to achieve certain specific objectives established by the Centers for Medicare & Medicaid Services. Thus far, the data standards related to advance care planning have been minimal, applying only to hospital patients aged 65 and older, but the evolution of meaningful use offers possibilities for expansion in various core areas, such as patient education and patient engagement. As noted earlier in this chapter, the ACA's meaningful use provisions for electronic health records do not require, and the major commercial electronic health records do not provide for, robust documentation of advance care planning, including advance directives, POLST, or information about designation of and contact information for a health care agent. Meaningful use stage 2 includes as an objective only to "record whether a patient 65 years old or older has an advance directive" (CMS, 2012c, p. 1); further, this is not considered a "core" objective, and it is relevant only for eligible hospitals and critical access hospitals, not for eligible professionals (CMS, 2012d,e). Final recommendations from the Health Information Technology Policy Committee for meaningful use stage 3 maintained this stage 2 objective; however, the policy committee is now

---

[35]Health Information Technology for Economic and Clinical Health (HITECH) Act, Title XIII of Division A and Title IV of Division B of the American Recovery and Reinvestment Act of 2009 (ARRA), Public Law 111-5, 111th Cong., 1st sess. (February 17, 2009).

recommending that it be a core objective for eligible hospitals and a menu objective for eligible professionals (HHS, 2014). (See also the discussion of research needs related to electronic health records in Chapter 5, as well as that chapter's recommendation.)

A PROPOSED LIFE CYCLE MODEL OF ADVANCE CARE PLANNING

As reflected in the standards of the National Framework and Preferred Practices for Palliative and Hospice Care Quality (NQF, 2006), discussed earlier, good advance care planning is not a one-time event, but should occur at appropriate decision points throughout life, roughly as detailed below (Benson and Aldrich, 2012; Bomba, 2005). The following life cycle model of advance care planning is based on these standards and practices, findings from the extant literature reviewed in this chapter, and the committee's expertise and expert judgment. Considering the aspects of advance care planning throughout the life cycle continuum normalizes the process and aims to avoid the emotional burden sometimes experienced by patients, families, and loved ones who have not adequately prepared for making end-of-life care decisions. This proposed model has implications for quality improvement programs, clinician training, public and patient education, and payment systems.

Milestone-Specific

Under the life cycle model proposed by the committee, an initial conversation about values and life goals is held at some key maturation point—such as obtaining a driver's license, turning 18, leaving home to go to school or into the military, or marriage (milestones when risks may change or the locus of responsibility shifts):

- The presumption is that the person is generally healthy and mentally competent, but like everyone is at risk for acute illness or injury and sudden (and possibly temporary) loss of capacity to make medical decisions.
- The purpose of the conversation at this point is to help normalize the advance care planning process by starting it early, to identify a health care agent, and to obtain guidance in the event of a rare catastrophic event.
- The consultation might be performed by a trained counselor, advanced practice nurse, physician assistant, or social worker.

Situation-Specific

Additional discussion of values and life goals is held, for example, with people in high-risk occupations; those involved in high-risk activities, including military training or deployment; and those with major genetic or congenital issues:

- Again, the presumption is that the person is in good health.
- The purpose is to ensure that a health care agent has been designated and to take into consideration any family issues (e.g., spouse, children).
- The consultation might be performed by a trained counselor, advanced practice nurse, physician assistant, or social worker.

As Part of Primary Care

Regular and periodic conversations are held with patients who do not have a serious disease regarding their values, goals, and preferences:

- This conversation can be led by a nonphysician.
- The choice of health care agent should be reviewed.

Initial Diagnosis of Chronic Illness (Disease Management)

Further discussion takes place at the initial diagnosis of a chronic life-limiting illness (although the end-point still may be years out):

- A physician should explain the diagnosis, the likely course of the illness, complications to watch for, and ways to slow the disease's progression.
- A nonphysician can ensure that a health care agent is named and encourage a conversation about what it means to be an agent and what patient-agent discussions should take place.

As Health Worsens (Case Management)

Discussion also takes place at turning points in the disease (major treatment changes; significant side effects or "turns for the worse"; onset of comorbidities):

- Members of the care team can participate in these discussions, which should also include the designated health care agent. As the disease worsens, family members may benefit from counseling and practical advice. Spiritual counseling can be offered.

- Patient and family should be asked how much information they want about prognosis and what to expect.

In the Final Year of Expected Life

Discussion takes place again when death would not be a surprise if it occurred in the next year:

- The opportunity for thoughtful POLST discussions is offered to increase the likelihood that preferences for care and treatment are accessible and honored.
- A "palliative care time out"—a required family meeting after a patient has been in intensive care for a certain number of days—is held so that everyone stops and reconsiders what is being done and why.
- Members of the interdisciplinary health care team work with the family and health care agent to support their role and potentially forestall complicated bereavement.
- Members of the interdisciplinary health care team obtain help for the family with practical matters.

Special Considerations for Seriously Ill Children

Children transitioning from childhood to adulthood should choose a health care agent. For minors with decision-making capacity near the end of life, according to the NQF standard, the child's views and preferences for medical care, including assent for treatment, should be documented and given appropriate weight in decision making (NQF, 2006; Dahlin, 2013). When the child's wishes differ from those of the adult decision maker, appropriate professional staff members should be made available for consultation and intervention.

RESEARCH NEEDS

A large body of research exists on advance directives—whether they have been created, whether they have been followed, and what impact they have on important outcomes of care. This literature is a principal reason that the usefulness of simple checkbox-style documents has come into question. Much less research has been conducted on the effectiveness of more thorough advance care planning conducted over time and tailored to immediate decisions as needed, as in the life cycle model described above. Also needed is further investigation into how advances in thinking about shared decision making and behavioral economics can be applied specifically in end-of-life situations. A focus on preparing people for in-the-moment decision making, rather than specifying exact treatment preferences, holds promise as well. With respect to the POLST paradigm and other community-wide efforts to encourage advance care planning, the research challenge is one of developing and validating best practices to ensure the integrity of these program models as they are diffused to other settings. Likewise, investigations should be initiated to determine the most effective ways in which electronic health records can support advance care planning.

Decision-making theory points to the various means used by individuals to arrive at important decisions; the stages of change theory described in this chapter is one such model. A better understanding of patient and family decision-making styles might help clinicians work with their patients more effectively and lead to decisions most relevant and appropriate to each patient. In addition, more information is needed on the way the care system respects, responds to, and sometimes shapes the decisions of patients and whether or in what ways this is affected by race, gender, income, literacy, insurance status, or other factors. Findings from such research should be useful in improving communication between clinicians and the full range of patients they serve. This type of research might lead to the development of appropriate decision supports as well.

Specific research needs include investigation into the effectiveness of strategies for advance care planning (versus advance directives) and their effects on achieving concordance with patients' informed preferences and quality of care. Specific needs relate also to

- the development of guidelines for pediatric and adolescent advance care planning;
- continued research toward understanding children's involvement in end-of-life decision making and comparative effectiveness studies of different approaches to decision support and communication;
- understanding of racial, ethnic, and cultural differences in advance care planning among nursing home residents;
- best practices and needs for different Asian, Hispanic, and South Asian populations;
- ways to improve shared decision making;
- the significance of and strategies for implementing choice architecture in advance care planning programs; and
- the most effective and cost-effective designs for financial incentives and reimbursement for clinicians to participate in advance care

planning, recognizing that doing so takes time and may require repeated consultations.

FINDINGS, CONCLUSIONS, AND RECOMMENDATION

Findings and Conclusions

This study yielded the following findings and conclusions on alignment of the care patients receive with the care they want.

Decision-Making Capacity

Most people nearing the end of life are not physically, mentally, or cognitively able to make their own decisions about care. Approximately 40 percent of adult medical inpatients, 44-69 percent of nursing home residents, and 70 percent of older adults facing treatment decisions are incapable of making those decisions themselves. Furthermore, the majority of these patients will receive acute hospital care from physicians who do not know them. As a result, advance care planning is essential to ensure that people receive care that reflects their values, goals, and preferences (Kim et al., 2002; Nelson et al., 2006; Raymont et al., 2004; Silveira et al., 2010).

Comfort-Focused Care Versus Acute Care

People who capture their preferences for care near the end of life most commonly, but not always, choose care that is focused on alleviating pain and suffering. Because the default mode of treatment is acute care in the hospital, however, a higher prevalence of advance care planning and medical orders will be more likely to achieve patient preferences (Billings, 2012; Mack et al., 2010b; Wright et al., 2008).

Implementation of Patient Wishes

Most people, even those who are older and have serious illnesses, do not complete advance directives, and even when these documents are completed, they rarely affect treatment decisions. They often are unavailable or difficult to interpret, and they may contradict the preferences of the family or clinicians. On the other hand, people who have had conversations about end-of-life care values, goals, and preferences (although they may not have completed formal advance directive documents) are less likely to receive unwanted treatment. Advance care planning should be considered a life-long process. Health care agents should be identified early in this process, and for people with advanced serious illnesses, POLST forms should be used (Ditto et al., 2006; Fried et al., 2007; Hammes et al., 2012; Hickman et al., 2011; Kelley et al., 2011; NQF, 2006). However, most people—particularly younger, poorer, minority, and less educated individuals—do not have conversations about end-of-life care. Clinicians need to recognize the multiple barriers to effective communication on these issues, initiate the conversation themselves, and take time and make the effort to ensure that patient and family decisions are made with adequate information and understanding (Clements, 2009; Curtis and Engelberg, 2011; Phipps et al., 2003; Sudore et al., 2010; Volandes et al., 2008a; Waite et al., 2003).

Lack of Clinician Communication Skills

The quality of communication between clinicians and patients who have advanced serious illnesses or are nearing death falls far short of the ideal, particularly with respect to discussing prognosis, dealing with emotional and spiritual concerns, and finding the right balance between hoping for the best and preparing for the worst. Advance care planning will not succeed without improved communication generally. Incentives, quality standards, and system support for the time required to conduct such conversations are necessary to promote improved communication that meets the standards expected by patients and families (Anderson et al., 2008; Back et al., 2003; Dias et al., 2003; Epstein and Street, 2007; NQF, 2006; Smith et al., 2013b).

> **Recommendation 2. Professional societies and other organizations that establish quality standards should develop standards for clinician-patient communication and advance care planning that are measurable, actionable, and evidence-based. These standards should change as needed to reflect the evolving population and health system needs and be consistent with emerging evidence, methods, and technologies. Payers and health care delivery organizations should adopt these standards and their supporting processes, and integrate them into assessments, care plans, and the reporting of health care quality. Payers should tie such standards to reimbursement, and professional societies should adopt policies that facilitate tying the standards to reimbursement, licensing, and credentialing to encourage**
>
> - **all individuals, including children with the capacity to do so, to have the opportunity to participate actively in their health care decision making throughout their lives and as they approach death, and receive medical and related social services consistent with their values, goals, and informed preferences;**
> - **clinicians to initiate high-quality conversations about advance care**

planning, integrate the results of these conversations into the ongoing care plans of patients, and communicate with other clinicians as requested by the patient; and

- clinicians to continue to revisit advance care planning discussions with their patients because individuals' preferences and circumstances may change over time.

REFERENCES

Abbott, C. H., H. G. Prigerson, and P. K. Maciejewski. 2013. The influence of patients' quality of life at the end of life on bereaved caregivers' suicidal ideation. *Journal of Pain and Symptom Management* [epub ahead of print].

AHRQ (Agency for Healthcare Research and Quality). 2010. *Service delivery innovation profile: Community-wide education, trained facilitators, and improved processes lead to more advance care planning, consistency between plans and end-of-life decisions, and low care costs.* http://www.innovations.ahrq.gov/content.aspx?id=2713 (accessed June 1, 2014).

Albrecht, G. L., and P. J. Devlieger. 1999. The disability paradox: High quality of life against all odds. *Social Science & Medicine* 48(8):977-988.

Allen, J. Y., W. E. Haley, B. J. Small, R. S. Schonwetter, and S. C. McMillan. 2013. Bereavement among hospice caregivers of cancer patients one year following loss: Predictors of grief, complicated grief, and symptoms of depression. *Journal of Palliative Medicine* 16(7):745-751.

American Bar Association. 2005. *Consumer's tool kit for health care advance planning.* 2nd ed. Washington, DC: American Bar Association Commission on Law and Aging.

American Bar Association. 2009. *Default surrogate consent statutes.* http://www.americanbar.org/content/dam/aba/migrated/aging/PublicDocuments/famcon_2009.authcheckdam.pdf (accessed June 30, 2014).

American Health Decisions. 1997. *The quest to die with dignity: An analysis of Americans' values, opinions and attitudes concerning end-of-life care.* Executive summary. http://www.ahd.org/The_Quest_to_Die_With_Dignity.html (accessed August 1, 2013).

American Lung Association. 2013. *Trends in COPD (chronic bronchitis and emphysema): Morbidity and mortality.* http://www.lung.org/finding-cures/our-research/trend-reports/copd-trend-report.pdf (accessed June 2, 2014).

Anderson, G. T. 2006. *What y'all gon' do with me?: The African-American spiritual and ethical guide to end of life care.* http://www.stu.ca/~spirituality/GloriaThomasAnderson-TheAfricanAmericanSpiritualandEthicalEndofLifeCareGuidepresentation2006.pdf (accessed June 2, 2014).

Anderson, W. G., S. C. Alexander, K. L. Rodriguez, A. S. Jeffreys, M. K. Olsen, K. I. Pollak, J. A. Tulsky, and R. M. Arnold. 2008. "What concerns me is..." Expressions of emotion by advanced cancer patients during outpatient visits. *Supportive Care in Cancer* 16(7):803-811.

Apatira, L., E. A. Boyd, G. Malvar, L. R. Evans, J. M. Luce, B. Lo, and D. B. White. 2008. Hope, truth, and preparing for death: Perspectives of surrogate decision makers. *Annals of Internal Medicine* 149(12):861-868.

Artnak, K. E. 2008. Ethics consultation in dual diagnosis of mental illness and mental retardation: Medical decision-making for community-dwelling persons. *Cambridge Quarterly of Healthcare Ethics* 17:239-246.

Azoulay, E., F. Pochard, N. Kentish-Barnes, S. Chevret, J. Aboab, C. Adrie, D. Annane, G. Bleichner, P. E. Bollaert, M. Darmon, T. Fassier, R. Galliot, M. Garrouste-Orgeas, C. Goulenok, D. Goldgran-Toledano, J. Hayon, M. Jourdain, M. Kaidomar, C. Laplace, J. Larché, J. Liotier, L. Papazian, C. Poisson, J. Reignier, F. Saidi, and B. Schlemmer. 2005. Risk of post-traumatic stress symptoms in family members of intensive care unit patients. *American Journal of Respiratory and Critical Care Medicine* 171(9):987-994.

Back, A. L., R. M. Arnold, and T. E. Quill. 2003. Hope for the best, and prepare for the worst. Medical writings. *Annals of Internal Medicine* 138(5):439-443.

Back, A. L., R. M. Arnold, W. F. Baile, K. A. Edwards, and J. A. Tulsky. 2010. When praise is worth considering in a difficult conversation. Perspectives. *Lancet* 376(9744):866-867.

Baer, J., M. Kutner, J. Sabatini, and S. White. 2009. *Basic reading skills and the literacy of America's least literate adults: Results from the 2003 National Assessment of Adult Literacy.* NCES 2009-481. Washington, DC: National Center for Education Statistics. http://nces.ed.gov/pubs2009/2009481.pdf (accessed February 10, 2014).

Balboni, T. A., L. C. Vanderwerker, S. D. Block, M. E. Paulk, C. S. Lathan, J. R. Peteet, and H. G. Prigerson. 2007. Religiousness and spiritual support among advanced cancer patients and associations with end-of-life treatment preferences and quality of life. *Journal of Clinical Oncology* 25(5):555-560.

Balboni, T., M. Balboni, M. E. Paulk, A. Phelps, A. Wright, J. Peteet, S. Block, C. Lathan, T. VanderWeele, and H. Prigerson. 2011. Support of cancer patients' spiritual needs and associations with medical care costs at the end of life. *Cancer* 117(23):5383-5391.

Balboni, T. A., M. Balboni, A. C. Enzinger, K. Gallivan, E. Paulk, A. Wright, K. Steinhauser, T. J. VanderWeele, and H. G. Prigerson. 2013. Provision of spiritual support to patients with advanced cancer by religious communities and associations with medical care at the end of life. *JAMA Internal Medicine* 173(12):1109-1117.

Barclay, S., N. Momen, S. Case-Upton, I. Kuhn, and E. Smith. 2011. End-of-life care conversations with heart failure patients: A systematic literature review and narrative synthesis. *British Journal of General Practice* 61(582):e49-e62.

Barnato, A. E., Z. Berhane, L. A. Weissfeld, C-C. H. Chang, W. T. Linde-Zwirble, and D. C. Angus. 2006. Racial variation in end-of-life intensive care use: A race or hospital effect? *Health Services Research* 41(6):2219-2237.

Barnato, A. E., C-C. H. Chang, O. Saynin, and A. M. Garber. 2007. Influence of race on inpatient treatment intensity at the end of life. *Journal of General Internal Medicine* 22(3):338-345.

Barnato, A. E., D. Mohan, J. Downs, C. L. Bryce, D. C. Angus, and R. M. Arnold. 2011. A randomized trial of the effect of patient race on physicians' intensive care unit and life-sustaining treatment decisions for an acutely unstable elder with end-stage cancer. *Critical Care Medicine* 39(7):1663-1669.

Bélanger, E., C. Rodríguez, and D. Groleau. 2010. Shared decision-making in palliative care: A systematic mixed studies review using narrative synthesis. *Palliative Medicine* 25(3):242-261.

Benson, W. F., and N. Aldrich. 2012. *Advance care planning: Ensuring your wishes are known and honored if you are unable to speak for yourself, critical issue brief.* Atlanta, GA: CDC. http://www.cdc.gov/aging/pdf/advanced-care-planning-critical-issue-brief.pdf (accessed June 1, 2014).

Berkman, N. D., S. L. Sheridan, K. E. Donahue, D. J. Halpern, A. Viera, K. Crotty, A. Holland, M. Brasure, K. N. Lohr, E. Harden, E. Tant, I. Wallace, and M. Viswanathan. 2011. *Health literacy interventions and outcomes: An updated systematic review.* Evidence Report/Technology Assessment No. 199. AHRQ Publication No. 11-E006. Rockville, MD: AHRQ.

Berlinger, N., B. Jennings, and S. M. Wolf. 2013. *The Hastings Center guidelines for decisions on life-sustaining treatment and care near the end of life.* 2nd ed. New York: Oxford University Press.

Billings, J. A. 2012. The need for safeguards in advance care planning. *Journal of General Internal Medicine* 27(5):595-600.

Blank, R. H. 2011. End-of-life decision making across cultures. *The Journal of Law, Medicine & Ethics* 39(2):201-214.

Block, S. D. 2013. *Assuring safe passage: Moving conversations about the end of life upstream.* Chicago, IL: The University of Chicago Department of Medicine Grand Rounds. http://medicine.uchicago.edu/grandrounds/assuring%20safe%20passage%20101513.ppt (accessed May 26, 2014).

Bluebond-Langner, M., J. B. Belasco, A. Goldman, and C. Belasco. 2007. Understanding parents' approaches to care and treatment of children with cancer when standard therapy has failed. *Journal of Clinical Oncology* 25(17):2414-2419.

Bomba, P. A. 2005. Advance care planning along the continuum. *The Case Manager* 16(2):68-72.

Bomba, P. A., and D. Vermilyea. 2006. Integrating POLST into palliative care guidelines: A paradigm shift in advance care planning in oncology. *Journal of the National Comprehensive Cancer Network* 4(8):819-829.

Bomba, P. A., M. Kemp, and J. S. Black. 2012. POLST: An improvement over traditional advance directives. *Cleveland Clinic Journal of Medicine* 79(7):457-464.

Bose-Brill, S., and T. R. Pressler. 2012. Commentary: Opportunities for innovation and improvement in advance care planning using a tethered patient portal in the electronic health record. *Journal of Primary Care & Community Health* 3(4):285-288.

Boyd, E. A., B. Lo, L. R. Evans, G. Malvar, L Apatira, J. M. Luce, and D. B. White. 2010. "It's not just what the doctor tells me": Factors that influence surrogate decision-makers' perceptions of prognosis. *Critical Care Medicine* 38(5):1270-1275.

Bruera, E., C. Sweeney, K. Calder, L. Palmer, and S. Benisch-Tolley. 2001. Patient preferences versus physician perceptions of treatment decisions in cancer care. *Journal of Clinical Oncology* 19(11):2883-2885.

Bruera, E., J. S. Willey, J. L. Palmer, and M. Rosales. 2002. Treatment decisions for breast carcinoma: Patient preferences and physician perceptions. *Cancer* 94(7):2076-2080.

Brugger, C., L. C. Breschi, E. M. Hart, M. Kummer, J. I. Lane, P. T. Morrow, F. L. Smith, W. L. Toffler, M. Beffel, J. F. Brehany, S. Buscher, and R. L. Marker. 2013. The POLST paradigm and form: Facts and analysis. *The Linacre Quarterly* 80(2):103-138.

Buck, H. G., and S. H. Meghani. 2012. Spiritual expressions of African Americans and whites in cancer pain. *Journal of Holistic Nursing* 30(2):107-116.

Burkle, C. M., P. S. Mueller, K. M. Swetz, C. C. Hook, and M. T. Keegan. 2012. Physician perspectives and compliance with patient advance directives: The role external factors play on physician decision making. *BMC Medical Ethics* 13:31.

Butow, P. N., R. F. Brown, S. Cogar, M. H. Tattersall, and S. M. Dunn. 2002. Oncologists' reactions to cancer patients' verbal cues. *Psycho-Oncology* 11(1):47-58.

Byock, I. 2013. This is personal! In *Trends in cancer care near the end of life: A Dartmouth Atlas of Health Care Brief,* edited by D. C. Goodman, N. E. Morden, C.-H. Chang, E. S. Fisher, and J. E. Wennberg. Lebanon, NH: The Dartmouth Atlas of Health Care. Pp. 5-8. http://www.dartmouthatlas.org/downloads/reports/Cancer_brief_090413.pdf (accessed September 6, 2013).

Caprio, T., and S. Gillespie. 2008. *Update on MOST facility implementation and quality improvement audits.* Presentation to the Monroe County MOLST Quality Forum. http://www.compassionandsupport.org/pdfs/news/MC_MOLST_Quaity_Forum_QI_Presentation.FINAL.ppt (accessed March 22, 2014).

Carlson, L. E., S. L. Groff, O. Maciejewski, and B. D. Bultz. 2010. Screening for distress in lung and breast cancer outpatients: A randomized controlled trial. *Journal of Clinical Oncology* 28(33):4884-4491.

Carlson, L. E., A. Waller, and A. J. Mitchell. 2012. Screening for distress and unmet needs in patients with cancer: Review and recommendations. *Journal of Clinical Oncology* 30(11):1160-1177.

Carr, D. 2011. *Why don't older adults prepare for the end of life? The social stratification of advance care planning.* Paper presented at Living in a High Inequality Regime Conference, Stanford University, Stanford, CA, November.

Carr, D. 2012a. Racial and ethnic differences in advance care planning: Identifying subgroup patterns and obstacles. *Journal of Aging and Health* 24(6):923-947.

Carr, D. 2012b. The social stratification of older adults' preparations for end-of-life health care. *Journal of Health and Social Behavior* 53(3):297-312.

Carr, D., and D. Khodyakov. 2007. Health care proxies: Whom do young old adults choose and why? *Journal of Health and Social Behavior* 48(2):180-194.

Carr, D., and S. M. Moorman. 2009. End-of-life treatment preferences among older adults: An assessment of psychosocial influences. *Sociological Forum* 24(4):754-778.

Castillo, L. S., B. A. Williams, S. M. Hooper, C. P. Sabatino, L. A. Weithorn, and R. L. Sudore. 2011. Lost in translation: The unintended consequences of advance directive law on clinical care. *Annals of Internal Medicine* 154(2):121-128.

Catholic Bishops of New York State. 2011. *Now and at the hour of our death: A Catholic guide to end-of-life decision-making.* http://www.nyscatholic.org/wp-content/uploads/2011/11/End-of-Life-booklet-final.pdf (accessed February 5, 2013).

CDC (Centers for Disease Control and Prevention). 2011. *Alzheimer's disease.* http://www.cdc.gov/aging/aginginfo/alzheimers.htm (accessed February 5, 2014).

CDC. 2012. Chronic obstructive pulmonary disease among adults—United States, 2011. *Morbidity and Mortality Weekly Report* 61(46):938-943.

CDC. 2013a. *Heart failure fact sheet.* http://www.cdc.gov/dhdsp/data_statistics/fact_sheets/fs_heart_failure.htm (accessed November 21, 2013).

CDC. 2013b. *Leading causes of death.* http://www.cdc.gov/nchs/fastats/leading-causes-of-death.htm (accessed June 2, 2014).

Ceronsky, L., and D. E. Weissman. 2011. Helping families in long-term care facing complex decisions: Applying the evidence about family meetings from other settings. *Annals of Long Term Care* 19(2):27-32.

CHCF (California HealthCare Foundation). 2012. *Final chapter: Californians' attitudes and experiences with death and dying.* http://www.chcf.org/~/media/MEDIA%20LIBRARY%20Files/PDF/F/PDF%20FinalChapterDeathDying.pdf (accessed August 7, 2013).

Chochinov, H. M., D. Tataryn, J. J. Clinch, and D. Dudgeon. 1999. Will to live in the terminally ill. *Lancet* 354(9181):816-819.

Christakis, N. A., and T. J. Iwashyna. 2003. The health impact of health care on families: A matched cohort study of hospice use by decedents and mortality outcomes in surviving, widowed spouses. *Social Science & Medicine* 57(3):465-475.

Christakis, N. A., and E. B. Lamont. 2000. Extent and determinants of error in physicians' prognoses in terminally ill patients: Prospective cohort study. *British Medical Journal* 320:469-473.

Clayton, J. M., P. N. Butow, R. M. Arnold, and M. H. N. Tattersall. 2005. Fostering coping and nurturing hope when discussing the future with terminally ill cancer patients and their caregivers. *Cancer* 103(9):1965-1975.

Clements, J. M. 2009. Patient perceptions on the use of advance directives and life prolonging technology. *American Journal of Hospice & Palliative Medicine* 26(4):270-276.

CMS (Centers for Medicare & Medicaid Services). 2012a. *Quick reference information: The ABCs of providing the initial preventive physical examination.* http://www.cms.gov/Outreach-and-Education/Medicare-Learning-Network-MLN/MLNProducts/downloads/MPS_QRI_IPPE001a.pdf (accessed October 17, 2013).

CMS. 2012b. *Medicare preventive services national provider call: The initial preventive physical exam and the annual wellness visit.* Presented on the MLN Connect National Provider Call, March 28. http://www.cms.gov/Outreach-and-Education/Outreach/NPC/Downloads/IPPE-AWV-NPC-Presentation.pdf (accessed November 22, 2013).

CMS. 2012c. *Stage 2 eligible hospital and critical access hospital meaningful use menu set measures: Measure 1 of 6.* http://www.cms.gov/Regulations-and-Guidance/Legislation/EHRIncentivePrograms/Downloads/Stage2_MeaningfulUseSpecSheet_TableContents_EPs.pdf (accessed June 2, 2014).

CMS. 2012d. *Stage 2 eligible hospital and critical access hospital (CAH) meaningful use core and menu objectives.* http://www.cms.gov/Regulations-and-Guidance/Legislation/EHRIncentivePrograms/Downloads/Stage2_MeaningfulUseSpecSheet_TableContents_EligibleHospitals_CAHs.pdf (accessed June 2, 2014).

CMS. 2012e. *Stage 2 eligible professional (EP) meaningful use core and menu objectives.* http://www.cms.gov/Regulations-and-Guidance/Legislation/EHRIncentivePrograms/Downloads/Stage2_MeaningfulUseSpecSheet_TableContents_EPs.pdf (accessed June 2, 2014).

CMS. 2014. *The official web site for the Medicare and Medicaid electronic health records (EHR) incentives programs.* http://www.cms.gov/Regulations-and-Guidance/Legislation/EHRIncentivePrograms/index.html?redirect=/ehrincentiveprograms (accessed June 1, 2014).

Colclough, Y. Y., and G. M. Brown. 2013. End-of-life treatment decision making: American Indians' perspective. *American Journal of Hospice & Palliative Medicine* [epub ahead of print].

Coleman, D. 2013. *Full written public comment: Disability related concerns about POLST.* http://www.notdeadyet.org/full-written-public-comment-disability-related-concerns-about-polst#_edn10 (accessed September 6, 2013).

Collins, S. P., P. S. Pang, G. C. Fonarow, C. W. Yancy, R. O. Bonow, and M. Gheorghiade. 2013. Is hospital admission for heart failure really necessary?: The role of the emergency department and observation unit in preventing hospitalization and rehospitalization. *Journal of the American College of Cardiology* 61(2):121-126.

Compassion and Support. 2008. *Medical Orders for Life-Sustaining Treatment (MOLST) Program: A POLST Paradigm Program: A Community-Wide End-of-Life/Palliative Care Initiative Project.* Poster presented to the Blue Cross Association Conference. http://www.compassionandsupport.org/pdfs/MOLST-poster.pdf (accessed May 29, 2014).

Compassion and Support. 2010. *Advance care planning: Know your choices, share your wishes. Maintain control, achieve peace of mind, and assure your wishes are honored.* http://www.compassionandsupport.org/pdfs/about/B-1576_Excellus_2010_Complete.pdf (accessed May 15, 2014).

Compassion and Support. 2013. *eMOLST program manual.* Vol. 10. http://www.compassionandsupport.org/pdfs/professionals/molst/eMOLSTProgramManual.pdf (accessed June 1, 2014).

Compassion and Support. 2014a. *About us.* https://www.compassionandsupport.org/index.php/about_us (accessed May 29, 2014).

Compassion and Support. 2014b. *eMOLST: Electronic Medical Orders for Life-Sustaining Treatment in New York State.* http://www.compassionandsupport.org/index.php/for_professionals/molst_training_center/emolst (accessed June 1, 2014).

Compassion and Support. undated-a. *EMS and MOLST pilot results.* http://www.compassion andsupport.org/pdfs/molst-training/ems-molst-pilot-results.pdf (accessed March 22, 2014).

Compassion and Support. undated-b. *eMOLST form completion (clinical) screenshots.* http:// www.compassionandsupport.org/pdfs/professionals/molst/eMOLSTFormCompletion Screenshots.pdf (accessed June 1, 2014).

The Conversation Project. 2013. *New survey reveals "conversation disconnect": 90 percent of Americans know they should have a conversation about what they want at the end of life, yet only 30 percent have done so.* News release. http://theconversationproject.org/ wp-content/uploads/2013/09/TCP-Survey-Release_FINAL-9-18-13.pdf (accessed September 18, 2013).

Cosgriff, J. A., M. Pisani, E. H. Bradley, J. R. O'Leary, and T. R. Fried. 2007. The association between treatment preferences and trajectories of care at the end-of-life. *Journal of General Internal Medicine* 22(11):1566-1571.

Cox, C., E. Cole, T. Reynolds, M. Wandrag, S. Breckenridge, and M. Dingle. 2006. Implications of cultural diversity in Do Not Attempt Resuscitation (DNAR) decision making. *Journal of Multicultural Nursing and Health* 12(1):20.

Curtis, J. R., and R. A. Engelberg. 2011. What is the "right" intensity of care at the end of life and how do we get there? Editorial. *Annals of Internal Medicine* 154(4):283-284.

Curtis, J. R., D. L. Patrick, R. A. Engelberg, K. Norris, C. Asp, and I. Byock. 2002. A measure of the quality of dying and death: Initial validation using after-death interviews with family members. *Journal of Pain and Symptom Management* 24(1):17-31.

Curtis, J. R., R. A. Engelberg, E. L. Nielsen, D. H. Au, and D. L Patrick. 2004. Patient-physician communication about end-of-life care for patients with severe COPD. *European Respiratory Journal* 24:200-205.

Dahlin, C., ed. 2013. *Clinical practice guidelines for quality palliative care.* 3rd ed. Pittsburgh, PA: National Consensus Project for Quality Palliative Care. http://www.hpna. org/multimedia/NCP_Clinical_Practice_Guidelines_3rd_Edition.pdf (accessed August 5, 2013).

Deep, K. S., A. Hunter, K. Murphy, and A. Volandes. 2010. "It helps me see with my heart": How video informs patients' rationale for decisions about future care in advanced dementia. *Patient Education and Counseling* 81(2):229-234.

Delaware Health and Social Services. 2012. *Medical Orders for Life-Sustaining Treatments (MOLST) form.* http://www.patientsrightscouncil.org/site/wp-content/uploads/2012/12/ Delaware_MOLST_11_12.pdf (accessed September 25, 2013).

Dellefield, M. E., and R. Ferrini. 2011. Promoting excellence in end-of-life care: Lessons learned from a cohort of nursing home residents with advanced Huntington Disease. *Journal of Neuroscience Nursing* 43(4):186-192.

DesHarnais, S., R. E. Carter, W. Hennessy, J. E. Kurent, and C. Carter. 2007. Lack of concordance between physician and patient: Reports on end-of-life care discussions. *Journal of Palliative Medicine* 10(3):728-740.

Detering, K. M., A. D. Hancock, M. C. Reade, and W. Silvester. 2010. The impact of advance care planning on end of life care in elderly patients: Randomised controlled trial. *British Medical Journal* 340:c1345.

Dias, L., B. A. Chabner, T. J. Lynch, Jr., and R. T. Penson. 2003. Breaking bad news: A patient's perspective. *The Oncologist* 8:587-596.

Ditto, P. H., J. A. Jacobson, W. D. Smucker, J. H. Danks, and A. Fagerlin. 2006. Context changes choices: A prospective study of the effects of hospitalization on life-sustaining treatment preferences. *Medical Decision Making* 26(4):313-322.

Dresser, R. 2013. *Taking care: Ethical caregiving in our aging society.* Presentation at meeting of the IOM Committee on Approaching Death: Addressing Key End-of-Life Issues, Houston, TX, July 22.

Durall, A., D. Zurakowski, and J. Wolfe. 2012. Barriers to conducting advance care discussions for children with life-threatening conditions. *Pediatrics* 129(4):e975-e982.

Edwards, A., N. Pang, V. Shiu, and C. Chan. 2010. Review: The understanding of spirituality and the potential role of spiritual care in end-of-life and palliative care: A meta-study of qualitative research. *Palliative Medicine* 24(8):753-770.

Edwards, J. D., S. S. Kun, R. J. Graham, and T. G. Keens. 2012. End-of-life discussions and advance care planning for children on long-term assisted ventilation with life-limiting conditions. *Journal of Palliative Care* 28(1):21-27.

El-Jawahri, A., L. J. Podgurski, A. F. Eichler, S. R. Plotkin, J. S. Temel, S. L. Mitchell, Y. Chang, M. J. Barry, and A. E. Volandes. 2010. Use of video to facilitate end-of-life discussions with patients with cancer: A randomized controlled trial. *Journal of Clinical Oncology* 28(2):305-310.

Elwyn, G., D. Frosch, A. E. Volandes, A. Edwards, and V. M. Montori. 2010. Investing in deliberation: A definition and classification of decision support interventions for people facing difficult health decisions. *Medical Decision Making* 30(6):701-711.

Epstein, A. S., A. E. Volandes, L. Y. Chen, K. A. Gary, Y. Li, P. Agre, T. T. Levin, D. L. Reidy, R. D. Meng, N. H. Segal, K. H. Yu, G. K. Abou-Alfa, Y. Y. Janjigian, D. P. Kelsen, and E. M. O'Reilly. 2013. A randomized controlled trial of a cardiopulmonary resuscitation video in advance care planning for progressive pancreas and hepatobiliary cancer patients. *Journal of Palliative Medicine* 16(6):623-631.

Epstein, R. M., and R. L. Street, Jr. 2007. *Patient-centered communication in cancer care: Promoting healing and reducing suffering.* NIH No. 07-6225. Bethesda, MD: National Cancer Institute.

Evans, L. R., E. A. Boyd, G. Malvar, L. Apatira, J. M. Luce, B. Lo, and D. B. White. 2009. Surrogate decision-makers' perspectives on discussing prognosis in the face of uncertainty. *American Journal of Respiratory and Critical Care Medicine* 179:48-53.

Fischer, S. M., A. Sauaia, S-J. Min, and J. Kutner. 2012. Advance directive discussions: Lost in translation or lost opportunities? *Journal of Palliative Medicine* 15(1):86-92.

Fischer, S. M., S. J. Min, L. Cervantes, and J. Kutner. 2013. Where do you want to spend your last days of life? Low concordance between preferred and actual site of death among hospitalized adults. *Journal of Hospital Medicine* 8(4):178-183.

Flannelly, K. J., L. L. Emanuel, G. F. Handzo, K. Galek, N. R. Silton, and M. Carlson. 2012. A national study of chaplaincy services and end-of-life outcomes. *BMC Palliative Care* 11:10.

Fowler, F. J., Jr., B. S. Gerstein, and M. J. Barry. 2013. How patient centered are medical decisions? Results of a national survey. *JAMA Internal Medicine* 173(13):1215-1221.

Frahm, K. A., L. M. Brown, and K. Hyer. 2012. Racial disparities in end-of-life planning and services for deceased nursing home residents. *Journal of the American Medical Directors Association* 13(9):819.e7-819.e11.

Fried, T. R., and J. R. O'Leary. 2008. Using the experiences of bereaved caregivers to inform patient- and caregiver-centered advance care planning. *Journal of General Internal Medicine* 23(10):1602-1607.

Fried, T. R., E. H. Bradley, V. R. Towle, and H. Allore. 2002. Understanding the treatment preferences of seriously ill patients. *New England Journal of Medicine* 346(14):1061-1066.

Fried, T. R., E. H. Bradley, and J. O'Leary. 2003. Prognosis communication in serious illness: Perceptions of older patients, caregivers, and clinicians. *Journal of the American Geriatrics Society* 51(10):1398-1403.

Fried, T. R., E. H. Bradley, and J. O'Leary. 2006. Changes in prognostic awareness among seriously ill older persons and their caregivers. *Journal of Palliative Medicine* 9(1):61-69.

Fried, T. R., J. O'Leary, P. Van Ness, and L. Fraenkel. 2007. Inconsistency over time in the preferences of older persons with advanced illness for life-sustaining treatment. *Journal of the American Geriatrics Society* 55(7):1007-1014.

Fried, T. R., C. Redding, M. Robbins, A. Palva, J. O'Leary, and L. Iannone. 2010. Stages of change for the component behaviors of advance care planning. *Journal of the American Geriatrics Society* 58(12):2329-2336.

Friedman, S., and D. Gilmore. 2007. Factors that impact resuscitation preferences for young people with severe developmental disabilities. *Intellectual and Developmental Disabilities* 45(2):90-97.

Fritch, J., S. Petronia, P. R. Helft, and A. Torke. 2013. Making decisions for hospitalized older adults: Ethical factors considered by family surrogates. *Journal of Clinical Ethics* 24(2):125-134.

Fromme, E. K., D. Zive, T. A. Schmidt, E. Olszewski, and S. W. Tolle. 2012. POLST registry do-not-resuscitate orders and other patient treatment preferences. Research letter. *Journal of the American Medical Association* 307(1):34-35.

Fromme, E. K., Zive, D., Schmidt, T. A., Cook, J. N. B., and Tolle, S. W. 2014. Association between Physician Orders for Life-Sustaining Treatment for scope of treatment and in-hospital death in Oregon. *Journal of the American Geriatrics Society* [epub ahead of print].

Fujimori, M., and Y. Uchitomi. 2009. Preferences of cancer patients regarding communication of bad news: A systematic literature review. *Journal of Clinical Oncology* 39(4):201-216.

Fujimori, M., T. Akechi, T. Morita, M. Inagaki, N. Akizuki, Y. Sakano, and Y. Uchitomi. 2007. Preferences of cancer patients regarding the disclosure of bad news. *Psycho-Oncology* 16:573-581.

Ganti, A. K., S. J. Lee, J. M. Vose, M. P. Devetten, R. G. Bociek, J. O. Armitage, P. J. Bierman, L. J. Maness, E. C. Reed, and F. R. Loberiza, Jr. 2007. Outcomes after hematopoietic stem-cell transplantation for hematologic malignancies in patients with or without advance care planning. *Journal of Clinical Oncology* 25(35):5643-5648.

Gao, W., M. I. Bennett, D. Stark, S. Murray, and I. J. Higginson. 2010. Psychological distress in cancer from survivorship to end of life care: Prevalence, associated factors and clinical implications. *European Journal of Cancer* 46(11):2036-2044.

Gardiner, C., M. Gott, N. Small, S. Payne, D. Seamark, S. Barnes, D. Halpin, and C. Ruse. 2009. Living with advanced chronic obstructive pulmonary disease: Patients concerns regarding death and dying. *Palliative Medicine* 23(8):691-697.

Garrido, M. M., E. L. Idler, H. Leventhal, and D. Carr. 2013. Pathways from religion to advance care planning: Beliefs about control over length of life and end-of-life values. *The Gerontologist* 53(5):801-816.

Garvie, P. A., J. He., J. Wang, L. J. D'Angelo, and M. E. Lyon. 2012. An exploratory survey of end-of-life attitudes, beliefs, and experiences of adolescents with HIV/AIDS and their families. *Journal of Pain and Symptom Management* 44(3):373-385.e29.

Gay, E. B., P. J. Pronovost, R. D. Bassett, and J. E. Nelson. 2009. The intensive care unit family meeting: Making it happen. *Journal of Critical Care* 24(4):629.e1-629.12.

Gill, C. J. 2010. No, we don't think our doctors are out to get us: Responding to the straw man distortions of disability rights arguments against assisted suicide. *Disability and Health Journal* 3:31-38.

Gillick, M. R. 2010. Reversing the code status of advanced directives? Editorial. *New England Journal of Medicine* 362(13):1239-1240.

Gillick, M. R. 2013. The critical role of caregivers in achieving patient-centered care. Viewpoint. *Journal of the American Medical Association* 310(6):575-576.

Go, A. S., D. Mozaffarian, V. L. Roger, E. J. Benjamin, J. D. Berry, W. B. Borden, D. M. Bravata, S. Dai, E. S. Ford, C. S. Fox, S. Franco, H. J. Fullerton, C. Gillespie, S. M. Hailpern, J. A. Heit, V. J. Howard, M. D. Huffman, B. M. Kissela, S. J. Kittner, D. T. Lackland, J. H. Lichtman, L. D. Lisabeth, D. Magid, G. M. Marcus, A. Marelli, E. R. Mohler, C. S. Moy, M. E. Mussolino, G. Nichol, N. P. Paynter, P. J. Schreiner, P. D. Sorlie, J. Stein, T. N. Turan, S. S. Virani, N. D. Wong, D. Woo, and M. B. Turner. 2013. Heart disease and stroke statistics—2013 update: A report from the American Heart Association. *Circulation* 127:e6-e245.

Godlee, F. 2013. Partnering with patients. *British Medical Journal* 346:f3153.

Goodman, D. C., N. E. Morden, C.-H. Chang, E. S. Fisher, and J. E. Wennberg. 2013. *Trends in cancer care near the end of life: A Dartmouth Atlas of Health Care Brief.* http://www. dartmouthatlas.org/downloads/reports/Cancer_brief_090413.pdf (accessed September 6, 2013).

Gordon, H. S., R. L. Street, Jr., B. F. Sharf, P. A. Kelly, and J. Souchek. 2006. Racial differences in trust and lung cancer patients' perceptions of physician communication. *Journal of Clinical Oncology* 24(6):904-909.

Gott, M., C. Gardiner, N. Small, S. Payne, D. Seamark, S. Barnes, D. Halpin, and C. Ruse. 2009. Barriers to advance care planning in chronic obstructive pulmonary disease. *Palliative Medicine* 23(7):642-648.

Gramling, R., S. A. Norton, S. Ladwig, M. Metzger, J. DeLuca, D. Gramling, D. Schatz, R. Epstein, T. Quill, and S. Alexander. 2013. Direct observation of prognosis communication in palliative care: A descriptive study. *Journal of Pain and Symptom Management* 45(2):202-212.

Greenberg, S. 2011. *A profile of older Americans: 2011.* http://www.aoa.gov/aoaroot/ aging_statistics/Profile/2011/docs/2011profile.pdf (accessed October 4, 2013).

Gruneir, A., V. Mor, S. Weitzen, R. Truchil, J. Teno, and J. Roy. 2007. Where people die: A multilevel approach to understanding influences on site of death in America. *Medical Care Research and Review* 64(4):351-378.

Gundersen Health System. 2014a. *Respecting choices: Advance care planning.* http://www. gundersenhealth.org/respecting-choices (accessed June 1, 2014).

Gundersen Health System. 2014b. *Respecting choices history/overview.* http://www.gundersen health.org/respecting-choices/about-us/history-and-overview (accessed June 1, 2014).

Gutierrez, K. M. 2012. Advance directives in an intensive care unit: Experiences and recommendations of critical care nurses and physicians. *Critical Care Nursing Quarterly* 35(4):396-409.

Halpern, S. D. 2012a. Shaping end-of-life care: Behavioral economics and advance directives. *Seminars in Respiratory and Critical Care Medicine* 33(4):393-400.

Halpern, S. D. 2012b. Young leaders: Employing behavioral economics and decision science in crucial choices at end of life. *Health Affairs* 31(12):2789-2790.

Halpern, S. D., P. A. Ubel, and D. A. Asch. 2007. Harnessing the power of default options to improve health care. Sounding board. *New England Journal of Medicine* 357(13): 1340-1344.

Halpern, S. D., G. Loewenstein, K. G. Volpp, E. Cooney, K. Vranas, C. M. Quill, M. S. McKenzie, M. O. Harhay, N. B. Gabler, T. Silva, R. Arnold, D. C. Angus, and C. Bryce. 2013. Default options in advance directives influence how patients set goals for end-of-life care. *Health Affairs* 32(2):408-417.

Hammes, B. J. 2003. Update on respecting choices: Four years on. *Innovations in End-of-Life Care* 5(2):1-6. http://www.rpctraining.com.au/module06/mod06_toolkit/Additional%20 references/Reference-4-3.pdf (accessed October 1, 2013).

Hammes, B. J., and B. L. Rooney. 1998. Death and end-of-life planning in one Midwestern community. *Archives of Internal Medicine* 158(4):383-390.

Hammes, B. J., J. Klevan, M. Kempf, and M. S. Williams. 2005. Pediatric advance care planning. *Journal of Palliative Medicine* 8(4):766-773.

Hammes, B. J., B. L. Rooney, J. D. Gundrum, S. E. Hickman, and N. Hager. 2012. The POLST program: A retrospective review of the demographics of use and outcomes in one community where advance directives are prevalent. *Journal of Palliative Medicine* 15(1):77-85.

Han, B., R. E. Remsburg, and T. J. Iwashyna. 2006. Differences in hospice use between black and white patients during the period 1992 through 2000. *Medical Care* 44(8):731-737.

Hargrave, B. 2013. New form adds some teeth to end-of-life care preferences. *USA Today*, August 5. http://www.usatoday.com/story/news/nation/2013/08/04/polst-paradigm-end-of-life-care-form-expanding-reach/2595889 (accessed June 2, 2014).

Heffner, J. E. 2011. Advance care planning in chronic obstructive pulmonary disease: Barriers and opportunities. *Current Opinion in Pulmonary Medicine* 17:103-109.

HHS (U.S. Department of Health and Human Services). 2008. *Advance directives and advance care planning: Report to Congress.* http://aspe.hhs.gov/daltcp/reports/2008/adcongrpt. htm (accessed August 7, 2013).

HHS. 2014. *Meaningful use stage 3 final recommendations.* http://www.healthit.gov/facas/sites/faca/files/HITPC_MUWG_Stage3_Recs_2014-04-01.pdf (accessed June 2, 2014).

Hickman, S. E., C. A. Nelson, A. H. Moss, B. J. Hammes, A. Terwilliger, A. Jackson, and S. W. Tolle. 2009. Use of the Physician Orders for Life-Sustaining Treatment (POLST) paradigm program in the hospice setting. *Journal of Palliative Medicine* 12(2):133-141.

Hickman, S. E., C. A. Nelson, N. A. Perrin, A. H. Moss, B. J. Hammes, and S. W. Tolle. 2010. A comparison of methods to communicate treatment preferences in nursing facilities: Traditional practices versus the Physician Orders for Life-Sustaining Treatment program. *Journal of the American Geriatrics Society* 58(7):1241-1248.

Hickman, S. E., C. A. Nelson, A. H. Moss, S. W. Tolle, N. A. Perrin, and B. J. Hammes. 2011. The consistency between treatments provided to nursing facility residents and orders on the Physician Orders for Life-Sustaining Treatment (POLST) form. *Journal of the American Geriatrics Society* 59(11):2091-2099.

Hinds, P. S., L. Oakes, and W. L. Furman. 2010. End-of-life decision-making in pediatric oncology. In *Oxford textbook of palliative nursing,* 3rd ed., edited by B. R. Ferrell and N. Coyle. New York: Oxford University Press. Pp. 1049-1063.

Hoyert, D. L., and J. Xu. 2012. Deaths: Preliminary data for 2011. *National Vital Statistics Reports* 61(6):1-52.

Hudson, P., K. Quinn, B. O'Hanlon, and S. Aranda. 2008. Family meeting in palliative care: Multidisciplinary clinical practice guidelines. *BMC Palliative Care* 7:12.

in der Schmitten, J., S. Rothärmel, C. Mellert, S. Rixen, B. J. Hammes, L. Briggs, K. Wegscheider, and G. Marckmann. 2011. A complex regional intervention to implement advance care planning in one town's nursing homes: Protocol of a controlled interregional study. *BMC Health Services Research* 11(14):1-9. http://www.biomedcentral. com/content/pdf/1472-6963-11-14.pdf (accessed October 1, 2013).

IOM (Institute of Medicine). 1997. *Approaching death: Improving care at the end of life.* Washington, DC: National Academy Press.

IOM. 2001. *Crossing the quality chasm: Improving the 21st century health care system.* Washington, DC: National Academy Press.

IOM. 2004. *Health literacy: A prescription to end confusion.* Washington, DC: The National Academies Press.

Jezewski, M. A., M. A. Meeker, L. Sessanna, and D. S. Finnell. 2007. The effectiveness of interventions to increase advance directive completion rates. *Journal of Aging and Health* 19(3):519-536.

Johnson, K. S., K. I. Elbert-Avila, and J. A. Tulsky. 2005. The influence of spiritual beliefs and practices on the treatment preferences of African Americans: A review of the literature. *Journal of the American Geriatrics Society* 53(4):711-719.

Johnson, K. S., M. Kuchibhatla, and J. A. Tulsky. 2008. What explains racial differences in the use of advance directives and attitudes toward hospice care? *Journal of the American Geriatrics Society* 56(10):1953-1958.

Johnson, K. S., M. Kuchibhatla, and J. A. Tulsky. 2011. Racial differences in location before hospice enrollment and association with hospice length of stay. *Journal of the American Geriatrics Society* 59(4):732-737.

Kagawa-Singer, M., and L. J. Blackhall. 2001. Negotiating cross-cultural issues at the end of life: "You got to go where he lives." *Journal of the American Medical Association* 286(23):2993-3001.

Kane, L. 2010. *Exclusive ethics survey results: Doctors struggle with tougher-than-ever dilemmas.* http://www.medscape.com/viewarticle/731485 (accessed September 6, 2013).

Karches, K. E., G. S. Chung, V. Arora, D. O. Meltzer, and F. A. Curlin. 2012. Religiosity, spirituality, and end-of-life planning: A single-site survey of medical inpatients. *Journal of Pain and Symptom Management* 44(6):843-851.

Karp, N., and E. Wood. 2003. *Incapacitated and alone: Health care decision making for unbefriended older people.* http://www.americanbar.org/content/dam/aba/administrative/law_aging/2003_Unbefriended_Elderly_Health_Care_Descision-Making7-11-03.authcheckdam.pdf (accessed February 10, 2014).

Kelley, A. S., N. S. Wenger, and C. A. Sarkisian. 2010. Opiniones: End of life care preferences and planning among older Latinos. *Journal of the American Geriatrics Society* 58(6):1109-1116.

Kelley, A. S., S. L. Ettner, S. Morrison, Q. Du, N. S. Wenger, and C. A. Sarkisian. 2011. Determinants of medical expenditures in the last 6 months of life. *Annals of Internal Medicine* 154(4):235-242.

Kim, M. K., and A. Alvi. 1999. Breaking the bad news of cancer: The patient's perspective. *Laryngoscope* 109(7, Pt. 1):1064-1067.

Kim, S. Y. H., J. H. T.Karlawish, and E. D. Cain. 2002. Current state of research on decision-making competence of cognitively impaired elderly persons. *American Journal of Geriatric Psychiatry* 10:151-165.

King, J., L. Yourman, C. Ahalt, C. Eng, S. J. Knight, E. J. Pérez-Stable, and A. K. Smith. 2012. Quality of life in late-life disability: "I don't feel bitter because I am in a wheelchair." *Journal of the American Geriatrics Society* 60(3):569-576.

Kirchhoff, K. T., B. J. Hammes, K. A. Kehl, L. A. Briggs, and R. L. Brown. 2010. Effect of a disease-specific planning intervention on surrogate understanding of patient goals for future medical treatment. *Journal of the American Geriatrics Society* 58(7):1233-1240.

Kirkpatrick, J. N., C. J. Guger, M. F. Arnsdorf, and S. E. Fedson. 2007. Advance directives in the cardiac care unit. *American Heart Journal* 154(3):477-481.

Kirsch, I., H. Braun, K. Yamamoto, and A. Sum. 2007. *America's perfect storm: Three forces changing our nation's future.* Princeton, NJ: Educational Testing Service. https://www.ets.org/Media/Research/pdf/PICSTORM.pdf (accessed July 14, 2014).

Klugman, C. M., and R. P. Usatine. 2012. An evaluation of two online advance directive programs. *American Journal of Hospice and Palliative Medicine* 30(7):657-663.

Knauft, E., E. L. Nielsen, R. A. Engelberg, D. L. Patrick, and J. R. Curtis. 2005. Barriers and facilitators to end-of-life care communication for patients with COPD. *Chest* 127(6):2188-2196.

Ko, E., and C. S. Berkman. 2010. Role of children in end-of-life treatment planning among Korean American older adults. *Journal of Social Work in End-of-Life & Palliative Care* 6(3-4):164-184.

Ko, E., and J. Lee. 2013. Completion of advance directives among low-income older adults: Does race/ethnicity matter? *American Journal of Hospice and Palliative Medicine* 31(3): 247-253.

Kohn, N. A., and J. A. Blumenthal. 2008. Designating health care decision-makers for patients without advance directives: A psychological critique. *Georgia Law Review* 42:1-40.

Kressel, L. M., and G. B. Chapman. 2007. The default effect in end-of-life medical treatment preferences. *Medical Decision Making* 27(3):299-310.

Kressel, L. M., G. B. Chapman, and E. Leventhal. 2007. The influence of default options on the expression of end-of-life treatment preferences in advance directives. *Journal of General Internal Medicine* 22:1007-1010.

Kutner, M., E. Greenberg, Y. Jin, C. Paulsen, and S. White. 2006. *The health literacy of America's adults: Results from the 2003 National Assessment of Adult Literacy*. NCES 2006-483. Washington, DC: National Center for Education Statistics. http://nces.ed.gov/pubsearch/pubsinfo.asp?pubid=2006483 (accessed November 18, 2013).

Lakin, J. R., E. Le, M. Mourad, H. Hollander, and W. G. Anderson. 2013. Incentivizing residents to document inpatient advance care planning. Research letter. *JAMA Internal Medicine* 173(17):1652-1654.

Lamont, E. B., and N. A. Christakis. 2003. Complexities in prognostication in advanced cancer: "To help them live their lives the way they want to." *Journal of the American Medical Association* 290(1):98-104.

Lannen, P., J. Wolfe, J. Mack, E. Onelov, U. Nyberg, and U. Kreicbergs. 2010. Absorbing information about a child's incurable cancer. *Oncology* 78:259-266.

LeBlanc, T. W., and J. A. Tulsky. in press. Communication with the patient and family. In *Oxford textbook of palliative medicine*, 5th ed., edited by N. Cherney, M. Fallon, S. Kaasa, R. Portenoy, and D. Currow. Oxford, England: Oxford University Press.

Lepore, M. J., S. C. Miller, and P. Gozalo. 2011. Hospice use among urban black and white U.S. nursing home decedents in 2006. *The Gerontologist* 51(2):251-260.

Limehouse, W. E., V. R. Feeser, K. J. Bookman, and A. Derse. 2012a. A model for emergency department end-of-life communications after acute devastating events—Part I: Decision-making capacity, surrogates, and advance directives. *Academic Emergency Medicine* 19(9):1068-1072.

Limehouse, W. E., V. R. Feeser, K. J. Bookman, and A. Derse. 2012b. A model for emergency department end-of-life communications after acute devastating events—Part II: Moving from resuscitative or end-of-life palliative treatment. *Academic Emergency Medicine* 19(11):1300-1308.

Lindqvist, G., and L. R. Hallberg. 2010. "Feelings of guilt due to self-inflicted disease": A grounded theory of suffering from chronic obstructive pulmonary disease (COPD). *Journal of Health Psychology* 15(3):456-466.

Lipkin, M. 2013. Shared decision making. Invited commentary. *JAMA Internal Medicine* 173(13):1204-1205.

Loewenstein, G. 2005. Hot-cold empathy gaps and medical decision making. *Health Psychology* 24(4):S49-S56.

Lotz, J. D., R. J. Jox, G. D. Borasio, and M. Führer. 2013. Pediatric advance care planning: A systematic review. *Pediatrics* 131(3):e873-e880.

Lyon, M. E., P. A. Garvie, R. McCarter, L. Briggs, J. He, and L. J. D'Angelo. 2009. Who will speak for me? Improving end-of-life decision-making for adolescents with HIV and their families. *Pediatrics* 123(2):e199-e206.

Lyon, M. E., S. Jacobs, L. Briggs, Y. I. Cheng, and J. Wang. 2013. Family-centered advance care planning for teens with cancer. *JAMA Pediatrics* 167(5):460-467.

Mack, J. W., and T. J. Smith. 2012. Reasons why physicians do not have discussions about poor prognosis, why it matters, and what can be improved. *Journal of Clinical Oncology* 30(22):2715-2717.

Mack, J. W., E. Paulk, K. Viswanath, and H. G. Prigerson. 2010a. Racial disparities in the outcomes of communication on medical care received near death. *Archives of Internal Medicine* 170(17):1533-1540.

Mack, J. W., J. C. Weeks, A. A. Wright, S. D. Block, and H. G. Prigerson. 2010b. End-of-life discussions, goal attainment, and distress at the end of life: Predictors and outcomes of receipt of care consistent with preferences. *Journal of Clinical Oncology* 28(7):1203-1208.

Mack, J. W., A. Cronin, N. Taback, H. A. Huskamp, N. L. Keating, J. L. Malin, C. C. Earle, and J. C. Weeks. 2012. End-of-life care discussions among patients with advanced cancer: A cohort study. *Annals of Internal Medicine* 156(3):204-210.

Majesko, A., S. Y. Hong, L. Weissfeld, and D. B. White. 2012. Identifying family members who may struggle in the role of surrogate decision maker. *Critical Care Medicine* 40(8):2281-2286.

Marco, C. A., E. S. Bessman, and G. D. Kelen. 2009. Ethical issues of cardiopulmonary resuscitation: Comparison of emergency physician practices from 1995 to 2007. *Academic Emergency Medicine* 16(3):270-273.

Martin, D. K., E. C. Thiel, and P. A. Singer. 1999. A new model of advance care planning: Observations from people with HIV. *Archives of Internal Medicine* 159:86-92.

Massachusetts Department of Public Health. 2011. *MOLST demonstration program: Recommendations for statewide expansion. Pilot results 2011.* http://www.mass.gov/eohhs/docs/dph/quality/healthcare/molst-final-results-2011.pdf (accessed October 1, 2013).

Matlock, D. D., T. A. E. Keech, M. B. McKenzie, M. R. Bronsert, C. T. Nowels, and J. S. Kutner. 2011. Feasibility and acceptability of a decision aid designed for people facing advanced or terminal illness: A pilot randomized trial. *Health Expectations* 1-11.

McCusker, M., L. Ceronsky, C. Crone, H. Epstein, B. Greene, J. Halvorson, K. Kephart, E. Mallen, B. Nosan, M. Rohr, E. Rosenberg, R. Ruff, K. Schlecht, and L. Setterlund. 2013. *Health care guideline: Palliative care for adults.* Bloomington, MN: Institute for Clinical Systems Improvement. https://www.icsi.org/_asset/k056ab/PalliativeCare.pdf (accessed May 29, 2014).

McDonagh, J. R., T. B. Elliott, R. A. Engelberg, P. D. Treece, S. E. Shannon, G. D. Rubenfeld, D. L. Patrick, and J. R. Curtis. 2004. Family satisfaction with family conferences about end-of-life care in the intensive care unit: Increased proportion of family speech is associated with increased satisfaction. *Critical Care Medicine* 32(7):1484-1488.

Meyer, H. 2011. Changing the conversation in California about care near the end of life. *Health Affairs* 30(3):390-393.

Mirarchi, F. L., L. A. Hite, T. E. Cooney, T. M. Kisiel, and P. Henry. 2008. TRIAD I: The realistic interpretation of advanced directives. *Journal of Patient Safety* 4(4):235-240.

Mirarchi, F. L., S. Kalantzis, D. Hunter, E. McCracken, and T. Kisiel. 2009. TRIAD II: Do living wills have an impact on pre-hospital lifesaving care? *Journal of Emergency Medicine* 36(2):105-115.

Mirarchi, F. L., E. Costello, J. Puller, T. Cooney, and N. Kottkamp. 2012. TRIAD III: Nationwide assessment of living wills and do not resuscitate orders. *Journal of Emergency Medicine* 42(5):511-520.

Mitchell, B. L., and L. C. Mitchell. 2009. Review of the literature on cultural competence and end-of-life treatment decisions: The role of the hospitalist. *Journal of the National Medical Association* 101(9):920-926.

Mitchell, S. L., J. M. Teno, D. K. Kiely, M. L. Shaffer, R. N. Jones, H. G. Prigerson, L. Volicer, J. L. Givens, and M. B. Hamel. 2009. The clinical course of advanced dementia. *New England Journal of Medicine* 361(16):1529-1538.

Morgan, P. A., J. S. de Oliveira, S. C. Alexander, K. I. Pollak, A. S. Jeffreys, M. K. Olsen, R. M. Arnold, A. P. Abernethy, K. L. Rodriguez, and J. A. Tulsky. 2010. Comparing oncologist, nurse, and physician assistant attitudes toward discussions of negative emotions with patients. *Journal of Physician Assistant Education* 21(3):13-17.

Morris, D. A., K. S. Johnson, N. Ammarell, R. M. Arnold, J. A. Tulsky, and K. E. Steinhauser. 2012. What is your understanding of your illness? A communication tool to explore patients' perspectives of living with advanced illness. *Journal of General Internal Medicine* 27(11):1460-1466.

Muni, S., R. A. Engelberg, P. D. Treece, D. Dotolo, and J. R. Curtis. 2011. The influence of race/ethnicity and socioeconomic status on end-of-life care in the ICU. *Chest* 139(5):1025-1033.

Murphy, K., A. Cooney, E. O. Shea, and D. Casey. 2009. Determinants of quality of life for older people living with a disability in the community. *Journal of Advanced Nursing* 65(3):606-615.

National POLST. 2012a. *About the National POLST Paradigm.* http://www.polst.org/about-the-national-polst-paradigm (accessed March 20, 2014).

National POLST. 2012b. *FAQ.* http://www.polst.org/advance-care-planning/faq (accessed June 1, 2014).

National POLST. 2012c. *How does POLST work?* http://www.polst.org/advance-care-planning/how-does-polst-work (accessed June 1, 2014).

National POLST. 2012d. *What is POLST?* http://www.polst.org/about-the-national-polst-paradigm/what-is-polst (accessed June 1, 2014).

National POLST. 2012e. *POLST and advance directives.* http://www.polst.org/advance-care-planning/polst-and-advance-directives (accessed June 1, 2014).

National POLST. 2012f. *Programs in your state.* http://www.polst.org/programs-in-your-state (accessed June 1, 2014).

NCCN (National Comprehensive Cancer Network). 2013. *Clinical practice guidelines in oncology—palliative care.* Version 2.2013. Fort Washington, PA: NCCN.

NCOA (National Council on Aging), United Healthcare, and USA Today. 2013. *The United States of aging survey.* http://www.ncoa.org/improve-health/community-education/united-states-of-aging/usa-survey-2013.html (accessed August 5, 2013).

Nease, R. F., S. G. Frazee, L. Zarin, and S. B. Miller. 2013. Choice architecture is a better strategy than engaging patients to spur behavior change. *Health Affairs* 32(2):242-249.

Nelson, J. E., D. C. Angus, L. A. Weissfeld, K. A. Puntillo, M. Danis, D. Deal, M. M. Levy, and D. J. Cook. 2006. End-of-life care for the critically ill: A national intensive care unit survey. *Critical Care Medicine* 34(10):2547-2553.

NHPCO (National Hospice and Palliative Care Organization). 2013. *Facts and figures: Hospice care in America.* Alexandria, VA: NHPCO.

Nicholas, L. H., K. M. Langa, T. J. Iwashyna, and D. R. Weir. 2011. Regional variation in the association between advance directives and end-of-life Medicare expenditures. *Journal of the American Medical Association* 306(13):1447-1453.

Nienstedt, J. C., J. F. Kinney, J. M. LeVoir, J. M. Quinn, P. D. Sirba, M. J. Hoeppner, and L. A. Piché. 2013. Stewards of the gift of life. *Minnesota Catholic Conference.* http://www.mncc.org/wp-content/uploads/2013/01/POLSTBrochure2013-21.pdf (accessed October 3, 2013).

Nilsson, M. E., P. K. Maciejewski, B. Zhang, A. A. Wright, E. D. Trice, A. C. Muriel, R. J. Friedlander, K. M. Fasciano, S. D. Block, and H. G. Prigerson. 2009. Mental health, treatment preferences, advance care planning, location, and quality of death in advanced cancer patients with dependent children. *Cancer* 115(2):399-409.

NNLM (National Network of Libraries of Medicine). 2013. *Health literacy.* http://nnlm.gov/outreach/consumer/hlthlit.html (accessed August 13, 2013).

NQF (National Quality Forum). 2006. *A national framework and preferred practices for palliative and hospice care quality.* http://www.qualityforum.org/Publications/2006/12/A_National_Framework_and_Preferred_Practices_for_Palliative_and_Hospice_Care_Quality.aspx (accessed August 5, 2013).

ODPHP (Office of Disease Prevention and Health Promotion). 2010. *National action plan to improve health literacy.* Washington, DC: HHS. http://www.health.gov/communication/hlactionplan/pdf/Health_Literacy_Action_Plan.pdf (accessed February 20, 2014).

Orleans, T., and E. F. Cassidy. 2011. Health and behavior. In *Health care delivery in the United States*, 10th ed., Ch. 7, edited by A. R. Kovner and J. R. Knickman. New York: Springer Publishing Company. Pp. 125-149.

Parker, R. M., M. S. Wolf, and I. Kirsch. 2008. Preparing for an epidemic of limited health literacy: Weathering the perfect storm. *Journal of General Internal Medicine* 23(8): 1273-1276.

Parks, S. M., L. Winter, A. J. Santana, B. Parker, J. J. Diamond, M. Rose, and R. E. Myers. 2011. Family factors in end-of-life decision-making: Family conflict and proxy relationship. *Journal of Palliative Medicine* 14(2):179-184.

Patel, K., D. J. A. Janssen, and R. J. Curtis. 2012. Advance care planning in COPD. *Respirology* 17(1):72-78.

Peteet, J. R., and M. J. Balboni. 2013. Spirituality and religion in oncology. *CA: A Cancer Journal for Clinicians* 63(4):280-289.

Pew Research Center. 2013. *Views on end-of-life medical treatments.* http://www.pewforum.org/2013/11/21/views-on-end-of-life-medical-treatments (accessed January 16, 2014).

Phelps, A. C., P. K. Maciejewski, M. Nilsson, T. A. Balboni, A. A. Wright, M. E. Paulk, E. Trice, D. Schrag, J. R. Peteet, S. D. Block, and H. G. Prigerson. 2009. Religious coping and use of intensive life-prolonging care near death in patients with advanced cancer. *Journal of the American Medical Association* 301(11):1140-1147.

Phipps, E., G. True, D. Harris, U. Chong, W. Tester, S. I. Chavin, and L. E. Braitman. 2003. Approaching the end of life: Attitudes, preferences, and behaviors of African-American and white patients and their family caregivers. *Journal of Clinical Oncology* 21(3):549-554.

Pollak, K. I., R. M. Arnold, A. S. Jeffreys, S. C. Alexander, M. K. Olsen, A. P. Abernethy, C. S. Skinner, K. L. Rodriguez, and J. A. Tulsky. 2007. Oncologist communication about emotion during visits with patients with advanced cancer. *Journal of Clinical Oncology* 25(36):5748-5752.

Prendergast, T. J. 2001. Advance care planning: Pitfalls, progress, promise. *Critical Care Medicine* 29(Suppl. 2):N34-N39.

President's Council on Bioethics. 2005. *Taking care: Ethical caregiving in our aging society.* https://bioethicsarchive.georgetown.edu/pcbe/reports/taking_care (accessed February 10, 2014).

Puchalski, C., and B. Ferrell. 2010. *Making health care whole: Integrating spirituality into patient care.* West Conshohocken, PA: Templeton Press.

Ratzan, S. C., and R. M. Parker. 2000. Introduction. In *National Library of Medicine current bibliographies in medicine: Health literacy*, edited by C. R. Selden, M. Zorn, S. C. Ratzan, and R. M. Parker. Bethesda, MD: National Institutes of Health. Pp. v-vi. http://www.nlm.nih.gov/archive//20061214/pubs/cbm/hliteracy.pdf (accessed February 10, 2014).

Raymont, V., W. Bingley, A. Buchanan, A. S. David, P. Hayward, S. Wessely, and M. Hotopf. 2004. Prevalence of mental incapacity in medical inpatients and associated risk factors: Cross-sectional study. *Lancet* 364(9443):1421-1427.

Reynolds, K. S., L. C. Hanson, M. Henderson, and K. E. Steinhauser. 2008. End-of-life care in nursing home settings: Do race or age matter? *Palliative and Supportive Care* 6(1):21-27.

Robinson, T. M., S. C. Alexander, M. Hays, A. S. Jeffreys, M. K. Olsen, K. L. Rodriguez, K. I. Pollak, A. P. Abernethy, R. Arnold, and J. A. Tulsky. 2008. Patient-oncologist communication in advanced cancer: Predictors of patient perception of prognosis. *Support Care Cancer* 16(9):1049-1057.

Rodgers, M., and T. Picchi. 2013. Testimony submitted on behalf of the Catholic Health Association to the IOM Committee on Approaching Death: Addressing Key End-of-Life Issues, Washington, DC.

Russell, B. J., and A. M. Ward. 2011. Deciding what information is necessary: Do patients with advanced cancer want to know all the details. *Cancer Management and Research* 3:191-199.

Ryan, C. 2013. *Language use in the United States: 2011.* https://www.census.gov/prod/2013pubs/acs-22.pdf (accessed May 29, 2014).

Sabatino, C. P. 2010. The evolution of health care advance planning law and policy. *Milbank Quarterly* 88(2):211-239.

Sahm, S., R. Will, and G. Hommel. 2005. Would they follow what has been laid down? Cancer patients' and healthy controls' views on adherence to advance directives compared to medical staff. *Medicine, Health Care and Philosophy* 8:297-305.

Schellinger, S., A. Sidebottom, and L. Briggs. 2011. Disease specific advance care planning for heart failure patients: Implementation in a large health system. *Journal of Palliative Medicine* 14(11):1224-1230.

Schenker, Y., M. Crowley-Matoka, D. Dohan, G. A. Tiver, R. M. Arnold, and D. B. White. 2012. I don't want to be the one saying "we should just let him die": Intrapersonal tensions experienced by surrogate decision makers in the ICU. *Journal of General Internal Medicine* 27(12):1657-1665.

Schmidt, T. A., E. A. Olszewski, D. Zive, E. K. Fromme, and S. W. Tolle. 2013. The Oregon Physician Orders for Life-Sustaining Treatment registry: A preliminary study of emergency medical services utilization. *Journal of Emergency Medicine* 44(4):796-805.

Schubart, J. R., B. H. Levi, F. Camacho, M. Whitehead, E. Farace, and M. J. Green. 2012. Reliability of an interactive computer program for advance care planning. *Journal of Palliative Medicine* 15(6):637-642.

Sessums, L. L., H. Zembrzuska, and J. L. Jackson. 2011. Does this patient have medical decision-making capacity. *Journal of the American Medical Association* 306(4):420-427.

Shah, A. B., R. P. Morrissey, A. Baraghoush, P. Bharadwaj, A. Phan, M. Hamilton, J. Kobashigawa, and E. R. Schwarz. 2013. Failing the failing heart: A review of palliative care in heart failure. *Reviews in Cardiovascular Medicine* 14(1):41-48.

Shapiro, S. P. 2012. Advance directives: The elusive goal of having the last word. *NAELA Journal* 8(2):205-232.

Sharp, S., D. Carr, and C. Macdonald. 2012. Religion and end-of-life treatment preferences: Assessing the effects of religious denomination and beliefs. *Social Forces* 91(1):275-298.

Shockney, L. D., and A. Back. 2013. Communicating with patients on treatment options for advanced disease. *Journal of the National Comprehensive Cancer Network* 11(5.5): 684-686.

Silveira, M. J., S. Y. H. Kim, and K. M. Langa. 2010. Advance directives and outcomes of surrogate decision making before death. *New England Journal of Medicine* 362(13): 1211-1218.

Smith, A. K., R. B. Davis, and E. L. Krakauer. 2007. Differences in the quality of the patient-physician relationship among terminally ill African-American and white patients: Impact on advance care planning and treatment preferences. 2007. *Journal of General Internal Medicine* 22(11):1579-1582.

Smith, A. K., L. C. Walter, Y. Miao, W. J. Boscardin, and K. E. Covinsky. 2013a. Disability during the last two years of life. *JAMA Internal Medicine* 173(16):1506-1513.

Smith, A. K., D. B. White, and R. M. Arnold. 2013b. Uncertainty—the other side of prognosis. *New England Journal of Medicine* 368(26):2448-2450.

Song, J., E. R. Ratner, M. M. Wall, D. M. Bartels, N. Ulvestad, D. Petroskas, M. West, A. M. Weber-Main, L Grengs, and L. Gelberg. 2010. Effect of an end-of-life planning intervention on the completion of advance directives in homeless persons: A randomized trial. *Annals of Internal Medicine* 153(2):76-84.

Stark, M., and J. J. Fins. 2013. What's not being shared in shared decision-making? *The Hastings Center Report* 43(4):13-16.

Stein, J. 2003. The ethics of advance directives: A rehabilitation perspective. *American Journal of Physical Medicine & Rehabilitation* 82(2):152-157.

Stein, R. A., L. Sharpe, M. L. Bell, F. M. Boyle, S. M. Dunn, and S. J. Clarke. 2013. Randomized controlled trial of a structured intervention to facilitate end-of-life decision making in patients with advanced cancer. *Journal of Clinical Oncology* 31(27):3403-3410.

Steinhauser, K. E., N. A. Christakis, E. C. Clipp, M. McNeilly, L. McIntyre, and J. A. Tulsky. 2000a. Factors considered important at the end of life by patients, family, physicians, and other care providers. *Journal of the American Medical Association* 284(19):2476-2482.

Steinhauser, K. E., E. C. Clipp, M. McNeilly, N. A. Christakis, L. McIntyre, and J. A. Tulsky. 2000b. In search of a good death: Observations of patients, families, and providers. *Annals of Internal Medicine* 132(10):825-832.

Steinhauser, K. E., C. I. Voils, E. C. Clipp, H. B. Bosworth, N. A. Christakis, and J. A. Tulsky. 2006. "Are you at peace?": One item to probe spiritual concerns at the end of life. *Archives of Internal Medicine* 166:101-105.

Sudore, R. L., and T. R. Fried. 2010. Redefining the "planning" in advance care planning: Preparing for end-of-life decision making. *Annals of Internal Medicine* 153:256-261.

Sudore, R. L., D. Schillinger, S. J. Knight, and T. R. Fried. 2010. Uncertainty about advance care planning treatment preferences among diverse older adults. *Journal of Health Communication* 15(Suppl. 2):159-171.

Sulmasy, D. P. 2009. Spirituality, religion, and clinical care. *Chest* 135(6):1634-1642.

Swindell, J. S., A. L. McGuire, and S. D. Halpern. 2010. Beneficent persuasion: Techniques and ethical guidelines to improve patients' decisions. *Annals of Family Medicine* 8(3):260-264.

Swindell, J. S., A. L. McGuire, and S. D. Halpern. 2011. Shaping patients' decisions. *Chest* 139(2):424-429.

Tang, S. T. 2003. When death is imminent: Where terminally ill patients with cancer prefer to die and why. *Cancer Nursing* 26(3):245-251.

Temel, J. S., J. A. Greer, A. Muzikansky, E. R. Gallagher, S. Admane, J. A. Jackson, C. M. Dahlin, C. D. Blinderman, J. Jacobsen, W. F. Pirl, J. A. Billinbs, and T. J. Lynch. 2010. Early palliative care for patients with metastatic non-small-cell lung cancer. *New England Journal of Medicine* 363(8):733-742.

Teno, J. M., A. Gruneir, Z. Schwartz, A. Nanda, and T. Wetle. 2007. Association between advance directives and quality of end-of-life care: A national study. *Journal of the American Geriatrics Society* 55(2):189-194.

Teno, J. M., P. L. Gozalo, J. P. Bynum, N. E. Leland, S. C. Miller, N. E. Morden, T. Scupp, D. C. Goodman, and V. Mor. 2013. Change in end-of-life care for Medicare beneficiaries: Site of death, place of care, and health care transitions in 2000, 2005, and 2009. *Journal of the American Medical Association* 309(5):470-477.

Toce, S., and M. A. Collins. 2003. The FOOTPRINTS model of pediatric palliative care. *Journal of Palliative Medicine* 6(6):989-1000.

Tompson, T. J. Benz, J. Agiesta, D. Junius, K. Nguyen, and K. Lowell. 2013. *Long-term care: Perceptions, experiences, and attitudes among Americans 40 or older.* http://www.apnorc.org/PDFs/Long%20Term%20Care/AP_NORC_Long%20Term%20Care%20Perception_FINAL%20REPORT.pdf (accessed August 7, 2013).

Topf, L., C. A. Robinson, and J. L. Bottorff. 2013. When a desired home death does not occur: The consequences of broken promises. *Journal of Palliative Medicine* 16(8):875-880.

Torke, A. M., M. Siegler, A. Abalos, R. M. Moloney, and G. C. Alexander. 2009. Physicians' experience with surrogate decision making for hospitalized adults. *Journal of General Internal Medicine* 24(9):1023-1028.

Towers, B. 1978. The impact of the California Natural Death Act. *Journal of Medical Ethics* 4(2):96-98.

Trice, E. D., and H. G. Prigerson. 2009. Communication in end-stage cancer: Review of the literature and future research. *Journal of Health Communication* 14(Suppl. 1):95-108.

Tuffrey-Wijne, I., and L. McEnhill. 2008. Communication difficulties and intellectual disability in end-of-life care. *International Journal of Palliative Nursing* 14(4):189-194.

Tulsky, J. A., G. S. Fischer, M. R. Rose, and R. M. Arnold. 1998. Opening the black box: How do physicians communicate about advance directives? *Annals of Internal Medicine* 129(6):441-449.

Venneman, S. S., P. Namor-Harris, M. Perish, and M. Hamilton. 2008. "Allow natural death" versus "do not resuscitate": Three words that can change a life. *Journal of Medical Ethics* 34:2-6.

Veysman, B. 2010. Shock me, tube me, line me. *Health Affairs* 29(2):324-326.

Vig, E. K., J. S. Taylor, H. Starks, E. K. Hopley, and K. Fryer-Edwards. 2006. Beyond substituted judgment: How surrogates navigate end-of-life decision-making. *Journal of the American Geriatrics Society* 54(11):1688-1693.

Vig, E. K., H. Starks, J. S. Taylor, E. K. Hopley, and K. Fryer-Edwards. 2007. Surviving surrogate decision-making: What helps and hampers the experience of making medical decisions for others. *Journal of General Internal Medicine* 22(9):1274-1279.

Volandes, A. E., M. Ariza, E. D. Abbo, and M. Paasche-Orlow. 2008a. Overcoming educational barriers for advance care planning in Latinos with video images. *Journal of Palliative Medicine* 11(5):700-706.

Volandes, A. E., M. Paasche-Orlow, M. R. Gillick, E. F. Cook, S. Shaykevich, E. D. Abbo, and L. Lehmann. 2008b. Health literacy not race predicts end-of-life care preferences. *Journal of Palliative Medicine* 11(5):754-762.

Volandes, A. E., G. H. Brandeis, A. D. Davis, M. K. Paasche-Orlow, M. R. Gillick, Y. Chang, E. S. Walker-Corkery, E. Mann, and S. L. Mitchell. 2012a. A randomized controlled trial of a goals-of-care video for elderly patients admitted to skilled nursing facilities. *Journal of Palliative Medicine* 15(7):805-811.

Volandes, A. E., T. T. Levin, S. Slovin, R. D. Carvajal, E. M. O'Reilly, M. L. Keohan, M. Theodoulou, M. Dickler, J. F. Gerecitano, M. Morris, A. S. Epstein, A. Naka-Blackstone, E. S. Walker-Corkery, Y. Chang, and A. Noy. 2012b. Augmenting advance care planning in poor prognosis cancer with a video decision aid: A pre-post study. *Cancer* 118(17):4331-4338.

Volandes, A. E., M. K. Paasche-Orlow, S. L. Mitchell, A. El-Jawahri, A. D. Davis, M. J. Barry, K. L. Hartshorn, V. A. Jackson, M. R. Gillick, E. S. Walker-Corkery, Y. Chang, L. López, M. Kemeny, L. Bulone, E. Mann, S. Misra, M. Peachey, E. D. Abbo, A. F. Eichler, A. S. Epstein, A. Noy, T. T. Levin, and J. S. Temel. 2013. Randomized controlled trial of a video decision support tool for cardiopulmonary resuscitation decision making in advanced cancer. *Journal of Clinical Oncology* 31(3):380-386.

Wachterman, M. W., E. R. Marcantonio, R. B. Davis, R. A. Cohen, S. S. Waikar, R. S. Phillips, and E. P. McCarthy 2013. Relationship between the prognostic expectations of seriously ill patients undergoing hemodialysis and their nephrologists. *JAMA Internal Medicine* 173(13):1206-1214.

Wagemans, A., H. van Schrojenstein Lantman-de Valk, I Proot, J. Metsemakers, I. Tuffrey-Wijne, and L. Curfs. 2013. The factors affecting end-of-life decision-making by physicians of patients with intellectual disabilities in the Netherlands: A qualitative study. *Journal of Intellectual Disability Research* 57(4):380-389.

Waite, K. R., A. D. Federman, D. M. McCarthy, R. Sudore, L. M. Curtis, D. W. Baker, E. A. Wilson, R. Hasnain-Wynia, M. S. Wolf, and M. K. Paasche-Orlow. 2013. Literacy and race as risk factors for low rates of advance directives in older adults. *Journal of the American Geriatrics Society* 61(3):403-406.

Walling, A., K. A. Lorenz, S. M. Dy, A. Naeim, H. Sanati, S. M. Asch, and N. S. Wenger. 2008. Evidence-based recommendations for information and care planning in cancer care. *Journal of Clinical Oncology* 26(23):3896-3902.

Washington, H. A. 2006. *Medical apartheid: The dark history of medical experimentation on black Americans from colonial times to the present.* New York: Anchor Books.

Weeks, J. C., P. J. Catalano, A. Cronin, M. D. Finkelman, J. W. Mack, N. L. Keating, and D. Schrag. 2012. Patients' expectations about effects of chemotherapy for advanced cancer. *New England Journal of Medicine* 367(17):1616-1625.

Welch, L. C., J. M. Teno, and V. Mor. 2005. End-of-life care in black and white: Race matters for medical care of dying patients and their families. *Journal of the American Geriatrics Society* 53(7):1145-1153.

Wendler, D., and A. Rid. 2011. Systematic review: The effects on surrogates of making treatment decisions for others. *Annals of Internal Medicine* 154(5):336-346.

Wenger, N. S., J. Citko, K. O'Malley, A. Diamant, K. Lorenz, V. Gonzalez, and D. M. Tarn. 2012. Implementation of physician orders for life sustaining treatment in nursing homes in California: Evaluation of a novel statewide dissemination mechanism. *Journal of General Internal Medicine* 28(1):51-57.

West, S. K., and M. Hollis. 2012. Barriers to completion of advance care directives among African Americans ages 25-84: A cross-generational study. *Omega* (Westport) 65(2): 125-137.

White, D. B., L. R. Evans, C. A. Bautista, J. M. Luce, and B. Lo. 2009. Are physicians' recommendations to limit life support beneficial or burdensome? Bringing empirical data to the debate. *American Journal of Respiratory and Critical Care Medicine* 180:320-325.

White, D. B., S. M. Cua, R. Walk, L. Pollice, L. Weissfeld, S. Hong, C. S. Landefeld, and R. M. Arnold. 2012. Nurse-led intervention to improve surrogate decision making for patients with advanced critical illness. *American Journal of Critical Care* 21(6):396-409.

WHO (World Health Organization). 2014. *Chronic respiratory diseases: Burden of COPD.* http://www.who.int/respiratory/copd/burden/en (accessed June 2, 2014).

Wicher, C. P., and M. A. Meeker. 2012. What influences African American end-of-life preferences? *Journal of Health Care for the Poor and Underserved* 23(1):28-58.

Wiener, L., E. Ballard, T. Brennan, H. Battles, P. Martinez, and M. Pao. 2008. How I wish to be remembered: The use of an advance care planning document in adolescent and young adult populations. *Journal of Palliative Medicine* 11(10):1309-1313.

Wiener, L., S. Zadeh, H. Battles, K. Baird, E. Ballard, J. Osherow, and M. Pao. 2012. Allowing adolescents and young adults to plan their end-of-life care. *Pediatrics* 130(5):897-905.

Wilson, C. J., J. Newman, S. Tapper, S. Lai, P. H. Cheng, F. M. Wu, and M. Tai-Seale. 2013. Multiple locations of advance care planning documentation in an electronic health record: Are they easy to find? *Journal of Palliative Medicine* 16(9):1089-1094.

Winter, L., M. P. Dennis, and B. Parker. 2007. Religiosity and preferences for life-prolonging medical treatments in African-American and white elders: A mediation study. *Omega* 56(3):273-288.

Wolfe, J., N. Klar, H. E. Grier, J. Duncan, S. Salem-Schatz, E. J. Emanuel, and J. C. Weeks. 2000. Understanding of prognosis among parents of children who died of cancer: Impact on treatment goals and integration of palliative care. *Journal of the American Medical Association* 284(19):2469-2475.

Wright, A. A., B. Zhang, A. Ray, J. W. Mack, E. Trice, T. Balboni, S. L. Mitchell, V. A. Jackson, S. D. Block, P. K. Maciejewski, and H. G. Prigerson. 2008. Associations between end-of-life discussions, patient mental health, medical care near death, and caregiver bereavement adjustment. *Journal of the American Medical Association* 300(14):1665-1673.

Yennurajalingam, S., A. Noguera, H. A. Parsons, I. Torres-Vigil, E. R. Duarte, A. Palma, S. Bunge, L. L. Palmer, M. O. Delgado-Guay, and E. Bruera. 2013a. A multicenter survey of Hispanic caregiver preferences for patient decision control in the United States and Latin America. *Palliative Medicine* 27(7):692-698.

Yennurajalingam, S., H. A. Parsons, S., E. R. Duarte, A. Palma, S. Bunge, L. L. Palmer, M. O. Delgado-Guay, J. Allo, and E. Bruera. 2013b. Decisional control preferences of Hispanic patients with advanced cancer from the United States and Latin America. *Journal of Pain and Symptom Management* 46(3):376-385.

Yung, V. Y., A. M. Walling, L. Min, N. S. Wenger, and D. A. Ganz. 2010. Documentation of advance care planning for community-dwelling elders. *Journal of Palliative Medicine* 13(7):861-867.

Zabora, J., K. BrintzenhofeSzoc, B. Curbow, C. Hooker, and S. Piantadosi. 2001. The prevalence of psychological distress by cancer site. *Psychooncology* 10(1):19-28.

Zaide, G. B., R. Pekmezaris, C. N. Nouryan., T. P. Mir, C. P. Sison, T. Liberman, M. L. Lesser, L. B. Cooper, and G. P. Wolf-Klein. 2013. Ethnicity, race, and advance directives in an inpatient palliative care consultation service. *Palliative and Supportive Care* 11(1):5-11.

Zaleskiewicz, T., A. Gasiorowska, and P. Kesebir. 2013. Saving can save from death anxiety: Mortality salience and financial decision-making. *PLoS ONE* 8(11):e79407.

Zettel-Watson, L., P. H. Ditto, J. H. Danks, and W. D. Smucker. 2008. Actual and perceived gender differences in the accuracy of surrogate decisions about life-sustaining medical treatment among older spouses. *Death Studies* 32(3):273-290.

Zhang, B., A. A. Wright, H. A. Huskamp, M. E. Nilsson, M. L. Maciejewski, C. C. Earle, S. D. Block, P. K. Maciejewski, and H. G. Prigerson. 2009. Health care costs in the last week of life: Associations with end of life conversations. *Archives of Internal Medicine* 169(5):480-488.

Zheng, N. T., D. B. Mukamel, T. Caprio, S. Cai, and H. Temkin-Greener. 2011. Racial disparities in in-hospital death and hospice use among nursing home residents at the end-of-life. *Medical Care* 49(11):992-998.

Zier, L. S., P. D. Sottile, S. Y. Hong, L. A. Weissfeld, and D. B. White. 2012. Surrogate decision makers' interpretation of prognostic information: A mixed-methods study. *Annals of Internal Medicine* 156(5):360-366.

Zilberberg, M. D., and A. F. Shorr. 2012. Economics at the end of life: Hospital and ICU perspectives. *Seminars in Respiratory and Critical Care Medicine* 33(4):362-369.

Zive, D. M., and T. A. Schmidt. 2012. *Pathways to POLST registry development: Lessons learned.* http://www.polst.org/wp-content/uploads/2012/12/POLST-Registry.pdf (accessed October 2, 2013).

ANNEX 3-1:
ADVANCE CARE PLANNING IN THE CONTEXT
OF COMMON SERIOUS CONDITIONS

For each of the four common serious conditions described in this appendix, all of which are leading causes of death in the United States, the failure to provide palliative care—important components of which are the setting of treatment goals and effective communication among patient, family, and clinicians—is a major shortcoming in the quality of care.

Heart Failure

Heart failure was the primary cause of more than 56,000 deaths in the United States in 2009 and was a contributing cause in 1 of every 9 deaths (274,000 deaths) (Go et al., 2013). About half of people who have heart failure die within 5 years of diagnosis (CDC, 2013a). The condition accounts for some 800,000 hospital admissions through the emergency department each year (Collins et al., 2013).[36]

Patients and families need good counseling so they understand the specific end-of-life quandaries raised by heart failure. These include the disease's unpredictability and the considerable risk of sudden death, which heightens the need to designate a health care agent and specify the circumstances under which permanent pacemakers or defibrillators should be deactivated (Shah et al., 2013).

A comprehensive review of almost 25 years of medical literature found little evidence of discussions between health care professionals and heart failure patients regarding care preferences, disease progression, or future care options (Barclay et al., 2011). The authors note the frequent lack of agreement between doctors and patients/family members regarding whether such discussions had occurred and the information that was exchanged (see also DesHarnais et al., 2007[37]; Kirkpatrick et al., 2007). Although some of these studies involved relatively small numbers of patients, consistent findings were that heart failure patients

- have mixed views about having these conversations, with some wanting a great deal of information and some wanting no details about their condition; and

---

[36]Heart failure hospitalizations are considered an ambulatory care–sensitive condition by the federal Agency for Healthcare Research and Quality: http://www.qualitymeasures.ahrq.gov/content.aspx?id=38562 (accessed December 16, 2014).

[37]The study by DesHarnais and colleagues (2007) involved 30 patients with heart failure (42 percent of the study population), as well as 41 patients with terminal cancer diagnoses.

- are most likely to want such conversations when they are unwell and in the hospital (a time when they may be least able to process information effectively).

In addition, health care professionals

- find establishing a diagnosis and prognosis for heart failure difficult, which complicates the task of explaining the condition to patients in a way that is not frightening and determining the appropriate timing for the discussion (Barclay et al., 2011);
- do not know patient preferences for pain control and place of death and the financial/religious considerations that factor into those preferences (DesHarnais et al., 2007); and
- tend to focus on immediate concerns of disease management, instead of viewing heart failure as a terminal illness (Barclay et al., 2011).

The articles reviewed by Barclay and colleagues (2011) indicate that patients value clinicians' communication skills, although many cardiology professionals believe they lack such skills. Clinicians' time pressures and manner and patients' reluctance to ask questions are among the identified barriers to conversation on these issues.

A heart failure–specific advance care planning model was tested in a Midwest health system (Schellinger et al., 2011). The model used the Respecting Choices program, discussed earlier in this chapter, and included a facilitated, in-depth interview with patients and their family/health care agents. Discussion tools completed during the disease-specific advance care planning interviews were scanned into patients' electronic health records. The study found no significant difference between patients among whom the model was used and a control group with respect to inpatient and emergency department admissions, although among patients who died, those who had completed their advance care planning were more than twice as likely to have been enrolled in hospice. The health system's management was sufficiently encouraged by this study's effectiveness in recruiting patients and achieving completion of advance directives to expand training in the model, improve the visibility of advance care planning information in the electronic health record, and continue implementation efforts.

Chronic Obstructive Pulmonary Disease (COPD)

COPD is the cause of significant morbidity and mortality worldwide (WHO, 2014). In the United States, it is the third leading cause of death (CDC, 2012), and accounted for 715,000 hospitalizations in 2011, approximately 65 percent of which were among adults aged 65 and older (American Lung Association, 2013). Like heart failure, COPD is a frequent cause of emergency hospitalizations, is progressive, has frightening and disabling symptoms (principally severe shortness of breath and anxiety), has an unpredictable trajectory, is associated with multiple comorbidities, and is a not infrequent cause of sudden death.

Few patients with COPD have discussed their end-of-life preferences with their physician (Heffner, 2011; Patel et al., 2012), and many do not know they have a life-limiting illness or even what that illness is (Gardiner et al., 2009). The barriers to greater advance care planning discussions resemble those for other medical conditions, with the added difficulty of multiple COPD phenotypes and multiple associated comorbid conditions that can affect the disease's course (Heffner, 2011; Patel et al., 2012).

Patients with COPD have given physicians low marks with respect to discussing the specific issues of prognosis, what dying might be like, and spirituality and religion, while at the same time acknowledging their general communication skills (willingness to listen and address patients' questions and concerns) (Curtis et al., 2004). Communication about care planning typically occurs in the crisis situation of an intensive care unit rather than in the primary care physician's office, with each discipline believing the conversation is someone else's responsibility (Gott et al., 2009).

COPD's acute exacerbations followed by partial recovery "lull physicians into thinking [advance care planning] can wait until a future date and clouds the definition of what constitutes 'end of life' because points of transition are so poorly recognizable" (Heffner, 2011, p. 105). In this unpredictable disease, models for in-the-moment decision making may be more useful than discussions about future preferences based on hypothetical outcomes (Patel et al., 2012).

Mental health issues that characterize COPD (and many other chronic, progressive conditions) further complicate advance care planning discussions. The link between cigarette smoking and COPD stimulates feelings of remorse, shame, and guilt, which decrease patients' motivation for engaging in advance care planning and suggest a need for psychological support and possible psychotherapeutic treatment (Heffner, 2011; Lindqvist and Hallberg, 2010).

Depression and anxiety are relatively common in chronic diseases, and are linked to increased health care utilization and higher disability rates. Depression also affects patients' choices about care and "leads to social isolation and loneliness, which are also experienced by patients' family caregivers," who may stop encouraging them to engage in advance care planning (Heffner, 2011, p. 106).

Cancer

Most of the research on advance care planning for patients with specific diseases has been conducted among patients with cancer, which is responsible for more than 500,000 U.S. deaths per year (CDC, 2013b). "Cancer is an emotionally laden, often disruptive, and sometimes tumultuous experience for patients, families and providers" (Walling et al., 2008, p. 3896). For that reason alone, an essential aspect of good oncology care is good communication about the disease, its path, and choices for treatment (Trice and Prigerson, 2009). (See also the section of this chapter on handling emotional encounters.)

Advance care planning is recommended for patients with cancer at several specific points: at diagnosis, at any subsequent key time when goal-oriented discussions are appropriate (e.g., when invasive procedures or new chemotherapy regimens are contemplated, when neurological symptoms or brain metastases appear, or upon admission to an intensive care unit), and before an expected death (Walling et al., 2008). Guidelines from the National Comprehensive Cancer Network and the National Consensus Project for Quality Palliative Care recommend that physicians have an advance care planning discussion with any patients who have "incurable" cancer and an expected life span of less than 1 year (Bomba and Vermilyea, 2006; Dahlin, 2013; NCCN, 2013).

Treatment preferences of patients with advanced cancer often are unexpressed and undiscussed (Mack et al., 2010b), and care often reflects "the prevailing styles of treatment in the regions and health care systems where they happen to receive cancer treatment" (Goodman et al., 2013, p. 1). If these discussions occur, evidence from large studies suggests they tend to occur late in the disease trajectory, when patients already are in decline, and during acute hospital admissions, whereas they might better be accomplished during less stressful outpatient visits (Mack et al., 2012).

However, patients who have end-of-life discussions of any kind are more likely than those who do not to receive care in accordance with their wishes, especially when those discussions take place relatively early in the course of the illness (Goodman et al., 2013). Compared with patients who do not have these discussions, those who do, as well as patients who understand they are terminally ill, are more likely to receive end-of-life care consistent with their preferences (Mack et al., 2010b). Those who have end-of-life discussions also have lower rates of ventilation, resuscitation, and admission to the intensive care unit and are more likely to enroll in hospice earlier; early hospice enrollment is associated with improved patient and caregiver quality of life (Wright et al., 2008).

Despite these benefits, while some people "set limits on the amount of discomfort and treatments they will accept," others "want all possible treatments to prolong life, regardless of discomfort" (Byock, 2013, p. 7). Ironically, it is possible that choosing intensive or life-extending treatment in the face of advanced disease does not always increase longevity (e.g., Mack et al., 2010b). In a highly regarded randomized controlled trial of early introduction of palliative care in metastatic lung cancer,[38] survival was actually longer in the patients who received palliative care and less chemotherapy (Temel et al., 2010).

The degree to which patients want to discuss end-of-life matters varies among individuals and families, over time, and in the face of changing circumstances, so that "the information preferences of a particular patient cannot be reliably predicted by demographic, cultural, or cancer-specific factors" (Russell and Ward, 2011, p. 191). Doctors are not accurate at guessing what those preferences will be; they must ask, although evidence suggests that this does not occur systematically. Mack and colleagues (2012) found that medical oncologists documented end-of-life discussions with only about one-quarter of their patients.

Dementias

Alzheimer's disease is the sixth leading cause of death in the United States and was the direct cause of more than 83,000 deaths in 2010 (CDC, 2013b), although pneumonia or other manifestations of frailty often are listed as the cause of death for people with Alzheimer's disease and dementia. Estimates are that nearly one-half of Americans aged 85 and older have Alzheimer's disease (CDC, 2011). More than one-half of patients with Alzheimer's disease (54 percent) lack decision-making capacity, and decisions about their care eventually end up being made by their health care agents or surrogates (Sessums et al., 2011).

Dementia differs from many other cognitive impairments in that the people afflicted went through a lifetime of making decisions and acquired the inability to continue doing so only with advancing age or the appearance of other chronic conditions. Thus, there presumably was a period of many years during which people with dementia would have been capable of expressing preferences for treatment.

Dementias are also different from many other conditions in that they typically are progressive. Huntington's disease, for example, is a progressive neurodegenerative disorder for which there is no disease-altering treatment and that eventually results in institutionalization. Because of the pattern of erratic and impulsive behavior early in the disease, those afflicted often

---

[38]In the Temel et al. (2010) study, palliative care specifically included the advance care planning activities of establishing goals of care and assisting with decision making regarding treatment.

lose the support of friends or family, and patients have difficulty expressing themselves verbally. In a study involving 53 specialized nursing home residents with Huntington's disease, one-quarter of the patients (or their representatives) requested cardiopulmonary resuscitation (Dellefield and Ferrini, 2011). By contrast, a study of 323 nursing home residents found that when health care agents understood the patient's poor prognosis and the clinical complications typical in advanced dementia, they were much less likely to authorize burdensome interventions, such as hospitalization, emergency room visits, tube feeding, or intravenous therapy (Mitchell et al., 2009). In this study, fewer than one in three of the health care agents had been counseled by a physician about these complications; even fewer (18 percent) had received prognostic information from a physician.

ANNEX 3-2:
OREGON PHYSICIAN ORDERS FOR
LIFE-SUSTAINING TREATMENT (POLST) FORM

HIPAA PERMITS DISCLOSURE TO HEALTH CARE PROFESSIONALS & ELECTRONIC REGISTRY AS NECESSARY FOR TREATMENT

Physician Orders for Life-Sustaining Treatment (POLST)

Follow these medical orders until orders change. Any section not completed implies full treatment for that section.

Patient Last Name:	Patient First Name:	Patient Middle Name:	Last 4 SSN:

Address: (street / city / state / zip):	Date of Birth: (mm/dd/yyyy) ___ / ___ / ___	Gender: ☐ M ☐ F

A Check One	**CARDIOPULMONARY RESUSCITATION (CPR):** *Unresponsive, pulseless, & not breathing.*
	☐ **Attempt Resuscitation/CPR** If patient is not in cardiopulmonary arrest, ☐ **Do Not Attempt Resuscitation/DNR** follow orders in **B** and **C**.

B Check One	**MEDICAL INTERVENTIONS:** *If patient has pulse and is breathing.*
	☐ **Comfort Measures Only**. Provide treatments to relieve pain and suffering through the use of any medication by any route, positioning, wound care and other measures. Use oxygen, suction and manual treatment of airway obstruction as needed for comfort. *Patient prefers no transfer to hospital* for life-sustaining treatments. *Transfer if comfort needs cannot be met in current location.* <u>Treatment Plan</u>: **Provide treatments for comfort through symptom management.**
	☐ **Limited Treatment**. In addition to care described in Comfort Measures Only, use medical treatment, antibiotics, IV fluids and cardiac monitor as indicated. No intubation, advanced airway interventions, or mechanical ventilation. May consider less invasive airway support (e.g. CPAP, BiPAP). *Transfer to hospital if indicated. Generally avoid the intensive care unit.* <u>Treatment Plan</u>: **Provide basic medical treatments.**
	☐ **Full Treatment**. In addition to care described in Comfort Measures Only and Limited Treatment, use intubation, advanced airway interventions, and mechanical ventilation as indicated. *Transfer to hospital* and/or intensive care unit if indicated. <u>Treatment Plan</u>: **All treatments including breathing machine.**
	Additional Orders: _____

C Check One	**ARTIFICIALLY ADMINISTERED NUTRITION:** *Offer food by mouth if feasible.*
	☐ Long-term artificial nutrition by tube. ☐ Defined trial period of artificial nutrition by tube. ☐ No artificial nutrition by tube.	*Additional Orders (e.g., defining the length of a trial period):* _____

D Must Fill Out	**DOCUMENTATION OF DISCUSSION: (REQUIRED)** *See reverse side for add'l info.*
	☐ Patient (If patient lacks capacity, must check a box below)
	☐ Health Care Representative (legally appointed by advance directive or court)
	☐ Surrogate defined by facility policy or Surrogate for patient with developmental disabilities or significant mental health condition (Note: Special requirements for completion- see reverse side)
	Representative/Surrogate Name: _____ Relationship: _____

E	**PATIENT OR SURROGATE SIGNATURE AND OREGON POLST REGISTRY OPT OUT**
	Signature: *recommended*	This form will be sent to the POLST Registry unless the patient wishes to opt out, if so check opt out box: ☐

F Must Print Name, Sign & Date	**ATTESTATION OF MD / DO / NP / PA (REQUIRED)**
	By signing below, I attest that these medical orders are, to the best of my knowledge, consistent with the patient's **current** medical condition and preferences.
	Print Signing MD / DO / NP / PA Name: *required*	Signer Phone Number:	Signer License Number: *(optional)*
	MD / DO / NP / PA Signature: *required*	Date: *required*	Office Use Only

SEND FORM WITH PATIENT WHENEVER TRANSFERRED OR DISCHARGED
SUBMIT COPY OF BOTH SIDES OF FORM TO REGISTRY IF PATIENT DID NOT OPT OUT IN SECTION E

© CENTER FOR ETHICS IN HEALTH CARE, Oregon Health & Science University.   2014

HIPAA PERMITS DISCLOSURE TO HEALTH CARE PROFESSIONALS & ELECTRONIC REGISTRY AS NECESSARY FOR TREATMENT

Information for patient named on this form   PATIENT'S NAME: _____

The POLST form is **always voluntary** and is usually for persons with serious illness or frailty. POLST records your wishes for medical treatment in your current state of health (states your treatment wishes if something happened tonight). Once initial medical treatment is begun and the risks and benefits of further therapy are clear, your treatment wishes may change. Your medical care and this form can be changed to reflect your new wishes at any time. No form, however, can address all the medical treatment decisions that may need to be made. An Advance Directive is recommended for all capable adults and allows you to document in detail your future health care instructions and/or name a Health Care Representative to speak for you if you are unable to speak for yourself. Consider reviewing your Advance Directive and giving a copy of it to your health care professional.

Contact Information (Optional)

Health Care Representative or Surrogate:	Relationship:	Phone Number:	Address:

Health Care Professional Information

Preparer Name:	Preparer Title:	Phone Number:	Date Prepared:

PA's Supervising Physician:	Phone Number:

Primary Care Professional:

Directions for Health Care Professionals

Completing POLST

- Completing a POLST is always voluntary and cannot be mandated for a patient.
- An order of CPR in Section A is incompatible with an order for Comfort Measures Only in Section B (will not be accepted in Registry).
- For information on legally appointed health care representatives and their authority, refer to ORS 127.505 - 127.660.
- Should reflect current preferences of persons with serious illness or frailty. Also, encourage completion of an Advance Directive.
- Verbal / phone orders are acceptable with follow-up signature by MD/DO/NP/PA in accordance with facility/community policy.
- Use of original form is encouraged. Photocopies, faxes, and electronic registry forms are also legal and valid.
- A person with developmental disabilities or significant mental health condition requires additional consideration before completing the POLST form; refer to *Guidance for Health Care Professionals* at www.or.polst.org.

Oregon POLST Registry Information

Health Care Professionals:	**Registry Contact Information:**	**Patients:**
(1) You are *required* to send a copy of both sides of this POLST form to the Oregon POLST Registry unless the patient opts out.	Phone: 503-418-4083 Fax or eFAX: 503-418-2161 www.orpolstregistry.org polstreg@ohsu.edu	Mailed confirmation packets from Registry may take four weeks for delivery.
(2) The following sections must be completed: • Patient's full name • Date of birth • MD / DO / NP / PA signature • Date signed	Oregon POLST Registry 3181 SW Sam Jackson Park Rd. Mail Code: CDW-EM Portland, Or 97239	**MAY PUT REGISTRY ID STICKER HERE:**

Updating POLST: A POLST Form only needs to be revised if patient treatment preferences have changed.

This POLST should be reviewed periodically, including when:

- The patient is transferred from one care setting or care level to another (including upon admission or at discharge), or
- There is a substantial change in the patient's health status.

If patient wishes haven't changed, the POLST Form does not need to be revised, updated, rewritten or resent to the Registry.

Voiding POLST: A copy of the voided POLST must be sent to the Registry unless patient has opted-out.

- A person with capacity, or the valid surrogate of a person without capacity, can void the form and request alternative treatment.
- Draw line through sections A through E and write "VOID" in large letters if POLST is replaced or becomes invalid.
- Send a copy of the voided form to the POLST Registry (**required** unless patient has opted out).
- If included in an electronic medical record, follow voiding procedures of facility/community.

For permission to use the copyrighted form contact the OHSU Center for Ethics in Health Care at orpolst@ohsu.edu or (503) 494-3965. Information on the Oregon POLST Program is available online at **www.or.polst.org** or at **orpolst@ohsu.edu**

SEND FORM WITH PATIENT WHENEVER TRANSFERRED OR DISCHARGED, SUBMIT COPY TO REGISTRY

4

Professional Education and Development

Education of health professionals who provide care to people nearing the end of life has improved substantially in several areas since the Institute of Medicine (IOM) reports *Approaching Death* (IOM, 1997) and *When Children Die* (IOM, 2003) were published. Most notably, hospice and palliative medicine has become established as a defined medical specialty, with 10 cosponsoring certification boards. Despite this progress, however, major educational deficiencies remain with respect to end-of-life care.

This chapter begins by summarizing progress made in professional education with respect to end-of-life care since the above two IOM reports were issued, as well as deficiencies that remain. It then describes impediments to teaching all physicians and nurses about palliative care. Removing these impediments would enhance basic palliative care as provided by clinicians who are not hospice and palliative medicine specialists. Next, the chapter describes the roles and preparation of palliative care team members, including specialists in palliative care in the professions of medicine, nursing, social work, pharmacy, and chaplaincy; rehabilitation therapists and direct care workers are also discussed. The chapter ends with the committee's findings, conclusions, and recommendation on creating change in professional education.

PROGRESS AND CONTINUING NEEDS

When Children Die recommends creating and testing end-of-life care curricula and educational experiences for all health care professionals who work with children and families, as well as specialty clinicians and palliative care specialists (IOM, 2003). *Approaching Death* includes a recommendation to raise palliative medicine to specialty or near-specialty status. The report's recommendation 5 says, in part, "Palliative care should become, if not a medical specialty, at least a defined area of expertise, education, and research" (IOM, 1997, pp. 9, 12; see also pp. 224-227). This important recommendation has been realized with the board certification of thousands of hospice and palliative medicine specialists drawn from other disciplines. Palliative care specialties have been developed as well for advanced practice nurses and registered nurses. A palliative care specialty has emerged in social work, and another is under way in chaplaincy. Nearly 100 hospice and palliative medicine fellowship programs, with the capacity to graduate some 200 fellows annually, have gained accreditation. Similar gains have occurred in nursing and social work. Clinical experiences in hospital-based palliative care and outpatient hospice have become more widely available. Other areas of progress include the following:

- *Faculty preparation*—Increasing numbers of faculty members have palliative care credentials. Since *Approaching Death* was published, important efforts to train faculty have included the Faculty Scholars Program for physicians and nurses and the Social Work Leadership Development Awards, both initiatives of the Open Society Institute's Project on Death in America (Open Society Institute, 2004). Such efforts have also included the End of Life/Palliative Education Resource Center (Medical College of Wisconsin, undated) and faculty recognition through the U.S. Department of Veterans Affairs (VA) Faculty Leader Project for Improved Care at the End of Life (Stevens et al., 1999). Two major ongoing continuing education programs—the Education in Palliative and End-of-life Care program and End-of-Life Nursing Education Consortium—together have trained thousands of physicians and nurses through a train-the-trainer approach.
- *Medical education*—Medical students today have greater exposure than before to end-of-life knowledge and skills in medical schools. Education in palliative care is offered in 99 percent of U.S. medical schools, usually as part of another course, and all medical schools offer some type of instruction on death and dying, although the average total instruction is a mere 17 hours in the 4-year curriculum (Dickinson, 2011). In a 2013 annual survey conducted by the Association of American Medical Colleges, nearly 80 percent of graduating medical students deemed the instruction they received

in palliative care and pain management appropriate, and about 20 percent thought it inadequate (AAMC, 2013).[1]

- *Professional infrastructure*—As reflected in many of the sources cited in this report, important research on palliative care has been published in first-tier journals, and several new peer-reviewed journals on palliative care have been launched. Moreover, the number of active organizations dedicated to the advancement of palliative care, partly through the setting or promotion of standards, has grown and now includes the American Academy of Hospice and Palliative Medicine, the Center to Advance Palliative Care, the National Hospice and Palliative Care Organization (formerly the National Hospice Organization), the Hospice and Palliative Nurses Association, and the Social Work Hospice and Palliative Care Network.
- *Knowledge base*—Major gains have been made in the knowledge base of palliative care. These gains are evidenced in palliative care textbooks (e.g., in medicine, Hanks et al. [2009] and Bruera et al. [2009]; in nursing, Ferrell and Coyle [2010]; and in pediatrics, Hinds et al. [2010], Wolfe et al. [2011], and Carter et al. [2011]), as well as in increased palliative care content in nonspecialty texts.

Despite these gains, however, two important deficiencies persist. First, these knowledge gains have not necessarily been matched by the transfer of knowledge to most clinicians caring for people with advanced serious illnesses. As was true at the time *Approaching Death* was published in 1997, the topic of death and dying does not have a strong presence in the medical school curriculum. Similarly, in the care of very sick children, many family physicians, pediatricians, and their counterparts and colleagues in nursing and social work have developed an expertise in palliative care, but the overall pattern of inattention to palliative and end-of-life care observed in *When Children Die* still appears to predominate in the pediatric world. To illustrate, a 2003 survey of 49 pediatric residents at the Children's Hospital of Pittsburgh found "minimal training, experience, knowledge, competence, and comfort in virtually all areas of palliative care for children," with no significant improvement in any of these areas from the first to the third year of training (Kolarik et al., 2006, p. 1952). Other studies have also found that physicians and other health professionals continue to experience mini-

---

[1]By contrast, in an earlier telephone survey of 1,751 U.S. medical students and residents, two-fifths said they felt unprepared to address dying patients' fears, to manage their own feelings about patients' deaths or help bereaved families, and to teach end-of-life care, and nearly half said dying patients were not considered good teaching cases (Sullivan et al., 2003).

mal or no training in palliative care for the pediatric population (Liben et al., 2008; Rapoport et al., 2013; Serwint et al., 2006).

The second major remaining deficiency involves the limited number of palliative care specialists. As noted in a later section of this chapter, approximately 6,500 physicians are board certified in hospice and palliative medicine. In 2010, the national shortage in this specialty was estimated to be between 6,000 and 18,000 physicians (Lupu and American Academy of Hospice and Palliative Medicine Workforce Task Force, 2010). In one sense, this shortage estimate could be interpreted as too high because it was based on a supply of only 4,400 palliative care specialists and on a model of demand reflecting staffing levels at "exemplar" institutions.[2] In another sense, the estimate could be interpreted as too low because it was not population based (or empirically determined). Moreover, it rested on an apparent assumption that people do not need, and present no demand for, specialty palliative care services outside of institutional settings.

However, many people outside of institutional settings do need what in this report is termed *basic palliative care* (see Box 1-2 in Chapter 1). Basic palliative care is vital because hospice and palliative medicine specialists will never be sufficient in number to provide regular face-to-face treatment of every person with an advanced serious illness. Hospice and palliative medicine specialists supplement, and do not replace, the palliative care services of clinicians in primary care and disease-oriented specialties.

I am a family physician who provides end-of-life care in a rural setting for patients, both at a nursing home and in their personal homes. As difficult as these situations can be, as medical providers we can provide a great deal of comfort walking patients and families through these end-of-life events by detailing how the events normally transpire. More important, though, is that we are able to provide mental and spiritual care for the patient and family. Once the patient and family realize they are in an end-of-life situation, they are almost always open to care options to help make the dying process meaningful and physically comfortable for the patient. *

---

*Quotation from a response submitted through the online public testimony questionnaire for this study. See Appendix C.

---

[2]In the cited study, the "exemplar" institutions used in modeling demand included three hospices and one academic medical center, and the estimate was based on the Center to Advance Palliative Care's recommended staffing level of one hospice and palliative medicine physician for every 12 patients (CAPC, 2014; Lupu and American Academy of Hospice and Palliative Medicine Workforce Task Force, 2010).

BOX 4-1
Domains of Clinical Competence in End-of-Life Care

Scientific and clinical knowledge and skills
- Symptom control and medication management
- Patient assessment and caregiver assessment
- Physical and emotional symptoms
- Advance care planning

Interpersonal skills and knowledge
- Communication
- Respecting patient and family choices (overlap with ethics)

Ethical and professional principles
- Doing good
- Avoiding harm
- Respecting patient and family choices (overlap with interpersonal skills)

Organizational skills
- How the clinician interacts with the system

Approaching Death (IOM, 1997) and *When Children Die* (IOM, 2003) specify the same four domains of clinical competency in palliative care: scientific and clinical knowledge; interpersonal skills and knowledge, ethical and professional principles, and organizational skills. These domains are as relevant today as they were when those earlier reports were produced. Box 4-1 summarizes these domains.

IMPEDIMENTS TO CHANGING THE CULTURE
OF CARE THROUGH EDUCATION

Health professions education can help transform the care of people with advanced serious illnesses. Indeed, far-reaching changes in how physicians, nurses, and other health professionals are educated and trained may be necessary to effect that transformation.

In the committee's judgment, three impediments in health professions education and development have obstructed coordination, compassion, and choice in end-of-life care. Interacting with each other, these impediments reinforce a general inadequacy in preparing physicians, nurses, and other health professionals to provide basic palliative care, and overcoming them would greatly improve the palliative care landscape. The three impediments are as follows:

- *Curriculum deficits:* The usual curricula of medical and nursing schools contain too little content on palliative care. Many physicians and nurses have entered practice with only a limited understanding of palliative care and generally are ill equipped to meet patients' basic palliative care needs.
- *Lack of interprofessional collaboration:* Education for medical professionals takes a generally siloed approach, whereas palliative care requires an interdisciplinary, team-based approach. Having been educated separately, physicians, nurses, and other health professionals have not had the opportunity to develop teamwork skills and attitudes.
- *Neglect of communication skills:* Communication skills are neglected in both the undergraduate (medical school) and graduate (internships, residencies, and fellowships) education of physicians, as well as in the preparation of nurses and other health professionals.

Curriculum Deficits

Undergraduate and Graduate Medical Education

In a major advance, the Liaison Committee on Medical Education now requires accredited U.S. and Canadian medical schools to teach end-of-life care.[3] To the extent that this policy is carried out, nearly all future physicians will be at least somewhat prepared to practice basic palliative care. However, the Liaison Committee's requirement is vague—it does not specifically mention palliative care, for example—and it does not appear to be rigorously enforced through specific standards or clear expectations. Perhaps partly as a consequence, end-of-life care, including principles and practices of palliative care and hospice and palliative medicine, still is not taught widely and intensively in U.S. medical schools.

As noted above, palliative care usually is offered only as part of another course. In a 2008 survey on palliative care in 128 U.S. medical schools, only 47 responded, and just 14 of these had a required course (Van Aalst-Cohen et al., 2008). A recent review found an "absence of sufficient formal classroom and clinical instruction" in palliative care and concluded that most

---

[3]Liaison Committee on Medical Education standard ED-13 states, in full: "The curriculum of a medical education program must cover all organ systems, and include the important aspects of preventive, acute, chronic, continuing, rehabilitative, and end-of-life care" (Liaison Committee on Medical Education, 2013, p. 10). This policy was initiated in 2000.

medical students learn about the subject largely informally, through "the 'hidden' curriculum."[4] In these authors' view, this hidden content often presents negative messages, such as "death is a medical failure," and there is no reason to assign students to dying patients because there is "nothing to learn" from them (Horowitz et al., 2014, p. 63).

When palliative care is taught, results can be impressive. A review of nine studies published in 1996-2006 found "a wide range of format structures and curriculum content," but the author notes that all of the studies "demonstrate that end-of-life educational curricula and clinical training improve the competency of medical students" (Bickel-Swenson, 2007, pp. 233-234). A qualitative assessment of the reflective written comments of 593 third-year medical students before and after taking a 32-hour didactic and experiential clerkship that included home hospice visits and inpatient hospice care found a 23 percent improvement in knowledge, a 56 percent improvement in students' feelings of competence, and a 29 percent decrease in their concerns (von Gunten et al., 2012).

Other examples of how hospice and palliative medicine content has been incorporated into medical school curricula include

- George Washington University's standardized patient case on palliative care in the second year, coupled with a course on medical interviewing and decision making;
- the University of Rochester's content on advance care planning, chronic pain management, and discussion of treatment goals provided in the first and second years, supplemented by a session on palliative care in a 2-week follow-up to a clinical rotation in the third year (Shaw, 2012);
- development of a 4-year integrated curriculum and establishment of an Office of Palliative Care by Northeast Ohio Medical University (Radwany et al., 2011); and
- the Association of American Medical Colleges' collaboration with the Coalition to Transform Advanced Care to identify relevant core competencies.[5]

---

[4]The "hidden curriculum" is expressed through institutional policies, evaluation activities, resource allocations, and institutional "slang," among other means (Hafferty, 1998). For further discussion and a personal view, see Liao (2014).

[5]Core competencies in geriatric education, identified by the Association of American Medical Colleges with support from the John A. Hartford Foundation, include some aspects of hospice and palliative medicine: pain management; the importance of interdisciplinary care; and psychological, social, and spiritual needs of patients with advanced serious illness and their families (Leipzig et al., 2009; see also Sanchez-Reilly and Ross, 2012, p. 118).

The need for a systematic approach to medical schools' commitment to hospice and palliative medicine has been described as follows:

> An educationally rich palliative care curriculum should include didactic and clinical experiences where learners observe the role-modeling of competent and compassionate palliative care and have supervised experiential opportunities. Improvements within individual schools/residencies still largely rely on the presence of an effective palliative medicine champion who combines commitment and vision, leadership skills, education skills, and clinical skills. To provide meaningful clinical experiences for learners and to mainstream palliative medicine[,] it is crucial to provide faculty development in primary palliative care skills to non-HPM faculty to ensure care for the growing population of complex chronically and seriously ill people. (Sanchez-Reilly and Ross, 2012, p. 120)

The structures of academic medical centers and cancer centers typically are rooted in more established specialties, impeding the ability of hospice and palliative medicine specialists to become educators. These structures also fail to facilitate interprofessional training. What appears to be needed is a core of board-certified hospice and palliative medicine specialists serving in appropriate departments or divisions as educators of medical students and residents and as liaisons with colleagues in other professions, especially nursing, social work, and chaplaincy. A few efforts have been made to train medical school faculty members in palliative care. The annual 2-week Program in Palliative Care Education and Practice at Harvard Medical School was rated as "transformative" by 82 percent of respondents who participated in 2000-2003 (Sullivan et al., 2005). The shortage of hospice and palliative medicine faculty may in part reflect the low levels of funding for palliative care research noted in Chapter 2, with faculty members' ability to attract research dollars being a high priority for medical schools.

One way to ensure attention to hospice and palliative medicine in the undergraduate curriculum, in graduate training, and in the minds of future physicians is to include more of this content in medical licensure and specialty board certification examinations. Currently, little hospice and palliative medicine content appears in the main licensure test, Step 3 of the United States Medical Licensing Examination. As the final phase of the physician licensure examination process, Step 3 centers on biomedical and clinical science and is open to all medical and osteopathic school graduates who have passed Steps 1 and 2. Authoritative content outlines provide an overview, or "blueprint," of the content for 15 areas of the Step 3 examination (United States Medical Licensing Examination, 2013). Although a few test questions related to specific disorders conceivably involve the terminal phases of illness, there is no blueprint for end-of-life care.

Sufficient hospice and palliative medicine content is also lacking in many board certification examinations in specialties in which basic palliative care is especially relevant. In oncology, end-of-life care and communication combined are only 2 percent of the entire examination (ABIM, 2013a). The closest thing to hospice and palliative medicine content in the cardiovascular recertification examination, taken by current cardiologists and other cardiovascular disease practitioners, is a topic called "ethics, malpractice, other" within a "miscellaneous" portion of the exam content that is only 1.5 percent of the entire examination (ABIM, 2013b). In the certification examination for general internal medicine, "palliative/end-of-life care" is 3 percent of the examination content (ABIM, 2013c).

Continuing Medical Education

Because many or most physicians have had little exposure to hospice and palliative medicine in their undergraduate and graduate education, efforts have been made to fill the gap through continuing medical education. Most notably, a program originally named Education for Physicians on End-of-life Care (EPEC) was developed in the late 1990s by the American Medical Association with support from the Robert Wood Johnson Foundation. EPEC has reached many physicians and other professionals through small-group training sessions and has as its mission "to educate all healthcare professionals in the essential clinical competencies of palliative care" (EPEC, 2013b).

EPEC uses a train-the-trainer approach to disseminate knowledge and improve skills. Participants rated the project highly from the beginning, and 92 percent of 200 physicians participating in EPEC training in 1999-2000 reported that they used its content in their teaching (Robinson et al., 2004). Since being renamed Education in Palliative and End-of-life Care, EPEC has developed numerous learning modules and now disseminates them through various venues—conferences, online learning, and specialized training, with didactic sessions, videotape presentations, interactive discussions, and practical exercises (CAPC, 2013). Nurse practitioners and other nonphysicians also take advantage of EPEC, making it an interdisciplinary training platform.

Illustrating EPEC's current scope, EPEC-Pediatrics has 23 core and 2 elective topics, taught through 20 distance learning modules and 6 1-day, in-person conference sessions (EPEC, 2013a). Since 2012, physicians and nurse practitioners have participated in "Become an EPEC-Pediatrics Trainer" workshops.[6] Caregivers, emergency medicine, long-term care, on-

---

[6]Personal communication, S. Friedrichsdorf, Children's Hospitals and Clinics of Minnesota, February 6, 2014.

cology, and veterans are among the many other subjects of EPEC training. EPEC has become essentially self-sustaining through participation fees, and it partners with diverse professional associations and other organizations, such as the National Cancer Institute (NCI, 2013).

Legislation in the state of California requires that most physicians obtain 12 hours of continuing education in pain management and end-of-life care.[7] State legislatures or medical licensing boards sometimes do require that physicians, as a condition of periodic relicensure, take continuing education courses on specified, socially pressing topics, although it is not clear that such continuing education mandates are effective in changing practice patterns.[8] However, among 81 physicians taking a course complying with the California requirement, two-thirds of 51 immediate respondents reported an interest in changing their practice patterns, and most (90 percent) of 31 respondents reported 4 months later that their practice patterns had indeed changed (Leong et al., 2010).

Interdisciplinary formats are a common feature of continuing education in communication related to end-of-life care. At Children's Hospital Boston, physicians participated with nurses, social workers, psychologists, and chaplains involved in pediatric critical care in a day-long interprofessional communication program (the Program to Enhance Relational and Communication Skills, or PERCS). The program was created by the Institute for Professionalism and Ethical Practice. In a survey of 110 participants, 106 responded immediately, and 57 of these returned a follow-up questionnaire 5 months later. Respondents were nearly unanimous in indicating that the course improved their skills and confidence in communication (Meyer et al., 2009).

In some cases, continuing education requirements may limit patient care. In 2012, for example, the U.S. Food and Drug Administration (FDA) adopted a risk evaluation and mitigation strategy for prescribing more than 30 extended-release and long-acting opioid analgesic medications that "strongly encourages" prescribers to take a continuing medical education course on opioid prescribing (FDA, 2013). The FDA supports making this education mandatory and linking it to prescriber registration with the Drug Enforcement Administration (American Pharmacists Association, 2012; FDA, 2013). Although prescribers of these frequently abused drugs certainly should be aware of the attendant risks (see IOM, 2011, pp. 142-

---

[7]California AB487 (2001), *Cal. Bus. & Prof. Code*, sec. 2190.5. This is a one-time requirement. Pathologists and radiologists are exempt. Exemptions may also be granted to physicians who are not engaged in direct patient care, do not provide patient consultations, or do not reside in California.

[8]For a meta-analysis of the outcome literature on continuing medical education, see Mansouri and Lockyer (2007).

148),[9] such a requirement might dissuade some clinicians from prescribing opioids at all, thereby limiting the availability of an important pain relief modality for people with advanced serious illnesses.

Nursing Education

Accreditation standards for undergraduate baccalaureate nursing programs, adopted by the American Association of Colleges of Nursing in 2008, specify that all baccalaureate nursing graduates should be prepared to "implement patient and family care around resolution of end-of-life and palliative care issues, such as symptom management, support of rituals, and respect for patient and family preferences" (AACN, 2008, p. 31). This mandate is analogous to the Liaison Committee on Medical Education standard noted above.

Historically, the lack of emphasis on palliative care seen in medical education appears to have been duplicated in nursing education. For example, registered nurse anesthetists received little training in palliative or end-of-life care as students, and a literature search involving preparation of certified registered nurse anesthetists found "no publications addressing the importance of incorporating elements of palliative care into nursing and nurse anesthesia practice" (Callahan et al., 2011, p. S15).

Oncology nurses were found to be so consistently distressed when communicating with patients and families about end-of-life care that development of a communication curriculum was considered necessary for use in early palliative care (Goldsmith et al., 2013). An examination of palliative care education for pediatric nurses showed that nurses entering practice "often were grossly unprepared to care for children and families in need of end-of-life care" (Malloy et al., 2006, p. 555). However, a survey of 279 pediatric nurses in Florida found "a good level of baseline knowledge of palliative care" (Knapp et al., 2009, p. 432), especially in cities with a pediatric palliative care program (Knapp et al., 2011).[10] In a 2006 survey in which 71 percent of baccalaureate nursing schools participated, 99 percent reported some offering on death and dying, but on average, these totaled less than 15 hours of instruction (Dickinson, 2007).

Several organizations have joined forces to train nursing school faculty and potential nursing mentors in palliative care. The End-of-Life Nursing Education Consortium (ELNEC) was initiated in 2000 with 4 years' sup-

---

[9]In a 2014 state of the state address devoted entirely to problems of addiction, Vermont Governor Peter Shumlin said that treatment for opiate addiction in his state increased by 770 percent, to 4,300 cases (or 1 in about every 150 residents), between 2000 and 2012 (Seelye, 2014). Nationwide opioid overdoses tripled in 20 years, causing 15,500 deaths in 2009 (CDC, 2013).

[10]A "concept analysis" of pediatric palliative nursing care is provided in Stayer (2012).

port from the Robert Wood Johnson Foundation. The ELNEC program is administered by the American Association of Colleges of Nursing and City of Hope National Medical Center. The National Cancer Institute began to train graduate nursing faculty members using ELNEC in 2002. ELNEC content consists of eight modules,[11] and participants receive a textbook, a 1,000-page syllabus, and other resource materials. More than 15,000 nurses and others, an estimated 11,500 of whom are nurse educators, had received ELNEC training by 2013. Besides the core ELNEC training, separate courses exist for oncology, pediatrics, critical care, geriatrics, veterans, public hospitals, and advanced practice registered nursing (ELNEC, 2013).

Examples exist in which palliative care is integrated into the undergraduate nursing curriculum. At the University of Rochester School of Nursing, topics roughly conforming to the eight ELNEC modules are included in a core end-of-life curriculum, and a hospice and palliative care elective is offered (University of Rochester Medical Center, 2013). At the University of California, San Francisco, School of Nursing, a course in palliative and end-of-life care recently became mandatory for many of the school's programs (Schwartz, 2012). In a very different approach, one nursing school offers a course on palliative and end-of-life care structured around three apprenticeships—in cognitive learning, clinical reasoning and know-how, and moral reasoning (Hold et al., 2014).

A major textbook in palliative nursing is divided into general principles, symptom assessment and management, the meaning of hope in the dying, spiritual care, special patient populations, end-of-life care across settings, pediatric palliative care, special issues for the nurse in end-of-life care, international models of palliative care, and a conclusion on a good death (Ferrell and Coyle, 2010). Another textbook is divided into caring for the whole person, social and professional issues, psychosocial considerations, and physical aspects of dying (Matzo and Sherman, 2010).

Schools of Public Health

Medical and nursing schools are not the only health professions education venues that find little room in their curricula for end-of-life and palliative care. In 2011-2013, only 3 of the 49 accredited U.S. schools of public health offered a course on end-of-life care policy. Another 6 public health schools offered some content on end-of-life concerns, but most of these offerings embedded this content in courses on aging policy and so did not consider the entire life span (Lupu et al., 2013). A curriculum on the topic

---

[11]The eight ELNEC modules are nursing care at the end of life; pain management; symptom management; ethical/legal issues; cultural considerations in end-of-life care; communication; loss, grief, and bereavement; and preparation for and care at the time of death.

has been developed under the auspices of the Foundation for Advanced Education in the Sciences at the National Institutes of Health, but it apparently has not been widely adopted.

Public health courses on end-of-life care could help lead future health care administrators and policy makers and their educators to incorporate principles of palliative care into health care systems. To illustrate, local, state, and national population health strategies could emphasize the quality of life of people with advanced serious illnesses, promote palliative care in health professions education, provide assistance to family caregivers, and ensure greater availability of bereavement services.

Cross-Cutting Considerations

As a clinical field in which communication is exceptionally important, palliative care lends itself to education approaches other than didactic lectures. Simulation techniques, experiential learning, role playing (with or without outside actors), team-building exercises, interdisciplinary seminars, use of social media, journal or research clubs, and other nontraditional or supplemental methods of learning all may be appropriate in building students' knowledge and skills. Educational approaches could include clerkships and other placements in hospices or other palliative or long-term care settings, interviews and conversations with patients and families, case studies involving unwanted or futile treatment, an opportunity to accompany a hospital chaplain on rounds, preparation and discussion of research papers, telehealth or telemedicine demonstrations, and exploration of attitudes toward health care in a minority community.

Perhaps more than most other clinical specialties, hospice and palliative medicine calls on clinicians to be flexible and embrace uncertainty, especially in prognosis. Health professionals involved in either basic or specialty palliative care must respond in timely and appropriate ways when advanced disease trajectories take an unexpected path. Hospice and palliative medicine's focus on maximizing patient comfort and quality of life requires a different mind-set on the part of the care team, and often, considerable creativity.

Lack of Interprofessional Collaboration

The development of high-functioning teams of health professionals is receiving increased attention. Forms of collaboration include *interprofessional*, or multiple professions working together toward a common goal, and *transdisciplinary*, or multiple professions working together under a shared model with a common language (IOM, 2013a). In this report, the term "interprofessional" education encompasses the concept of transdisciplinary education. In these and other collaborative arrangements, physicians and other participating health professionals subordinate their own interests to the interests of the team and evince core humanistic values, such as honesty and integrity, caring and compassion, altruism and empathy, respect for others, and trustworthiness (IOM, 2013a; Swick, 2000).

Professional education can encourage or obstruct interprofessional collaboration. It can foster team-building skills, such as communication, and important team-supporting attributes, such as trust and a focus on results. George Thibault, president of the Josiah Macy Jr. Foundation, suggested at a recent IOM workshop that team-based competencies should be a core goal of health professions education, and a theme of that workshop was the importance of leadership, including educational leadership, to effect such a cultural change (IOM, 2013b).

In reality, however, most health professions education is siloed. According to a Macy Foundation report, for example, "medical education inculcates physicians with a 'captain of the ship' attitude[,] which can impair interprofessional collaboration" (Josiah Macy Jr. Foundation, 2011, p. 6). Nursing education, too, is "very siloed," relying on a preponderance of theory classes unconnected to practical realities (IOM, 2010, p. 20). According to authors of a nursing-oriented review of interprofessional education, "Despite some successes in educating the different disciplines collaboratively, the degree of interdisciplinary education at present is insufficient and sporadic. Within the nursing curriculum, the content for teamwork is present, but the evidence for education of disciplines together is sparse" (Newhouse and Spring, 2010, p. 2).

Interprofessional collaboration is a key feature of palliative care, which, as emphasized in Chapter 2, is largely a team enterprise. Siloed education fosters attitudes that can lead team members to struggle over jurisdictional turf, misunderstand each other's processes and objectives, fail to listen to or anticipate the concerns of other disciplines, avoid collective responsibility, and allow individual interests to interfere with patient and family interests.

Palliative care training, by contrast, "is oriented to teams rather than individuals," especially in Palliative Care Leadership Centers, established in 2004 through the Center to Advance Palliative Care with initial support from the Robert Wood Johnson Foundation. These centers provide education programs geared to eight types of health care settings,[12] followed by a year-long mentoring program. The education programs include a core program, consultancy-based programs oriented to a developing or recently established palliative care program, and a pediatrics program

---

[12]The eight types of settings used by the leadership centers are integrated health systems, community hospitals, hospices, academic medical centers, cancer centers, children's hospitals, U.S. Department of Veterans Affairs (VA) facilities, and safety-net hospitals (CAPC, undated).

(CAPC, undated). Further, interprofessional fellowships in palliative care have been established by the VA as part of that agency's commitment to palliative care.

Neglect of Communication Skills

Clinicians' skill in communicating with patients and families is a key aspect of end-of-life and palliative care, as noted in Chapter 2 and discussed at length in Chapter 3. As a pair of palliative care experts recently commented, "Foremost, clinicians and students in the health professions need better training in basic palliative care competencies, especially communication skills" (Block and Billings, 2014, p. 1700). Research on health professionals' communication skills has focused primarily on physicians, for whom the need may be greatest. This section likewise focuses on the development of physician communication skills, but the committee believes that the development of these skills also is important for nurses and other health professionals.

Effective physician communication in end-of-life situations has been described as follows:

> good communication in palliative medicine adopts a modern, patient-centered, biopsychosocial-spiritual framework, and focuses on eliciting patient concerns, identifying their agenda, providing complete information, but doing so in a way that allows patients and families to digest what they hear. It is respectful, empathic, inclusive, and efficient, seeks to elicit patients' goals and preferences, and to match these to an individualized plan of care. (LeBlanc and Tulsky, in press)

These authors also observe that "communication behaviors are readily measurable, teachable, and learnable" (LeBlanc and Tulsky, in press).

Hospice and palliative medicine specialists are not alone in needing knowledge and skill in communicating with patients and families facing the end of life. Primary care clinicians, of course, but also oncologists, cardiologists, nephrologists, intensivists, emergency physicians, hospitalists, surgeons, and other clinicians must effectively sound out, listen, ask, inform, come to agreement, comfort, and in other ways achieve communication success with patients and family members as part of basic palliative care. Even radiologists, anesthesiologists, pain specialists, and physical medicine specialists have occasion to communicate effectively with patients with advanced serious illnesses and their families.

Nonetheless, physician shortcomings in communication, especially an apparent unwillingness to discuss the full range of treatment options for people with advanced serious illnesses, are well documented. According to Wright and colleagues (2008, p. 1672), "Physicians . . . often avoid

EOL [end-of-life] conversations, communicate euphemistically, are overly optimistic, or delay discussions until patients are close to death." Interviews with 196 physicians caring for 70 patients who died in a hospital revealed that 86 percent of the physicians reported knowing death was imminent, but only 11 percent reported personally speaking with patients about the possibility of dying (Sullivan et al., 2007). Shah and colleagues (2013) report that many cardiologists and primary care physicians do not discuss options with patients with heart failure, partly out of a fear of destroying hope.

A long line of studies has established that communication skills can be taught effectively to physicians at numerous points in their educational careers:

- A communication intervention course led internal medicine residents to significant improvements in delivering bad news (Alexander et al., 2006).
- A communication training course led oncology fellows to improvements in comfort level and skill with difficult conversations (Back et al., 2003).
- Similarly, a course in teaching communication skills led medical school faculty members to greater comfort level and skill in teaching communication skills (Back et al., 2009).
- Seminal UK research showed that courses in communication skills led senior oncologists to improvements in confidence and behavior in communication, initially and at 3 and 12 months (Fallowfield et al., 1998, 2002, 2003).
- Three weekly sessions with an expert facilitator and a simulated patient or caregiver led "junior doctors" working in Australian hospitals to improvements in communication skills and greater confidence in communicating about end-of-life problems (Clayton et al., 2013).
- A three-pronged approach led house officers in a medical intensive care unit rotation to improvements in confidence in conducting family conferences; delivering bad news; and discussing do-not-resuscitate orders, comfort care, withdrawal of life-sustaining treatment, and advance directives (Seoane et al., 2012).
- Instruction sessions on communication for first- and second-year medical students at the Warren Alpert Medical School of Brown University were rated highly by students for their effectiveness in enhancing communication skills and helping students gain perspective on and appreciate the complexities of health care situations (Shield et al., 2011).

Although these results show that good communication can be taught, there appears to be a dearth of medical faculty members actually teaching the subject. To fill this deficit, faculty training programs in communication have emerged. One such program is Oncotalk Teach, offered to oncology faculty through faculty retreats and distance learning (Back et al., 2009). In another example, 33 physicians in diverse specialties at a comprehensive cancer center participated in a communications workshop; afterward, three-fourths reported feeling comfortable with facilitating training workshops in communication skills (Bylund et al., 2008).

Nevertheless, the medical literature offers a paucity of information about medical schools' efforts to redress students' communication difficulties (Wiskin et al., 2013), and many of these efforts appear to be relatively modest. They include, for example, two communication interventions for third-year students at the Yale School of Medicine: a 3.5-hour workshop in communicating difficult news; and an assignment, including preparation of a written report, on communication and other problems in a single patient's end-of-life care as part of a clinical clerkship (Ellman and Fortin, 2012).

Graduate medical education also does not typically emphasize development of communication skills. In a survey of 89 pediatric residents, for example, all but one said acquiring effective communication skills during their residency was a priority, but only 19 percent felt confident in discussing end-of-life issues with patients and families, 23 percent felt confident in speaking with children about serious illness, and 27 percent felt confident in giving bad news (Rider et al., 2008).

Communication in the advance care planning context also is not widely taught. To the extent that future physicians learn about advance care planning, the topic typically is covered in medical ethics courses, and according to one group of researchers, "formal curricula on advance directives are not commonly offered by residency programs." These researchers conducted a survey of 59 internal medicine and family medicine residents in Texas. Nearly half of the respondents said they did not have "sufficient knowledge of advance directives, given my years of training" (Colbert et al., 2010, p. 280). Some new approaches are emerging. For example, a facilitated quality improvement workshop for internal medicine residents increased confidence with advance care planning for patients who were not English proficient (Tung et al., 2013). Chapter 3 provides additional detail on communication challenges, including those related to advance care planning.

ROLES AND PREPARATION OF PALLIATIVE
CARE TEAM MEMBERS

Palliative care team members include physician specialists in hospice and palliative medicine, palliative nursing specialists, hospice and palliative care social workers, pharmacists, and chaplains. Others with important roles include rehabilitation therapists, direct care workers, and family members.

Physician Specialists in Hospice and Palliative Medicine

For patients who receive specialty (versus basic) palliative care, the hospice and palliative medicine specialist is responsible for managing all diagnostic and treatment services related to comfort and relief of symptoms. This role, although it differs somewhat from setting to setting, is comparable to that of the hospice medical director, who, under the Medicare Hospice Benefit, "has responsibility for the medical component of the hospice's patient care program."[13]

Because of their relatively low numbers, hospice and palliative medicine specialists typically function as consultants rather than as direct care providers. Despite this predominantly consultative role, it appears reasonable, in the committee's view, for patients who are referred to specialty palliative care services to expect to be seen by a qualified palliative care physician at some point, similar to the expectation when a patient enrolls in hospice. A personal encounter can help reassure patients that care is being well managed and is truly patient-centered. Even the physician's touch can be reassuring (Verghese et al., 2011). Likewise, personal encounters enhance physicians' understanding of the patient's condition and personality and thereby potentially improve clinical decisions and coordination of care.

Following considerable growth in hospice and palliative medicine training over the past decade, there were 107 accredited fellowship programs in 39 states plus the District of Columbia in the 2014-2015 academic year (ACGME, 2014). What factors lead a physician to enter this field? In a survey of 62 fellows conducted in July 2009, 63 percent said they did not feel prepared to manage dying patients, and 41 percent felt regret about the care they delivered. While 59 percent had no exposure to hospice and palliative medicine in medical school, 61 percent were exposed to it during residency training (Legrand and Heintz, 2012).

The increase in postgraduate training has been accompanied by changes in the certification process for physicians seeking to demonstrate competence in this field. In the 10-year period ending in 2006, the American Board of Hospice and Palliative Medicine certified more than 2,100 physicians (NHPCO, 2006). Then in September 2006, the new field received formal recognition when the American Board of Medical Specialties (ABMS) approved the creation of hospice and palliative medicine as a subspecialty. At that point, physicians certified by the previous, less formal process

---

[13]42 CFR 418.102(d).

received "grandfathered" certification status for a period of 10 years after their initial certification. The ABMS examination has been offered every 2 years since 2008. In 2012, the examination pass rate was 82 percent, and 3,368 candidates passed (ABEM, 2013). Beginning in 2014, completion of an accredited hospice and palliative medicine fellowship is a prerequisite for certification.

ABMS sponsors the hospice and palliative medicine certification examination with the participation of 10 certification boards. As Table 4-1 shows, two boards—the American Board of Internal Medicine and American Board of Family Medicine—account for 88 percent of all certifications among a total complement of about 6,400 hospice and palliative medicine specialists.

To ensure continuing competence, the ABMS certification must be renewed every 10 years. The recertification requirements of continuing education, training, and examinations are similar to those of other ABMS certifications. The recertification examination, administered by the American Board of Internal Medicine on behalf of all 10 cosponsoring boards, is administered simultaneously to all eligible physicians.

For osteopathic physicians, the American Osteopathic Boards of Family Medicine, Internal Medicine, Neurology and Psychiatry, and Physical Medicine and Rehabilitation offer a Certificate of Added Qualification (and peri-

TABLE 4-1 Physicians Board-Certified in Hospice and Palliative Medicine Through the American Board of Medical Specialties, by Specialty Board, 2008-2012

Sponsoring Board	Number Certified	Percentage
Internal Medicine	3,974	62
Family Medicine	1,631	26
Pediatrics	210	3
Anesthesiology	111	2
Psychiatry and Neurology	104	2
Emergency Medicine	94	1
Obstetrics and Gynecology	68	1
Radiology	62	1
Surgery	62	1
Physical Medicine and Rehabilitation	40	1
TOTAL	6,356	100

SOURCES: Personal communication, S. McGreal, marketing and communications specialist, ABMS, February 4, 2014; ABEM, 2013; ABFM, 2013; ABIM, 2013d; ABP, 2013; ABPMR, 2013; ABPN, 2013; ABS, 2013.

odic recertification) in hospice and palliative medicine. From 2009 to 2013, all doctors of osteopathy (DOs) who obtained board certification in any specialty were permitted to participate in the hospice and palliative medicine osteopathic certification examination, but as of 2014, only candidates from these four boards will be eligible. As of 2012, 174 DOs held osteopathic certification in hospice and palliative medicine. This figure comprises 118 family physicians, 48 internists, 3 emergency physicians, 2 neurologist-psychiatrists, 2 surgeons, and 1 physical medicine-rehabilitation specialist (Gross and Bell, 2013). DOs also may qualify for ABMS certification.

The total number of physicians certified in hospice and palliative medicine is not readily apparent. One source estimates there were 5,000 board-certified hospice and palliative medicine specialists in 2013 (Quill and Abernathy, 2013), but as Table 4-1 reveals, the actual number was at least 25 percent higher. Complications entailed in computing an accurate total include the lack of data on how many physicians who became certified in the pre-2006 process have not yet been certified through the ABMS process but are still practicing. Taken together, however, data from Table 4-1 and the osteopathic certification process suggest a total of more than 6,500 board-certified hospice and palliative medicine specialists in the United States. This figure amounts to about 0.8 percent of all practicing U.S. physicians (KFF, 2014).

In May 2014, the Hospice Medical Director Certification Board administered the first certification exam directed explicitly at the unique clinical and administrative skills and knowledge required in a hospice setting. With no prerequisite fellowship for this focused certification, the aim is to raise the bar for physicians who may work closely with hospices but are not seeking extensive tertiary training (HMDCB, 2013).

One important dimension of the adequacy of the supply of hospice and palliative medicine specialists is race/ethnicity. The committee did not find data on the racial/ethnic composition of the nation's supply of board-certified hospice and palliative medicine physicians. In the survey of 62 fellows noted at the beginning of this section, however, none were African American (Legrand and Heintz, 2012). Greater success in recruiting minority physicians into hospice and palliative medicine would likely make palliative care more attractive and accessible to minority patients and families (see Chapter 3) and would enhance cultural competence within the specialty.

Hospice and Palliative Nursing Specialists

Nurses play especially vital roles in care at the end of life. One important role is serving as a patient advocate, ensuring that patients and families receive culturally sensitive care and sufficient pain management and relief of other symptoms (Hebert et al., 2011). A review of 44 articles from 10 countries found that hospital nurses aid in the decision-making process near the end of life by serving as information brokers, supporters, and advocates, and have sets of strategies for accomplishing each of these roles. Additional research would aid in understanding how these roles and strategies link to patient and family member outcomes (Adams et al., 2011).

The goal of hospice and palliative care nursing "is to promote and improve the patient's quality of life through the relief of suffering along the course of illness, through the death of the patient, and into the bereavement period of the family" (ANA, 2010b, p. 5; ANA and HPNA, 2007, p. 1). Palliative nurses who are registered nurses assess patients for their palliative care needs, including relief of pain and other symptoms and spiritual and social needs. They manage symptoms such as pain, anorexia/cachexia, constipation, dehydration, nausea and vomiting, diarrhea, delirium, dyspnea, lymphedema, ascites (accumulation of excess fluid in the peritoneal cavity), pruritus (itching), various oral conditions, fatigue, and other conditions. Further, they coordinate care, anticipate and attend to emergencies, and provide psychosocial care (Bruera et al., undated). Coordination, communication with families, collaboration, and patient advocacy all characterize nursing—in palliative care, in end-of-life care, and in general (ANA, 2010a).

Nursing has seven different specialty certifications in palliative care as offered by the National Board for Certification of Hospice and Palliative Nurses, geared to different levels of education and areas of training and experience. Nurses with the most training are the advanced certified hospice and palliative nurses—nurse practitioners or clinical nurse specialists who deliver care similar to that delivered by physician specialists in hospice and palliative medicine. However, state scope-of-practice laws and regulations may impose some restrictions on practice for these nurses, such as a requirement that advanced practice nurses have formal physician backup protocols or strict limits on nurses' prescribing authority.

The group with the least amount of training is the certified hospice and palliative nursing assistants who provide bedside care, such as assistance with activities of daily living, under the supervision of a registered nurse. Certified nursing assistants help implement care plans, identify impacts on quality of life, document patient and family responses, and demonstrate other competencies (HPNA, 2009).

Table 4-2 summarizes all seven palliative nursing certification programs, which were established between 1994 and 2004. To ensure continuing competence, they require recertification within 4 years (NBCHPN®, 2014).

Palliative nursing is an increasingly well-established field. An authoritative roster of nursing education programs in palliative care lists 15 programs

TABLE 4-2 Nursing Certifications in Palliative Care

Type of Certification	Eligibility	Number Certified*
Advanced certified hospice and palliative nurse	Master's degree in nursing from an advanced practice palliative care accredited education program, or certain equivalences	943
Certified hospice and palliative nurse	License to practice registered nursing; 2 years of experience in hospice or palliative care recommended	11,878
Certified hospice and palliative pediatric nurse	License to practice registered nursing; 2 years of experience caring for children with life-limiting illnesses recommended	160
Certified hospice and palliative licensed nurse	Practical/vocational nursing license; 2 years of experience as a licensed practical nurse in hospice or palliative care recommended	1,022
Certified hospice and palliative nursing assistant	2,000 practice hours in hospice or palliative care under supervision of a registered nurse in the past 2 years	3,843
Certified hospice and palliative care administrator	2 years of full-time experience within the past 3 years in an administrative role in an area covered by the examination, or equivalent	273
Certified in perinatal loss care	Professional degree (such as registered nurse) and 2 years of full-time experience in the past 3 years in perinatal loss care and/or bereavement support	62

*Numbers certified are current as of April 2014.
SOURCES: NBCHPN®, 2014; Personal communication, S. L. Schafer, director of certification, NBCHPN®, February 5, 2014.

at the master's or doctoral level, with the eastern, southern, midwestern, and western regions of the country each being represented by at least two programs (HPNA, 2013).

Reflecting growth in the specialty, the Hospice and Palliative Nurses Association now claims 11,000 members, primarily hospice and palliative nurses, such as certified hospice and palliative nurses. The association, the certification board, and the Hospice and Palliative Nurses Foundation have joined in the Alliance for Excellence in Hospice and Palliative Nursing, which advocates on behalf of the field. The alliance's concerns include patient access, ensuring patient choice, patient-centered interdisciplinary care, acknowledgment of the role of nurses, and enabling advanced certified hospice and palliative nurses to practice to the full extent of their training instead of being restricted by state scope-of-practice laws (Alliance for Excellence in Hospice and Palliative Nursing, 2013). Another practice concern is the low staffing levels in units that provide end-of-life care, which do not take into account patients' spiritual and emotional needs, the importance of having a nurse at the bedside at the time of death, and a nurse's need for some respite after a patient dies (Douglas, 2012).

Hospice and Palliative Care Social Workers

The role of social workers in end-of-life care often focuses on self-determination, including bioethics consultation and advance care planning. Additional competencies include resource linkage (such as discharge planning), case management (for care coordination), and advocacy. Social workers are particularly concerned about the end-of-life needs of vulnerable individuals (NASW, 2004). They often are part of palliative care teams in hospitals, nursing homes, and hospices, and even may work in emergency departments (Lawson, 2012). Others work in social service agencies to provide community-based social supports for patients and families, such as assistance with transportation, income support, and enrollment in health plans.

In recent years, the profession of social work has developed standards, certifications, and advanced levels of training for those providing support to people approaching death:

- Since 2008, the National Association of Social Workers (NASW) has offered specialty certification in hospice and palliative care at the level of advanced certified hospice and palliative care social worker for licensed social workers who hold a master's degree in social work, have at least 2 years' experience in hospice and palliative care, and have acquired at least 20 hours of related continuing education.
- Since 2009, certification at the level of certified hospice and palliative care social worker has been available to licensed social workers who hold a bachelor's degree in social work, have at least 3 years' experience in hospice and palliative care, and have acquired at least 20 hours of related continuing education.

These two credentials are among 18 advanced practice specialty credentials offered by NASW as of 2014. All require biannual renewal (NASW, 2014).

Another organization, the Board of Oncology Social Work Certification, offers advanced specialty credentials for master's degree social workers involved in oncology. While oncology encompasses a separate specialty from hospice and palliative care, this certification requires experience in oncology, palliative care, or end-of-life care (Board of Oncology Social Work Certification, 2014).

Partly with support from the Project on Death in America, many colleges and universities have developed specific courses and postdegree certificate programs for social workers in palliative and end-of-life care (Walsh-Burke and Csikai, 2005). That project was also instrumental in establishing the Social Work Hospice and Palliative Care Network, an ongoing enterprise "created to bridge the gaps in social work's access to information, knowledge, education, training, and research in hospice and palliative care" (Social Work Hospice and Palliative Care Network, 2014). The network was partly a product of two Social Work Summits on End-of-Life and Palliative Care, held in 2005 and 2006 (Blacker et al., undated).

Many hospice and palliative care social workers practice in hospice. Under the Centers for Medicare & Medicaid Services' hospice conditions of participation, hospice social workers must hold a master's degree in social work; hold a bachelor's degree in social work and have 1 year of experience in a health care setting; or hold a bachelor's degree in a related social science discipline, have 1 year of experience in a health care setting, and work under the supervision of a social worker holding a master's degree in social work (CMS, 2008, Section 418.114(b)(3)). In a survey of 1,169 hospice and palliative care social workers, most reported being engaged in communicating the psychosocial needs of patients and families to other members of the care team and in assessing patients' and family members' grief and bereavement needs; few held NASW certification (Weisenfluh and Csikai, 2013).

NASW's Standards for Palliative and End of Life Care cover ethics and values; knowledge; assessment; intervention/treatment planning; attitude and self-awareness; empowerment and advocacy; documentation; interdisciplinary teamwork; cultural competence; continuing education; and supervision, leadership, and training (NASW, 2004). A major textbook in social work palliative care includes sections on specific settings of care, components of practice (screening, assessment, intervention), population-specific practice, collaboration, "Regional Voices from a Global Perspective," ethics, and professional issues (Altilio and Otis-Green, 2011).

Pharmacists

The role of pharmacists in palliative care and hospice includes

- assessing the appropriateness of medication orders and helping to ensure the timely administration of effective medicine,
- counseling and educating other palliative care team members about medication therapy,
- educating patients and family caregivers about the administration and use of medications,
- ensuring the availability of compounding of unusual medications,
- addressing patient and family financial concerns relating to medications,
- ensuring safe and legal disposal of medications after death, and
- communicating with regulatory authorities as appropriate (ASHP, 2002).

Given that symptom management for people who have advanced serious illnesses or are nearing the end of life relies heavily on the use of medications, pharmacists can play a key role in the interdisciplinary palliative care team. In 2002, a statement of the American Society of Health-System Pharmacists (ASHP) on the role of the pharmacy profession in hospice and palliative care highlighted pharmacists' responsibilities and scope of practice. Pharmacists, said the statement, have a pivotal role to play in improving pain management, including "patient specific monitoring for drug therapy outcomes, recommending alternative drug products and dosage forms, minimizing duplicative and interacting medications, compounding medications extemporaneously, improving drug storage and transportation, and educating staff, patients, and families about the most efficient ways of handling and using medications" (ASHP, 2002, p. 1772).

Although pharmacy school accreditation standards do not require separate courses in end-of-life care for pharmacy students, concepts associated with pain management and palliative care are part of curriculum standards in pharmacotherapy (ACPE, 2011). A 2012 survey of education in pharmacy schools found an average of 6.2 hours devoted to teaching students about death and dying, an increase from 3.9 hours in 2001 (Dickinson, 2013; Herndon et al., 2003). The 2012 survey also found that 82 percent of pharmacy schools offered coursework on end-of-life care for pharmacists.

Pharmacy school graduates are eligible for a year-long post-graduate (PGY1) residency in pharmacy practice, community pharmacy, or managed care pharmacy. Individuals who wish to gain further specialization can enroll in a second year of residency (PGY2). ASHP serves as the recognizing body for pharmaceutical residency programs, a role that includes monitoring the implementation of the Resident Matching Program. In 2014, 26 distinct types of PGY2 specialty programs were available, including one in pain management and palliative care. Within this one specialty, 11 individual programs are available in the United States. Most of these programs offer only one position per program, so a total complement of only 13 pain management and palliative care positions was available during the 2014 match (National Matching Services, 2014). However, pharmacists need not complete a pain management and palliative care residency program to work in palliative care. A recent survey of pharmacists in that field found that only 23 percent had completed a PGY1 residency, and just 5 percent had completed a PGY2 residency (Latuga et al., 2012).

The Board of Pharmacy Specialties (BPS) offers certification in eight specialties, as well as two areas that provide an Added Qualification credential. As recently as 2011, BPS considered adding pain and palliative medicine as a specialty, but it has yet to do so (BPS, 2011).

Chaplains

Chaplaincy services tend to be the most visible means of meeting the spiritual care needs of patients with advanced serious illnesses. Spiritual care is one of eight domains of quality palliative care identified by the National Consensus Project for Quality Palliative Care (Dahlin, 2013), and accreditation standards require hospitals and home health agencies to accommodate all patients' religious and spiritual needs (Joint Commission, 2008).

Although spiritual care can be provided by physicians,[14] nurses, social workers, other clergy, practitioners of integrative medicine, and lay people, it is the special domain of chaplains. In health care institutions, chaplains typically strive to serve people of many different denominations.

Chaplains perform spiritual assessments of patients and families, formulate spiritual treatment plans, consult with other palliative care team members or outside clergy to ensure that spiritual needs are adequately met, and provide direct services to patients and families. A consensus conference on spiritual palliative care developed a set of recommendations that emphasizes spiritual assessment, responses to spiritual distress, and timely access to chaplaincy services (Puchalski et al., 2009).

About two-thirds of U.S. hospitals have chaplains, and in hospitals with palliative care programs, their duties may include serving palliative care patients. Hospital chaplains conduct spiritual assessments; provide

---

[14]In a 2005 survey of 363 family medicine residents, 96 percent agreed (and 60 percent of these strongly agreed) they would discuss spirituality with a patient on request (Saguil et al., 2011).

empathetic listening along with life review and emotional assistance; and when asked, lead prayer and religious observances (Jankowski et al., 2011). As one example of the scope of services that may be provided, a chaplaincy program at the Methodist Hospital System in Houston trains staff in the system's spiritual environment of caring and when to call in a chaplain, provides direct services to patients, and conducts community outreach (Millikan, 2013).

In a nationwide study of hospital patients who died between 2001 and 2005, the presence of chaplaincy services was associated with a 4 percent lower rate of hospital mortality and a 6 percent higher rate of hospice enrollment, after controlling for geographic variables, hospital type and size, population density, socioeconomic status, and presence of a palliative care program (Flannelly et al., 2012).

A study of family members of 284 deceased residents of long-term care facilities in four states found that 87 percent of residents had received spiritual care from one source or another. Family members of residents who did receive spiritual care rated the quality of care received in the last month of life higher than did other family members (Daaleman et al., 2008; see also Daaleman, 2010). One impediment to spiritual care may be that the privacy provisions of the Health Insurance Portability and Accountability Act of 1996 appear to exclude spiritual and religious healing from the definition of health care. As a result, clergy who are not on a hospital (or nursing home) staff cannot readily determine which of their congregants are patients there (Tovino, 2005).

Chaplaincy services are a required element of hospice care under the Medicare Hospice Benefit. Hospice and palliative care chaplains sometimes perform the role of clergy for people near the end of life who do not have a regular religious affiliation (Vitello, 2008).

Chaplains are certified by the Board of Chaplaincy Certification Inc., an affiliate of the 4,500-member Association of Professional Chaplains. This workforce appears small compared with the potential need. The general certification examination covers 29 areas of competency and exists on two levels: board certified chaplain (BCC) and associate certified chaplain (ACC). Both levels require an undergraduate degree, ordination or commission to function as a chaplain, a letter of endorsement from a recognized faith group, and 2,000 hours of work experience. Additional BCC qualifications are 72 credit hours in a graduate theological program and four units of clinical pastoral education. Additional ACC qualifications are 48 credit hours in a graduate theological program and two units of clinical pastoral education (BCCI, 2013).

Specialty certification in palliative care (BCC-PCC) was introduced in 2013 as the first in an expected series of specialty chaplaincy certifications. Part of the purpose of palliative care specialty certification is to help chaplains become fully recognized and functioning members of palliative care teams (APC, 2013).

Other Roles

Rehabilitation Therapists

Several categories of rehabilitation therapists are active in the care of people with advanced serious illnesses, including palliative care:

- Occupational therapists help patients perform activities of daily living by dressing, bathing, and ensuring safety. They further assist with instrumental activities of daily living through meal preparation and home management. They facilitate rest and sleep, play, and social and family interaction (AOTA, 2011).
- Physical therapists provide services involving home safety, pain management, training in the use of medical equipment, caregiver education, patient positioning, energy conservation, breathing techniques, strengthening, balance reeducation, gait training, transfer training, and discharge planning (Cruz, 2013).
- Speech-language pathologists help relieve communication impairments and swallowing difficulties (Pollens, 2004).

Direct Care Workers

According to an IOM report on workforce needs for an aging population, direct care workers "are the primary providers of paid hands-on care, supervision, and emotional support for older adults in the United States" (IOM, 2008, p. 199).[15] Direct care workers often provide assistance with activities of daily living and serve the patient at the bedside morning, noon, and night in nursing homes, private homes, and other nonhospital settings. The category of direct care workers consists of nursing assistants, home health aides, and personal care aides.

Direct care is not established as a profession, and workers often are foreign born (23 percent in 2010) and constitute an almost invisible corps of essential health care personnel. In 2008, there already were more than 3 million direct care workers, and a workforce of 4.3 million is forecast for 2018—a projected increase of more than 40 percent in 10 years (PHI,

---

[15]The term "direct care worker" in this context differs from some other uses of the term. In other contexts, the term may cover not only aides but also many nurses and other health professionals who provide services to patients directly, rather than through consultations, administration, or other indirect ways.

2011). About 90 percent are women, and 45 percent are African American or Hispanic (IOM, 2008).

Many direct care workers are employed by nursing homes, hospices, home health agencies, or continuing care residential communities, and others are hired by families and paid out of pocket for services provided in the home. Because pay rates are low and many jobs are part-time, nearly half of direct care workers are eligible for public assistance. A recent U.S. Department of Labor regulation would bring direct care workers under minimum wage legislation (Lopez, 2013). The federal government sets training requirements for nursing assistants and home health aides who work in nursing homes and home health agencies certified for Medicare and Medicaid. For other types of direct care workers, states may set requirements (PHI, 2011). Under the Affordable Care Act, nursing homes are required to provide in-service training to nursing assistants on dementia and resident abuse (CMS, 2011).

Given low pay rates and other negative aspects of many direct care jobs, as well as projected increases in demand associated with the aging population, the IOM report cited above recommends that state Medicaid programs increase direct-care pay rates and fringe benefits. It also recommends state and federal action to increase minimum training standards, including establishment of 120 hours of training (compared with the current 75 hours) as a minimum requirement (IOM, 2008, Recommendations 5-1 and 5-2).

Family Members

Family members, even those who may not be fully engaged as family caregivers, play vital roles on the palliative care team. They support the patient. They advocate for the patient to ensure that needs are being met and obvious errors are avoided. They assist with medication acquisition and administration, especially in home-based care. They inform professional care team members about patient preferences and personal traits. They contribute to, and help patients understand, the treatment plan and how it is being implemented. And they participate in transitions from one setting to another. As described in Chapter 2, family caregivers (with "family" defined broadly) have a dual presence on the palliative care team, both serving as the main provider of services from hour to hour and requiring support services themselves.

FINDINGS, CONCLUSIONS, AND RECOMMENDATION

Findings

This study yielded the following findings on creating change in professional education to improve the quality of end-of-life care.

Growth of Palliative Care Specialties

Since the IOM report *Approaching Death* (IOM, 1997) was published, hospice and palliative medicine has become established as a defined medical specialty, with 10 cosponsoring certification boards, and as a certification of added qualification in four osteopathic specialties. As a result, more than 6,500 physicians are now board certified in this specialty. Certification programs in palliative care have also been established for seven levels of nursing, two levels of social work, and chaplaincy[16],[17] (ABEM, 2013; ABFM, 2013; ABIM, 2013d; ABMS, 2012; ABP, 2013; ABPN, 2013; ABS, 2013; APC, 2013; Gross and Bell, 2013; NASW, 2014; NBCHPN®, 2014).

Palliative Care in the Curriculum

In medical schools, the curriculum is required to cover end-of-life care, but the average total offering is only 17 hours over the 4 years, and there usually is no required course. Baccalaureate nursing programs are similarly required to include end-of-life care, but the average total offering was most recently determined to be less than 15 hours (AACN, 2008; Dickinson, 2007, 2011; Liaison Committee on Medical Education, 2013; Van Aalst-Cohen et al., 2008).

Palliative Care Content in Medical Licensure and Certification Examinations

Palliative care content in medical licensure and non–hospice and palliative medicine certification examinations appears limited. Palliative and end-of-life care is not among the 15 areas blueprinted for Step 3 of the United States Medical Licensing Examination. End-of-life care and communication account for only 2 percent of the content of the oncology certification examination. The entire subject of "ethics, malpractice, other"—which conceivably could include some aspects of palliative care—accounts for only

---

[16]Personal communication, S. McGreal, marketing and communications specialist, ABMS, February 4, 2014.

[17]Personal communication, S. L. Schafer, director of certification, NBCHPN®, February 5, 2014.

0.5 percent of the content of the cardiovascular recertification examination (ABIM, 2013a,b; United States Medical Licensing Examination, 2013).

Continuing Education in Palliative Care

Continuing education in palliative care includes two well-established programs that use a train-the-trainer approach: Education in Palliative and End-of-life Care (EPEC), primarily for physicians and advanced practice nurses, and the End-of-Life Nursing Education Consortium (ELNEC) for nurses (CAPC, 2013; ELNEC, 2013; EPEC, 2013b).

Supply of Hospice and Palliative Medicine Specialists

A shortage of 6,000-18,000 hospice and palliative medicine specialists has been estimated. This estimate is based on assumptions involving hospital-based services only (Lupu and American Academy of Hospice and Palliative Medicine Workforce Task Force, 2010).

Professions and Other Groups Providing Palliative Care

Palliative care providers include *physicians* (both hospice and palliative medicine specialists and clinicians who provide basic palliative care); *nurses* (including advanced certified hospice and palliative nurses, certified hospice and palliative nurses, and nonpalliative nurses); *social workers* (including advanced certified hospice and palliative care social workers and certified hospice and palliative care social workers); *pharmacists*; *chaplains*; *rehabilitation therapists* (physical therapists, occupational therapists, and speech-language pathologists); *direct care workers* (nursing assistants, home health aides, and personal care aides); and *family members* (ABMS, 2012; ANA and HPNA, 2007; AOTA, 2011; ASHP, 2002; Cruz, 2013; HPNA, 2009; IOM, 2008; Latuga et al., 2012; Lawson, 2012; PHI, 2011; Pollens, 2004; Puchalski et al., 2009; Weisenfluh and Csikai, 2013; see also Chapter 2).

Conclusions

The major improvement in the education of health professionals who provide care to people nearing the end of life has been the establishment of the specialty of hospice and palliative medicine, along with the establishment or growth of palliative care specialties in nursing and social work. Three remaining problems are insufficient attention to palliative care in medical and nursing school curricula, educational silos that impede the development of interprofessional teams, and deficits in equipping physicians (and possibly nurses and other health professionals) with sufficient communication skills.

To serve patients who are not currently hospitalized or do not require specialty palliative care (and their families), there is a need for "basic" or "primary" palliative care. As defined in Chapter 1 (see Box 1-2), basic palliative care is provided by physicians who are not hospice and palliative medicine specialists (such as general internists, family physicians, general pediatricians, oncologists, cardiologists, nephrologists, hospitalists, emergency physicians, anesthesiologists, intensivists, psychiatrists, and surgeons), along with colleagues in other health professions. The three problems noted above contribute to a general inadequacy in preparing health professionals to provide basic palliative care.

> **Recommendation 3. Educational institutions, credentialing bodies, accrediting boards, state regulatory agencies, and health care delivery organizations should establish the appropriate training, certification, and/or licensure requirements to strengthen the palliative care knowledge and skills of all clinicians who care for individuals with advanced serious illness who are nearing the end of life.**

Specifically,

- all clinicians across disciplines and specialties who care for people with advanced serious illness should be competent in basic palliative care, including communication skills, interprofessional collaboration, and symptom management;
- educational institutions and professional societies should provide training in palliative care domains throughout the professional's career;
- accrediting organizations, such as the Accreditation Council for Graduate Medical Education, should require palliative care education and clinical experience in programs for all specialties responsible for managing advanced serious illness (including primary care clinicians);
- certifying bodies, such as the medical, nursing, and social work specialty boards, and health systems should require knowledge, skills, and competency in palliative care;
- state regulatory agencies should include education and training in palliative care in licensure requirements for physicians, nurses, chaplains, social workers, and others who provide health care to those nearing the end of life;
- entities that certify specialty-level health care providers should create pathways to certification that increase the number of health

care professionals who pursue specialty-level palliative care training; and

- entities such as health care delivery organizations, academic medical centers, and teaching hospitals that sponsor specialty-level training positions should commit institutional resources to increasing the number of available training positions for specialty-level palliative care.

REFERENCES

AACN (American Association of Colleges of Nursing). 2008. *The essentials of baccalaureate education for professional nursing practice.* Washington, DC: AACN. https://www.aacn. nche.edu/education-resources/BaccEssentials08.pdf (accessed February 10, 2014).

AAMC (Association of American Medical Colleges). 2013. *Medical school graduation questionnaire. 2013 all schools summary report.* https://www.aamc.org/download/350998/ data/2013gqallschoolssummaryreport.pdf (accessed March 17, 2014).

ABEM (American Board of Emergency Medicine). 2013. *Annual report, 2012-2013.* East Lansing, MI: ABEM. https://www.abem.org/public/docs/default-source/publication-documents/2012-13-annual-report.pdf?sfvrsn=8 (accessed January 31, 2014).

ABFM (American Board of Family Medicine). 2013. *Diplomate statistics.* Lexington, KY: ABFM. https://www.theabfm.org/about/stats.aspx (accessed December 4, 2013).

ABIM (American Board of Internal Medicine). 2013a. *Medical oncology: Certification examination blueprint.* Philadelphia, PA: ABIM. http://www.abim.org/pdf/blueprint/ medon_cert.pdf (accessed November 29, 2013).

ABIM. 2013b. *Cardiovascular disease: Maintenance of certification examination blueprint.* Philadelphia, PA: ABIM. http://www.abim.org/pdf/blueprint/card_moc.pdf (accessed November 29, 2013).

ABIM. 2013c. *Internal medicine: Certification examination blueprint.* Philadelphia, PA: ABIM. http://www.abim.org/pdf/blueprint/im_cert.pdf (accessed November 29, 2013).

ABIM. 2013d. *Number of certificates issued—all candidates.* Philadelphia, PA: ABIM. http:// www.abim.org/pdf/data-candidates-certified/all-candidates.pdf (accessed December 3, 2013).

ABMS (American Board of Medical Specialties). 2012. *2012 ABMS certificate statistics.* Chicago, IL: ABMS.

ABP (American Board of Pediatrics). 2013. *Number of diplomate certificates granted through December 2012.* Chapel Hill, NC: ABP. https://www.abp.org/ABPWebStatic/?anticache =0.1225979424765275#murl%3D%2FABPWebStatic%2FaboutPed.html%26surl%3D %2Fabpwebsite%2Fstats%2Fnumdips.htm (accessed December 3, 2013).

ABPMR (American Board of Physical Medicine and Rehabilitation). 2013. *Examination statistics.* Rochester, MN: ABPMR. https://www.abpmr.org/candidates/exam_statistics. html (accessed December 3, 2013).

ABPN (American Board of Psychiatry and Neurology, Inc.). 2013. *Initial certification statistics.* Buffalo Grove, IL: ABPN. http://www.abpn.com/cert_statistics.html (accessed December 4, 2013).

ABS (American Board of Surgery). 2013. *Diplomate totals.* Philadelphia, PA: ABS. http://www. absurgery.org/default.jsp?statsummary (accessed December 3, 2013).

ACGME (Accreditation Council for Graduate Medical Education). 2014. *Number of accredited programs for the current academic year (2014-2015), United States.* Chicago, IL: ACGME. https://www.acgme.org/ads/Public/Reports/Report/3 (accessed April 14, 2014).

ACPE (Accreditation Council for Pharmacy Education). 2011. *Accreditation standards and guidelines for the professional program in pharmacy leading to the doctor of pharmacy degree.* Chicago, IL: ACPE. https://www.acpe-accredit.org/pdf/FinalS2007Guidelines2.0.pdf (accessed January 27, 2014).

Adams, J. A., D. E. Bailey, Jr., R. A. Anderson, and S. L. Docherty. 2011. Nursing roles and strategies in end-of-life decision making in acute care: A systematic review of the literature. *Nursing Research and Practice* 527834.

Alexander, S. C., S. A. Keitz, R. Sloane, and J. A. Tulsky. 2006. A controlled trial of a short course to improve residents' communication with patients at the end of life. *Academic Medicine* 81(11):1008-1012.

Alliance for Excellence in Hospice and Palliative Nursing. 2013. Comments submitted by the Hospice and Palliative Nurses Association to the Institute of Medicine (IOM) Committee on Transforming Care at the End of Life. Pittsburgh, PA: Hospice and Palliative Nurses Association.

Altilio, T., and S. Otis-Green, eds. 2011. *The Oxford textbook of palliative social work.* Cary, NC, and New York: Oxford University Press.

American Pharmacists Association. 2012. *FDA approves final ER/LA opioid analgesic REMS.* Washington, DC: American Pharmacists Association. http://www.pharmacist.com/fda-approves-final-erla-opioid-analgesic-rems (accessed November 25, 2013).

ANA (American Nurses Association). 2010a. *Nursing's social policy statement: The essence of the profession.* Silver Spring, MD: ANA.

ANA. 2010b. *Registered nurses' roles and responsibilities in providing expert care and counseling at the end of life.* Position statement. Silver Spring, MD: ANA.

ANA and HPNA (Hospice and Palliative Nurses Association). 2007. *Hospice and palliative care nursing: Scope and standards of practice.* Silver Spring, MD: ANA.

AOTA (American Occupational Therapy Association). 2011. *The role of occupational therapy in palliative care.* Bethesda, MD: AOTA. http://www.aota.org/~/media/Corporate/Files/AboutOT/Professionals/WhatIsOT/PA/Facts/FactSheet_PalliativeCare.ashx (accessed August 24, 2013).

APC (Association of Professional Chaplains). 2013. *The Association of Professional Chaplains introduces palliative care specialty certification.* News release. May 1. Schaumburg, IL: APC. http://www.professionalchaplains.org/Files/news/pr_palliative_care_specialty_certification.pdf (accessed August 6, 2014).

ASHP (American Society of Health-System Pharmacists). 2002. ASHP statement on the pharmacist's role in hospice and palliative care. *American Journal of Health-System Pharmacy* 59:1770-1773.

Back, A. L., R. M. Arnold, J. A. Tulsky, W. F. Baile, and K. A. Fryer-Edwards. 2003. Teaching communication skills to medical oncology fellows. *Journal of Clinical Oncology* 21(12):2433-2436.

Back, A. L., R. M. Arnold, W. F. Baile, J. A. Tulsky, G. E. Barley, R. D. Pea, and K. A. Fryer-Edwards. 2009. Faculty development to change the paradigm of communication skills teaching in oncology. *Journal of Clinical Oncology* 27(7):1137-1141.

BCCI (Board of Chaplaincy Certification Inc.). 2013. *BCCI certification.* Schaumburg, IL: APC. http://bcci.professionalchaplains.org/content.asp?pl=25&contentid=25 (accessed December 3, 2013).

Bickel-Swenson, D. 2007. End-of-life training in U.S. medical schools: A systematic literature review. *Journal of Palliative Medicine* 10(1):229-235.

Blacker, S., G. H. Christ, and S. Lynch. undated. *Charting the course for the future of social work in end-of-life and palliative care: A report on the 2nd Social Work Summit on End-of-life and Palliative Care.* The Social Work in Hospice and Palliative Care Network. http://www.swhpn.org/monograph.pdf (accessed January 31, 2014).

Block, S. D., and J. A. Billings. 2014. A need for scalable outpatient palliative care interventions. *Lancet* [epub ahead of print].

Board of Oncology Social Work Certification. 2014. *Oncology Social Work Certification (OSW-C) requirements.* http://oswcert.org/?page_id=161 (accessed April 14, 2014).

BPS (Board of Pharmacy Specialties). 2011. *BPS approves ambulatory care designation; explores new specialties in pain and palliative care, critical care and pediatrics.* Washington, DC: BPS. http://www.bpsweb.org/news/pr_041911.cfm (accessed January 24, 2014).

Bruera, E., L. Higginson, C. Ripamonti, and C. von Gunten, eds. 2009. *Textbook of palliative medicine.* London, England: Hodder Arnold.

Bruera, E., M. T. San-M. Arregui, N. L. Schuren, and K. Swint, eds. undated. *MD Anderson's guide to supportive and palliative care for nurses.* Houston: The University of Texas MD Anderson Cancer Center.

Bylund, C. L., R. F. Brown, B. L. di Ciccone, T. T. Levin, J. A. Gueguen, C. Hill, and D. W. Kissane. 2008. Training faculty to facilitate communication skills training: Development and evaluation of a workshop. *Patient Education and Counseling* 70(3):430-436.

Callahan, M. F., S. Breakwell, and R. Suhayda. 2011. Knowledge of palliative and end-of-life care by student registered nurse anesthetists. *American Association of Nurse Anesthetists Journal* 79(4):S15-S20.

CAPC (Center to Advance Palliative Care). 2013. *Education for Physicians on End-of-life Care (EPEC).* New York: CAPC. http://www.capc.org/palliative-care-professional-development/Training/education-for-physicians-on-end-of-life-care-epec (accessed November 25, 2013).

CAPC. 2014. *Staffing a palliative care program.* New York: CAPC. http://www.capc.org/building-a-hospital-based-palliative-care-program/implementation/staffing (accessed January 26, 2014).

CAPC. undated. *Palliative Care Leadership Centers: PCLC overview.* New York: CAPC. http://www.capc.org/palliative-care-leadership-initiative/overview (accessed November 30, 2013).

Carter, B. S., M. Levetown, and S. E. Friebert, eds. 2011. *Palliative care for infants, children, and adolescents: A practical handbook.* 2nd ed. Baltimore, MD: The Johns Hopkins University Press.

CDC (Centers for Disease Control and Prevention). 2013. *Saving lives and protecting people: Preventing prescription painkiller overdoses.* http://www.cdc.gov/injury/about/focus-rx.html (accessed February 11, 2014).

Clayton, J. M., P. N. Butow, A. Waters, R. C. Laidsaar-Powell, A. O'Brien, F. Boyle, A. L. Back, R. M. Arnold, J. A. Tulsky, and M. H. Tattersall. 2013. Evaluation of a novel individualized communication skills training intervention to improve doctors' confidence and skills in end-of-life communication. *Palliative Medicine* 27(3):236-243.

CMS (Centers for Medicare & Medicaid Services). 2008. *Conditions of participation: Hospice care (418.3-418.116).* http://www.cms.gov/Regulations-and-Guidance/Legislation/CFCsAndCoPs/Hospice.html (accessed January 16, 2014).

CMS. 2011. *Mandate of Section 6121 of the Affordable Care Act for nurse aide training in nursing homes.* http://www.cms.gov/Medicare/Provider-Enrollment-and-Certification/SurveyCertificationGenInfo/downloads/SCLetter11_35.pdf (accessed December 4, 2013).

Colbert, C. Y., C. Mirkes, P. E. Ogden, M. E. Herring, C. Cable, J. D. Myers, A. R. Ownby, E. Boisaubin, I. Murguia, M. A. Farnie, and M. Sadoski. 2010. Enhancing competency in professionalism: Targeting resident advance directive education. *Journal of Graduate Medical Education* 2(2):278-282.

Cruz, M. L. 2013. *Patient-centered care: How physical therapy can help patients who need palliative care.* Advance Health Care Network for Physical Therapy and Rehab Medicine. http://physical-therapy.advanceweb.com/Features/Articles/Patient-Centered-Care.aspx (accessed August 24, 2013).

Daaleman, T. 2010. *Families rank end-of-life care higher when spiritual care received.* http://www.nacc.org/vision/May_June_2010/ru.asp (accessed December 3, 2013).

Daaleman, T. P., C. S. Williams, V. L. Hamilton, and S. Zimmerman. 2008. Spiritual care at the end of life in long-term care. *Medical Care* 46(1):85-91.

Dahlin, C., ed. 2013. *Clinical practice guidelines for quality palliative care.* 3rd ed. Pittsburgh, PA: National Consensus Project for Quality Palliative Care. http://www.hpna.org/multimedia/NCP_Clinical_Practice_Guidelines_3rd_Edition.pdf (accessed December 3, 2013).

Dickinson, G. E. 2007. End-of-life and palliative care issues in medical and nursing schools in the United States. *Death Studies* 31(8):713-726.

Dickinson, G. E. 2011. Thirty-five years of end-of-life issues in U.S. medical schools. *American Journal of Hospice and Palliative Care* 28(6):412-417.

Dickinson, G. E. 2013. End-of-life and palliative care education in U.S. pharmacy schools. *American Journal of Hospice and Palliative Medicine* 30(6):532-535.

Douglas, K. S. 2012. Staffing for end of life: Challenges and opportunities. *Nursing Economics* 30(3):167-169, 178.

Ellman, M. S., and A. H. Fortin, VI. 2012. Benefits of teaching medical students how to communicate with patients having serious illness: Comparison of two approaches to experiential, skill-based, and self-reflective learning. *Yale Journal of Biology and Medicine* 85(2):261-270.

ELNEC (End-of-Life Nursing Education Consortium). 2013. *End-of-Life Nursing Education Consortium (ELNEC) fact sheet.* Washington, DC: AACN.

EPEC (Education in Palliative and End-of-life Care). 2013a. *EPEC—pediatrics.* Chicago, IL: EPEC. http://epec.net/epec_pediatrics.php?curid=6 (accessed November 25, 2013).

EPEC. 2013b. *EPEC: Education in Palliative and End-of-life Care.* Chicago, IL: EPEC. http://epec.net (accessed November 25, 2013).

Fallowfield, L., M. Lipkin, and A. Hall. 1998. Teaching senior oncologists communication skills: Results from phase 1 of a comprehensive longitudinal program in the United Kingdom. *Journal of Clinical Oncology* 16(5):1961-1968.

Fallowfield, L., V. Jenkins, V. Farewell, J. Saul, A. Duffy, and R. Eves. 2002. Efficacy of a cancer research UK communications skills training model for oncologists: A randomized controlled trial. *Lancet* 359(9307):650-656.

Fallowfield, L., V. Jenkins, V. Farewell, and I. Silis-Trapala. 2003. Enduring impact of communications skills training: Results of a 12-month follow-up. *British Journal of Cancer* 89(8):1445-1449.

FDA (U.S. Food and Drug Administration). 2013. *Questions and answers: FDA approves a Risk Evaluation and Mitigation Strategy (REMS) for extended-release and long-acting (ER/LA) opioid analgesics.* http://www.fda.gov/Drugs/DrugSafety/InformationbyDrugClass/ucm309742.htm (accessed November 25, 2013).

Ferrell, B. R., and N. Coyle, eds. 2010. *Oxford textbook of palliative nursing.* 3rd ed. New York: Oxford University Press. http://global.oup.com/academic/product/oxford-textbook-of-palliative-nursing-9780195391343?cc=us&lang=en&tab=toc (accessed December 2, 2013).

Flannelly, K. J., L. L. Emanuel, G. F. Handzo, K. Galek, N. R. Silton, and M. Carlson. 2012. A national study of chaplaincy services and end-of-life outcomes. *BMC Palliative Care* 11:10.

Goldsmith, J., B. Ferrell, E. Lyles-Wittenberg, and S. L.Ragan. 2013. Palliative care communication in oncology nursing. *Clinical Journal of Oncology Nursing* 17(2):163-167.

Gross, C., and E. C. Bell. 2013. AoA specialty board certification. *Journal of the American Osteopathic Association* 113(4):339-342.

Hafferty, F. W. 1998. Beyond curriculum reform: Confronting medicine's hidden curriculum. *Academic Medicine* 73(4):403-407.

Hanks, G., N. I. Cherny, N. A. Christakis, M. Fallon, S. Kaasa, and R. K. Portenoy, eds. 2009. *Oxford textbook of palliative medicine.* 4th ed. Oxford, England: Oxford University Press.

Hebert, K., H. Moore, and J. Rooney. 2011. The nurse advocate in end-of-life care. *Ochsner Journal* 11(4):325-329.

Herndon, C. M., K. Jackson, D. S. Fike, and T. Woods. 2003. End-of-life care education in United States pharmacy schools. *American Journal of Hospice and Palliative Care* 20(5):340-344.

Hinds, P. S., L. Oakes, and W. L. Furman. 2010. End-of-life decision-making in pediatric oncology. In *Oxford textbook of palliative nursing,* edited by B. R. Ferrell and N. Coyle. New York: Oxford University Press.

HMDCB (Hospice Medical Director Certification Board). 2013. *Hospice Medical Director Certification Board.* http://www.hmdcb.org (accessed August 26, 2014).

Hold, J. L., E. N. Ward, and B. J. Blake. 2014. Integrating professional apprentices into an end-of-life course. *Journal of Nursing Education* 53(2):112-115.

Horowitz, R., R. Gramling, and T. Quill. 2014. Palliative care education in U.S. medical schools. *Medical Education* 48(1):59-66.

HPNA (Hospice and Palliative Nurses Association). 2009. *Hospice and palliative nursing assistant competencies.* Pittsburgh, PA: HPNA. https://www.hpna.org/PicView.aspx?ID=287 (accessed January 31, 2014).

HPNA. 2013. *Graduate program listing.* Pittsburgh, PA: HPNA. http://www.hpna.org/DisplayPage.aspx?Title=Graduate%20Program%20Listing (accessed January 24, 2014).

IOM (Institute of Medicine). 1997. *Approaching death: Improving care at the end of life.* Washington, DC: National Academy Press.

IOM. 2003. *When children die: Improving palliative and end-of-life care for children and their families.* Washington, DC: The National Academies Press.

IOM. 2008. *Retooling for an aging America: Building the health care workforce.* Washington, DC: The National Academies Press.

IOM. 2010. *A summary of the February 2010 Forum on the Future of Nursing Education: Workshop summary.* Washington, DC: The National Academies Press.

IOM. 2011. *Relieving pain in America: A blueprint for transforming prevention, care, education, and research.* Washington, DC: The National Academies Press.

IOM. 2013a. *Establishing transdisciplinary professionalism for improving health outcomes: Workshop summary.* Washington, DC: The National Academies Press.

IOM. 2013b. *Interprofessional education for collaboration: Learning how to improve health from interprofessional models across the continuum of education to practice: Workshop summary.* Washington, DC: The National Academies Press.

Jankowski, K. R. B., G. F. Handzo, and K. J. Flannelly. 2011. Testing the efficacy of chaplaincy care. *Journal of Health Care Chaplaincy* 17:100-125.

Joint Commission. 2008. *Standards FAQs (hospital manual and home care manual).* Oakbrook Terrace, IL: Joint Commission. http://www.jointcommission.org/standards_information/jcfaq.aspx (accessed July 26, 2013).

Josiah Macy Jr. Foundation. 2011. *Ensuring an effective physician workforce for the United States: Recommendations for reforming graduate medical education to meet the needs of the public—the second of two conferences—the content and format of GME.* New York: Josiah Macy Jr. Foundation. http://macyfoundation.org/docs/macy_pubs/Macy_GME_Report,_Aug_2011.pdf (accessed November 30, 2013).

KFF (The Henry J. Kaiser Family Foundation). 2014. *State health facts: Total professionally active physicians.* http://kff.org/other/state-indicator/total-active-physicians (accessed March 11, 2014).

Knapp, C. A., V. Madden, H. Wang, K. Kassing, C. Curtis, P. Sloyer, and E. A. Shenkman. 2009. Paediatric nurses' knowledge of palliative care in Florida: A quantitative study. *International Journal of Palliative Nursing* 15(9):432-439.

Knapp, C. A., V. Madden, H. Wang, K. Kassing, C. Curtis, P. Sloyer, and E. A. Shenkman. 2011. Pediatric nurses' attitudes toward hospice and pediatric palliative care. *Journal of Pediatric Nursing* 37(3):121-126.

Kolarik, R. C., G. Walker, and R. M. Arnold. 2006. Pediatric resident education in palliative care: A needs assessment. *Pediatrics* 117(6):1949-1954.

Latuga, N. M., R. G. Wahler, and S. V. Monte. 2012. A national survey of hospice administrator and pharmacist perspectives on pharmacist services and the impact on medication requirements and cost. *American Journal of Hospice and Palliative Care* 29(7):546-554.

Lawson, R. 2012. Palliative social work in the emergency department. *Journal of Social Work in End of Life and Palliative Care* 8(2):120-134.

LeBlanc, T. W., and J. A. Tulsky. in press. Communication with the patient and family. In *Oxford textbook of palliative medicine*, 5th ed., edited by N. Cherney, M. Fallon, S. Kaasa, R. Portenoy, and D. Currow. Oxford, England: Oxford University Press.

Legrand, S. B., and J. B. Heintz. 2012. Palliative medicine fellowship: A study of resident choices. *Journal of Pain and Symptom Management* 43(3):558-568.

Leipzig, R. M., L. Granville, D. Simpson, M. B. Anderson, K. Sauvigne, and R. P. Soriano. 2009. Keeping granny safe on July 1: A consensus on minimum geriatrics competencies for graduating medical students. *Academic Medicine* 84(5):604-610.

Leong, L., J. Ninnis, N. Slatkin, M. Rhiner, L. Schroeder, B. Pritt, J. Kagan, T. Ball, and R. Morgan. 2010. Evaluating the impact of pain management (PM) education on physician practice patterns: A continuing medical education (CME) outcomes study. *Journal of Cancer Education* 25(2):224-228.

Liaison Committee on Medical Education. 2013. *Functions and structure of a medical school: Standards for accreditation of medical education programs leading to the M.D. degree.* Chicago, IL: American Medical Association, and Washington, DC: Association of American Medical Colleges. https://www.lcme.org/publications/functions2013june.pdf (accessed November 26, 2013).

Liao, J. M. 2014. Speaking up about the dangers of the hidden curriculum. *Health Affairs* 33(1):168-171.

Liben, S., D. Papadatou, and J. Wolfe. 2008. Paediatric palliative care: Challenges and emerging ideas. *Lancet* 371(9615):852-864.

Lopez, R. 2013. Minimum wage, overtime protections extended to direct care workers. *Los Angeles Times*, September 17. http://www.latimes.com/business/money/la-fi-mo-direct-care-workers-labor-rules-20130917,0,4108023.story (accessed September 18, 2013).

Lupu, D., and American Academy of Hospice and Palliative Medicine Workforce Task Force. 2010. Estimate of current hospice and palliative medicine physician workforce shortage. *Journal of Pain and Symptom Management* 40(6):899-911.

Lupu, D., C. Deneszczuk, T. Leystra, R. McKinnon, and V. Seng. 2013. Few U.S. public health schools offer courses on palliative and end-of-life care policy. *Journal of Palliative Medicine* 16(12):1582-1587.

Malloy, P., B. Ferrell, R. Virani, K. Wilson, and G. Uman. 2006. Palliative care education for pediatric nurses. *Journal of Pediatric Nursing* 32(6):555-561.

Mansouri, M., and J. Lockyer. 2007. A meta-analysis of continuing medical education effectiveness. *Journal of Continuing Education in the Health Professions* 27(1):6-15.

Matzo, M., and D. W. Sherman. 2010. *Palliative care nursing: Quality care to the end of life.* 3rd ed. New York: Springer Publishing. http://books.google.com/books?hl=en&lr =&id=rTexGiX5bqoC&oi=fnd&pg=PR7&dq=advanced+practice+nurse+hospice+pallia tive+education+programs&ots=cHxHd5Md19&sig=M_IPplucY4ROMOXs9z6Zg8b6_ lU#v=onepage&q=advanced%20practice%20nurse%20hospice%20palliative%20 education%20programs&f=false (accessed December 2, 2013).

Medical College of Wisconsin. undated. *End of life/palliative education resource center: Advancing end-of-life care through an online community of educational scholars.* Milwaukee, WI: Medical College of Wisconsin. http://www.eperc.mcw.edu/EPERC.htm (accessed January 25, 2014).

Meyer, E. C., D. E. Sellers, D. M. Browning, K. McGuffie, M. Z. Solomon, and R. D. Truog. 2009. Difficult conversations: Improving communication skills and relational abilities in health care. *Pediatric Critical Care Medicine* 10(3):352-359.

Millikan, C. R. 2013. *Spirituality in Healthcare.* Presentation at Meeting of the IOM Committee on Approaching Death: Addressing Key End-of-Life Issues, Houston, TX, July 22.

NASW (National Association of Social Workers). 2004. *NASW standards for palliative and end of life care.* Washington, DC: NASW. https://www.socialworkers.org/practice/ bereavement/standards/standards0504New.pdf (accessed January 31, 2014).

NASW. 2014. *NASW professional social work credentials and advanced practice specialty credentials.* Washington, DC: NASW. https://www.socialworkers.org/credentials/list.asp (accessed January 8, 2014).

National Matching Services. 2014. *ASHP resident matching program for positions beginning in 2014: Summary of programs and positions offered and filled for the 2014 match.* Toronto, Ontario, and Lewiston, NY: National Matching Services, Inc. https://natmatch. com/ashprmp/stats/2013summpos.html (accessed April 29, 2014).

NBCHPN® (National Board for Certification of Hospice and Palliative Nurses). 2013. *National Board for Certification of Hospice and Palliative Nurses (NBCHPN®).* Pittsburgh, PA: NBCHPN®. http://www.nbchpn.org (accessed December 2, 2013).

NBCHPN®. 2014. *Certifications offered.* http://www.nbchpn.org/DisplayPage.aspx?Title= Certifications%20Offered (accessed August 18, 2014).

NCI (National Cancer Institute). 2013. *EPEC^{TM}-O: Palliative care educational materials.* http://www.cancer.gov/cancertopics/cancerlibrary/epeco/selfstudy (accessed November 25, 2013).

Newhouse, R. P., and B. Spring. 2010. Interdisciplinary evidence-based practice: Moving from silos to synergy. *Nursing Outlook* 58(6):309-317.

NHPCO (National Hospice and Palliative Care Organization). 2006. *Physician board certification in hospice and palliative medicine (HPM).* http://www.nhpco.org/palliative-care/ physician-certification (accessed August 26, 2014).

Open Society Institute. 2004. *Transforming the culture of dying: The Project on Death in America.* New York: Project on Death in America. http://www.opensocietyfoundations. org/sites/default/files/a_transforming.pdf (accessed January 25, 2014).

PHI (Paraprofessional Healthcare Institute). 2011. *Who are direct-care workers?* New York: PHI. http://phinational.org/sites/phinational.org/files/clearinghouse/PHI%20FactSheet3_ singles.pdf (accessed December 4, 2013).

Pollens, R. 2004. Role of the speech-language pathologist in palliative hospice care. *Journal of Palliative Medicine* 7(5):694-702.

Puchalski, C., B. Ferrell, R. Virani, S. Otis-Green, P. Baird, J. Bull, H. Chochinov, G. Handzo, H. Nelson-Becker, M. Prince-Paul, K. Pugliese, and D. Sulmasy. 2009. Improving the quality of spiritual care as a dimension of palliative care: The report of the Consensus Conference. *Journal of Palliative Medicine* 12(10):885-904.

Quill, T. E., and A. P. Abernethy. 2013. Generalist plus specialist palliative care—creating a more sustainable model. *New England Journal of Medicine* 368(13):1173-1175.

Radwany, S. M., E. J. Stovsky, D. M. Frate, K. Dieter, S. Friebert, B. Palmisano, and M. Sanders. 2011. A 4-year integrated curriculum in palliative care for medical undergraduates. *American Journal of Hospice and Palliative Medicine* 28(8):528-535.

Rapoport, A., C. Obwanga, G. Sirianni, S. Lawrence Librach, and A. Husain. 2013. Not just little adults: Palliative care physician attitudes toward pediatric patients. *Journal of Palliative Medicine* 16(6):675-679.

Rider, E. A., K. Volkan, and J. P. Hafler. 2008. Pediatric residents' perceptions of communication competencies: Implications for teaching. *Medical Teacher* 30(7):e208-e217.

Robinson, K., S. Sutton, C. F. von Gunten, F. D. Ferris, N. Molodyko, J. Martinez, and L. L. Emanuel. 2004. Assessment of the Education for Physicians on End-of-life Care (EPEC) project. *Journal of Palliative Medicine* 7(5):637-645.

Saguil, A., A. L. Fitzpatrick, and G. Clark. 2011. Are residents willing to discuss spirituality with patients? *Journal of Religion and Health* 50(2):279-288.

Sanchez-Reilly, S., and J. S. Ross. 2012. Hospice and palliative medicine: Curriculum evaluation and learner assessment in medical education. *Journal of Palliative Medicine* 15(1):116-122.

Schwartz, A. 2012. Is this palliative care's moment? *Science of caring.* http://scienceofcaring. ucsf.edu/acute-and-transitional-care/palliative-cares-moment (accessed November 30, 2013).

Seelye, K. Q. 2014. In annual speech, Vermont governor shifts focus to drug abuse. *The New York Times,* January 8.

Seoane, L., D. A. Bourgeois, C. M. Blais, R. B. Rome, H. H. Luminais, and D. E. Taylor. 2012. Teaching palliative care in the intensive care unit: How to break the news. *Ochsner Journal* 12(4):312-317.

Serwint, J. R., L. E. Rutherford, and N. Hutton. 2006. Personal and professional experiences of pediatric residents concerning death. *Journal of Palliative Medicine* 9(1):70-81.

Shah, A. B., R. P. Morrissey, A. Baraghoush, P. Bharadwaj, A. Phan, M. Hamilton, J. Kobashigawa, and R. R. Schwarz. 2013. Failing the failing heart: A review of palliative care in heart failure. *Reviews in Cardiovascular Medicine* 14(1):41-48.

Shaw, G. 2012. New opportunities for palliative care in medical education. *AAMC Reporter,* July. Washington, DC: Association of American Medical Colleges. https://www.aamc.org/ newsroom/reporter/july2012/297224/palliative-care.html (accessed November 20, 2013).

Shield, R. R., I. Tong, M. Tomas, and R. W. Besdine. 2011. Teaching communication and compassionate care skills: An innovative curriculum for pre-clerkship medical students. *Medical Teacher* 33(8):e408-e416.

Social Work Hospice and Palliative Care Network. 2014. *Welcome to the network.* http:// www.swhpn.org (accessed January 31, 2014).

Stayer, D. 2012. Pediatric palliative care: A conceptual analysis for pediatric nursing practice. *Journal of Pediatric Nursing* 27(4):350-356.

Stevens, D. P., D. H. Jones, J. A. Salerno, and B. J. Ryan. 1999. A strategy for improvement in care at the end of life: The VA Faculty Leaders Project. *Journal of Palliative Medicine* 2(1):5-7.

Sullivan, A. M., M. D. Lakoma, and S. D. Block. 2003. The status of medical education in end-of-life care. *Journal of General Internal Medicine* 18(9):685-695.

Sullivan, A. M., M. D. Lakoma, J. A. Billings, A. S. Peters, S. D. Block, and PCEP Core Faculty. 2005. Teaching and learning end-of-life care: Evaluation of a faculty development program in palliative care. *Academic Medicine* 80(7):657-668.

Sullivan, A. M., M. D. Lakoma, R. K. Matsuyama, L. Rosenblatt, R. M. Arnold, and S. D. Block. 2007. Diagnosing and discussing imminent death in the hospital: A secondary analysis of physician interviews. *Journal of Palliative Medicine* 10(4):882-893.

Swick, H. M. 2000. Toward a normative definition of medical professionalism. *Academic Medicine* 75(6):612-616. http://medprof.bjmu.edu.cn/xsqy/57_towards%20a%20normative%20definition%20of%20medical%20professionalis.pdf (accessed November 30, 2013).

Tovino, S. A. 2005. Hospital chaplaincy under the HIPAA privacy rule: Health care or "just visiting the sick"? *Scholarly Works*, paper 392. Las Vegas: University of Nevada, Las Vegas, William S. Boyd School of Law. http://scholars.law.unlv.edu/facpub/392 (accessed January 25, 2014).

Tung, E. E., M. L. Wieland, B. P. Verdoorn, K. F. Mauck, J. A. Post, M. R. Thomas, J. B. Bundrick, T. M. Jaeger, S. S. Cha, and K. G. Thomas. 2013. Improved resident physician confidence with advance care planning after an ambulatory clinic intervention. *American Journal of Hospital Palliative Care* 31(3):275-280.

United States Medical Licensing Examination. 2013. *Step 3: Content outlines*. Washington, DC: Federation of State Medical Boards, and Philadelphia, PA: National Board of Medical Examiners. http://www.usmle.org/step-3/#outlines (accessed November 29, 2013).

University of Rochester Medical Center. 2013. *Palliative care program: Nursing programs*. Rochester, NY: University of Rochester Medical Center. http://www.urmc.rochester.edu/medicine/palliative-care/education/nurse.cfm (accessed November 29, 2013).

Van Aalst-Cohen, E. S., R. Riggs, and I. R. Byock. 2008. Palliative care in medical school curricula: A survey of United States medical schools. *Journal of Palliative Medicine* 11(9):1200-1202.

Verghese, A., E. Brady, C. C. Kapur, and R. I. Horwitz. 2011. The bedside evaluation: Ritual and reason. *Annals of Internal Medicine* 155(8):550-554.

Vitello, P. 2008. Hospice chaplains take up bedside counseling. *New York Times*, October 28. http://www.nytimes.com/2008/10/29/nyregion/29hospice.html?pagewanted=all&_r=0 (accessed September 20, 2013).

von Gunten, C. F., P. Mullan, R. A. Nelesen, M. Soskins, M. Savoia, G. Buckholz, and D. E. Weissman. 2012. Development and evaluation of a palliative medicine curriculum for third-year medical students. *Journal of Palliative Medicine* 15(11):1198-1217.

Walsh-Burke, K., and E. L. Csikai. 2005. Professional social work education in end-of-life care: Contributions of the Project on Death in America's Social Work Leadership Development program. *Journal of Social Work in End-of-Life and Palliative Care* 1(2):11-26.

Weisenfluh, S. M., and E. L. Csikai. 2013. Professional and educational needs of hospice and palliative care social workers. *Journal of Social Work in End-of-Life and Palliative Care* 9(1):58-73.

Wiskin, C., E. M. Doherty, M. von Fragstein, A. Laidlaw, and H. Salisbury. 2013. How do United Kingdom (UK) medical schools identify and support undergraduate medical students who "fail" communication assessments? A national survey. *BMC Medical Education* (July):95.

Wolfe, J., P. Hinds, and B. M. Sourkes. 2011. *Textbook of interdisciplinary pediatric palliative care*. Philadelphia, PA: Elsevier Saunders.

Wright, A. A., B. Zhang, A. Ray, J. W. Mack, E. Trice, T. Balboni, S. L. Mitchell, V. A. Jackson, S. D. Block, P. K. Maciejewski, and H. G. Prigerson. 2008. Associations between end-of-life discussions, patient mental health, medical care near death, and caregiver bereavement adjustment. *Journal of the American Medical Association* 300(14):1665-1673.

5

Policies and Payment Systems to Support High-Quality End-of-Life Care

Financial incentives built into the programs that most often serve people with advanced serious illnesses—Medicare and Medicaid—encourage providers to render more services and more intensive services than are necessary or beneficial, and the lack of coordination among programs leads to fragmented care, with all its negative consequences. In short, the current health care system increases risks to patients and creates avoidable burdens on them and their families. Meanwhile, the practical but essential day-to-day support services, such as caregiver training, nutrition services, and medication management, that would allow people near the end of life to live in safety and comfort at home—where most prefer to be—are not easily arranged or paid for.

The U.S. health care system is in a state of rapid change. The impact of these shifting programs and incentives—and both their beneficial and unintended negative consequences—on Americans nearing the end of life should not be overlooked. Appropriate measurement and accountability structures are needed to ensure that people nearing the end of life will benefit under changing program policies. In assessing how the U.S. health care system affects Americans near the end of life, the committee focused on evidence that the current system is characterized by fragmentation and inefficiency, inadequate treatment of pain and other distressing symptoms, frequent transitions among care settings, and enormous and growing care responsibilities for families.

While the committee focused on improving the quality of care for people with serious advanced illnesses who may be approaching death, it also was attentive to the need to control spending throughout the U.S.

263

health care system. Likewise, most new health program proposals for the last several decades, up to and including the 2010 Patient Protection and Affordable Care Act (ACA), have tried to balance increasing access and improving the quality of care with managing costs. Indeed, decades of experience with the nation's flagship health care programs—Medicaid for low-income Americans (including those who "spend down" their life savings to become eligible) and Medicare for those aged 65 and older and persons with disabilities—suggest that improving the quality of care can reduce costs.

For those nearing the end of life, better quality of care through a range of new delivery models has repeatedly been shown to reduce the need for frequent 911 calls, emergency department visits, and unnecessary urgent hospitalizations. Evidence suggests that palliative care, hospice, and various care models that integrate health care and social services may provide high-quality end-of-life care that can reduce the use of expensive hospital- and institution-based services, and have the potential to help stabilize and even reduce health care costs for people near the end of life. The resulting savings could be used to fund highly targeted and carefully tailored social services for both children and adults (Komisar and Feder, 2011; Unroe and Meier, 2013), improving patient care while protecting and supporting families. This chapter describes those opportunities.

The U.S. health care system is a complex mix of individual profession-als, acute and long-term care facilities, dozens of ancillary services, payers, vendors, and many other components. Making a potentially cost-saving change in one area, regardless of how theoretically sound it may be, may create a response elsewhere in the system that prevents overall savings from being achieved. For that reason, piecemeal reforms will not work, and com-prehensive approaches are needed.

The committee notes that many positive aspects of the nation's current evolving health care system—the opportunities it affords for patients to choose providers and treatments, the growing number of quality initiatives, its investment in research and technology, and the commitment of large numbers of professionals and institutions to care for the frailest and sickest Americans—could be lost in draconian or ill-considered cost-containment measures, such as stinting on needed and beneficial care. For that reason, the committee focused on the system changes that would not only serve the needs of the sickest patients and their families but also, as a result of bet-ter quality, lead to more efficient, affordable, and sustainable practices. To this end, much can be learned from existing successful programs and care delivery models that could be applied more widely.

In May 2013 testimony before the House Committee on Ways and

Means Subcommittee on Health, Alice Rivlin[1] began with an interesting question and arrived at an even more interesting answer:

> Why reform Medicare? The main reason for reforming Medicare is *not* that the program is the principal driver of future federal spending increases, although it is. The main reason is *not* that Medicare beneficiaries could be receiving much better coordinated and more effective care, although they could. The most important reason is that Medicare is big enough to move the whole American health delivery system away from fee-for-service reimbursement, which rewards volume of services, toward new delivery structures, which reward quality and value. Medicare can lead a revolution in health care delivery that will give *all* Americans better health care at sustainable cost. (Rivlin, 2013)

Rivlin's remarks highlight the two issues facing Medicare and the U.S. health sector as a whole—costs and quality. These two intertwined issues pervaded this study.

The poorer quality of care and higher costs that result from lack of service coordination, risky and repeated transitions across settings and programs, and fragmented and siloed delivery and payment systems affect large numbers of Americans, including those nearing the end of life. Although it is too early to predict the ultimate effects of the ACA, it is not too soon to start calling for accountability and transparency in care near the end of life to ensure that the goals of health care reform are realized for the most vulnerable and sickest beneficiaries.

This chapter describes systemic shortcomings in U.S. health care that hinder high-quality, compassionate, and cost-effective care for people of all ages near the end of life and their families. The chapter begins by summarizing the quality and cost challenges that must be faced in efforts to redesign policies and payment systems to support high-quality end-of-life care. It then provides background information on the most important programs responsible for financing and organizing U.S. health care and the perverse incentives in those programs that affect people near the end of life. Next, the chapter examines the gap between the services these programs pay for and what patients nearing the end of life and their families want and need. The chapter then turns to opportunities and initiatives to address the shortfalls and gaps in the current system and the concomitant need to establish greater transparency and accountability in the delivery of care near the end of life. After outlining research needs, the chapter ends with the commit-

---

[1] Alice Rivlin is Leonard D. Schaeffer chair in health economics at the Brookings Institution, a visiting professor at the Public Policy Institute of Georgetown University, and director of Brookings' Engelberg Center for Health Care Reform. She recently served as a member of the President's Debt Commission, was founding director of the Congressional Budget Office, served as Office of Management and Budget director, and was Federal Reserve vice-chair.

tee's findings, conclusions, and recommendations on policies and payment systems to support high-quality end-of-life care.

THE QUALITY CHALLENGES

Americans of any age who have a serious and potentially life-limiting medical condition—from infants with a devastating genetic disorder, to young adults brain-injured in an automobile crash, to frail older people with multiple chronic diseases—can experience a system that is structured and financed to provide costly interventions, high-tech services, and crisis and emergency care. This system is experienced by many thousands of people. What requires close examination and reform is how those resources are spent and whether they are well matched to the values, goals, wishes, and needs of patients and families. Current evidence suggests they are not.

The health care payment system in the United States is different from that in other wealthy, industrialized nations and has resulted from the nation's unique politics and history. The U.S. system rewards the volume of medical procedures and therapies provided, and typically neither recognizes nor pays for the day-to-day, long-term services and supports—such as a companion to help with dressing, bathing, and eating—that are needed by people with advanced serious illnesses and their families (Feder et al., 2000; MedPAC, 2011; Rivlin, 2013). As noted in Chapter 2, given an informed choice, most people would prefer to have these ongoing needs met in their homes and communities. Because they often cannot, they routinely and repeatedly resort to 911 calls, emergency department visits, and hospitalizations that are neither beneficial nor wanted (Meier, 2011). This is poor-quality care, and it is extremely expensive.

People with advanced serious illnesses and multiple chronic conditions share certain needs independent of their diagnosis, stage of illness, or age. They have a high prevalence of pain and other distressing symptoms that adversely affect function and quality of life. They are at high risk of functional dependency, and the majority, like more than 60 percent of the costliest 5 percent of Medicare beneficiaries, require help from another person in meeting basic needs on a daily basis. Many suffer from cognitive impairments, such as dementia or delirium, and from other mental health problems, such as depression and anxiety—problems that require specialized attention and intervention. Meeting such needs places enormous burdens—physical, emotional, practical, and financial—on their families and especially, as discussed in Chapter 2, on family caregivers.

In this context, the committee believes a major reorientation of Medicare and Medicaid is needed to craft a system of care that is properly designed to address the central needs of nearly all Americans nearing the end of life. This reorientation will require recognizing the root causes of high utilization of the system (such as exhausted family caregivers); designing services to address those causes (such as round-the-clock access to advice by telephone); reallocating funding away from preventable or unwanted acute/specialist/emergency care to support more appropriate services; and reducing the financial incentives that drive reliance on the riskiest, least suitable, and most costly care settings—the emergency department, the hospital, and the intensive care unit. Fundamentally, services must be tailored to the evolving needs of seriously ill individuals and families so as to provide a positive alternative to costly acute care and to help these patients remain safely at home, if that is their preference. Such tailoring of services would benefit far more people than attempting to reduce services for those in predictably imminent danger of dying.

THE COST CHALLENGES

Forty years ago, U.S. national health care expenditures totaled $75 billion, or 7.2 percent of the nation's gross domestic product (GDP); by 1990, they totaled 10 times that amount—$724 billion—or 12.5 percent of GDP; and just 22 years later, in 2012, they totaled $2.8 trillion, or about 17.2 percent of GDP, having risen some $100 billion between 2011 and 2012 (Martin et al., 2014).[2]

With by far the largest budget of any department in the federal government and a program scope that "touches the lives of virtually every American" (IOM, 2009, pp. 21-23), the U.S. Department of Health and Human Services (HHS) exerts enormous influence over health care in America. That influence is exerted chiefly through Medicare and Medicaid, and the cost challenges in the Medicare and Medicaid programs are of urgent and long-standing concern to policy analysts across the political spectrum (Altman and Shactman, 2011, p. 345; Moffit and Senger, 2013; Robillard, 2013).

The National Commission on Fiscal Responsibility and Reform called federal health spending the nation's "single largest fiscal challenge over the long run" (National Commission on Fiscal Responsibility and Reform, 2010, p. 36). Medicare and Medicaid have grown exponentially since their establishment almost 50 years ago, and their rules and structure have done much to shape care for the seriously ill and those who are dying. Financial pressure on federal health spending has several causes:

---

[2]The $2.79 trillion figure includes expenditures for personal health care ($2.36 trillion), government administration ($33 billion), net cost of health insurance ($164 billion), and government public health activities ($75 billion), as well as $160 billion in noncommercial research, structures, and equipment.

- *Medicare and Medicaid are expensive.* The two programs cost a combined $994 billion in 2012,[3] or about 36 percent of total U.S. national health expenditures, and are projected to cost $1.125 trillion in 2014 (Cuckler et al., 2013). By consuming a large and growing portion of public spending, Medicare and Medicaid may crowd out needed investments in education, the environment, housing, infrastructure such as roads and bridges, alleviation of poverty, and other areas, which together arguably have a greater effect than medical care on population health.
- *Expenditures for the two programs continue to rise and are projected to account for an increasing share of the economy.* Although overall growth in U.S. health expenditures has slowed in recent years, spending on Medicare grew by almost one-third between 2007 and 2012 (from $432.8 billion to $572.5 billion) and on Medicaid by about 30 percent (from $326.2 billion to $421.2 billion) (Martin et al., 2014). Medicare trustees project that the cost of the program will grow from 3.6 percent of the nation's GDP in 2012 to 5.6 percent in 2035 (Boards of Trustees, Federal Hospital Insurance and Federal Supplementary Medical Insurance Trust Funds, 2013), while Medicaid expenditures are expected to more than double between 2013 and 2022, from $265 billion to $536 billion, especially with expansions in eligibility under the ACA (Elmendorf, 2013).
- *The population is changing.* The aging of baby boomers (those born between 1946 and 1964) and the growing number of Americans who are living longer but with substantial burdens of chronic disease put pressure on both Medicare (health services) and Medicaid (long-term care). Older people are the population group most likely to have chronic conditions leading to functional dependency, and spending on patients of all ages with chronic conditions accounts for 84 percent of health care costs (Moses et al., 2013).[4]
- *Family caregiving has its limits.* Older Americans' reliance on family members—whose care was valued at $450 billion in 2009—to serve as caregivers may be difficult to sustain (Feinberg et al., 2011). About one-half (45 percent) of American women aged 75 and older live alone, and their children, if they have any, may be unable to leave their own jobs to take on the caregiving role (AoA, 2013). A loss of family caregiving capacity would increase demand for services paid for by both Medicare and Medicaid.

---

[3]The sum of Medicare ($572.5 billion); Medicaid, federal ($237.9 billion); and Medicaid, state and local ($183.3 billion) (Martin et al., 2014).

[4]The Medicare-eligible population is 14 percent of the U.S. population and 40 percent of the population incurring high health care costs (see Appendix E).

- *The proportional tax base for the programs is shrinking.* The ratio of elderly Americans to working-age Americans, who pay the taxes that fund Medicare and Medicaid, is shifting. In 1990, there were 21 Americans aged 65 and older for every 100 working-age Americans (Bureau of the Census, 2013); the projection for 2030 is 38 Americans 65 and older for every 100 of working age. An ever-smaller proportion of working Americans will be asked to contribute to health care for people at all income levels, including those with large incomes and substantial financial assets.[5]
- *The pay-as-you-go system has its limits.* Despite popular misconceptions, Medicare is funded by current contributions and revenues. In general, beneficiaries have not fully "paid in" during their working years for the benefits they later "take out" (Jacobson, 2013). In 2010, for example, a one-income, average-wage couple took out more than $6.00 in Medicare benefits for every $1.00 paid in (Steuerle and Quakenbush, 2012).

Analysts differ in their views on the relative importance of the various factors implicated in the rise in federal expenditures on health care:

- One recent analysis suggests that most increases in health care costs since 2000 have not been the result of population factors, such as aging or demand for services, but of high prices (especially for hospital care), the cost of drugs and medical devices, and administrative costs (Moses et al., 2013). These authors conclude that higher prices accounted for some 91 percent of the increase between 2000 and 2011. Average prices for everything from pharmaceuticals to surgeries are dramatically higher in the United States than in other countries (Klein, 2013).
- Other analyses attribute growth in health care costs to a larger mix of factors. The Bipartisan Policy Center (2012), for example, cites 13 major contributors to costs,[6] emphasizing that none of them exists in isolation and that policy interventions must address multiple cost drivers.

---

[5]Although higher-income beneficiaries pay somewhat more for their Part B (physician) coverage.

[6]The 13 cost contributors are fee-for-service reimbursement; fragmentation in care delivery; administrative burden; population aging, rising rates of chronic disease, and comorbidities; advances in medical technology; tax treatment of health insurance; insurance benefit design; lack of transparency about cost and quality to inform consumer choice; cultural biases that influence care utilization; changing trends in market consolidation; high unit prices of medical services; the legal and regulatory environment; and the structure and supply of the health professional workforce.

- Based on a series of workshops on lowering health care costs and improving outcomes, an Institute of Medicine (IOM) committee concluded that almost 31 percent of 2009's total health care costs could have been avoided by eliminating unnecessary services, inefficiently delivered services, excess administrative costs, prices that were too high, missed prevention opportunities, and fraud (IOM, 2010a, Box S-2).

Because of these economic realities, recommendations simply to increase total Medicare or Medicaid expenditures—say, to add new benefits for people with advanced serious illnesses without reducing costs elsewhere—are unlikely to be accepted. Conversely, proposals that demonstrably reduce costs as a result of improving the quality of care may be far better received by policy makers of all political persuasions.

U.S. health spending has grown more slowly than expected since the recent recession, a trend that has persisted. The slowdown has been attributed to a number of factors, including less new technology, greater patient cost sharing, and increased efficiency of providers (Ryu et al., 2013). If the trend continues, public-sector health care spending through 2021 will be substantially lower than projected, some analysts believe, and "bring much-needed relief throughout the economy" (Cutler and Sahni, 2013, p. 848). Others are less optimistic and believe the fundamental structural, marketplace, pricing, and demographic causes of cost growth remain unchanged (Bipartisan Policy Center, 2012).

Despite the above analyses, people in their last year of life are widely believed to be a main driver of excess health care spending. As described in the background paper prepared for this study by Aldridge and Kelley (see Appendix E), however, people in the last year of life account for just under 13 percent of total annual U.S. health care spending.[7] Although the top 5 percent of health care spenders account for 60 percent of all health care costs, almost 90 percent of that costliest 5 percent are not in their last year of life. Since 1978, expenditures for Medicare beneficiaries in the last year of life—many of whom have multiple chronic conditions and dementia— have held steady at just over one-quarter of all Medicare expenditures (see Appendix E). In light of this analysis, the oft-expressed concern about "excess spending in the last year of life" distracts from the real drivers of U.S. health care expenditures overall, such as those described above, or those

---

[7]This estimate is based on 2011 Health and Retirement Study data on cost of care in the last year of life paid by Medicare, adjusted to account for costs paid by other sources (Medicaid, 10 percent; out of pocket, 18 percent; other, including private payers, 11 percent). The per person estimate that resulted was then applied to all 2011 deaths to arrive at a total. A limitation of this approach is that it excludes information on the non-Medicare population; however, the majority of costs in the last year of life are covered by Medicare.

of the Medicare program in particular. Those drivers include the system incentives described in this chapter, which not only push people toward use of the expensive acute care system as a substitute for inadequate community and social services but also, by being so costly, inhibit expansion of those services.

FINANCING AND ORGANIZATION OF END-OF-LIFE CARE

The IOM reports *Approaching Death* (1997) and *When Children Die* (2003) acknowledge the importance of the U.S. health care system in securing the care needed by dying adults and children and the "complex and often confusing organizational, financial, and regulatory arrangements that link health care professionals and institutions with each other and with governments, insurers, and other organizations" (IOM, 2003, p. 181). The present report revisits many of these entrenched problems. (Appendix B provides an overview of progress on the two previous reports' recommendations.)

Over the past five decades, Congress has established an array of programs intended to meet the health care needs of older and low-income Americans:

- Medicare, the largest program, covers Americans aged 65 and older, people with permanent disabilities receiving Social Security Disability Income, and those with one of several specific life-threatening conditions. As noted, Medicare is federally funded by current revenue.
- Medicaid covers pregnant women, children, adults with dependent children, people with disabilities, the low-income elderly, and in some states the "medically needy"[8] (KFF, 2013a). Although people commonly think of Medicaid as a program for poor children and their parents, fully 30 percent of the program's 2011 expenditures (approximately $125 billion) was for long-term care. Medicaid is financed jointly by the federal government and the states. The federal government allows the states wide administrative latitude, which results in great variability in benefits and eligibility among states.
- The nearly 10 million Americans who receive both Medicare and Medicaid benefits are termed "dual-eligible." A recent study of 10 years of data on the extent and causes of people "spending down"

---

[8]States that have "medically needy" programs allow people whose income exceeds usual Medicaid eligibility thresholds to enroll if their income minus medical expenses meets the eligibility standard (http://www.medicare.gov/your-medicare-costs/help-paying-costs/medicaid/medicaid.html [accessed December 16, 2014]).

their assets to become eligible for Medicaid found that almost 10 percent of the non-Medicaid population aged 50 and older became Medicaid eligible by the end of the study. Almost two-thirds of Medicaid recipients became eligible by spending down, and people who spent down had substantially lower incomes and fewer assets to begin with—a finding "inconsistent with the common assumption that . . . people who spend down are predominantly middle class" (Wiener et al., 2013, p. ES-2).

The dual-eligible population faces special challenges because the separately created and managed health and social programs under Medicare and Medicaid are not coordinated and contain perverse eligibility and coverage incentives. These financial incentives create waste and result in patients moving back and forth between care settings (and payment options) not for medical reasons, but to maximize provider reimbursements. The result is care that is both poor quality and very costly. The ACA created a new Medicare-Medicaid Coordination Office, described later in this chapter, in an attempt to address these challenges.

Table 5-1 briefly summarizes the principal programs available to meet the needs of people with serious advanced illnesses and their families. The paper by Huskamp and Stevenson in Appendix D provides additional detail, as does the series of "Payment Basics" papers available on the website of the Medicare Payment Advisory Commission (MedPAC, an independent congressional agency, http://www.medpac.gov). The detailed regulations

TABLE 5-1 Major Health and Social Programs Available to People with Serious Advanced Illnesses

Program	Number of Americans Who Benefit	Principal Services Covered[a]	Program Payments (FY 2012 unless noted)
Traditional Medicare[b] (federal)			
Medicare Part A	49.4 million (2012)	Primarily acute inpatient hospital care (90 days per illness episode), skilled nursing facility stays, and other services	$139 billion
Medicare Part B	44 million (2010)	Physician visits and other health professional services	$102 billion

TABLE 5-1 Continued

Program	Number of Americans Who Benefit	Principal Services Covered[a]	Program Payments (FY 2012 unless noted)
Medicare Advantage Program	14.4 million (2013)	Part A and Part B benefits managed by local and regional health plans, with other services (hospice, drug coverage) optional, often for an additional premium	$123 billion
Medicare Part D	36 million (2013)	Outpatient drug expenses through prescription drug plans (deductibles and cost sharing apply, except for low-income Americans)	$54 billion
Medicare Hospice Benefit (under Part A)	1.2 million (2011)	Hospice-provided services related to a terminal illness	$14 billion (2011)
Medicare Home Health Care (under Parts A and B)	3.4 million (2011)	Skilled care at home: nursing; physical, occupational, or speech therapy; medical social work; home health aide services	$21 billion
Medicaid (federal and state)			
Medicaid Health Insurance	14.8 million elderly people and people with disabilities (2013)	Inpatient and outpatient hospital care, physician and other professional services, and laboratory and radiology; all states except Oklahoma cover hospice care	$272 billion (2011)
Long-Term Care Assistance	4.4 million adults (2011)	Nursing home and home health care	$125 billion (2011)
Assistance to Medicare Beneficiaries	9.4 million Medicare beneficiaries	Medicare premiums and cost sharing, as well as uncovered services (especially long-term care) for "dual-eligible" people	$115 billion (2011)

continued

TABLE 5-1 Continued

Program	Number of Americans Who Benefit	Principal Services Covered[a]	Program Payments (FY 2012 unless noted)
U.S. Department of Veterans Affairs (VA)[c]			
Medical Care	5.6 million veteran patients	Medical care, including long-term care, home care, respite care, and hospice/palliative care	$46 billion (2012)
Private Insurance			
Usually through Employment-Related Plans for Employees and Retirees	149 million nonelderly	Wide variation in coverage; almost 8 percent of hospice patients' care is paid for by private insurance, compared with 84 percent paid for by the Medicare Hospice Benefit	$917 billion
Medicare Supplemental Insurance	10.2 million	Mostly costs not covered by Medicare, such as deductibles, co-insurance, and co-payments	Information not available
Long-Term Care Insurance	10 percent of the elderly	Nursing home and other long-term care services, depending on the policy	4 percent of long-term care expenses

NOTES:

[a]Does not include some services, administration, public health, and investment.

[b]Some people receive benefits under more than one program.

[c]The VA's medical care category includes costs of medical services, medical administration, facility maintenance, educational support, research support, and other overhead items, but does not include costs of construction or other nonmedical support (http://www.va.gov/vetdata/Expenditures.asp [accessed December 16, 2014]).

SOURCES: MedPAC (payment basics): http://www.medpac.gov; Huskamp and Stevenson (see Appendix D); Medicare Part A and Medicaid enrollees: Kaiser Family Foundation, *State Health Facts* (KFF, 2014); Medicare Part B: CMS "Medicare Enrollment: National Trends" (CMS, undated-a; KFF, 2013a); Medicaid Long-Term Care Assistance: AARP Public Policy Institute (2013), KFF (2013a); Private insurance: Martin et al. (2014); Medicare Supplemental Insurance: AHIP (2013); Long-Term Care Insurance: NBER (undated).

pertaining to these programs run to thousands of pages, and many of their key features are changing as a result of the ACA. As an example, the number of enrollees in the Medicaid program will rise substantially under the act as many states extend coverage to newly eligible residents (most of whom formerly lacked health insurance).

Medicare is the chief payer of care for people aged 65 and older with advanced serious illnesses and those who elect hospice. The committee calculated that in 2009, approximately 80 percent of U.S. deaths occurred among people covered by Medicare. This share has grown since the publication of *Approaching Death* (IOM, 1997), when Medicare covered approximately 70 percent of deaths (IOM, 1997, p. 155).

Medicaid is the most significant payer for care of low-income children with life-limiting conditions, and it paid more than two-fifths of the nation's total bill for nursing home and other long-term care services in 2010 (KFF, 2013a,b). Additional funding for long-term care services comes from Medicare (for post-acute care), the Social Services Block Grant, the VA, Older Americans Act programs, the U.S. Department of Housing and Urban Development, other state programs, private insurance, and out-of-pocket spending. Families pay out of pocket for many expenses incurred in the last years of life. In a study of 3,209 Medicare beneficiaries, total health care expenditures in the 5 years before death not covered by insurance plans amounted to $38,688 for individuals and $51,030 for couples in which one spouse dies. For one-quarter of the families studied, these expenditures amounted to more than total household assets (Kelley et al., 2013b). Note that high out-of-pocket costs and severe financial impacts are not limited to families with elderly decedents. Recent research has highlighted the economic hardship—including work disruptions, income loss, and increased poverty—among families of children who have advanced cancer and those who die (Bona et al., 2014; Dussel et al., 2011).

One way or another, however, Medicare and Medicaid cover the great majority of people in the last years of life, present identifiable problems, and are clearly amenable to change through federal action. Consequently, this chapter focuses on these two programs.

PERVERSE INCENTIVES AND PROGRAM MISALIGNMENT

At the system level, the financial incentives driving the volume of services delivered and leading to fragmentation in the nation's health care system are among the most significant contributors to unnecessarily high costs (Kamal et al., 2013). According to Elhauge (2010, p. 8), "The current payment system perversely provides disincentives for any provider to invest in coordination or care that might lessen the need of patients for health care, because . . . such investments result in fewer payments for medical or hospital services." These perverse incentives have led to a series of disconnected, siloed service programs, each with different payment, eligibility, and benefit rules and requirements.

Rigid silos of covered services are difficult for program managers, health care facilities, clinicians, and families to overcome when trying to meet the needs of a particular patient. In fact, one of the most burdensome problems patients and family caregivers face is the lack of coordination and communication among different components of the health care system. Not knowing whom to call or who is in charge of a patient's care is deeply frustrating and adds unnecessary stress to already difficult situations (National Direct Service Workforce Resource Center, 2011). Default reliance on the emergency care system and on 911 calls adds risk of harm, burden, and cost. Table 5-2 summarizes how the financial incentives of public programs affect people with serious advanced illnesses.

Absent incentives and mechanisms for true integration across program eligibility, benefits, and financing, it will be impossible to achieve an effectively functioning continuum of care for people with advanced serious illnesses. This situation is in sharp contrast to the IOM's "new rules to redesign and improve care," which emphasize customization based on patient needs, with the patient, not the health system, as the source of control (IOM, 2001, pp. 61-62). Technical, political, and attitudinal barriers must be overcome to integrate funding streams and end cost shifting among programs. Whether recent health care reforms will be able to sufficiently realign current incentives remains to be seen.

Payer Policies and Costs of Care

Since Medicare's inception nearly half a century ago, doctors and hospitals have been reimbursed for the care they provide on the basis of fees for services performed. (Figure 5-1 shows a breakdown of Medicare benefit payments by type of service for 2012.) Fee-for-service payments reward the volume, not the quality, of services delivered. They remain the dominant financing model in U.S. health care despite a rising proportion of Americans in capitated health plans, including Medicare managed care (Medicare Advantage), and the growing number of salaried physicians (Kane and Emmons, 2013).

Generous fee-for-service payments give physicians incentives to—even in the final weeks of life—provide high-intensity, high-cost services, consult multiple subspecialties, order tests and procedures, and hospitalize patients. And because referring patients to hospice reduces the income of some other providers, the fee-for-service system discourages timely referrals to hospice. A study of more than 286,000 randomly selected fee-for-service Medicare beneficiaries who died in 2009 found that although 42 percent

TABLE 5-2 How Financial Incentives in Public Programs Affect People with Serious Advanced Illnesses

Program	General Payment Approach	Financial Incentives	Effects on People with Serious Advanced Illnesses
Medicare Part A (hospitals)	Fee-for-service, based on patient's diagnosis and hospital's cost experience	(1) Higher payments for more intensive services are an incentive to provide services and procedures; (2) fixed, diagnosis-based payments for an inpatient stay encourage early discharge, often to a skilled nursing facility	(1) May encourage overuse of services, even when nonbeneficial; (2) frail, very sick people experience multiple transfers from one care setting to another and increased rehospitalization rates
Medicare Part A (skilled nursing facilities)	Payment of a fixed per diem based on the seriousness of a resident's condition	Patients cannot receive both skilled nursing and hospice care for the same condition; basing payment on patient acuity in theory encourages providers to capture the entirety of patients' needs (although quality concerns remain)	30 percent of Medicare beneficiaries receive "rehabilitative" care in a skilled nursing facility in the last 6 months of life, almost always after a hospital discharge
Medicare Part A (Medicare Hospice Benefit)	For 97 percent of days, hospices receive an all-inclusive per diem payment, not adjusted for case mix or setting or for outlier cases	(1) The hospice benefit is limited to people who have an expected prognosis of 6 months or less if the disease runs the expected course and who agree to forgo curative treatment for the terminal condition; (2) the program was designed mainly for care in the home (where room and board are not an issue) and does not take into account variable needs over time	(1) Survival is difficult to predict, and the limit creates "an artificial distinction between potentially life-prolonging and palliative therapies" (see Appendix D) as well as a psychological barrier to accepting hospice care; (2) if care is too complex for the home, transfer to a hospital and discharge to skilled nursing may appear to be the best option unless patients also have Medicaid (which pays for nursing homes)

continued

TABLE 5-2 Continued

Program	General Payment Approach	Financial Incentives	Effects on People with Serious Advanced Illnesses
Medicare Part B (physicians)	Fee-for-service	Encourages clinicians to provide more services and treatments	Excessive, high-intensity, and burdensome care that may not be wanted is provided in the last months and weeks of life
Medicare Part C (Medicare Advantage)	Capitation	(1) Plans are rewarded for efforts to manage chronic diseases effectively; (2) when patients enroll in hospice, they revert to fee-for-service Medicare	(1) Unnecessary and unwanted treatments, services, and hospitalizations may be reduced; (2) plans may be encouraged to promote hospice enrollment among high-need, high-cost patients
Medicare Part D (drugs)	Administered prices	Prescription drug costs are controlled	Less expensive products, often generic forms, are used when available
Medicaid Long-Term and Nursing Home Care	Acuity score assigned to each resident	(1) The acuity score method reduces incentives to avoid people with costly conditions; (2) Medicaid's lower reimbursement for nursing home care is an incentive to hospitalize dual-eligible residents and return them to the facility under the higher-paying Medicare skilled nursing benefit	(1) Unknown (2) Individuals discharged from the hospital back to the nursing home under the skilled nursing benefit cannot receive hospice care concurrently for the same condition; a 2011 analysis suggested one-quarter of the hospitalizations for dual-eligible beneficiaries in the year studied (2005) were preventable, being due largely to the financial incentives for nursing homes to make these transfers (Segal, 2011)

TABLE 5-2 Continued

Program	General Payment Approach	Financial Incentives	Effects on People with Serious Advanced Illnesses
Medicaid Home Health	For people eligible for nursing facility services; benefits vary	Intended to prevent excessively long periods of nursing home care	Unknown
Administration for Community Living (ACL)	$1.34 billion budget in 2013 for programs addressing health and independence, caregiver support, and Medicare improvements	Examples include elder rights services, the Alzheimer's Disease Supportive Services Program, long-term care information, a family caregiver support program, nutrition services, and some support services	ACL's goal is to increase access to community supports for older Americans and people with disabilities; it administers programs authorized under the Older Americans Act and Developmental Disabilities Assistance and Bill of Rights Act

SOURCES: Appendix D; effects of skilled nursing facility benefit: Aragon et al. (2012), Segal (2011); ACL: http://www.acl.gov/About_ACL/Organization/Index.aspx (accessed December 16, 2014).

were enrolled in hospice at the time of their death, fully 28 percent were under hospice care for 3 days or less. More than 40 percent of late enrollments in hospice were preceded by an intensive care unit stay (Teno et al., 2013). The authors further compared these 2009 rates with patterns of care for similar numbers of Medicare beneficiaries in 2000 and 2005. Over the decade, the tendency to provide hospital and intensive care near the end of life appeared to be increasing.

Both liberals and conservatives find fault with the fee-for-service payment system (Capretta, 2013). The National Commission on Physician Payment Reform, established by the Society of General Internal Medicine in 2012, concluded that fee-for-service reimbursement is the most important cause of high health care costs and expenditures. The first of the commission's 12 recommendations says, "Over time, payers should largely eliminate stand-alone fee-for-service payment to medical practices because of its inherent inefficiencies and problematic financial incentives" (Schroeder and Frist, 2013, p. 2029).

Nevertheless, fee-for-service is expected to remain a continuing and significant payment approach for many years to come (Wilensky, 2014). While Medicare and other payers will reimburse accountable care organizations (ACOs) established under the ACA through a graduated capitation

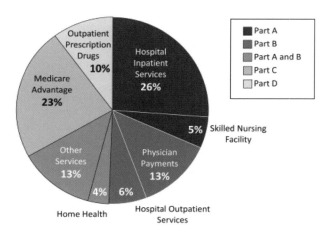

Total Benefit Payments = $536 billion

NOTE: Excludes administrative expenses and is net of recoveries. *Includes hospice, durable medical equipment, Part B drugs, outpatient dialysis, ambulance, lab services, and other services.
SOURCE: Congressional Budget Office (CBO) Medicare Baseline, February 2013.

FIGURE 5-1 Medicare benefit payments by type of service, 2012.
SOURCE: KFF, 2012. Reprinted with permission from The Henry J. Kaiser Family Foundation.

approach, ACOs in turn will use fee-for-service methods to pay many physicians. The act therefore includes provisions to improve the fee-for-service system, revising the physician fee schedule and better reflecting the relative value of resources expended (Ginsburg, 2012).

The Hospital Environment

Hospital Care

As noted in *Approaching Death* (IOM, 1997, p. 96), "curing disease and prolonging life are the central missions of [hospitals]. Hospital culture often regards death as a failure." While hospital and intensive care undoubtedly saves the lives of a great many otherwise healthy people, it is not necessarily useful—and is, to the contrary, harmful—for people with advanced and irreversible chronic illnesses. Yet it is hospital care, not community- or home-based care, that consumes the largest share of Medicare spending for patients in the final phase of life: fully 82 percent of all 2006 Medicare spending during the last 3 months of life was for hospital care, despite the known risks and costs of such care and despite widespread patient preferences, noted in earlier chapters of this report, for less intensive and more home-based services (Lakdawalla et al., 2011).

The transitions between care sites—from hospital to home or nursing home and back again—encouraged, as discussed earlier in this chapter, by the current payment system, put patients at risk (Davis et al., 2012). Resulting higher rates of infection, medical errors, delirium, and falls are collectively captured by the term "burdensome transitions" (see Chapter 2), and they are increasingly common near the end of life. Earlier death may also result from these transitions. The average (mean) number of transitions from one site of care to another in the last 90 days of life increased from 2.1 per decedent in 2000 to 3.1 in 2009, and more than 14 percent of these took place in the last 3 days of life (Teno et al., 2013). This high rate of transitions between care settings is costly and inconsistent with high-quality care.

Emergency Services

When emergency medical services (EMS) providers respond to a 911 call for a Medicare patient, they are required under current Centers for Medicare & Medicaid Services (CMS) policies (generally followed by private insurers as well) to transport the patient to a hospital as a condition for being paid for their response. As a result, patients who might better be served by a palliative care home visit or a trip to a primary care clinician, if such services were available, end up being treated in an emergency department (Alpert et al., 2013).[9] Pain and other unmanaged symptoms prompt many of these visits.

Fifty percent of older Americans visit the emergency department in their last month of life, and 75 percent do so in the last 6 months of life; in 77 percent of cases, the visit results in hospitalization (Smith et al., 2012). Approximately 1.1 million EMS transports are covered by Medicare annually, at a cost of some $1.3 billion.

Unnecessary and burdensome EMS transports represent poor-quality care for people with advanced serious illnesses. When they present at the emergency department, they may be admitted to inpatient care because of an unclear diagnosis; the severity of symptom distress; caregiver concerns; and, most important, a lack of prior clarification of achievable goals for care. Emergency departments are experiencing a growing number of visits by elderly patients whose mix of serious medical conditions, cognitive impairments, functional dependencies, complex medication regimens, and

---

[9]Recent growth in hospital admissions has been attributed entirely to emergency department admissions, which increased by 2.7 million between 2003 and 2009 (Kellermann et al., 2013).

caregiver exhaustion make high-quality emergency care extremely difficult (Hwang et al., 2013).

Many terminally ill patients return to the emergency department because they have not been informed and do not know that they are dying or that there are no effective treatments for their underlying disease (Mitchell et al., 2009). They may be unaware of care alternatives, such as physician house calls, community-based palliative care, or hospice. If EMS providers had more options available to them—other than not being paid—when they respond to overwhelmed caregivers who have panicked and called 911, emergency transfers to hospitals might be avoided. Communities are testing new approaches to training and paying EMS personnel to assess and intervene with soluble problems at home, such as a fall without evidence of injury, rather than routinely transporting all patients who call 911 to the emergency department. Improved "geriatric emergency services" and other models for providing more in-home care and forestalling 911 calls are being tested (Hwang et al., 2013).

The use of emergency services near the end of life is not limited to elderly individuals. Parents of uninsured or publicly insured children with serious illnesses often face delays in obtaining physician appointments and end up seeking care in the emergency department, or they may be referred there by their primary care clinician (Rhodes et al., 2013). In some parts of the country, critically ill children are stabilized at a general emergency department, where experience in recognizing a rapidly worsening condition may be lacking, before transfer to a specialized children's hospital for further care (Chamberlain et al., 2013).

Medicaid reimbursement policies, such as lesser payment for ambulatory versus emergency department care, give hospitals incentives that favor care in the emergency department instead of the hospital's primary care or pediatric clinic (Chamberlain et al., 2013). Finally, once a child is in the care system, fee-for-service reimbursement and the greater malpractice litigation concerns associated with pediatric care may create incentives to overtest and overtreat (Greve, 2011).

The Ambulatory Care Environment

Physician Services

As the gatekeepers for almost all other services, physicians are among the most important players in end-of-life care. Under Medicare, beneficiaries may see a physician as many times as they wish during a year. However, they may be responsible for a 20 percent co-payment for every visit after paying the deductible of $147 (as of 2014). Part B Medicare imposes no restrictions on the type or number of physicians a beneficiary may visit (CMS, undated-c).

Physicians' end-of-life care often fails to meet the needs of patients and families because some clinicians may

- provide care that is overly specialized and does not address the multiplicity of a patient's diseases or the emotional, spiritual, family, practical, and support service needs of patients and their caregivers;
- continue disease treatments beyond the point when they are likely to be effective;
- fail to adequately address pain and other discomfort that often accompanies serious chronic illnesses and the dying process; and
- fail to have compassionate and caring communication with patients and family members about what to expect and how to respond as disease progresses (Weiner and Cole, 2004; Yabroff et al., 2004).

These problems have numerous causes. Shortcomings in physician education regarding end-of-life care are covered in Chapter 4. In addition, the overall culture of medicine is focused on curing acute medical problems. Reflecting and reinforcing this tendency, the financing structure of Medicare and other insurance programs rewards the performance of a high volume of services and the administration of well-reimbursed treatments and procedures rather than encouraging the provision of palliative and comfort care.

As noted earlier, the general financial incentive within fee-for-service is to see as many patients as possible and to perform multiple procedures. In addition, Congress in 1989 created a physician fee structure of "relative value scales" that takes into account primarily physician time, intensity of service, malpractice insurance, and a geographic factor. Medicare, Medicaid, and many private insurers use this system, which also financially rewards more complex specialty procedures without regard to patient benefit or cost (MedPAC, 2011). At the same time, the system undervalues the evaluation and management services necessary to help patients and families understand what to expect, to explain the pros and cons of treatment options, and to establish goals for care as a disease evolves (Kumetz and Goodson, 2013).

Annual increases in Medicare's reimbursements to physicians are, in theory, tied to growth in the nation's GDP. This adjustment method, established by Congress via the Balanced Budget Act of 1997 and called the "sustainable growth rate" (SGR), was intended to be cost-saving. Opposition to limiting physician fee increases has been so strong, however, that

Congress has not imposed these controls since 2002.[10] Medicare payment rates for physicians already are about one-fifth lower than private insurance rates (Hackbarth, 2009), and any large additional reduction could lead many physicians to stop accepting new Medicare beneficiaries into their practices (MedPAC, 2011). Because the SGR approach could jeopardize older Americans' access to care, it is politically unpalatable, and because it fails to incentivize higher-quality care or control health care spending, it is deemed unrealistic and outmoded (Guterman et al., 2013; Hackbarth, 2013; MedPAC, 2011). Discussion of its repeal continues.

Other Services

Although Medicare does not cap beneficiaries' hospital admissions or medical and surgical procedures, it does cap payments for ancillary services that might substantially benefit certain people nearing the end of life—often more so than acute care and procedures. Such services may forestall hospitalizations, help people better manage daily activities, and improve both health status and quality of life (Eva and Wee, 2010; Farragher and Jassal, 2012). Limitations on rehabilitation services (including those that aid in mobility, swallowing, and communication) may therefore have unintended adverse consequences for both quality of care and health care costs if patients' remediable problems are not addressed.

Depression, anxiety, and other mental health issues are a significant concern at the end of life and may combine with cognitive problems to cloud a person's last months. Federal rules implementing mental health parity legislation have erased most long-standing differences between coverage of mental health and other health services for patients with Medicaid and those covered by large group health insurance plans (SAMHSA, 2013); Medicare will reimburse outpatient mental health treatment (therapy and medication management) at parity with other Part B services beginning in 2014.[11] Whether mental health services will actually become available re-

---

[10]The SGR distorts the Congressional Budget Office's (CBO's) estimates of future health care costs. CBO is required to base its estimates on current law, and the SGR is current law, even though it is unenforced. In discussing future federal health spending, the Simpson-Bowles commission said, "These projections likely understate [the] true amount, because they count on large phantom savings—from a scheduled 23 percent cut in Medicare physician payments [in 2012; larger thereafter] that will never occur" (National Commission on Fiscal Responsibility and Reform, 2010, p. 36). The commission made reforming the SGR its first recommendation in the health arena.

[11]In addition, drug plans operating under Medicare Part D must cover certain classes of drugs, including antidepressants and antipsychotics. Certain intensive mental health services—such as psychiatric rehabilitation and psychiatric case management—are not covered (Bazelon Center for Mental Health Law, 2012).

mains to be seen, however, as many mental health care providers (including psychiatrists) do not accept insurance at all (Bishop et al., 2014).

The Managed Care Environment

Managed care was developed and tested in the early 1970s as a way of improving the quality and affordability of health care through capitated, integrated provider networks; an emphasis on disease prevention; utilization review for high-cost services; and other means. In the approach's simplest formulation, managed care organizations receive capitated payments—that is, an annual fixed dollar amount for each individual enrolled in the plan (i.e., per capita).[12] For that fee, enrollees receive all their physician care, hospital care, emergency services, and many other covered benefits, depending on what is included in a specific plan. The managed care organization negotiates with providers to achieve reasonable charges and contracts with (or even hires) physicians. Capitation, in theory, switches incentives toward keeping enrollees healthy and avoiding costly overtreatment.

Medicare Part C (Medicare Advantage) plans are managed care plans offered by private insurance companies that cover all Part A and Part B services. In 2012, Medicare Advantage accounted for 23 percent of all Medicare expenditures (see Figure 5-1). Unlike Medicare fee-for-service, Medicare Advantage gives physicians a financial incentive to recommend hospice for patients nearing the end of life because when plan members enroll in hospice, fee-for-service Medicare becomes the payer. This hospice "carve-out" makes it attractive for a plan to shift patients likely to be high-cost from its rolls to the Medicare Hospice Benefit, but also decreases the incentive for the plan to develop high-quality palliative care services (see Appendix D).

In general, health insurance, including managed care programs, may contain disincentives to enroll people who are the very sickest and costliest. Such initiatives require careful risk stratification and monitoring to ensure adequate access and protection for these beneficiaries.

Just as Medicare, through Medicare Advantage, has embraced managed care partly as a way to avoid the costs of unnecessary hospitalizations, Medicaid has embraced managed care partly to avoid unnecessary nursing home admissions. Ideally, these capitated environments should provide models of care and financing that best meet the needs of program beneficiaries, especially those eligible for both Medicare and Medicaid

---

[12]Payments might include some adjustments, such as for patient age and health status or local cost of living. The Balanced Budget Act of 1997 included risk adjustment, based on patients' diagnoses, to encourage managed care organizations to enroll the sickest Medicare beneficiaries.

(CMS, 2013b). However, the development of policies for implementing and ensuring the quality of managed care options for the dual-eligible population is hampered by significant data limitations, including a lack of timely Medicaid data and comprehensive information about dual eligibles enrolled in Medicare Advantage plans (Gold et al., 2012).

An evaluation of nine state programs of integrated care for dually eligible beneficiaries, performed for MedPAC, identified several additional barriers to the development of managed care programs:

- Enrolling beneficiaries in managed care is problematic because of a lack of awareness of such programs, which may contribute to opposition from providers, beneficiary advocates, and others.
- Structural design problems include administrative leadership (through Medicare Advantage rather than state Medicaid programs), complications in providing patients with social supports and behavioral health services, and uncertainty regarding whether to create separate programs for people under age 65.
- Conflicting Medicare and Medicaid eligibility, coverage, and provider rules complicate state efforts to initiate such programs (Verdier et al., 2011).

Despite these barriers, models of managed care for dually eligible individuals have shown promise, even if they have not been widely replicated. The Evercare model, implemented in five nursing homes (Atlanta, Baltimore, Boston, Colorado [Denver/Colorado Springs], and Tampa) and involving more than 3,600 patients (half enrolled in Evercare, half receiving usual care), offered a capitated package of Medicare-covered services and intensive primary care by nurse practitioners for long-stay, frail, chronically ill nursing home patients. Services included customized care planning, coordination, and delivery. Evercare paid nursing homes an extra fee for "intensive service days" to handle cases that might otherwise have required hospitalization; this measure contributed to a 50 percent reduction in the hospitalization rate for enrollees compared with the usual care group. For those who were hospitalized, stays were shorter for the Evercare group. Evercare enrollees also had one-half the rate of emergency room visits of the usual care group and received more physician visits and mental health services (Kane et al., 2002).

Similarly, an 18-month cohort study of 323 residents with advanced dementia in 22 Boston-area nursing homes found that managed care enrollees had higher rates of do-not-hospitalize orders, primary care visits, and nurse practitioner visits and lower rates of burdensome transitions and hospitalizations for acute illnesses compared with traditional fee-for-service Medicare beneficiaries—all suggesting higher-quality care. Rates of survival, comfort, and other outcomes did not differ significantly between the two groups (Goldfeld et al., 2013).

Finally, the Program of All-inclusive Care for the Elderly (PACE) offers a comprehensive service package designed to avoid nursing home placements. The program was established as a type of provider for Medicare and Medicaid through the Balanced Budget Act of 1997. PACE serves primarily dual-eligible individuals with chronic illnesses who are aged 55 and older. It uses a centralized, nonprofit provider model rather than a looser network of independent practitioners to provide medical and other clinical services along with the kinds of supportive and personal care services discussed later in this chapter—such as meals, transportation to day centers or other facilities, and in-home modifications.

In 2014, 31 states offered the PACE program. Data from 95 of the nation's 103 PACE projects indicate they serve a total of slightly more than 31,000 people (National PACE Association, 2014). Thus, the PACE program remains small, and its effectiveness in serving the specific needs of the population requiring palliative care or those nearing the end of life has not been established (Huskamp et al., 2010; see also Appendix D). Moreover, a recent analysis found that, although PACE improves quality by effectively integrating acute care and long-term community supports and reducing hospitalizations, it has not reduced Medicare expenditures for beneficiaries with substantial long-term care needs, perhaps because capitation rates have been set too high (Brown and Mann, 2012).

The slow rate of PACE expansion has been attributed to regulatory and financial constraints, poor understanding of the program among referral sources, competition, and rigid structural characteristics of the program model (Gross et al., 2004). PACE is a comprehensive approach, and it requires a sophisticated infrastructure. Enabling PACE to be implemented more widely might require designing ways to expand it to the non-Medicaid population, as well as other measures (Hirth et al., 2009).

The Palliative Care and Hospice Environment

A full description of the services involved in and benefits of palliative care, including hospice, is provided in Chapter 2. This section addresses the costs of palliative care and hospice compared with usual care and the policies that regulate the organization and provision of palliative care and hospice services.

Palliative Care

Palliative care programs focus on relieving the medical, emotional, social, practical, and spiritual problems that arise in the course of a serious illness. Many seriously ill people—not just those nearing the end of life— can benefit from palliative care, and it can be provided in many settings, including the home and the nursing home. In hospitals, palliative care teams work alongside treating physicians to provide an added layer of support for patients and their families, focusing on expert symptom management, skilled communication about what to expect, and planning for care beyond the hospital. As discussed in Chapter 2, hospital-based palliative care has grown significantly in the past two decades (CAPC, 2011, 2013).

Palliative care is sometimes viewed as an alternative to what has been termed "futile care"—that is, interventions that are unlikely to help patients or be of marginal benefit and may harm them. Although identifying which treatments are of marginal benefit may be subjective, a study conducted in one academic medical center found that critical care clinicians themselves believed almost 20 percent of their patients received care that was definitely (10.8 percent) or probably (8.6 percent) futile (Huynh et al., 2013). These opinions were based on four principal rationales: the burden on the patient greatly outweighed the benefits, the treatment could never achieve the patient's goals, death was imminent, and the patient would never be able to survive outside the critical care unit. The total annual cost of futile treatment for the 123 (10.8 percent of) patients who received futile care was estimated at $2.6 million.

At the age of 84, my mother arrived at the emergency room [ER] in significant pain. During the preceding 3 weeks, she had contacted her health care provider several times about nausea and been assured it was not significant. Within 36 hours of arriving at the hospital, she was diagnosed with severely metastasized cancer, especially the liver and including her bones. Even though the source of the cancer had not yet been identified and no one had discussed the reasonableness of pursuing treatment, a port was installed in her chest for chemotherapy, "just in case." In the next couple of days, as further testing was done, she had an instance of unstable heartbeat and was taken to ICU, where she was given medication and her heart rate returned to normal. The hospital cardiologist assured us her heart was not a problem, but that he would see her every day while she remained in the hospital. Why? All medical staff consistently pushed ahead with an attitude that chemotherapy WOULD be pursued, that they would get her well enough to go home and return for outpatient chemo, and no one ever raised the issue of whether such an approach would be futile. My sister and I had to press the doctor intensely to get him to acknowledge that even with chemo, her life expectancy was well less than a year.

Her condition did not improve over her stay, and 1 week later she decided not to pursue treatment (after several bouts of explosive diarrhea and an inability to get out of bed) and went home in hospice care. She died 2 weeks to the day after going to the ER. Even when leaving the hospital, they did not suggest the end was imminent. She had a great deal of testing, implantation of a PIC [peripherally inserted central catheter] line, and yet no reasonable analysis of the value of further care from anyone. *

---

*Quotation from a response submitted through the online public testimony questionnaire for this study. See Appendix C.

The committee agrees with Parikh and colleagues' (2013, p. 2348) opinion that while "cost savings are never the primary intent of providing palliative care to patients with serious illnesses . . . it is necessary to consider the financial consequences of serious illness." Much of the spending on the sickest Medicare beneficiaries is attributable to hospital care. Hospitals with specialty palliative care services have been able to reduce their expenditures through shorter lengths of stay in the hospital and in intensive care and lower expenditures on imaging, laboratory tests, and costly pharmaceuticals. In addition, patients receiving hospital-based palliative care have been shown to have longer median hospice stays than patients receiving usual care (Gade et al., 2008; Morrison et al., 2008; Starks et al., 2013).

Most studies comparing the costs of palliative and usual care have been conducted in the hospital setting, but the differing approaches, methods, and rigor of these studies make their findings difficult to compare. Nevertheless, research using robust methods to assess many of the more mature U.S. palliative care programs shows a pattern of savings and demonstrates the substantial excess costs associated with usual care (see Tables 5-3 and 5-4). A 2012 Canadian literature review[13] similarly found that hospital-based palliative care teams reduce hospital costs by $7,000 to $8,000 per patient and reduce the cost of end-of-life care by 40 percent or more (Hodgson, 2012).

Palliative care provided in nonhospital settings has also been found to yield cost savings. A systematic review examined studies of palliative care—cohort studies (34), randomized controlled trials (5), nonrandomized trials (2), and others (5)—published between 2002 and 2011 and conducted variously in hospital-based, home-based, and other program settings. Two-

---

[13]In 2012, the Canadian government allocated $3 million over 3 years to support the development and implementation of a framework for community integrated hospice and palliative care models. The Way Forward initiative is led by the Quality End-of-Life Care Coalition of Canada and managed by the Canadian Hospice Palliative Care Association.

TABLE 5-3 Randomized Controlled Trials Comparing the Costs of Palliative and Usual Care

Study (Period Studied)	Number of Patients and Setting	Excess Cost of Usual Care	Other Findings
Gade et al., 2008 (2002-2003)	517 patients in three hospitals receiving interdisciplinary palliative care services (275 patients) or usual care (237)	Excess 6-month post-hospital discharge costs of $4,855 for each usual care patient (p = 0.001)	Greater patient satisfaction with the care experience and provider communication in the palliative care than in the usual care group; also median hospice stays of 24 versus 12 days, respectively
Brumley et al., 2007 (2002-2004)	145 late-stage patients who received in-home palliative care versus 152 who received usual care in two group-model health maintenance organizations in two states	Excess costs of $7,552 for each usual care group member (p = 0.03)	Palliative care recipients were 2.2 times more likely than usual care recipients to die at home and had fewer emergency department visits and hospitalizations; survival differences between the two groups disappeared after data were adjusted for diagnosis, demographics, and severity of illness (Personal communication, S. Enguidanos, University of Southern California, February 25, 2014)
Greer et al., 2012 (2006-2009)	151 patients with metastatic non-small-cell lung cancer receiving usual outpatient oncologic care with or without early palliative care comanagement	Excess overall costs of $2,282 per patient among those receiving usual care only	Patients receiving early palliative care had significantly higher quality of life, experienced fewer depressive symptoms, were less likely to receive chemotherapy within 2 weeks of death, had earlier hospice enrollment, and survived 2.7 months longer

TABLE 5-4 Observational Studies Comparing the Costs of Palliative and Usual Care

Study (Description)	Number of Patients and Setting	Excess Cost of Usual Care	Other Findings
Morrison et al., 2008 (observational study using propensity score matching, 2002-2004)	4,908 patients who received palliative care consultations and 20,551 who received usual care in eight geographically and structurally diverse hospitals	Excess total costs of $2,642 for each usual care patient discharged alive (p = 0.02) and $6,896 for each who died in the hospital (p = 0.001)	Intensive care unit (ICU), imaging, laboratory, and pharmacy costs were higher among the usual care patients
Morrison et al., 2011 (observational study using propensity score matching, Medicaid-only patients, 2004-2007)	475 patients who received palliative care consultations and 1,576 who received usual care in four diverse urban New York State hospitals	Excess costs of $4,098 for each usual care patient discharged alive (p <0.05) and $7,563 for each who died in the hospital (p <0.05)	Patients receiving palliative care consultation were more likely than usual care patients to be discharged to hospice (30 percent versus 1 percent) and less likely to die in intensive care (34 percent versus 58 percent)
Starks et al., 2013 (observational study using propensity score matching, 2005-2008)	1,815 patients who received palliative care consultation and 1,790 comparison patients from two academic medical center hospitals	Excess costs of $2,141 for usual care patients with lengths of stay of 1-7 days (p = 0.001) and $2,870 for usual care patients with lengths of stay of 8-30 days (p = 0.012)	Some differences between palliative care and usual care groups remained
Penrod et al., 2010 (observational study, 2004-2006)	606 veterans who received palliative care and 2,715 who received usual care in five U.S. Department of Veterans Affairs (VA) hospitals	Excess costs of $464 per day for usual care patients (p = 0.001)	Instrumental variables method used to account for unmeasured selection into treatment bias (Stukel et al., 2007)

thirds of the studies were based in the United States, and the remainder were conducted internationally, in widely differing health systems. The authors found that, although the studies used a broad variety of utilization, cost, and outcome measures and employed different specialist palliative care models, palliative care was "most frequently found to be less costly relative to comparator groups, and in most cases, the difference in cost is statistically significant" (Smith et al., 2014, p. 1).

A recent review of published, peer-reviewed outcomes research on nonhospice outpatient palliative care, which included four randomized interventions and a number of nonrandomized studies, concluded that outpatient palliative care produced overall health care savings resulting from avoidance of expensive interventions. The authors suggest that such savings are "especially important in systems of shared cost/risk, integrated health systems, and accountable care organizations" (Rabow et al., 2013, p. 1546).

Community-based pediatric palliative care has also been found to produce positive patient and family outcomes, as well as cost savings (Gans et al., 2012), or at least to be relatively low cost (Bona et al., 2011).

These data across varying types of studies and care settings indicate potential savings from palliative care consultation and comanagement in hospitals and suggest savings in other settings as well. Additional research is needed before firm conclusions can be drawn on the impact of palliative care delivery on total health care spending.

Hospice Care

The Medicare Hospice Benefit is the one public insurance program intended specifically to serve beneficiaries within the last few months of life. Under this benefit, the enrolled beneficiary pays no charge for services received except for small deductibles for drugs and respite care. Most services are provided in the patient's home by visiting nurses, with variable additional support from physicians, social workers, personal care aides, and others. For fiscal year 2014, Medicare's daily hospice reimbursement rates were as follows: for routine home care, $156.06; for continuous home care, $910.78; for general inpatient care, $694.19; and for inpatient respite care, $161.42 (HHS and CMS, 2013).[14] In addition, the total amount of Medicare payments a hospice provider is allowed to receive in a single year is capped according to a defined formula.

As described in Chapter 2, hospice services produce many benefits for patients and families. Matched cohort studies demonstrate that hospice

---

[14]Minus a two percentage point reduction to the market basket update for hospices that fail to submit the required quality data.

care enhances the quality of care, helps patients avoid hospitalizations and emergency visits, prolongs life in certain groups of patients, improves caregivers' well-being and recovery, and in some reports appears to reduce total Medicare spending for patients with a length of hospice service of under 105 days (Kelley et al., 2013a).[15]

Enrollment disincentives Built into the Medicare Hospice Benefit and its payment rules are several policies that are intended to manage program costs but may work against the needs of patients with advanced serious illnesses and their families. Two eligibility requirements meant to limit the number of people who qualify for the hospice benefit are

- an expected prognosis of 6 months or less if the disease runs the expected course, as certified by two physicians[16]; and
- an agreement, signed by the beneficiary, to give up Medicare coverage for further treatments aimed at achieving a cure.

For many patients, these criteria have discouraged use of the benefit until the final days or hours of life and, according to *Approaching Death*, exclude "many [people] who might benefit from hospice services" (IOM, 1997, p. 169). The ban on "curative" treatments may also disadvantage patients with organ failure, for whom life-prolonging and palliative treatments—such as diuretics for people with heart failure—often are the same. In addition, physicians, patients, and family members alike may be unwilling to accept a prognosis of a few months—particularly given the uncertainty in predicting mortality for diseases other than cancer—or to abandon cure-oriented treatment (Fishman et al., 2009). These factors contribute to the brevity of hospice stays: the median length of stay in hospice is 18 days, and fully 30 percent of hospice beneficiaries are enrolled for less than 1 week. Still, the number of Medicare beneficiaries enrolling in the Medicare Hospice Benefit more than doubled between 2000 and 2011, from 0.5 million to more than 1.2 million (MedPAC, 2013).

Some hospice champions contend that the 6-month limit and the ban on cure-oriented treatments make the Medicare Hospice Benefit "a legal barrier to improving integration and collaboration across the health system" (Jennings and Morrissey, 2011, p. 304). In a survey of nearly 600

---

[15]Methodological difficulties in analyses of hospice savings include the lack of controlling for selection bias (that is, people who choose hospice care may be different in some way from those who do not) and the impact on the data of both very-long-stay patients and those discharged alive after very long stays, who may have been more appropriate candidates for long-term care programs rather than hospice.

[16]In reality, patients are able to receive hospice services for longer than 6 months if, at the end of the period, they receive a physician recertification of the 6-month prognosis.

hospices, 78 percent were found to restrict enrollment in some way, such as by declining to admit patients with ongoing disease treatment needs or without a family caregiver at home (Aldridge Carlson et al., 2012). Small hospices are especially likely to restrict enrollment (Wright and Katz, 2007).

---

*I am a registered nurse case manager, certified in palliative nursing, working with hospice patients in their homes. I think the single most effective change that could be brought about would be to extend the hospice benefit to a 1-year prognosis rather than the current 6 months. This may allow for a strengthening of the role of palliative care much earlier in the trajectory of life-limiting illnesses, particularly those for which the expected course is more certain, such as some cancers. I think the earlier the concept of palliative care is introduced, the less intimidating the "end-of-life" connotation of hospice will be. A patient's course would feel more of a continuum, rather than the abrupt shift from treatment to "hopelessness" that now exists. Just last week, I had a visit with a woman who had been referred to hospice by her oncologist, and she was very frightened that her death was imminent, even though it is not. Her family was equally upset with the physician for frightening the patient so.**

---

*Quotation from a response submitted through the online public testimony questionnaire for this study. See Appendix C.

Payment policies The flat daily rate allowed for by the Medicare Hospice Benefit—which means the hospice receives the same amount regardless of how many, or how few, services it provides on a given day—is coming under scrutiny. The methodology and mix of services used to calculate the daily rate "have not been recalibrated since initiation of the benefit in 1983" (MedPAC, 2013, p. 263), and are inadequate for some hospice programs to cover important services (e.g., palliative radiation, intrathecal delivery of opiates).

Lengths of stay Hospice services have evolved toward serving the two tails of the longevity curve: a large number of beneficiaries enrolled only a few days before death and a large number of very-long-stay patients, with hospice, in effect, serving as an alternative (and one more generously reimbursed) to the provision of long-term care in other settings. In some cases, long stays occur because patients improve under hospice care and outlive their original 6-month prognosis.

The high proportion of short stays in hospice is troubling on quality-of-care grounds, while growth in very long hospice stays is troubling on cost management grounds. The concern arises that incentives in the payment system may be encouraging some providers "to pursue business models that maximize profit by enrolling patients more likely to have long stays," some of whom may not meet hospice eligibility criteria (MedPAC, 2013, p. 265). This pattern, which is more common among for-profit hospice providers (Aldridge Carlson et al., 2012), is also believed to explain some hospices' high rates of "live discharges" for long-stay patients as the facility approaches its aggregate annual cap on Medicare reimbursements.

A concern is the enrollment in hospice of cognitively impaired nursing home residents. As a result of this trend, the *mean* length of stay for Medicare hospice patients, which was 48 days in 1998, was 86 days in 2011 (CMS, 2013a; MedPAC, 2013). In 2009, the longest average stays were for patients with Alzheimer's disease (106 days) and Parkinson's disease (105 days). By comparison, patients with lung cancer had average stays of 45 days and those with breast cancer 59 days (CMS, 2013a). Among the 10 percent of patients with stays longer than 6 months, the average length of stay in 2011 was 241 days (MedPAC, 2013).

The dominant and countervailing trend of notable concern, however—affecting at least 30 percent of all hospice beneficiaries—is stays that are too short. According to hospice industry figures, the *median* length of stay in hospice has steadily fallen, from 21.3 days in 2008 to 18.7 days in 2012 (NHPCO, 2009, 2013), which means that half of hospice patients have stays shorter than 18.7 days.

To the extent that the Medicare Hospice Benefit is being used for people with questionable eligibility as a de facto palliative care supplement to long-term care benefits under state Medicaid programs, the costs of the Medicare Hospice Benefit are raised artificially, and the costs of this care are transferred to the federal government. MedPAC has recommended closer program monitoring to forestall this potential misuse, and greater scrutiny is occurring (U.S. Department of Justice, 2013). Oversight is considered especially appropriate for the approximately 10 percent of hospices that exceed their benefit cap (MedPAC, 2013, p. 275).

The background paper prepared for this study by Huskamp and Stevenson (see Appendix D) reviews several potential or proposed changes to the Medicare Hospice Benefit that would affect hospice-related financial incentives and realign hospice services. Some of these changes were included in the ACA (see also Huskamp et al., 2010).

The Long-Term Care Environment

People with multiple chronic diseases and frailty need a variety of long-term services and supports that can improve the quality of their lives, potentially forestall the need for emergency visits and hospitalizations, and reflect individual and family desires for care at home for as long as possible.

Someone turning age 65 today has almost a 70 percent chance of needing some type of long-term care services and supports in their remaining years (HHS, 2014), yet few (only about 10 percent of the elderly) have private long-term care insurance. The low uptake of existing private long-term care insurance options may be attributable in part to the availability of Medicaid, which provides means-tested "public insurance to many households . . . who could otherwise afford and would be interested in private insurance coverage" (Senate Commission on Long-Term Care, 2013, p. 23), and the lack of long-term care insurance requires many people to deplete their assets to become Medicaid eligible.[17] The need for new public and private long-term care insurance options that would stabilize the financial future of Americans—a neglected corollary to addressing long-term care services and their financing (IOM, 2013e; Wiener et al., 2013)—is beyond the scope of this report.

Only one-third of elderly Americans have sufficient assets to pay for 1 year of nursing home care, which in 2012 averaged $81,030 for a semi-private room and $90,520 for a private room (National Health Policy Forum, 2013). Home-based care is less expensive, but still costly. Four hours per day of homemaker and home health aide services, 7 days per week, costs from $28,000 to $31,000 per year, and such services are not always available. It is no wonder, then, that long-term care has been called "the largest uninsured risk faced by the older population" (Norton, 2013; Spillman, 2012, p. 239).

Many families are caught in the middle: they are too "well off" for Medicaid, but unable to pay out of pocket to meet their personal care needs. This is another reason for relying on the acute care system of 911 calls, emergency departments, and hospitals when care needs become overwhelming. Unlike long-term services and supports, these much more costly acute care services are covered by Medicare.

Medicare's benefit structure reflects patients' health care needs as generally understood when the program was created nearly a half-century ago. Today, health and the use of health care services are understood as being influenced by a broad range of factors beyond those addressed by health professionals or traditionally covered by health insurers. There are many

---

[17]These assets do not include a person's home. As long as a house serves as the "principal place of residence" of a Medicaid applicant (or spouse or certain other close relatives), it is not factored into the Medicaid eligibility determination, regardless of its value (HHS, 2005, p. 2).

ways to improve quality of life and comfort for people with advanced serious illnesses and lessen the burden on their family caregivers (Topf et al., 2013) while preventing predictable crises. The resulting savings in costly emergency visits, hospitalizations, and even long-term nursing home care could be redirected toward underfunded and badly needed long-term services and supports (Unroe and Meier, 2013).

We got hospice when my mother-in-law died, but only for 2 weeks. She declined steadily for 2 years before her death, as we bounced back and forth between hospital, nursing home, and home (with private-paid caregivers). It was a bad way to go, with much pain, suffering, and expense for her and our family. There were too many barriers to getting the care she needed. Medicare pays for all types of care that is unbeneficial (911 trips to the hospital, certain tests, treatments, medications, surgeries, and skilled nursing home stays for rehab, etc.). But it will not pay for the care people actually need during chronic, progressive illness—custodial care, comfort care, nursing care. We need to fix this.*

---

*Quotation from a response submitted through the online public testimony questionnaire for this study. See Appendix C.

Institutional Long-Term Care

Medicare provides little payment for long-term services and supports, including personal assistance with activities of daily living (e.g., bathing, dressing, toileting, eating, transferring, and medication management). Medicare's sole contribution to nursing home care is in paying for short-term skilled nursing services aimed at rehabilitation following hospitalization and for short-term home health care for the homebound with a "skilled need." Post-acute care accounts for about 21 percent of all spending on long-term services and supports (KFF, 2013b), and its goal is to return beneficiaries to the highest possible level of functioning. In one analysis, almost one-third of Medicare beneficiaries used the skilled nursing benefit in their last 6 months of life, and 1 in 11 died while enrolled in that benefit. Many such patients may be too frail or ill to return home and would be well served if the benefit included a stronger palliative care component and allowed concurrent hospice care (Aragon et al., 2012).

The rehabilitation mission of skilled nursing facilities may conflict with patients' medical condition and goals, especially in the last months of life, when hospice or palliative care may be better matched to their needs. The decision to place a patient in a skilled nursing program may be based not on a clinical need for rehabilitative services or patient preferences but on built-in financial incentives. Some families are unable to provide home care for a patient in rapidly deteriorating health, but at hospital discharge they must make a difficult choice. They can choose Medicare payment for 100 days of room and board and "rehabilitative" care in a skilled nursing facility, but if they want hospice care and do not qualify for Medicaid, they will have to pay out of pocket for nursing home room and board (Aragon et al., 2012).

People covered by the skilled nursing facility benefit cannot be enrolled simultaneously in hospice unless the two services are treating totally unrelated medical conditions. Nursing homes and skilled nursing facilities have an incentive to keep people in post-acute care as long as possible instead of enrolling them in hospice because once patients are referred to hospice, they must shift from the generously reimbursed (by Medicare) skilled nursing benefit to the poorly reimbursed (by Medicaid) long-term care benefit.

Nursing homes have an incentive to hospitalize residents repeatedly so as to make them eligible once again for the higher-paying skilled nursing facility program. Indeed, there is some evidence of disproportionately high rates of potentially avoidable hospitalizations among dual-eligible residents in skilled nursing facilities and nursing homes (942 per 1,000 person years for skilled nursing facility residents and 338 per 1,000 person years for nursing home residents). By contrast, people living in the community had markedly lower rates of potentially avoidable hospitalization (250 per 1,000 person years for those receiving Medicaid-paid home- and community-based services, and only 88 per 1,000 person years for those not receiving those services) (Segal, 2011). A growing literature is finding that many hospitalizations for patients with dementia, in particular, are avoidable and a potential source of system savings (Grabowski and O'Malley, 2014).[18] As noted earlier, moreover, frequent transitions between the nursing home and hospital and back again are burdensome to patients and have been associated with increased rates of feeding tube insertions, intensive care unit stays, pressure ulcers, and late enrollment in hospice for residents with advanced cognitive and functional impairments (Gozalo et al., 2011).

From the standpoint of financially strapped state Medicaid programs and providers, the cost shift to Medicare and the transfer of patients back and forth between skilled nursing facilities and hospitals has obvious appeal. From the standpoint of the quality of care for patients and families and the nation's total health care spending, it reflects both poor quality and enormous costs.

---

[18]For example, the Evercare managed care demonstration program enhanced advance care planning, provided nurse practitioner care, and altered financial incentives, producing fewer preventable hospitalizations and improved survival with no diminution in the quality of care (Kane et al., 2004).

Home- and Community-Based Care

Because state rules governing Medicaid do not universally draw Medicare's line between health services and support services, Medicaid is the main source of payment for the latter. Additional funding for these services comes through Medicaid's Home and Community Based Services program.

By 2009, 3.3 million people were participating in Medicaid's Home and Community Based Services program, a 60 percent increase in participation since 2000 (National Health Policy Forum, 2013). AARP policy analysts are among those who have encouraged states to invest in this program, making their case primarily on the grounds of cost-effectiveness (AARP Public Policy Institute, 2008). As more people age into their 70s, 80s, and 90s and need daily help, the demand for long-term care services, including in-home home health services, will continue to rise (Employment Benefit Research Institute, 2012). In this context, state Medicaid programs are giving increasing attention to "rebalancing" efforts aimed at reducing their long-standing institutional bias (Kassner, 2013)—that is, shifting long-term services and supports from expensive institutional settings, mainly nursing homes, to people's homes. As illustrated in Box 5-1, however, while such shifts may make sense from the standpoint of both patient desires and program integrity, they need to be undertaken with some caution.

"During the late 1970s and early 1980s, the federal government sponsored a series of randomized, controlled . . . demonstrations to test the cost-effectiveness of home and community-based services as a substitute for nursing home care" (ASPE, 2000, p. 10). The National Channeling Demonstration, funded by the Health Care Financing Administration (HCFA),[19] Administration on Aging (AoA), and the Office of the Assistant Secretary for Planning and Evaluation (ASPE), tested two models for financing and delivering home- and community-based services (Kemper, 1988). HCFA and the National Center for Health Services Research (NCHSR)[20] sponsored more than a dozen state- or region-specific demonstrations. Major findings from these projects were as follows:

- Targeting program enrollment to those at highest risk of nursing home placement saves money.
- Home- and community-based services programs can achieve budget neutrality with narrow targeting to the highest-risk groups, low average benefit levels (taking into account the availability of informal supports), and an emphasis on high-quality services.

---

[19]HCFA is now the Centers for Medicare & Medicaid Services.
[20]NCHSR was a predecessor to the Agency for Healthcare Research and Quality.

BOX 5-1
Learning from Past Institution-to-Community Shifts

Experience with the community mental health services movement of several decades ago suggests that the shift from institutional to community care should be closely monitored. In the 1960s and 1970s, the nation's large, old-fashioned, and underperforming mental hospitals were closed or greatly reduced in size, and responsibility for former residents' continuing service needs was shifted to community service providers that were neither adequately prepared nor funded to assume this responsibility (Lyons, 1984). Setting these former patients adrift without appropriate support was a largely avoidable tragedy that contributed significantly to poor-quality care, high incarceration and hospitalization rates, and the rise of substance abuse and homelessness (Baum and Burnes, 1993; Yoon et al., 2013).

- Data limitations make designing and conducting research that truly measures cost-effectiveness—as distinct from "cost shifting" from one program to another, from state to federal funds, and from formal to informal care—nearly impossible. Cost-effectiveness studies of these programs typically use only Medicaid expenditure data and do not consider the impacts of other programs such as Medicare and Social Security Insurance.

A recent report summarizing analyses from 38 states, conducted between 2005 and 2012, found consistently lower average costs for home- and community-based care than for institutional long-term care. In 2008 in California, for example, "per recipient spending on nursing facilities was three times higher than for HCBS [home- and community-based services] ($32,406 for nursing facility care versus $9,129 for HCBS)" (Fox-Grage and Walls, 2013, pp. 6-7). However, many states cap the number of people who can enroll in the Home and Community Based Services program, and some states maintain waiting lists for the program; testimony to the Senate Commission on Long-Term Care suggests that nearly half a million people are on these lists (Senate Commission on Long-Term Care, 2013, p. 16). While the state studies varied in approach and should be replicated by independent researchers, they are important in contributing to state decisions about program policy.

The cost impact of home- and community-based services is almost always measured only in terms of Medicaid expenditures. However, analysts have repeatedly observed the need for a broader analytic framework along several dimensions. For example, capturing the true cost side of the equation requires consideration of the services' impact on other public programs, such as Medicare, Supplemental Security Income, and the Supplemental Nutrition Assistance Program (SNAP). These comprehensive analyses of expenditures and savings have not been carried out because acquiring the necessary data is too difficult and expensive. In addition, cost estimates need to take into account the dollar value of unpaid care provided by family caregivers.[21] Even if it were possible to assess costs adequately, estimating the benefits (effectiveness) and quality gains of these programs reliably presents an additional set of methodological challenges.

Movement toward alternatives to nursing homes is also supported by federal policy makers. In its 2013 report, the Senate Commission on Long-Term Care, established in 2012, urged a shift away from nursing homes and toward home care (Senate Commission on Long-Term Care, 2013). Likewise, the Administration for Community Living, an HHS agency that includes the Administration on Aging and Administration on Intellectual and Developmental Disabilities, emphasizes community options for the elderly (Administration for Community Living, 2013).

Yet while a wide variety of community-based providers try to help people needing long-term services and supports, the financing and organization of these services and supports create barriers to access. "The network of providers to deliver this support is complex, multifaceted, specialized, isolated from other services providers, and confusing to the average consumer," reported the Senate Commission on Long-Term Care (2013, p. 14). Rarely do service providers assess a patient's and family's overall needs so that they can arrange for the right set of services; instead, patients and families have access to what is funded by some mix of federal, state, and local sources, each with its own eligibility rules, limits, and procedures. Just finding out about available services and resources is a significant challenge.

An especially serious problem is the structural and financial isolation of the system for long-term services and supports from the health services sector. As a result, the planning and organization of the two are separate when patients are in transition across settings, and there are few incentives to integrate or streamline the two sets of services, despite their obvious interdependence and potential synergies.

One possible way to bridge the gap between these two service sectors for some patients and families is through community-based palliative care programs. As Huskamp and Stevenson (see Appendix D) note, "palliative care can be introduced at any point during the course of a serious advanced illness when a patient and family needs [sic] help to manage symptoms and maximize quality of life." Insurance coverage for hospice—under Medi-

---

[21]For example, a study of family caregiving for community-dwelling elders in the last year of life estimated the value of these services as between $22,500 and $42,400 (in 2002), which the authors note equaled the cost of a home aide (Rhee et al., 2009).

care, Medicaid, and many commercial insurance plans—is the dominant financing mechanism for community-based palliative care. Models aimed at bridging the gap, such as community-based palliative care, medical homes, house calls or home-based primary care programs, and PACE, have demonstrated effectiveness in improving value (improved quality leading to lower acute care spending) (Grabowski, 2006; Kamal et al., 2013; Komisar and Feder, 2011; Unroe and Meier, 2013).

Finally, if efforts to rebalance nursing home and home- and community-based care are to succeed and more seriously ill people are to be cared for in their homes, home- and community-based care will need to encompass certain medical and quasi-medical services. These services include

- case management;
- round-the-clock access to a clinician for advice;
- mental health services;
- respite care;
- comprehensive interdisciplinary primary care;
- medication management; and
- support for basic activities of daily living—eating, bathing, dressing, toileting, and transferring (into and out of bed, a chair, a wheelchair)—through personal care aides.

Matching Services to Needs for Dual-Eligible Individuals

The nearly 10 million Americans who are dually eligible for both Medicare and Medicaid present a particular challenge to the current care system. These individuals tend to make up the sickest, frailest, poorest, and highest-cost population served by the two programs (Brown and Mann, 2012).

Because dual-eligible individuals are either 65 and older or permanently disabled and because they are poorer than the general population, they often have significant long-term care needs (CBO, 2013). As Table 5-5 shows, they account for a significant proportion (roughly one-third) of expenditures for each program. Some 65 percent of Medicaid spending for this group is for long-term care (Young et al., 2013). Over the years, a

TABLE 5-5 Dual-Eligible People in Medicare and Medicaid, 2010

Indicator	Medicare	Medicaid
Share of beneficiaries who are eligible for both programs	1 in 5	1 in 6
Program expenditures for people eligible for both	33%	36%

SOURCE: Young et al., 2013.

number of initiatives, including a new effort under the ACA described later in this chapter, have been aimed at improving both quality of care and efficiency for this high-risk population by encouraging care in the community rather than in nursing homes.

Health care spending by dual-eligible individuals varies considerably. Two in five people receiving both Medicare and Medicaid generated lower expenditures than other Medicare beneficiaries, while one in five accounted for three-fifths of all dual-eligible spending. Fewer than 1 percent of individuals cost both Medicare and Medicaid high amounts; most individuals are high cost for only one of the programs (Coughlin et al., 2012). These findings suggest that dual-eligible individuals living in nursing homes might be good candidates for palliative care and care management intended to prevent avoidable hospitalizations, while others, living in the community, would be good candidates for a medical home or other entity that coordinates and integrates social and medical supports. Program savings resulting from such interventions are most likely to occur among people who have functional dependencies, frailty, and/or dementia in the context of one or more chronic diseases.

Efforts to produce Medicare and Medicaid savings in covering dually eligible people have centered on the twin strategies of enrollment in managed care programs, such as PACE, and use of care management to coordinate care (as discussed further below). However, many of these efforts have failed to target those at highest risk and as a result, have not produced the desired savings, although they "provide strong evidence that care management might be effective at reducing costs for some subgroups of dual eligibles, such as *those with severe chronic illnesses or at high risk for hospitalization*" [emphasis added] (Brown and Mann, 2012, p. 4).

Organization of Services

As described in Chapter 2, significant problems and burdens accompany each transfer of a seriously ill patient from one care setting to another, and the large number of such transfers as patients near the end of life has been documented (Teno et al., 2013). Each such transfer runs the risk of

- poor communication between settings and inadequate transfer of records, including advance directives (which results in, for example, inadequate information about self-care or perplexing changes in instructions; redundant tests; duplicate, confusing, or conflicting prescriptions and medication errors; and increased risk of falls, infection, and delirium—any of which can harm patients and lead to additional hospitalizations) (Press et al., 2013);

- poor communication between providers across settings, impeding primary physicians' ability to properly manage patients under their care; and
- confusion among patients and family members regarding what to do, which provider is responsible for what, and whom to consult when things go wrong.

Better coordination of care is widely perceived as essential to improving patient outcomes. Not only are people nearing the end of life often treated in several settings, but also they (and their families) interact with numerous physicians and other health professionals, are prescribed multiple medications and treatments that may interact in undesirable ways or be difficult to administer properly, and face logistical problems in accessing care when they need such basic services as transportation. In a conclusion still valid today, the 2001 IOM report *Crossing the Quality Chasm* notes that one serious consequence of the poorly organized U.S. health system is the "layers of processes and handoffs that patients and families find bewildering and clinicians view as wasteful" (IOM, 2001, p. 28). A renewed focus on discharge planning, continued access to care and support after discharge, medication reconciliation, and avoidance of rehospitalizations could improve continuity across settings in a patient-centered, family-oriented way (Coleman et al., 2006).

Conversely, inadequate care coordination results in avoidable medical complications and unnecessary hospital readmissions, which by themselves cost Medicare some $15 billion per year (Tilson and Hoffman, 2012). In the case of seriously ill children, for example, the lack of after-hours coverage in physician offices impels some working parents to seek whatever care is available, and that is found in costly hospital emergency departments (Chamberlain et al., 2013).

To the extent any organized attempt at coordination takes place outside of hospice, it is typically through "disease management" or more comprehensive "care management" programs. Often these programs entail assignment of a specially trained nurse or other health professional to help a patient with complex needs navigate the system across service providers. The success of these programs is highly variable, depending on their ability to select the most appropriate patients, meet needs around the clock, align supportive and medical services, and flexibly adjust the intensity of service to changing patient and family needs. Additional key program features are assessment of and support for family caregiver needs; round-the-clock access by phone; consistent relationships and communication among the care coordination team staff, patients, families, and medical providers; integrated assessment and delivery of both medical and social services; and generation and mobilization of needed long-term services and supports (Bass et al., 2013; Brown et al., 2012; Peikes et al., 2012) (see also the discussion of social services below). If care management initiatives that include such support services can produce savings when serving people with severe chronic illnesses or a high probability of hospital admission, they may also be well suited to people in the final phase of life before they become eligible for hospice.

A 15-program randomized controlled trial of the Medicare Coordinated Care Demonstration identified six features that appeared to be central to the limited number of coordination efforts that saved money:

- frequent face-to-face contact between the patient and the care coordinator;
- occasional face-to-face contact between the patient's physicians and the care coordinator;
- the care coordinator's functioning as the "communications hub" for the patient's practitioners;
- use of evidence-based patient education interventions;
- comprehensive medication management; and
- a timely, comprehensive response to transitions between care settings, such as discharge from a hospital to post-acute care (Brown et al., 2012).

A review of studies on the effectiveness of disease management efforts within the Medicaid program reveal additional themes:

- Disease management programs were most effective in improving quality of care and achieving cost-effectiveness for the sickest patients, including those with comorbidities, underscoring the importance of targeting interventions to those most likely to benefit from them.
- Although in-person care management was the costliest intervention, it also was the most effective with high-risk patients, while less intensive management was appropriate for lower-risk patients.
- Projects that used data mining and predictive modeling to stratify patients by disease severity and risk were "particularly successful in designing and delivering [disease management] programs across chronic disease groups" (Freeman et al., 2011, p. 35).

The studies reviewed varied greatly in the medical conditions and program designs addressed and in the kinds and quality of data collected. Nor were they specifically looking at the needs of patients near the end of life. However, the general profile of patients with functional dependency, with multiple chronic diseases and comorbidities, and at risk of hospitalization and emergency visits was relatively consistent across studies and mirrors the circumstances of people who may be nearing the end of life.

Beneficial outcomes of successful care coordination found in these studies included improved medication adherence, reduced hospitalizations and readmissions, reduced emergency visits, and fewer unnecessary medications. And disease management programs that reduced hospitalizations by only 10 percent were able to cover their associated program costs (Freeman et al., 2011). Other meta-analyses have likewise noted improvements in the quality of care but have produced less persuasive evidence on reduced health care utilization, except successes in lowering the risk of hospitalization, and on health care savings (Mattke et al., 2007). However, improvements in quality of care that are achieved without increasing costs can be considered successes when such high-risk, high-need recipients are being served.

In summary, clinician engagement and targeting and tailoring of social services and their integration with the medical care delivery system appear to be essential elements of successful disease and care management models (Freeman et al., 2011; Meyer and Smith, 2008).

Geographic Variations in Service Utilization and Costs

Studies of the costs of care in the last months of life have revealed marked differences in the utilization and costs of treatments from one geographic area to another and from one hospital to another. These differences are attributable in part to local variations in the supply and prices of medical resources (e.g., doctors, nursing home rehabilitation, home care agencies, hospitals, drugs, medical devices, and procedures) (Commonwealth Fund Commission on a High Performance Health System, 2013) and to a lesser extent to patient and family characteristics and preferences (Prigerson and Maciejewski, 2012).

Medicare payments vary widely among and within localities. Per capita Medicare spending (that is, the average amount Medicare pays out per beneficiary) varies more than two-fold among different regions of the country, mainly as the result of differences in the volume of services provided. The greatest influences on volume differences are the regional supply of physicians and available hospital beds (Dartmouth Atlas of Health Care, 2013).

An IOM committee recently determined that variation in Medicare spending across and within geographic areas is explained mainly by differences in spending for post-acute care, including subacute rehabilitation in skilled nursing facilities, long-term acute care facilities for ventilator-dependent Medicare beneficiaries, and home health agencies. If these spending variations were eliminated, overall spending variation would drop by 73 percent (IOM, 2013a). This finding has important implications for the care of people with serious advanced illnesses. The management of transitions from one setting to another may be a more important cost driver than has previously been recognized, and "a growing body of evidence leads to the conclusion that clinical and financial integration best positions health care systems to manage the continuum of care for their complex populations efficiently" (IOM, 2013a, p. 18).

Financial incentives for nursing homes to hospitalize dually eligible residents (and then to obtain Medicare's higher post-acute care skilled nursing benefit) are similar nationwide; however, state-level data reveal dramatic variations in preventable hospitalizations for nursing home residents. The lowest rate of such hospitalizations (65 per 1,000 person years) is found in Alaska, and the highest (231 per 1,000 person years) in Louisiana, although this analysis does not control for differences in population health across states (Segal, 2011). In one consensus of experts, expressed as a percentage of hospitalizations, a median of 19 percent of hospitalizations of all long-stay nursing home residents are considered potentially avoidable, with a range across states of 7-31 percent (Commonwealth Fund, 2013).

Variation in spending does not appear to be related to differences in quality of care provided or in care outcomes. After an extensive review of the literature, the IOM committee studying geographic variation in Medicare spending found no relationship between quality-of-care indicators and what Medicare paid for services. If people with chronic illnesses who live in higher-spending areas had better outcomes in terms of survival or quality of life, one could argue that similar resources should be expended in other locales; however, this is not the case (Dartmouth Atlas of Health Care, 2013; Wennberg et al., 2008).

To the extent that excessive services do not benefit (and may harm) patients, they represent wasteful and unnecessary expenditures, and therefore significant opportunities for both better-quality care and cost savings. Clearly, in the current environment, with abundant evidence of poor-quality care and national health expenditures continuing to rise, marked geographic and interinstitutional variations in expenditures may be a good focus for analysis of both shortfalls in quality and excess service provision.

THE GAP BETWEEN SERVICES PAID FOR AND WHAT PATIENTS AND FAMILIES WANT AND NEED

As noted throughout this report, an approach that enabled more people to remain in their homes or home-like settings in the final stages of life would better align with the preferences of many patients and families than the current system. And a significant barrier to improving the quality of end-of-life care and controlling costs is that the mix of services currently delivered and paid for fails to provide for precisely those needs that drive repeated reliance on the emergency and acute care systems: round-the-clock access to meaningful help, house calls and home care, caregiver support, and long-term services and supports. Although some states have used the demonstration and waiver authorities under Medicare and Medicaid to create a more comprehensive continuum of services for the elderly and people who have disabilities, the nation is far from achieving an easily accessible, reliable system of care for people who have advanced serious illnesses and are nearing the end of life. Clearly, significant changes in the approach to service delivery would be needed to effectively integrate traditional medical care and social services.

Impact of Social Services on Health Outcomes

Abundant evidence reveals the powerful role of social and behavioral factors in health and health spending in contexts other than end-of-life care (Farley, 2009; Marmor et al., 1994; McGinnis and Foege, 1993; U.S. Burden of Disease Collaborators, 2013). Research conducted over several decades has established that health care in itself plays a much smaller role in the health of a population than a range of other factors related to behavior and socioeconomic status. Indeed, recent analyses attribute the paradoxically high rate of health care spending and inferior health outcomes in the United States relative to other developed countries to the lack of integration of health and social support programs (Bradley and Taylor, 2013; Shier et al., 2013). Despite its position roughly in the middle in terms of total social[22] and medical spending per capita, the United States ranks 27th out of 40 nations in life expectancy, according to data from the Organisation for Economic Co-operation and Development (OECD). And while the United States is roughly in the middle relative to other OECD countries in *total* health and social services spending as a percentage of GDP,[23] the ratio of social services spending to health services spending is markedly lower relative to other nations. These different spending patterns may reflect countries' different histories, cultures, attitudes toward social spending, and political milieus.

In a changing health care landscape, new tools, approaches, and payment models are making it easier and more advantageous than ever for

---

[22] The OECD social expenditure database includes nations' expenditures for such programs as pensions and retirement, home health, and other benefits for the elderly; pensions, sick leave, residential care, and rehabilitation for people with disabilities; and family allowances and maternity leave (OECD, 2014).

[23] The figure for the United States is 25.4 percent. By comparison, the figure for Sweden is 33.2 percent and for Ireland is 18.2 percent. At the bottom for spending in these two categories are Chile, Estonia, Korea, Mexico, and Turkey, each of which spends a total of 15 percent of GDP or less in these two categories.

providers and health systems to meet the social needs of their patients (Bachrach et al., 2014). Interventions that address patients' social needs have been shown to positively impact patient outcomes and satisfaction with care.

The committee supports the expansion of social support for people with advanced chronic illnesses with functional debility and careful assessment of ongoing pilot programs focused on doing so (Shier et al., 2013). Much can be learned from those efforts about the impact of these services on health, as well as the means chosen to determine clients' service needs, establish eligibility, manage costs, and ensure quality, all of which can guide future programming.

The Importance of Social Services

In this report, the term "social services" refers to a rather modest but essential set of services not generally considered part of health care. A core list of commonly needed services includes the following:

- caregiver training and support,
- retrofitting of the home for safety and mobility,
- meals and nutrition services,
- family respite, and
- transportation.

Some of these services are provided through Medicare Advantage plans and through Medicaid. Some could be provided through expansion of the Older Americans Act, which currently is underfunded to meet its potential. And some could be provided through relatively low-cost, volunteer-staffed efforts if they were implemented effectively with training, oversight, and coordination with a person's needs. For example, health insurance counseling, legal and financial counseling, and bill payment services currently are offered by many community organizations through volunteers, consumer credit counseling programs, and representative payee programs. Volunteerism is a long-standing component of hospice.

Social services may be especially important for the sickest and most vulnerable individuals in a population, whose multiple chronic conditions, pain and other serious symptoms, functional dependency, cognitive impairment and other mental illnesses, frailty, and high family caregiver burden (Smith et al., 2010; Walke et al., 2006) converge to drive the high use of health care services (Komisar and Feder, 2011). Adequate and relatively inexpensive social services could lower demand for expensive health care services for some people nearing the end of life. For example, providing adequate caregiver training, eliminating safety risks in the home, or providing nutrition services could prevent many situations that lead to 911 calls, emergency department visits, and hospitalizations (Bachrach et al., 2014; Shier et al., 2013). In addition, sufficient support for caregivers at home might prevent the burnout that leads to those calls, visits, and hospitalizations, as well as to long-term institutionalization (AoA, undated; Reinhard et al., 2012).

Some social services could be provided through replication of successful private-sector models in populations served by managed care organizations and, eventually under the ACOs encouraged under the ACA. In this way, as different approaches to providing, tailoring, and targeting social services demonstrated their effectiveness, successful models could be expanded to cover additional population groups and to include additional services. At present, one of the most promising groups in which to expand these models is the dual-eligible population, for whom both great need and funding mechanisms exist.

How would such a service expansion be paid for? The potential savings that would result in the areas of hospital care and emergency services could exceed the cost of expanded social services. In addition, some social services themselves might produce net savings. For example, providing an elderly person daily meals is much less costly than the medical crisis and nursing home placement that result from the consequences of malnutrition (Thomas and Mor, 2013); likewise, providing an air conditioner for an elderly person with asthma is much less expensive than repeat hospitalizations.

Whatever menu of social services is available, at the top of the list should be an assessment of patient and family needs, resources, home environment, and receptivity to assistance (Feinberg, 2012), as well as aid in accessing appropriate benefits. The Senate Commission on Long-Term Care recommended "development and implementation of a standardized assessment tool that can produce a single care plan across care settings for an individual with cognitive or functional limitations" (Senate Commission on Long-Term Care, 2013, p. 43). This approach is the essence of patient-centeredness.

Many of the services listed above (and discussed in the following subsections) may not be needed every day, and they support the caregiver as well as the patient. Keeping the family confident, rested, informed about what to expect and how to handle it, and emotionally supported is essential to maintaining a seriously ill patient in the home. Through the grants to states provided by the National Family Caregiver Support Program under the Older Americans Act, social services are received by only about 700,000 caregivers annually. States work in partnership with area agencies on aging and other local community-service providers to offer information about and assistance in obtaining available services; individual counseling, organization of support groups, and evidence-based caregiver training; respite care;

and limited supplemental services. The Administration on Aging's national caregiver surveys indicate that these services improve caregiving and "can reduce caregiver depression, anxiety, and stress and enable them to provide care longer, thereby avoiding or delaying the need for costly institutional care" (AoA, undated).

Caregiver Training and Support

As described in Chapter 2, family caregivers are essential in managing the health and social service needs of patients still living at home and bear a strong burden in doing so. Training in the responsibilities of caregiving can help. In a large online survey of a nationally representative sample of almost 1,700 people caring for family members with multiple health problems, almost half of respondents said the training they received had positive effects on the care recipient, including avoiding nursing home placement (p <0.05). Yet such training is, at best, scanty. Some 47 percent of caregivers had never received any training regarding medication management[24]; 42 percent reported they had to learn wound care on their own; and 37 percent believed more training would be helpful. (These data apply to all caregivers, not just those caring for a family member near the end of life.)

Retrofitting of the Home for Safety and Mobility

Publicly funded health programs generally do not cover home modifications for safety and wheelchair access, for example. The home can be a dangerous place for patients who are frail or at risk of injuries and for the growing number of patients with progressive cognitive disorders. (Fully 80 percent of the care of people with Alzheimer's disease is provided "free" by family and friends [Horvath et al., 2013].) A randomized controlled efficacy trial of an intervention designed to give informal caregivers easy-to-read information and resources to minimize home injuries found significantly less risky behavior and fewer injuries (p ≤0.000) among members of the intervention group compared with controls. Because of the high costs of care for frail elders who experience falls, wandering, injuries in fires, and so on, even "small effect sizes translate into clinically relevant findings" (Horvath et al., 2013, p. 6).[25]

---

[24]Medication management included administering intravenous fluids and injections. Most care recipients took several medications: almost half took 5-9 different prescription medications, almost 20 percent took 10 or more prescription medications, and almost three-quarters took one or more over-the-counter drugs or supplements as well (Reinhard et al., 2012).

[25]The intervention was designed to require little, if any, professional staff time, and not counting the occasional need for a piece of specialized equipment, such as a tub transfer bench, the cost per family of the Home Safety Toolkit booklet and sample items was $210.

Meals and Nutrition Services

Buying food, cooking, and preparing meals are essential daily activities that become more difficult when one is caring for someone with an advanced serious illness living at home. Forty-one percent of caregivers in the AARP survey cited above were involved in preparing food for special diets, suggesting a need for nutrition counseling. This task involves more than "help with meals" and may include meal planning and cooking, more complicated and expensive food shopping, precise measurement, and laborious feeding for patients who have trouble swallowing. More than one-half of family caregivers surveyed found mealtime tasks difficult to carry out (Reinhard et al., 2012).

As a striking example of the impact of social services, results of a recent study suggest that among ostensibly "low-need" people aged 60 and older, home-delivered meals could mean the difference between living at home and needing nursing home placement (Thomas and Mor, 2013).[26] For almost 60 percent of the study subjects, home-delivered meals provided at least half of their daily food intake. The analysis revealed that if every state increased the number of seniors receiving home-delivered meals by a mere 1 percent, the resultant decline in the number of nursing home residents would yield initial savings to state Medicaid programs overall of more than $109 million per year. Ten states would save more than $3 million, and half would save at least $1 million.

The fragility of the nation's food programs for the elderly was demonstrated by the 2013 cuts to the nutrition programs under the Older Americans Act resulting from the federal budget sequestration. These programs expected to lose $41 million in federal funding, equivalent to the cost of 19 million meals (MOWAA, undated).

Family Respite

The shift to encouraging care at home cannot be accomplished successfully without addressing the concomitant need to support family caregivers. Burnout "is the point at which caregivers are often no longer able to continue in their caring roles and care recipients are at greatest risk of institutionalization" (Lilly et al., 2012, p. 104). Much has been written about the problem of caregiver burden and burnout, but the programmatic changes and investments that would prevent and ameliorate the problem fall short. The Senate Commission on Long-Term Care made detailed

---

[26] Among those included in this study, 70 percent were at least 75; 40 percent needed help with bathing, dressing, eating, using the toilet, and transferring into or out of a bed or chair; and 85 percent needed help with light housework, taking medications, managing money, and shopping for groceries.

recommendations about ways to strengthen supports for family caregivers (Senate Commission on Long-Term Care, 2013, p. 51).

Transportation

The accretion of family needs not adequately addressed in the community can influence the decision to admit a person to long-term care. An analysis of factors affecting that decision, conducted within the Connecticut Home Care Program for Elders (which serves approximately 14,000 state residents aged 65 and older), identified a lack of transportation for both medical and nonmedical purposes as one of these factors (Robison et al., 2012). Existing programs for meeting this need often have limitations, such as not transporting people across county or other jurisdictional lines, not providing assistance in lifting or transferring the patient from home to vehicle along with the transportation, or permitting patients to be accompanied by only certain categories of support personnel.

A proven approach to meeting this fundamental need was tested in the Cash and Counseling demonstration program, which directed cash to disabled beneficiaries with which to hire and direct their own workers.[27] The program served Medicaid recipients with a range of disabilities across the age spectrum, not specifically the end-of-life population. In a randomized trial, this program showed that moderate to large reductions in unmet transportation needs could be accomplished and that participants were highly satisfied with the transportation assistance received (Carlson et al., 2007). The Cash and Counseling program is now active in 15 states.

Comprehensive Approaches

A review of seven innovative U.S. care models suggests ways in which social issues facing people with complex medical needs can be addressed (Shier et al., 2013).[28] The individual projects used different designs and collected different data, yet all showed a number of positive outcomes, including "encouraging indications that greater attention to social supports may benefit patients and payers alike" (Shier et al., 2013, p. 547). All of

---

[27]The Cash and Counseling program allowed participants to purchase a range of services. Under the program, participants "appeared to receive care at least as good as that provided by agencies, in that they had the same or an even lower incidence of care-related health problems" (Carlson et al., 2007, p. 481).

[28]The models are the Vermont Blueprint for Health, Senior Care Options (Boston), Health-Care Partners Comprehensive Care Program (California), Mercy Health System (Pennsylvania), Geriatric Resources for Assessment and Care of Elders (GRACE) (Indianapolis, Indiana), Care Management Plus (Utah), and the Enhanced Discharge Planning Program (Chicago, Illinois).

the programs conducted baseline health and social assessments, developed individualized care plans, and made referrals to or arranged for social services. They used interdisciplinary care teams, closely involved primary care clinicians, and used electronic records. Most also used standardized intervention protocols, provided specialized training for service providers, and conducted ongoing monitoring. As these models and others develop under the ACA, their impact on both the quality and costs of care may provide insights to inform the development of new programs.

THE CHANGING HEALTH CARE SYSTEM: FINANCING AND ORGANIZATION

The financing and organization of the U.S. health care system are undergoing significant changes that have major implications for end-of-life care. These changes are resulting from the ACA, as well as from private-sector payment initiatives and state policies.

Changes Under the Affordable Care Act

Changes in financial incentives and organizational arrangements resulting from the ACA could have wide-ranging effects on Americans nearing the end of life. Specific opportunities arise from the new arrangements that involve risk sharing by Medicare providers, including ACOs, patient-centered medical homes, and bundled payments, as well as recently instituted penalties for 30-day readmissions, hospital mortality, and poor patient experience scores. These and other innovations under the ACA have spurred interest, discussed earlier, in meeting the needs of the nation's sickest and most vulnerable patients in their own homes and communities as an alternative to costly emergency department visits, hospital stays, and institutional care.[29]

In addition, the new CMS Innovation Center has the broad goal of working toward better care for patients, healthier communities, and lower costs through improvements in the system of care. The center's priorities are testing new payment and service delivery models, evaluating results and promoting best practices, and working with diverse stakeholders to develop new models for testing.

---

[29]For a detailed list of the ACA provisions affecting a related area—cancer care—see IOM (2013d, pp. 85-90). For detailed information that includes citations of specific statutory provisions, see Meier (2011, pp. 367-369).

Expansion of Home- and Community-Based Services

To accelerate the long-term trend of expanding home- and community-based services, described earlier, the ACA originally included a Community Living Assistance Services and Supports (CLASS) Act, which would have instituted a voluntary, national, federally administered long-term care insurance program. Implementation of this program was abandoned in 2011 because of persistent concerns about its costs and sustainability (Appleby and Carey, 2011).

Nevertheless, the ACA attempts to counter Medicaid's continuing institutional bias by supporting home- and community-based services (Miller, 2012). For example, the Balancing Incentive Payments program provides grants to states for increasing access to noninstitutional care. The "Money Follows the Person" Rebalancing Demonstration Grants program has been strengthened and expanded. By the end of 2012, it had helped only a small number of people—around 31,000—with chronic conditions and disabilities transition from institutions to the community. It now has the participation of 44 states and the District of Columbia (CMS, undated-b).

The Financial Alignment Initiative

Among the most important provisions of the ACA with the potential to effect major changes in care for people with serious advanced illnesses and to generate cost savings is the establishment of the federal Medicare-Medicaid Coordination Office. This office is charged with facilitating the integration and alignment of federal Medicare and state Medicaid funding into a single source of financial support (CMS, 2013c). The office's State Demonstrations to Integrate Care for Dual Eligible Individuals program, starting in 15 states, is aimed at breaking down payment silos by providing funds from both programs to an insurer or provider group that agrees to accept risk or participate in shared savings, and that may then match these dollars to patients' social and medical needs (CMS, 2012; Gore and Klebonis, 2012). This merging of funding streams creates an opportunity and an incentive for state Medicaid programs to seek efficiencies in care delivery for dual-eligible individuals, as opposed to the problematic cost and care shifting that currently occurs.

In a separate Financial Alignment Initiative, CMS will test two models that can be used by states to better integrate primary, acute, behavioral health, and long-term services and supports for Medicare-Medicaid beneficiaries:

- Under the capitated model, a state, CMS, and a health plan enter into a three-way contract, and the plan receives a prospective blended Medicare and Medicaid payment to provide comprehensive, coordinated care.

- Under the managed fee-for-service model, a state and CMS enter into an agreement by which the state can benefit from savings resulting from initiatives designed to improve quality and reduce costs for both Medicare and Medicaid (CMS, 2014a).

Not all states are expected to participate in this program, and those that do may find it difficult to coordinate medical and long-term services and supports for the highest-risk participants. At present, individuals who enroll in hospice are excluded from these alignment projects.

Bundled Payments

Another policy trend is the development and promotion of alternatives to fee-for-service reimbursement so as to "maximize good clinical outcomes, enhance patient and physician satisfaction and autonomy, and provide cost-effective care," as well as to promote evidence-based care (Rich et al., 2012; Schroeder and Frist, 2013, p. 2029). A prime example is the development of bundled payment approaches that cover episodes of care. Instead of reimbursing each provider separately, bundled payment systems pay a single price for a bundle of defined and related services from multiple providers associated with a single episode of care. In theory, bundled payments eliminate incentives to maximize reimbursement that were artifacts of the siloed payment system. Depending on which community-based services are included in the bundle, they may reduce cost shifting between Medicare and Medicaid. They are also expected to provide new incentives for greater care coordination and increased efficiency.

At present, CMS's Bundled Payments for Care Improvement Initiative specifically excludes hospice services (CMS, 2013d). These services may eventually be included in appropriate bundles if ways can be found to risk-adjust for the hospice population (Dobson et al., 2012).

The committee notes that new payment approaches have almost always been accompanied by unintended consequences as those affected seek to maximize revenues under the different rules and arrangements. Bundled payments could create perverse incentives affecting health care expenditures, such as incentives to increase the volume of bundled episodes and to make greater use of services not included in the bundle. They could also lead to problems in quality and access, such as stinting on care or selecting against patients with higher likely costs (Feder, 2013; Weeks et al., 2013; Wilensky, 2014). Various strategies for forestalling these potential negative effects are being discussed (see Appendix D).

Accountable Care Organizations

The ACA encourages the development of ACOs, which CMS describes as

groups of doctors, hospitals, and other health care providers, who come together voluntarily to give coordinated high quality care to their Medicare patients. The goal of coordinated care is to ensure that patients, especially the chronically ill, get the right care at the right time, while avoiding unnecessary duplication of services and preventing medical errors. (CMS, 2013e)

Under the Shared Savings Program, Medicare will continue to pay individual providers and suppliers for specific items and services as it currently does under the Medicare fee-for-service payment system. In addition, CMS will develop a performance measurement benchmark for each ACO to determine whether it qualifies to receive shared savings (or, for "pioneer" ACOs [see below] that have elected to accept responsibility for losses, whether the ACO will be held accountable for those losses). The benchmark is an estimate of what the total Medicare Parts A and B fee-for-service expenditures would have been absent the ACO and will take into account beneficiary characteristics and other factors that may affect health care service needs (the benchmark does not take into account the social environment or functional status of the patient, except that he or she is eligible for Medicaid) (CMS, 2013e). This feature is complicated by the fact that ACOs cannot prevent enrollees from seeking care from providers that are not part of the ACO.

ACOs update the original health maintenance organization concept and could prove extremely helpful to people with advanced serious illnesses given the importance of effective care coordination to high-quality care, as discussed earlier (Berwick, 2011). Medicare offers several ACO programs:

- As of December 2013, the Medicare Shared Savings Program included more than 360 ACOs serving more than 5.3 million Medicare beneficiaries. ACOs and Medicare share any savings they achieve by lowering the growth in health care costs and must meet established standards for high-quality care.
- The Advance Payment ACO Model is a supplementary incentive program for selected participants in the Shared Savings Program. It involves 35 smaller ACOs (rural and physician based) that lack access to capital for investing in infrastructure and care coordination. These ACOs receive an advance on the shared savings they are expected to earn that reflects both fixed and variable start-up costs.

- Beginning in 2012, the Medicare program initiated demonstrations that entailed contracting with a subset of pioneer ACOs, enabling them to move more rapidly from a shared savings to a population-based payment model (see Appendix D). These pioneer ACOs must assume the risk for any losses they incur (that is, if their cost increases exceed those of regular fee-for-service Medicare in their locale); however, if their cost increases fall below those of fee-for-service Medicare by a statistically significant amount, they share those savings with the Medicare Trust Fund in the form of bonus payments.

In 2011, almost one-third of patients in the full complement of ACOs were aged 80 or older, and the average (mean) age was 73.5. Sixteen to 17 percent of enrollees were eligible for Medicaid. Diabetes was their most common chronic condition, affecting around 30 percent (Epstein et al., 2014).

In their first year of operations, the 32 pioneer ACO plans did achieve some measurable quality improvements and had mixed financial results. Overall, they saw a 0.3 percent cost growth for their nearly 670,000 beneficiaries, compared with a 0.8 percent cost growth in fee-for-service Medicare in the same local markets. Savings were not evenly distributed across plans, with 18 achieving below-budget spending and 14 experiencing above-budget spending (Patel and Lieberman, 2013). Seven of the plans abandoned participation in the pioneer program and switched to the regular Medicare Shared Savings Program, and two abandoned their ACO efforts entirely, in part because of their objections to the program's quality metrics and administrative complexity.

Because these programs and markets are in transition, it is too early to make more than a preliminary judgment about the impact of ACOs on health care quality and costs. Nonetheless, experience to date suggests that the ACO model remains attractive to many providers, and that most are achieving both quality improvements and some reductions in cost growth. Overall first-year savings for the nearly 670,000 beneficiaries participating in the pioneer ACO program were estimated at $155.4 million (L&M Policy Research, 2013). These gains were made despite the program's being "incredibly ambitious, even for the most advanced health systems" (Damore and Champion, 2013).

Proposed ACO improvements include new CMS policies to encourage more physicians and Medicare beneficiaries to participate, perhaps by raising Medicare premiums for nonparticipating beneficiaries, and improving ACOs' ability to manage care (Lieberman, 2013). A specific problem for people with advanced serious illnesses is that beneficiaries placed in post-acute care or institutional settings following hospitalization may no longer belong (or be "attributable") to the ACO if those settings are not participants in the ACO. As a result, ACA-related efforts to coordinate care could omit a vulnerable and costly population.

Other Provisions of the Affordable Care Act

Hospice and home care Changes to hospice under the ACA include a demonstration program on value-based purchasing and a demonstration program to study concurrent care for Medicare beneficiaries. CMS announced in March 2014 that it will allow up to 30 hospices to participate in a 3-year concurrent care program starting in summer 2014 (CMS, 2014b). "Concurrent care" would allow Medicare hospice patients to continue receiving cure-oriented treatments. Under one provision of the act that has been implemented, children enrolled in hospice and covered by Medicaid now can obtain simultaneous disease treatment (Rau, 2013).

Medicare payments for both hospice and home care are being reduced. Hospice payments will decline by 11.8 percent over the next decade—this despite the claims of advocates that hospice's highly labor-intensive model does not lend itself to the productivity (and savings) gains possible in other components of the health care system.[30] For home care, reductions have been instituted for standard episode payments, unusually costly "outlier" cases, and annual updates. Reduced payments to these community providers may have implications for access to and quality of care for beneficiaries as smaller programs close and larger ones gain incentives to stint on costly treatments.

Pay-for-performance In accordance with the principle of pay-for-performance, the ACA penalizes hospitals that experience higher-than-expected readmission rates within 30 days of patient discharge. This policy places a premium on discharge planning and coordination of posthospitalization care, but it also could hurt inner-city public hospitals that treat sicker and poorer patients with fewer family or community resources (Press et al., 2013). Physicians, too, are under greater pressure to provide value, as defined by conformance with both quality measures and cost controls.

Gaps in the Affordable Care Act

From the standpoint of care of patients with advanced serious illnesses, the ACA has several noteworthy gaps:

---

[30]This cut is in addition to a phase-out of the Budget Neutrality Adjustment Factor used to calculate the Medicare hospice wage index, and will result in an additional reduction in hospice reimbursement of approximately 4.2 percent (NHPCO, undated).

- It does not measure or reward greater access to coordinated, compassionate care for people with advanced serious illnesses. At present, moreover, it specifically excludes hospice beneficiaries from some of the major innovations under the act, which means opportunities to learn from—and improve—their care experiences are being lost.
- MedPAC has explored carving in hospice care under Medicare Advantage plans, thereby making them responsible for hospice costs (Harrison and Neuman, 2013). Doing so might pave the way for concurrent care, which at present remains a gap under the ACA.
- The act is not required to include home-based palliative care as a covered service.
- The act does not improve prospects for a more effective or financially stable long-term care system that better matches patient and family needs with social services.
- The act establishes no mechanism for reimbursing clinicians for the extensive and repeated conversations necessary to engage in advance care planning with patients and families or for requiring that they honor patients' preferences regarding end-of-life care.[31]

The ACA is not the last word in this round of health care reform, just as Medicare was not the last word in health care financing for the elderly in 1966 (Skocpol, 2010). Even since the new law's enactment, health policy experts have proposed changes,[32] some of which could have a positive effect on care at the end of life if they

- were flexible and comprehensive, tailoring the mix and intensity of services to patient and family needs as they evolve over time;
- improved accessibility, reaching underserved populations and enabling early palliative care for those not imminently dying by

---

[31]Excellus BlueCross BlueShield has established an enhanced reimbursement program for physicians trained to conduct more thorough advance care planning discussions for seriously ill patients. This program recognizes the amount of time needed for such discussions and the fact that more than a single discussion may be required (http://www.compassionand support.org/index.php/for_professionals/molst_training_center/provider_training [accessed December 16, 2014]).

[32]One proposal would create a new Medicare option called "Medicare Essential." This proposal would combine Medicare Parts A, B, and D and supplemental "Medigap" coverage to save costs, improve coordination of care, and promote shared decision making (Davis et al., 2013). Another proposal, developed by the Bipartisan Policy Center's Health Care Cost Containment Initiative, would establish Medicare Networks as a more full-service alternative to ACOs (Daschle et al., 2013). A new Medicare Comprehensive Care program would be established under another major reform proposal, which would also seek to make Medicaid more "person-focused" (Antos et al., 2013).

establishing required standards for accreditation and participation in Medicare or Medicaid;

- provided for high-quality medical care in the community, through, for example, telemonitoring, round-the-clock access to a nurse, and medication management;
- provided nonmedical support services, including those described earlier in this chapter; and
- entailed measurement of quality of care for those with advanced serious illnesses, multiple chronic conditions, frequent transitions, and functional impairments to ensure accountability and transparency.

Private-Sector Payment Initiatives

Many reform efforts focused on care of people with advanced serious illnesses are taking place in the private sector. Private insurers and managed care plans are free to experiment broadly with strategies for reducing their costs by affecting the behavior of both enrollees and providers, whereas government programs generally focus only on the latter. A frequent shortcoming is the lack of rigorous independent evaluation of these private initiatives in terms of access, quality, and costs.

One of the most promising initiatives coming out of the private sector—one that meets at least the first three principles on the above list—is concurrent care, a model that allows patients to receive hospice-like services and disease treatments at the same time. This model avoids the perceived "terrible choice" between conventional treatment and comfort measures. Examples of the concurrent care approach include the following:

- Highmark, Inc. (Pittsburgh, Pennsylvania) has a program titled Advanced Illness Services: Enhancing Care at End of Life, which serves very ill Medicare Advantage beneficiaries who live at home, use outpatient department services, and wish to receive palliative care. Patients with an approximately 1-year prognosis receive up to 10 mainly consultative home or outpatient visits by hospice or palliative care professionals concurrently with disease treatment.
- Blue Cross Blue Shield of Michigan expanded hospice eligibility to patients with a life expectancy of up to 12 months rather than the usual 6, and permits concurrent care (BCBSM, 2009).
- Kaiser-Permanente deploys an interdisciplinary in-home palliative care team to provide concurrent care. The team includes physicians, nurses, and social workers, supplemented as needed by chaplains (if desired); bereavement coordinators; home health aides; pharmacists; dietitians; physical, occupational, and speech therapists; and

volunteers. A study of the impact of this model found that patients were satisfied with the care they received, and the likelihood of dying at home increased, while emergency department visits and hospitalizations declined. The result was significantly lower costs, after controlling for survival, age, severity of illness, and primary disease (Brumley et al., 2007).[33]

- Sutter Health, based in northern California, has developed an Advanced Illness Management program to coordinate palliative care across settings, including hospitals, physician offices, and patients' homes. The program also seeks to boost hospice utilization and duration. Initial evaluation results included improved satisfaction on the part of patients, families, and physicians, as well as substantial savings. In this program, African American and white patients were equally likely to choose hospice (Meyer, 2011). The Sutter approach retains fee-for-service reimbursement (AHRQ, 2013).
- Aetna's concurrent care model, which has been in place for about a decade, uses a comprehensive case management approach. Nurse care managers with special training in palliative care work with Medicare Advantage and commercially insured beneficiaries having a prognosis of about 12 months. They coordinate care, provide education and support, and help in symptom management. Beneficiary and family satisfaction is high. Hospice utilization was more than double for the case management group (70 percent) compared with a control group of patients (30 percent) (Spettell et al., 2009). Medical costs for people in the program were approximately $17,161—22 percent less than costs for a matched historical control population ($22,030) (Krakauer et al., 2009).

State Policies

The committee did not review in detail opportunities for states to improve systems of care for people nearing the end of life. Clearly, however, state actions in a number of domains can affect the quality, availability, and costs of care for people with advanced serious illnesses and nearing death (Christopher, 2003). Many states have initiated coalitions to contribute to policy reform at the state level and have engaged in a variety of activities

---

[33]In this study, researchers found a strong trend toward shorter survival in the palliative care group (196 days versus 242 days), potentially attributable to undetected problems with randomization between the palliative care and usual care groups, how patient preferences may have changed over time, or closer adherence to patient preferences in the palliative care group. This result is in conflict with other research indicating longer survival in palliative care programs (Temel et al., 2010; see Chapter 2), and further evaluation of the program model may be necessary to explain this finding.

to improve clinical care, program administration, and professional education; increase access to quality end-of-life care; increase the proportion of people in the state who have engaged in advance care planning; and support a range of public policies to further these efforts. Twenty-four state and local coalitions were funded under the Robert Wood Johnson Foundation's Community-State Partnerships to Improve End-of-Life Care program (RWJF, 2004).

Other examples of state policies that can have a significant effect on end-of-life care include

- rules affecting Medicaid eligibility and benefits;
- rules governing state Medicaid managed care programs;
- low Medicaid reimbursements that make it difficult for recipients to obtain physician care;
- regulation and oversight of health facilities (for example, nursing homes, hospice, home health programs, and hospitals), including certificate-of-need programs;
- regulation of emergency medical services;
- scope-of-practice laws that limit the roles and responsibilities of, for example, nurse practitioners;
- programs and policies that support patients at home and their caregivers;
- laws enabling Physician Orders for Life-Sustaining Treatment (POLST; see Chapter 3) or otherwise covering advance care planning; and
- approaches to malpractice enforcement conveying the impression that providers must "do everything for a patient."

Although there is evidence that concerns about malpractice liability affect physician practices, including, for example, their adherence to patients' advance directives (see Chapter 3), some physicians' anxiety about being sued may not be based in fact. A Congressional Budget Office study estimated that broad malpractice reforms would reduce national health care spending by only 0.5 percent (CBO, 2009). To encourage physicians to honor informed patient and family preferences for care at home, states could establish "safe harbors" protecting clinicians from liability in cases in which unwanted treatments are avoided in accordance with advance care plans. In general, fear of malpractice litigation should not be a compelling practical reason to refuse to honor patients' preferences. Family lawsuits against physicians who honored a patient's preference for less aggressive care are virtually nonexistent (Meisel, 2013), and to the contrary, are most likely to occur when a patient or family does not feel respected or heard by a physician.

THE NEED FOR GREATER TRANSPARENCY
AND ACCOUNTABILITY

The IOM report *HHS in the 21st Century* (IOM, 2009) includes the recommendation that the agency improve accountability, which the report describes as requiring a systematic approach encompassing the establishment of critical, measurable goals and clear lines of responsibility; regular reporting and assessment to gauge progress; and corrective action as needed. The report suggests that this management approach is relevant across HHS, within a framework that defines who is accountable to whom and for what purpose. At no time is attention to these tasks more important than when a fundamental overhaul of policy has been initiated, as has occurred with the passage and implementation of the ACA.

As this chapter has shown, past policy initiatives embedded in Medicare, Medicaid, and other federal programs have had many unintended negative consequences—mainly in the forms of perverse and misaligned incentives and uncoordinated services—that have hampered high-quality care for people who have advanced serious illnesses and are nearing the end of life. A time of change is a time to attempt to do better—to establish whether the system is providing value for current patients and to support continued improvements in care for patients in the future. The urgency of undertaking this effort rests on the confluence of three major trends impelling change: the rising complexity and fragmentation of modern health care, unsustainable cost increases, and outcomes that do not reflect the system's potential (IOM, 2013b).

The concept of value reflects a relationship between quality and costs. A high-value health care intervention is one that is that markedly improves quality at low cost (for example, immunizations). A low-value intervention is one that is of little to no benefit (or even harmful) and is high cost. In the current context, it is clear that recurrent hospitalizations for nursing home residents with advanced dementia are of low value. Improving value in health care is of growing importance to federal and state policy makers in light of the demonstrably poor quality of care despite high Medicare, Medicaid, and other health care expenditures.

Value improvement for clinicians often means having diagnostic and treatment tools and strategies that increase confidence in the effectiveness of their services. To communities and employers, improving value may mean keeping workers who are family caregivers and their care recipients healthier and more productive at lower cost, freeing up funds for infrastructure, education, and other important community activities. And for patients and families, improving value often involves helping them avoid bankruptcy and meeting their personal goals for care and for living as independently as possible, even with a serious chronic condition (IOM, 2010b). The value of a particular service or program is also important to these groups because spending a great deal on one form of care may leave few resources for other services or programs that might be more beneficial.

Although different actors in the health care system define value differently, the fundamental calculus for value in health care is the health outcome achieved per dollar spent to achieve it:

> If all [health] system participants have to compete on value, value will improve dramatically. As simple and obvious as this seems to be, however, improving value has not been the central goal of the participants in the system. The focus instead has been on minimizing short-term costs and battling over who pays what. The result is that many of the strategies, organizational structures, and practices of the various actors in the system are badly misaligned with value for the patient. (Porter and Teisberg, 2006, p. 4)

Many health policy experts are comfortable speaking in terms of benefit-cost ratios, cost-effectiveness, and comparative effectiveness, but clinicians usually are not trained to think in these terms.[34] Simply making clinicians more aware of the cost implications of their clinical recommendations for individual patients may be unlikely to affect their decision making without addition support from clinical guidelines that incorporate a value perspective (Ubel et al., 2012).

In the context of value and the desire of policy makers, professionals, and the public to close the gap between the health system's potential performance and its current shortcomings, "accurate, reliable, and valid measurements are a prerequisite for achieving and assessing progress in areas such as improving the quality of health care delivered to patients, reporting on the status of the health care system, and developing payment policies and financial incentives that reward improvement" (IOM, 2013c, p. 2). In general, "quality measures provide objective descriptors of the consequences of care and transform the nebulous concept of 'good medicine' into a measurable discipline" (IOM, 2013d, p. 272). A number of important quality measures relevant to end-of-life care already exist, as discussed in Chapter 2. The National Quality Measures Clearinghouse contains almost 200 measures coded as related to end-of-life care. Despite the number and scope of the existing measures relating to palliative and end-of-life care, there remain important omissions and limitations to existing measures. Most of the listed measures are either disease- or setting-specific; good measures that apply to the highest-cost, highest-risk individuals—those

---

[34]The quality-adjusted life-years (QALYs) metric commonly used to assess the benefits of an intervention must be used with care in the end-of-life context (Yang and Mahon, 2011, p. 1197).

with multiple chronic conditions and/or functional decline who receive care across many settings—are lacking. Few of these quality measures, however, have been integrated into CMS's value-based purchasing programs, so they as yet have no role in improving care. It would be valuable to assess other ways, aside from value-based purchasing, of effecting improvements in care, as well as the extent to which CMS's value-based purchasing programs improve care. Public reporting mechanisms for quality measures related to end-of-life care would be useful as well.

Improving the quality of care for Americans nearing the end of life, then, will require the development and implementation of new measures that, for example,

- are more patient-oriented and include population groups with multiple conditions receiving care across multiple settings;
- include demographic groups that are typically underserved;
- measure quality for a broader spectrum of patients, including people enrolled in Medicare Advantage, Medicaid managed care, and hospice and those residing in nursing homes;
- take into account a broader array of patient and family needs, particularly those related to the social services discussed in this chapter;
- measure the adequacy of support for informed choice by patients and families;
- enable assessment of system performance with respect to advance care planning, shared decision making, and provision of spiritual support, all now defined variably across programs and research efforts;
- track whether care provided accords with patients' values, goals, and informed preferences; and
- capture the full array of costs of care near the end of life, including out-of-pocket expenditures and those associated with informal caregiving.

Prioritization among existing and new quality measures and indicators is likely to be an important future endeavor (Meltzer and Chung, 2014).

RESEARCH NEEDS

Learning health care organizations generate and use accurate, timely, and up-to-date evidence that helps ensure that patients receive the care they need when they need it (IOM, 2007). System learning can take place—and is needed—at the level of the individual clinical practice, the health care institution, the payer, and various levels of government, from entities as small as a neighborhood health center to those as large as CMS. The measures described above are essential for conducting research that can provide actionable feedback to clinicians, payers, and managers and create a learning health care organization.

In advocating more effective and meaningful efficiency measures and incentives, Neuberg (2009, p. 132) says, "It is not sufficient to simply reward savings and hope that quality and outcomes are maintained." With good measures of quality of care for people nearing the end of life, important research questions such as the following can be answered:

- How can models of end-of-life care whose effectiveness has been demonstrated be diffused and adopted more widely?
- Do the savings in hospital costs achieved by palliative care hold true for total health care costs? Do they do so if social services are added to the mix?
- How are changes in the organization and financing of the health care system affecting the nature, quality, and costs of care for patients near the end of life? Are there unintended negative consequences, and especially, has the risk of undertreatment increased?
- What are the out-of-pocket expenses, costs, and economic impact for caregivers for people near the end of life, and what social services could help minimize and manage those costs?
- How can geographic variation in intensity of services be reduced to promote access to the best care without under- or overtreatment?
- What are the experiences of patients with advanced serious illnesses enrolled in Medicare Advantage and Medicaid managed care programs, and how do they compare with those of patients having fee-for-service coverage?
- What meaningful-use criteria relating to end-of-life care need to be developed so that emerging electronic health records will collect adequate data on this care?
- What are the most effective ways to tailor and target support services to specific patients and families to meet both their evolving needs and the requirement for program sustainability?
- How can patients, families, and the public best contribute to decisions about the design of end-of-life services, and are their views taken into account?
- Why is the risk for a malpractice action still feared by some clinicians when it is so low?

Moving forward in these areas will require efforts beyond what the ACA has accomplished. In some unintended ways, the ACA may even worsen care for people with serious advanced illnesses if it launches demonstrations involving bundled payments for discrete episodes of care without integrating long-term services and supports, or if it focuses on transitional care programs that are hospital-centric rather than truly community based (Naylor et al., 2012).

Health services research is needed to help organizations learn how to effect better transitions between hospitals; post-acute care settings, especially nursing homes; and homes. For example, it would be useful to determine the relative contribution of financial incentives, communication gaps, and resource shortages to the care provided to nursing home residents with dementia and to the causes of multiple hospitalizations for preventable conditions.

Other areas worthy of serious investigation that would directly benefit health care organizations, as suggested by the discussion in this chapter, would document the contribution of social services to quality care, and reimbursement approaches that support palliative care at home and in the hospital with full continuity between them. Benefiting patients, families, and providers would be research on approaches for attracting more members of vulnerable minority populations to hospice and ways to improve services for dual-eligible people.

Because of the profound realignment in the U.S. health care system currently under way, meaningful research is needed that is both timely and actionable. Such research can identify important modifications and refinements to these evolving financial and organizational strategies before they become firmly established and more difficult to change. The growing availability of data from electronic health records should facilitate these research efforts.

Finally, information about key end-of-life measures and the results of research need to be made broadly available so that all interested parties can learn from them; can maintain accountability; and can maximize efforts to ensure that end-of-life care is compassionate, high-quality, and affordable for all.

FINDINGS, CONCLUSIONS, AND RECOMMENDATION

Findings

This study yielded the following findings on policies and payment systems to support high-quality end-of-life care.

Fundamental Redesign of Medicare and Medicaid

Incentives under fee-for-service Medicare result in more use of services (for example, hospital days, intensive care, emergency care), more transitions among care settings that are a burden on patients, and late enrollment in hospice, all of which jeopardize the quality of end-of-life care and add to its costs. In addition, payment silos contribute to fragmentation of care, hinder coordination across providers, and encourage inappropriate utilization (Aragon et al., 2012; Davis et al., 2012; Gozalo et al., 2011; Grabowski and O'Malley, 2014; Segal, 2011; Teno et al., 2013).

Integration of Health Care and Social Services

Evaluations of programs that integrate health care and long-term social services indicate that the additional supports may reduce hospitalizations and health care costs while improving enrollees' quality of life. What makes such programs financially sustainable is an appropriate reimbursement level, along with careful targeting of services to individuals at highest risk of health care utilization (including hospitalization and nursing home placements) and tailoring of the services to individual/family needs as they evolve over time. Successful existing models need to be implemented more widely (Brown and Mann, 2012; Brown et al., 2012; Senate Commission on Long-Term Care, 2013; Unroe and Meier, 2013).

Expansion of Palliative Care

Palliative care interventions, including hospice, are effective in improving important patient outcomes, providing care more consonant with most patients' and families' informed preferences, and potentially reducing the costs for both public and private payers by avoiding unnecessary hospitalizations and use of intensive care. Changes throughout the health care system are needed to increase incentives for providing comprehensive palliative care (Brumley et al., 2007; Gade et al., 2008; Krakauer et al., 2009; Meyer, 2011; Morrison et al., 2008, 2011; Penrod et al., 2010; Rabow et al., 2013).

Increased Transparency and Accountability

Changes in the payment system under the ACA, as well as any future changes specifically affecting Americans nearing the end of life, need to be carefully monitored for their effects—intended and unintended—on this highly vulnerable population. To this end, relevant quality standards and actionable measures are needed (IOM, 2013b,c; Naylor et al., 2012).

Conclusions

At present, the U.S. health care system is ill designed to meet the needs of patients near the end of life and their families. The system is geared to providing acute care aimed at curing disease, but not at providing the comfort care most people near the end of life prefer. The financial incentives built into the programs that most often serve people with advanced serious illnesses—Medicare and Medicaid—are not well coordinated, and the result is fragmented care that increases risks to patients and creates avoidable burdens on them and their families. From a system perspective, fragmented, uncoordinated care and unwanted and unnecessary acute care services—which in the current system constitute "default care"—are extremely costly. At the same time, many of the practical, day-to-day social services that would allow people near the end of life to live in safety and comfort at home, where most prefer to be—such as caregiver training and support, meals and nutrition services, and family respite—are not easily arranged or paid for. The palliative care model and other care models that integrate health and social services, when properly implemented, may improve quality of care and reduce the use of expensive services, and could potentially help stabilize and even reduce increases in health care costs for people near the end of life.

Many aspects of the U.S. health care system are changing, and these and future changes may have both beneficial and unintended negative consequences for Americans of all ages near the end of life. For that reason, efforts to ensure the transparency and accountability of the programs that serve this population will need to be scrupulously monitored. Much can be learned from existing successful programs and care delivery models—such as palliative care—that merit rapid expansion.

> **Recommendation 4. Federal, state, and private insurance and health care delivery programs should integrate the financing of medical and social services to support the provision of quality care consistent with the values, goals, and informed preferences of people with advanced serious illness nearing the end of life. To the extent that additional legislation is necessary to implement this recommendation, the administration should seek and Congress should enact such legislation. In addition, the federal government should require public reporting on quality measures, outcomes, and costs regarding care near the end of life (e.g., in the last year of life) for programs it funds or administers (e.g., Medicare, Medicaid, the U.S. Department of Veterans Affairs). The federal government should encourage all other payment and health care delivery systems to do the same.**

Specifically, actions should

- provide financial incentives for
  - medical and social support services that decrease the need for emergency room and acute care services,
  - coordination of care across settings and providers (from hospital to ambulatory settings as well as home and community), and
  - improved shared decision making and advance care planning that reduces the utilization of unnecessary medical services and those not consistent with a patient's goals for care;
- require the use of interoperable electronic health records that incorporate advance care planning to improve communication of individuals' wishes across time, settings, and providers, documenting (1) the designation of a surrogate/decision maker, (2) patient values and beliefs and goals for care, (3) the presence of an advance directive, and (4) the presence of medical orders for life-sustaining treatment for appropriate populations; and
- encourage states to develop and implement a Physician Orders for Life-Sustaining Treatment (POLST) paradigm program in accordance with nationally standardized core requirements.

Medical and social services provided should accord with a person's values, goals, informed preferences, condition, circumstances, and needs, with the expectation that individual service needs and intensity will change over time. High-quality, comprehensive, person-centered, and family-oriented care will help reduce preventable crises that lead to repeated use of 911 calls, emergency department visits, and hospital admissions, and if implemented appropriately, should contribute to stabilizing aggregate societal expenditures for medical and related social services and potentially lowering them over time.

REFERENCES

AARP Public Policy Institute. 2008. A balancing act: State long-term care reform. *In Brief* 161. http://assets.aarp.org/rgcenter/il/inb161_ltc.pdf (accessed January 29, 2013).

AARP Public Policy Institute. 2013. *Medicaid: A program of last resort for people who need long-term services and supports.* http://www.aarp.org/content/dam/aarp/research/public_policy_institute/health/2013/medicaid-last-resort-insight-AARP-ppi-health.pdf (accessed August 19, 2014).

Administration for Community Living. 2013. *New models of community care for older adults and people with disabilities.* http://www.acl.gov/About_ACL/FederalInitiatives/CommunityCare.aspx (accessed November 29, 2013).

AHIP (America's Health Insurance Plans). 2013. *Trends in Medigap coverage and enrollment.* http://ahip.org/Trends-Medigap-Coverage-Enroll2012 (accessed August 19, 2014).

AHRQ (Agency for Healthcare Research and Quality). 2013. *Effective palliative care programs require health system change.* http://www.innovations.ahrq.gov/content.aspx?id=3742 (accessed July 16, 2013).

Aldridge Carlson, M. D., C. L. Barry, E. J. Cherlin, R. McCorkle, and E. H. Bradley. 2012. Hospices' enrollment policies may contribute to underuse of hospice care in the United States. *Health Affairs* 31(12):2690-2697.

Alpert, A., K. G. Morganti, G. S. Margolis, J. Wasserman, and A. L. Kellermann. 2013. Giving EMS flexibility in transporting low-acuity patients could generate substantial Medicare savings. *Health Affairs* 32(12):2142-2148.

Altman, S., and D. Shactman. 2011. *Power, politics, and universal health care.* Amherst, NY: Prometheus Books.

Antos, J., K. Baicker, M. Chernew, D. Crippen, D. Cutler, T. Daschle, F. de Brantes, D. Goldman, G. Hubbard, B. Kocher, M. Leavitt, M. McClellan, P. Orszag, M. Pauly, A. Rivlin, L. Schaeffer, D. Shalala, and S. Shortell. 2013. *Bending the curve: Person-centered health care reform: A framework for improving care and slowing health care cost growth.* Washington, DC: The Brookings Institution.

AoA (Administration on Aging). 2013. *A profile of older Americans: 2013.* http://www.aoa.gov/AoARoot/Aging_Statistics/Profile/2013/docs/2013_Profile.pdf (accessed August 6, 2014).

AoA. undated. *National Family Caregiver Support Program (OAA Title IIIE).* http://www.aoa.gov/aoa_programs/hcltc/caregiver/index.aspx (accessed February 3, 2014).

Appleby, J., and M. A. Carey. 2011. CLASS dismissed: Obama administration pulls plug on long-term care program. *Kaiser Health News*, October 14. http://www.kaiserhealthnews.org/Stories/2011/October/14/CLASS-Act-Implementation-Halted-By-Obama-Administration.aspx (accessed January 5, 2014).

Aragon, K., K. Covinsky, Y Miao, W. J. Boxcardin, L. Flint, and A. Smith. 2012. Medicare post-hospitalization skilled nursing benefit in the last six months of life. *Archives of Internal Medicine* 172(20):1573-1579.

Bachrach, D., Pfister, H., Wallis, K., and Lipson, M. 2014. *Addressing patients' social needs: An emerging business case for provider investment.* Washington, DC: Manatt Health Solutions. http://www.commonwealthfund.org/~/media/files/publications/fund-report/2014/may/1749_bachrach_addressing_patients_social_needs_v2.pdf (accessed May 29, 2014).

Bass, D. M., K. S. Judge, A. L. Snow, N. L. Wilson, R. Morgan, W. J. Looman, C. A. McCarthy, K. Maslow, J. A. Moye, R. Randazzo, M. Garcia-Maldonado, R. Elbein, G. Odenheimer, and M. E. Junik. 2013. Caregiver outcomes of partners in dementia care: Effect of a care coordination program for veterans with dementia and their family members and friends. *Journal of the American Geriatrics Society* 61(8):1377-1386.

Baum, A. S., and D. W. Burnes. 1993. *A nation in denial: The truth about homelessness.* Boulder, CO: Westview Press.

Bazelon Center for Mental Health Law. 2012. *Medicare.* http://www.bazelon.org/Where-We-Stand/Access-to-Services/Medicare.aspx (accessed December 5, 2013).

BCBSM (Blue Cross Blue Shield of Michigan). 2009. *Blue Cross Blue Shield of Michigan expands hospice services.* News release. August 26. Detroit, MI: BCBSM. http://www.bcbsm.com/content/microsites/blue-cross-blue-shield-of-michigan-news/en/index/news-releases/2009/august-2009/blue-cross-blue-shield-of-michigan-expands-hospice-services.html (accessed July 15, 2013).

Berwick, D. M. 2011. Making good on ACOS' promise—The final rule for the Medicare Shared Savings Program. *New England Journal of Medicine* 365(19):1753-1756.

Bipartisan Policy Center. 2012. *What is driving U.S. health care spending? America's unsustainable health care cost growth.* http://bipartisanpolicy.org/sites/default/files/BPC%20 Health%20Care%20Cost%20Drivers%20Brief%20Sept%202012.pdf (accessed December 2, 2013).

Bishop, T. F., M. J. Press, S. Keyhani, and H. A. Pincus. 2014. Acceptance of insurance by psychiatrists and the implications for access to mental health care. *JAMA Psychiatry* 71(92):176-181.

Boards of Trustees, Federal Hospital Insurance and Federal Supplementary Medical Insurance Trust Funds. 2013. *2013 annual report of the boards of trustees of the federal hospital insurance and supplementary medical insurance trust funds.* http://downloads.cms.gov/ files/TR2013.pdf (accessed August 12, 2014).

Bona, K., J. Bates, and J. Wolfe. 2011. Massachusetts' Pediatric Palliative Care Network: Successful implementation of a novel state-funded pediatric palliative care program. *Journal of Palliative Medicine* 14(11):1217-1223.

Bona, K., V. Dussel, L. Orellana, T. Kang, R. Geyer, C. Feudtner, and J. Wolfe. 2014. Economic impact of advanced pediatric cancer on families. *Journal of Pain and Symptom Management* 47(3):594-603.

Bradley, E. H., and L. A. Taylor. 2013. *The American health care paradox: Why spending more is getting us less.* New York: Public Affairs.

Brown, R., and D. R. Mann. 2012. *Best bets for reducing Medicare costs for dual eligible beneficiaries: Assessing the evidence.* Issue Brief. Menlo Park, CA: KFF.

Brown, R. S., D. Peikes, G. Peterson, J. Schore, and C. M. Razafindrakoto. 2012. Six features of Medicare coordinated care demonstration programs that cut hospital admissions of high-risk patients. *Health Affairs* 31(6):1156-1165.

Brumley, R., S. Enguidanos, P. Jamison, R. Seitz, N. Morgenstern, S. Saito, J. McIlwane, K. Hillary, and J. Gonzalez. 2007. Increased satisfaction with care and lower costs: Results of a randomized trial of in-home palliative care. *Journal of the American Geriatrics Society* 55(7):993-1000.

Bureau of the Census. 2013. *Aging in the United States: Past, present, and future.* http://www. census.gov/population/international/files/97agewc.pdf (accessed July 4, 2013).

CAPC (Center to Advance Palliative Care). 2011. America's care of serious illness: *A state-by-state report card on access to palliative care in our nation's hospitals.* New York: CAPC. http://reportcard.capc.org/pdf/state-by-state-report-card.pdf (accessed September 19, 2013).

CAPC. 2013. *Growth of palliative care in U.S. hospitals: 2013 snapshot.* http://www.capc.org/ capc-growth-analysis-snapshot-2013.pdf (accessed January 27, 2014).

Capretta, J. C. 2013. *The role of Medicare fee-for-service in inefficient health care delivery.* Washington, DC: American Enterprise Institute. http://www.aei.org/papers/health/ entitlements/medicare/the-role-of-medicare-fee-for-service-in-inefficient-health-care-delivery (accessed July 1, 2013).

Carlson, B. L., L. Foster, S. B. Dale, and R. Brown. 2007. Effects of Cash and Counseling on personal care and well-being. *Health Services Research* 42(1, Part 2):467-487.

CBO (Congressional Budget Office). 2009. *Letter to the Honorable Orrin G. Hatch.* http:// www.cbo.gov/sites/default/files/cbofiles/ftpdocs/106xx/doc10641/10-09-tort_reform.pdf (accessed July 11, 2013).

CBO. 2013. *Dual-eligible beneficiaries of Medicare and Medicaid: Characteristics, health care spending, and evolving policies.* http://www.cbo.gov/sites/default/files/cbofiles/ attachments/44308_DualEligibles.pdf (accessed July 7, 2013).

Chamberlain, J. M., S. Krug, and K. N. Shaw. 2013. Emergency care for children in the United States. *Health Affairs* 32(12):2109-2115.

Christopher, M. 2003. *Championing end-of-life care policy change.* http://www.rwjf.org/content/dam/files/legacy-files/article-files/2/State_Initiatives_EOL19.pdf (accessed January 9, 2014).

CMS (Centers for Medicare & Medicaid Services). 2012. *State demonstrations to integrate care for dual eligible individuals.* http://www.cms.gov/Medicare-Medicaid-Coordination/Medicare-and-Medicaid-Coordination/Medicare-Medicaid-Coordination-Office/State DemonstrationstoIntegrateCareforDualEligibleIndividuals.html (accessed December 2, 2013).

CMS. 2013a. *Medicare hospice data trends, 1998-2009.* http://www.cms.gov/Medicare/Medicare-Fee-for-Service-Payment/Hospice/Medicare_Hospice_Data.html (accessed May 30, 2014).

CMS. 2013b. *Guidance to states using 1115 demonstrations or 1915(b) waivers for managed long-term services and supports programs.* http://www.medicaid.gov/Medicaid-CHIP-Program-Information/By-Topics/Delivery-Systems/Downloads/1115-and-1915b-MLTSS-guidance.pdf (accessed July 5, 2013).

CMS. 2013c. *About the Medicare-Medicaid Coordination Office.* http://www.cms.gov/Medicare-Medicaid-Coordination/Medicare-and-Medicaid-Coordination/Medicare-Medicaid-Coordination-Office (accessed December 2, 2013).

CMS. 2013d. *Bundled payments for care improvement initiative: General information.* http://innovation.cms.gov/initiatives/Bundled-Payments (accessed January 30, 2014).

CMS. 2013e. *Accountable care organizations.* Baltimore, MD: CMS. http://www.cms.gov/Medicare/Medicare-Fee-for-Service-Payment/ACO/index.html?redirect=/aco (accessed May 17, 2013).

CMS. 2014a. *Financial alignment initiative.* http://www.cms.gov/Medicare-Medicaid-Coordination/Medicare-and-Medicaid-Coordination/Medicare-Medicaid-Coordination-Office/Financial AlignmentInitiative/FinancialModelstoSupportStatesEffortsinCareCoordination.html (accessed January 30, 2014).

CMS. 2014b. *Medicare Care Choices Model.* http://innovation.cms.gov/initiatives/Medicare-Care-Choices (accessed August 12, 2014).

CMS. undated-a. *Medicare enrollment: National trends, 1966-2010.* http://www.cms.gov/Research-Statistics-Data-and-Systems/Statistics-Trends-and-Reports/MedicareEnrpts/index.html?redirect=/MedicareEnRpts (accessed January 31, 2014).

CMS. undated-b. *Money follows the person.* http://www.medicaid.gov/Medicaid-CHIP-Program-Information/By-Topics/Long-Term-Services-and-Support/Balancing/Money-Follows-the-Person.html (accessed January 30, 2014).

CMS. undated-c. *Medicare 2014 costs at a glance.* http://www.medicare.gov/your-medicare-costs/costs-at-a-glance/costs-at-glance.html#collapse-4809 (accessed May 14, 2014).

Coleman, E. A., C. Parry, S. Chalmers, and S. Min. 2006. The care transitions intervention: Results of a randomized controlled trial. *Archives of Internal Medicine* 166(17):1822-1828.

Commonwealth Fund. 2013. *Potentially avoidable hospital admissions among vulnerable Medicare beneficiaries.* http://www.commonwealthfund.org/Charts/Report/Low-Income-Scorecard/Potentially-Avoidable-Hospital-Admissions-among-Vulnerable-Medicare-Beneficiaries.aspx (accessed January 4, 2014).

Commonwealth Fund Commission on a High Performance Health System. 2013. *Confronting costs: Stabilizing U.S. health spending while moving toward a high performance health care system.* New York: Commonwealth Fund Commission on a High Performance Health System. http://www.commonwealthfund.org/~/media/Files/Publications/Fund%20 Report/2013/Jan/1653_Commission_confronting_costs_web_FINAL.pdf (accessed February 22, 2014).

Coughlin, T. A., T. A. Waidmann, and L. Phadera. 2012. Among dual eligibles, identifying the highest-cost individuals could help in crafting more targeted and effective responses. *Health Affairs* 31(5):1083-1091.

Cuckler, G. A., A. M. Sisko, S. P. Keehan, S. D. Smith, A. J. Madison, J. A. Poisal, C. J. Wolfe, J. M. Lizonitz, and D. A. Stone. 2013. National health expenditure projections, 2012-22: Slow growth until coverage expands and economy improves. *Health Affairs* 32(10):1820-1831.

Cutler, D. M., and N. R. Sahni. 2013. If slow rate of health care spending growth persists, projections may be off by $770 billion. *Health Affairs* 32(5):841-850.

Damore, J., and W. Champion. 2013. *The Pioneer ACO first year results: A fuller picture.* http://healthaffairs.org/blog/2013/07/17/the-pioneer-aco-first-year-results-a-fuller-picture (accessed November 26, 2013).

Dartmouth Atlas of Health Care. 2013. *Reflections on variations.* Lebanon, NH: Dartmouth College, The Dartmouth Institute for Health Policy and Clinical Practice. http://www.dartmouthatlas.org/keyissues/issue.aspx?con=1338 (accessed June 27, 2013).

Daschle, T., P. Domenici, W. Frist, and A. Rivlin. 2013. Prescription for patient-centered care and cost containment. *New England Journal of Medicine* 369(5):471-474.

Davis, K., C. Schoen, and S. Guterman. 2013. Medicare essential: An option to promote better care and curb spending growth. *Health Affairs* 32(5):900-909.

Davis, M. M., M. Devoe, D. Kansagara, C. Nicolaidis, and H. Englander. 2012. "Did I do as best as the system would let me?" Healthcare professional views on hospital to home care transitions. *Journal of General Internal Medicine* 27(12):1649-1656.

Dobson, A., J. E. DaVanzo, S. Heath, M. Shimer, G. Berger, A. Pick, K. Reuter, A. El-Gamil, and N. Manolov. 2012. *Medicare payment bundling: Insights from claims data and policy implications.* Vienna, VA: Dobson/DaVanzo & Associates, LLC.

Dussel, V., K. Bona, J. A. Heath, J. M. Hilden, J. C. Weeks, and J. Wolfe. 2011 Unmeasured costs of a child's death: Perceived financial burden, work disruptions, and economic coping strategies used by American and Australian families who lost children to cancer. *Journal of Clinical Oncology* 29(8):1007-1013.

Elhauge, E., ed. 2010. *The fragmentation of U.S. health care: Causes and solutions.* New York: Oxford University Press.

Elmendorf, D. 2013. *How have CBO's projections of spending for Medicare and Medicaid changed since the August 2012 baseline?* http://www.cbo.gov/publication/43947 (accessed November 26, 2013).

Employment Benefit Research Institute. 2012. *Effects of nursing home stays on household portfolios.* Issue Brief 372. Washington, DC: Employment Benefit Research Institute. http://www.ebri.org/publications/ib/index.cfm?fa=ibDisp&content_id=5078 (accessed July 6, 2013).

Epstein, A. M., A. K. Jha, E. J. Orav, D. L. Liebman, A. J. Audet, M. A. Zezza, and S. Guterman. 2014. Analysis of early accountable care organizations defines patient, structural, cost and quality-of-care characteristics. *Health Affairs* 33(1):95-102.

Eva, G., and B. Wee. 2010. Rehabilitation in end-of-life management. *Current Opinion in Supportive and Palliative Care* 4(3):158-162.

Farley, T. A. 2009. Reforming health care or reforming health? Editorial. *American Journal of Public Health* 99(4):588-590.

Farragher, J., and S. V. Jassal. 2012. Rehabilitation of the geriatric dialysis patient. *Seminars in Dialysis* 25(6):649-656.

Feder, J. 2013. Bundle with care—Rethinking Medicare incentives for post-acute care services. *New England Journal of Medicine* 369(5):400-401.

Feder, J., H. L. Komisar, and N. Niefeld. 2000. Long-term care in the United States: An overview. *Health Affairs* 19(3):40-56.

Feinberg, L. 2012. *Assessing family caregiver needs: Policy and practice considerations.* Washington, DC: AARP Public Policy Institute.

Feinberg, L., S. C. Reinhard, A. Houser, and R. Choula. 2011. *Valuing the invaluable: 2011 update—The growing contribution and costs of family caregiving.* Washington, DC: AARP, Public Policy Institute. http://assets.aarp.org/rgcenter/ppi/ltc/i51-caregiving.pdf (accessed August 27, 2013).

Fishman, J., P. O'Dwyer, H. L. Lu, H. Henderson, D. A. Asch, and D. J. Casarett. 2009. Race, treatment preferences, and hospice enrollment: Eligibility criteria may exclude patients with the greatest needs for care. *Cancer* 115(3):689-697.

Fox-Grage, W., and Walls, J. 2013. *State studies find home and community-based services to be cost-effective.* http://www.aarp.org/content/dam/aarp/research/public_policy_institute/ltc/2013/state-studies-find-hcbs-cost-effective-spotlight-AARP-ppi-ltc.pdf (accessed December 2, 2013).

Freeman, R., K. M. Lybecker, and D. W. Taylor. 2011. *The effectiveness of disease management programs in the Medicaid population.* Hamilton, Ontario, Canada: The Cameron Institute. http://www.fightchronicdisease.org/sites/fightchronicdisease.org/files/docs/Main%20Report%20-%20The%20effectiveness%20of%20DMPs%20in%20the%20Medicaid%20Pop%202011.pdf (accessed December 5, 2013).

Gade, G., I. Venohr, D. Conner, K. McGrady, J. Beane, R. H. Richardson, M. P. Williams, M. Liberson, M. Blum, and R. Della Penna. 2008. Impact of an inpatient palliative care team: A randomized control trial. *Journal of Palliative Medicine* 11(2):180-190.

Gans, D. G. Kominski, D. H. Roby, A. L. Diamant, X. Chen, W. Lin, and N. Hohe. 2012. Better outcomes, lower costs: Palliative care program reduces stress, costs of care for children with life-threatening conditions. *Policy Brief UCLA Center for Health Policy Research* PB2012-3:1-8.

Ginsburg, P. B. 2012. Fee-for-service will remain a feature of major payment reforms, requiring more changes in Medicare physician payment. *Health Affairs* 31(9):1977-1983.

Gold, M. R., G. A. Jacobson, and R. L. Garfield. 2012. There is little experience and limited data to support policy making on integrated care for dual eligibles. *Health Affairs* 31(6):1176-1184.

Goldfeld, K. S., D. C. Grabowski, D. J. Caudry, and S. L. Mitchell. 2013. Health insurance status and the care of nursing home residents with advanced dementia. *JAMA Internal Medicine* 173(22):2047-2053.

Gore, S., and J. Klebonis. 2012. *Financial alignment models for Medicare-Medicaid enrollees: Considerations for reimbursement.* Technical Assistance Brief. http://www.chcs.org/usr_doc/Payment_and_Reimbursement_FINAL.pdf (accessed January 28, 2014).

Gozalo P., J. Teno, S. L. Mitchell, J. Skinner, J. P. Bynum, D. Tyler, and V. Mor. 2011. End-of-life transitions among nursing home residents with cognitive issues. *New England Journal of Medicine* 365(13):1212-1221.

Grabowski, D. C. 2006. The cost-effectiveness of noninstitutional long-term care services: Review and synthesis of the most recent evidence. *Medical Care Research and Review* 63(1):3-28.

Grabowski, D. C., and A. J. O'Malley. 2014. Use of telemedicine can reduce hospitalizations of nursing home residents and generate savings for Medicare. *Health Affairs* 33(2):244-250.

Greer, J., P. McMahon, A. Tramontano, E. Gallagher, W. F. Pirl, V. Jackson, and J. S. Temel. 2012. Effect of early palliative care on health care costs in patients with metastatic NSCLC. *Journal of Clinical Oncology* 30(Suppl., abstract 6004).

Greve, P. 2011. Pediatrics: A unique and volatile risk. *Journal of Healthcare Risk Management* 31(2):19-29.

Gross, D. L., H. Temkin-Greener, S. Kunitz, and D. B. Mukamel. 2004. The growing pains of integrated health care for the elderly: Lessons from the expansion of PACE. *Milbank Quarterly* 82(2):257-282.

Guterman, S., M. A. Zezza, and C. Schoen. 2013. *Paying for value: Replacing Medicare's sustainable growth rate formula with incentives to improve care.* New York: Commonwealth Fund. http://www.commonwealthfund.org/Publications/Issue-Briefs/2013/Mar/Paying-for-Value-Replacing-Medicares-Sustainable-Growth-Rate.aspx (accessed July 1, 2013).

Hackbarth, G. M. 2009. *Report to the Congress: Medicare payment policy. Statement before the Subcommittee on Health, Committee on Ways and Means, House of Representatives.* Washington, DC: MedPAC. http://www.medpac.gov/documents/Mar09_March%20 report%20testimony_WM%20FINAL.pdf (accessed July 29, 2013).

Hackbarth, G. M. 2013. *Moving forward from the sustainable growth rate system.* Washington, DC: MedPAC. http://www.medpac.gov/documents/04102013_MedPAC_updated_ SGR_letter.pdf (accessed July 1, 2013).

Harrison, S., and K. Neuman. 2013. *Medicare managed care topics.* http://www.medpac.gov/ transcripts/MA_topics11_13l.pdf (accessed January 9, 2014).

HHS (U.S. Department of Health and Human Services). 2000. *Cost-effectiveness of home and community based services.* http://aspe.hhs.gov/daltcp/reports/2000/costeff.htm (accessed August 29, 2013).

HHS. 2005. *Medicaid treatment of the home: Determining eligibility and repayment for long-term care.* http://aspe.hhs.gov/daltcp/reports/hometreat.htm (accessed February 21, 2014).

HHS. 2014. *Long term care: The basics.* http://longtermcare.gov/the-basics/how-much-care-will-you-need (accessed August 13, 2014).

HHS and CMS. 2013. Medicare program; FY 2014 hospice wage index and payment rate update; hospice quality reporting requirements; and updates on payment reform; final rule. *Federal Register* 78:152. http://www.gpo.gov/fdsys/pkg/FR-2013-08-07/pdf/2013-18838.pdf (accessed January 31, 2014).

Hirth, V., J. Baskins, and M. Dever-Bumba. 2009. Program of All-Inclusive Care (PACE): Past, present, and future. *Journal of the American Medical Directors Association* 10(3): 155-160.

Hodgson, C. 2012. *Cost-effectiveness of palliative care: A review of the literature.* http://www. hpcintegration.ca/media/36290/TWF-Economics-report-Eng-final-webmar7.pdf (accessed May 17, 2014).

Horvath, K. J., S. A. Trudeau, J. L. Rudolph, P. A. Trudeau, M. E. Duffy, and D. Berlowitz. 2013. Clinical trial of a home safety toolkit for Alzheimer's disease. *International Journal of Alzheimer's Disease* 1-11. http://www.hindawi.com/journals/ijad/2013/913606 (accessed November 27, 2013).

Huskamp, H. A., D. G. Stevenson, M. E. Chernew, and J. P Newhouse. 2010. A new Medicare end-of-life benefit for nursing home residents. *Health Affairs* 29(1):130-135.

Huynh, T. N., E. C. Kleerup, J. F. Wiley, T. D. Savitsky, D. Guse, B. J. Garber, and N. S. Wenger. 2013. The frequency and cost of treatment perceived to be futile in critical care. *JAMA Internal Medicine* 173(20):1887-1894.

Hwang, U., M. N. Shah, J. H. Han, C. R. Carpenter, A. L. Siu, and J. G. Adams. 2013. Transforming emergency care for older adults. *Health Affairs* 32(12):2116-2121.

IOM (Institute of Medicine). 1997. *Approaching death: Improving care at the end of life.* Washington, DC: National Academy Press.

IOM. 2001. *Crossing the quality chasm: A new health system for the 21st century.* Washington, DC: National Academy Press.

IOM. 2003. *When children die: Improving palliative and end-of-life care for children and their families.* Washington, DC: The National Academies Press.

IOM. 2007. *The learning healthcare system: Workshop summary.* Washington, DC: The National Academies Press.

IOM. 2009. *HHS in the 21st century: Charting a new course for a healthier America.* Washington, DC: The National Academies Press.

IOM. 2010a. *The healthcare imperative: Lowering costs and improving outcomes.* Washington, DC: The National Academies Press.

IOM. 2010b. *Value in health care: Accounting for cost, quality, safety, outcomes, and innovation.* Washington, DC: The National Academies Press.

IOM. 2013a. *Variation in health care spending: Target decision making, not geography.* Washington, DC: The National Academies Press.

IOM. 2013b. *Best care at lower cost: The path to continuously learning health care in America.* Washington, DC: The National Academies Press.

IOM. 2013c. *Core measurement needs for better care, better health, and lower costs: Counting what counts.* Washington, DC: The National Academies Press.

IOM. 2013d. *Delivering high-quality cancer care: Charting a new course for a system in crisis.* Washington, DC: The National Academies Press.

IOM. 2013e. *Financing long-term services and supports for individuals with disabilities and older adults.* Washington, DC: The National Academies Press.

Jacobson, L. 2013. Medicare and Social Security: What you paid in compared with what you get. *PolitiFact,* February 1. http://www.politifact.com/truth-o-meter/article/2013/feb/01/medicare-and-social-security-what-you-paid-what-yo (accessed July 5, 2013).

Jennings, B., and M. B. Morrissey. 2011. Health care costs in end-of-life and palliative care: The quest for ethical reform. *Journal of Social Work in End-of-Life and Palliative Care* 7:300-317.

Kamal, A. H., D. C. Currow, C. S. Ritchie, J. Bull, and A. P. Abernethy. 2013. Community-based palliative care: The natural evolution for palliative care delivery in the U.S. *Journal of Pain and Symptom Management* 46(2):254-264.

Kane, C. K., and D. W. Emmons. 2013. *New data on physician practice arrangements: Private practice remains strong despite shifts toward hospital employment.* Chicago, IL: American Medical Association. http://www.ama-assn.org/resources/doc/health-policy/prp-physician-practice-arrangements.pdf (accessed February 22, 2014).

Kane, R. L., G. Keckhafer, and J. Robst. 2002. *Evaluation of the Evercare Demonstration Program: Final report.* http://www.cms.gov/Medicare/Demonstration-Projects/DemoProjects EvalRpts/downloads/Evercare_Final_Report.pdf (accessed February 22, 2014).

Kane, R. L., S. Flood, B. Bershadsky, and G. Keckhafer. 2004. Effect of an innovative Medicare managed care program on the quality of care for nursing home residents. *Gerontologist* 44(1):95-103.

Kassner, E. 2013. *Home- and community-based services: The right place and the right time.* http://blog.aarp.org/2013/08/19/home-and-community-based-services-the-right-place-and-the-right-time (accessed December 2, 2013).

Kellermann, A. L., R. Y. Hsia, C. Yeh, and K. G. Morgani. 2013. Emergency care: Then, now, and next. *Health Affairs* 32(12):2069-2074.

Kelley, A. S., Deb, P., Du, Q., Carlson, M. D. A., and Morrison, R. S. 2013a. Hospice enrollment saves money for Medicare and improves care quality across a number of different lengths-of-stay. *Health Affairs* 32(3):552-561.

Kelley, A. S., K. McGarry, S. Fahle, S. M. Marshall, Q. Du, and J. S. Skinner. 2013b. Out-of-pocket spending in the last five years of life. *Journal of General Internal Medicine* 28(2):304-309.

Kemper, P. 1988. The evaluation of the National Long Term Care Demonstration. 10. Overview of the findings. *Health Services Research* 23(1):161-174.

KFF (The Henry J. Kaiser Family Foundation). 2012. *Medicare at a glance.* http://kff.org/medicare/fact-sheet/medicare-at-a-glance-fact-sheet (accessed July 2, 2013).

KFF. 2013a. *Medicaid: A primer. Key information on the nation's health coverage program for low-income people.* Menlo Park, CA: KFF, Kaiser Commission on Medicaid and the Uninsured. http://kaiserfamilyfoundation.files.wordpress.com/2010/06/7334-05.pdf (accessed August 7, 2014).

KFF. 2013b. A short look at long-term care for seniors. *Journal of the American Medical Association* 310(8):786.

KFF. 2014. *State health facts.* http://kff.org/medicare/state-indicator/total-medicare-beneficiaries (accessed January 31, 2014).

Klein, E. 2013. 21 graphs that show America's health-care prices are ludicrous. Wonkblog. *The Washington Post,* March 26. http://www.washingtonpost.com/blogs/wonkblog/wp/2013/03/26/21-graphs-that-show-americas-health-care-prices-are-ludicrous (accessed November 27, 2013).

Komisar, H. L., and J. Feder. 2011. *Transforming care for Medicare beneficiaries with chronic conditions and long-term care needs: Coordinating care across all services.* Washington, DC: Georgetown University. http://www.cahpf.org/docuserfiles/georgetown_trnsfrming_care.pdf (accessed December 2, 2013).

Krakauer, R., C. M. Spettell, L. Reisman, and M. J. Wade. 2009. Opportunities to improve the quality of care for advanced illness. *Health Affairs* 28(5):1357-1359.

Kumetz, E. A., and J. D. Goodson. 2013. The undervaluation of evaluation and management professional services: The lasting impact of current procedural terminology code deficiencies on physician payment. *Chest* 144(3):740-745.

L & M Policy Research. 2013. *Evaluation of CMMI Accountable Care Organization Initiatives.* Washington, DC: L & M Policy Research.

Lakdawalla, D. N., D. P. Goldman, A. B. Jena, and D. B. Agus. 2011. *Medicare end-of-life counseling: A matter of choice.* Washington, DC: American Enterprise Institute. http://www.aei.org/article/health/entitlements/medicare/medicare-end-of-life-counseling-a-matter-of-choice (accessed July 2, 2013).

Lieberman, S. M. 2013. Reforming Medicare through "Version 2.0" of accountable care. *Health Affairs* 32(7):1258-1264.

Lilly, M. B., C. A. Robinson, S. Holtzman, and J. L. Botorff. 2012. Can we move beyond burden and burnout to support the health and wellness needs of family caregivers to persons with dementia? *Health and Social Care in the Community* 20(1):103-112.

Lyons, R. D. 1984. How release of mental patients began. *The New York Times.* http://www.nytimes.com/1984/10/30/science/how-release-of-mental-patients-began.html?pagewanted=1 (accessed December 3, 2013).

Marmor, T. R., M. L. Barer, and R. G. Evans. 1994. *Why are some people healthy and others not? The determinants of health of populations.* Piscataway, NJ: Aldine Transaction.

Martin, A. B., M. Hartman, L. Whittle, A. Catlin, and the National Health Expenditure Accounts Team. 2014. National health spending in 2012: Rate of health spending growth remained low for the fourth consecutive year. *Health Affairs* 33(1):67-77.

Mattke, S., M. Seid, and S. Ma. 2007. Evidence for the effect of disease management: Is $1 billion a year a good investment? *American Journal of Managed Care* 13(12):670-676. http://www.allhealth.org/briefingmaterials/AJMC-Mattke-1131.pdf (accessed February 22, 2014).

McGinniss, J. M., and W. H. Foege. 1993. Actual causes of death in the United States. *Journal of the American Medical Association* 270(18):2207-2212.

MedPAC (Medicare Payment Advisory Commission). 2011. *The sustainable growth rate system: Policy considerations for adjustments and alternatives.* http://www.medpac.gov/chapters/jun11_ch01.pdf (accessed May 15, 2014).

MedPAC. 2013. *Report to Congress: Medicare payment policy.* http://www.medpac.gov/documents/Mar13_entirereport.pdf (accessed December 1, 2013).

Meier, D. E. 2011. Increased access to palliative care and hospice services: Opportunities to improve value in health care. *Milbank Quarterly* 89(3):343-380.

Meisel, A. 2013. Presentation at Meeting of the IOM Committee on Approaching Death: Addressing Key End-of-Life Issues, Houston, TX, July 22.

Meltzer, D., and J. W. Chung. 2014. The population value of quality indicator reporting: A framework for prioritizing health care performance measures. *Health Affairs* 33(1):132-139.

Meyer, H. 2011. Changing the conversation in California about care near the end of life. *Health Affairs* 30(3):390-393.

Meyer, J., and B. M. Smith. 2008. *Chronic disease management: Evidence of predictable savings.* http://www.idph.state.ia.us/hcr_committees/common/pdf/clinicians/savings_report.pdf (accessed January 30, 2014).

Miller, E. A. 2012. The Affordable Care Act and long-term care: Comprehensive reform or just tinkering around the edges? *Journal of Aging & Social Policy* 24(2):101-117.

Mitchell, S. L., J. M. Teno, D. K. Kiely, M. L. Shaffer, R. N. Jones, H. G. Prigerson, L. Volicer, J. L. Givens, and M. B. Hamel. 2009. The clinical course of advanced dementia. *New England Journal of Medicine* 361(16):1529-1538.

Moffit, R. E., and A. Senger. 2013. *Medicare's rising costs—and the urgent need for reform.* Washington, DC: The Heritage Foundation. http://www.heritage.org/research/reports/2013/03/medicares-rising-costsand-the-urgent-need-for-reform (accessed July 25, 2013).

Morrison, R. S., J. D. Penrod, B. Cassel, M. Caust-Ellenbogen, A. Litke, L. Spragens, D. E. Meier. 2008. Cost savings associated with U.S. hospital palliative care consultation programs. *Archives of Internal Medicine* 168(16):1783-1790.

Morrison, R. S., J. Dietrich, S. Ladwig, T. Quill, J. Sacco, J. Tangeman, and D. E. Meier. 2011. Palliative care consultation teams cut hospital costs for Medicaid beneficiaries. *Health Affairs* 30(3):454-463.

Moses, H., D. H. M. Matheson, E. R. Dorsey, B. P. George, D. Sadoff, S. Yoshimura. 2013. The anatomy of health care in the United States. *Journal of the American Medical Association* 310(18):1947-1963.

MOWAA (Meals on Wheels Association of America). undated. *Federal cuts hurt our nation's most vulnerable seniors.* http://www.mowaa.org/document.doc?id=533 (accessed May 15, 2014).

National Commission on Fiscal Responsibility and Reform. 2010. *The moment of truth: Report of the National Commission on Fiscal Responsibility and Reform.* http://www.momentoftruthproject.org/sites/default/files/TheMomentofTruth12_1_2010.pdf (accessed February 7, 2014).

National Direct Service Workforce Resource Center. 2011. *Building capacity and coordinating support for family caregivers and the direct service workforce.* White Paper. http://www.medicaid.gov/Medicaid-CHIP-Program-Information/By-Topics/Long-Term-Services-and-Support/Workforce/Downloads/cms-leadership-summit-on-family-white-paper.pdf (accessed February 7, 2014).

National Health Policy Forum. 2013. *The basics: National spending for long-term services and supports (LTSS), 2011.* Washington, DC: The George Washington University. https://www.nhpf.org/uploads/announcements/Basics_LTSS_02-01-13.pdf (accessed July 30, 2013).

National PACE Association. 2014. *PACE in the states.* http://www.npaonline.org/website/download.asp?id=1741&title=PACE_in_the_States (accessed May 7, 2014).

Naylor, M. D., E. T. Kurtzman, D. C. Grabowski, C. Harrington, M. McClellan, and S. C. Reinhard. 2012. Unintended consequences of steps to cut readmissions and reform payment may threaten care of vulnerable older adults. *Health Affairs* 31(7):1623-1631.

NBER (National Bureau of Economic Research). undated. *The market for long-term care insurance.* http://www.nber.org/bah/winter05/w10989.html (accessed August 19, 2014).

Neuberg, G. W. 2009. The cost of end-of-life care: A new efficiency measure falls short of AHA/ACC standards. *Circulation: Cardiovascular Quality and Outcomes* 2:127-133.

NHPCO (National Hospice and Palliative Care Organization). 2009. *NHPCO facts and figures: Hospice care in America.* Alexandria, VA: NHPCO.

NHPCO. 2013. *NHPCO's facts and figures: Hospice care in America.* Alexandria, VA: NHPCO.

NHPCO. undated. *The Medicare hospice benefit.* http://www.nhpco.org/sites/default/files/public/communications/Outreach/The_Medicare_Hospice_Benefit.pdf (accessed November 27, 2013).

Norton, A. 2013. *Many Americans worry about cost of long-term care: Poll.* http://health.usnews.com/health-news/news/articles/2013/09/30/many-americans-worry-about-cost-of-long-term-care-poll (accessed December 3, 2013).

OECD (Organisation for Economic Co-operation and Development). 2014. *Social expenditure—aggregated data.* http://stats.oecd.org/Index.aspx?DataSetCode=SOCX_AGG (accessed August 19, 2014).

Parikh, R. B., R. A. Kirch, T. J. Smith, and J. S. Temel. 2013. Early specialty palliative care—translating data in oncology into practice. *New England Journal of Medicine* 369(24):2347-2351.

Patel, K., and S. Lieberman. 2013. *Taking stock of initial year one results for Pioneer ACOs.* http://healthaffairs.org/blog/2013/07/25/taking-stock-of-initial-year-one-results-for-pioneer-acos (accessed November 26, 2013).

Peikes, D., G. Peterson. R. S. Brown, S. Graff, and J. P. Lynch. 2012. How changes in Washington University's Medicare Coordinated Care Demonstration pilot ultimately achieved savings. *Health Affairs* 31(6):1216-1226.

Penrod, J. D., P. Deb, C. Dellenbaugh, J. F. Burgess, C. W. Zhu, C. L. Christiansen, C. A. Luhrs, T. Cortez, E. Livote, V. Allen, and R. S. Morrison. 2010. Hospital-based palliative care consultation: Effects on hospital cost. *Journal of Palliative Medicine* 13(8):973-979.

Porter, M. E., and E. O. Teisberg. 2006. *Redefining health care: Creating value-based competition on results.* Boston, MA: Harvard Business School Press.

Press, M. J., D. P. Scanlon, A. M. Ryan, J. Zhu, A. S. Navathe, J. N. Mittler, and K. G. Volpp. 2013. Limits of readmission rates in measuring hospital quality suggest the need for added metrics. *Health Affairs* 32(6):1083-1091.

Prigerson, H. G., and P. K. Maciejewski. 2012. Dartmouth Atlas: Putting end-of-life care on the map, but missing psychosocial detail. *Journal of Supportive Oncology* 10(1):25-28.

Rabow, M., E. Kvale, L. Barbour, J. B. Cassel, S. Cohen, V. Jackson, C. Luhrs, V. Nguyen, S. Rinaldi, D. Stevens, L. Spragens, and D. Weissman. 2013. Moving upstream: A review of the evidence of the impact of outpatient palliative care. *Journal of Palliative Medicine* 16(12):1540-1549.

Rau, J. 2013. Medicare lags in project to expand hospice. *Kaiser Health News*, May 9. http://www.kaiserhealthnews.org/stories/2013/may/09/medicare-delays-experiment-on-hospice-and-curative-care.aspx (accessed January 7, 2014).

Reinhard, S. C., C. Levine, and S. Samis. 2012. *Home alone: Family caregivers providing complex chronic care.* Washington, DC: AARP Public Policy Institute. http://www.aarp.org/content/dam/aarp/research/public_policy_institute/health/home-alone-family-caregivers-providing-complex-chronic-care-rev-AARP-ppi-health.pdf (accessed February 22, 2014).

Rhee, Y., H. B. Degenholtz, A. T. Lo Sasso, and L. L. Emanuel. 2009. Estimating the quantity and economic value of family caregiving for community-dwelling older persons in the last year of life. *Journal of the American Geriatrics Society* 57(9):1654-1659.

Rhodes, K. V., J. Bisgaier, C. C. Lawson, D. Soglin, S. Krug, and M. Van Haitsma. 2013. "Patients who can't get an appointment go to the ER": Access to specialty care for publicly insured children. *Annals of Emergency Medicine* 61(4):394-403.

Rich, E. C., T. Lake, and C. S. Valenzano. 2012. *Paying wisely: Reforming incentives to promote evidence-based decisions at the point of care.* Princeton, NJ: Mathematica Policy Research, Inc.

Rivlin, A. K. 2013. *Why reform Medicare? The President's and other bipartisan proposals to reform Medicare.* Testimony before the U.S. House of Representatives Committee on Ways and Means, Subcommittee on Health, May 21. http://www.brookings.edu/research/testimony/2013/05/21-bipartisan-medicare-reform-rivlin (accessed December 6, 2013).

Robillard, K. 2013. Report: New Alan Simpson-Erskine Bowles plan. *POLITICO*, February 19. http://www.politico.com/story/2013/02/report-new-simpson-bowles-plan-87769.html (accessed July 25, 2013).

Robison, J., N. Shugrue, M. Porter, R. Fortinsky, L. A. Curry. 2012. Transition from home care to nursing home: Unmet needs in a home-and community-based program for older adults. *Journal of Aging and Social Policy* 24(3):251-270.

RWJF (Robert Wood Johnson Foundation). 2004. *Community-state partnerships to improve end-of-life care: An RWJF national program.* Princeton, NJ: RWJF. http://www.rwjf.org/content/dam/farm/reports/program_results_reports/2004/rwjf69596 (accessed June 2, 2014).

Ryu, A. J., T. B. Gibson, M. R. McKellar, and M. E. Chernew. 2013. The slowdown in health care spending in 2009-11 reflected factors other than the weak economy and thus may persist. *Health Affairs* 32(5):835-840.

SAMHSA (Substance Abuse and Mental Health Services Administration). 2013. *Mental health parity and addiction equity.* http://beta.samhsa.gov/health-reform/parity (accessed December 5, 2013).

Schroeder, S. A., and W. Frist. 2013. Phasing out fee-for-service payment. *New England Journal of Medicine* 368(21):2029-2031.

Segal, M. 2011. Dual eligible beneficiaries and potentially avoidable hospitalizations. *Policy Insight Brief.* http://www.cms.gov/Research-Statistics-Data-and-Systems/Statistics-Trends-and-Reports/Insight-Briefs/downloads/PAHInsightBrief.pdf (accessed January 4, 2014).

Senate Commission on Long-Term Care. 2013. *Report to the Congress.* http://www.chhs.ca.gov/OLMDOC/Agenda%20Item%206-%20Commission%20on%20Long-Term%20Care-%20Final%20Report%209-26-13.pdf (accessed December 2, 2013).

Shier, G., M. Ginsburg, J. Howell, P. Volland, and R. Golden. 2013. Strong social support services, such as transportation and help for caregivers, can lead to lower health care use and costs. *Health Affairs* 32(3):544-550.

Skocpol, T. 2010. The political challenges that may undermine health reform. *Health Affairs* 29(7):1288-1292.

Smith, A. K., I. S. Cenzer, S. J. Knight, K. A. Puntillo, E. Widera, B. A. Williams, W. J. Boscardin, and K. E. Covinsky. 2010. The epidemiology of pain during the last two years of life. *Annals of Internal Medicine* 153(9):563-569.

Smith, A. K., E. McCarthy, E. Weber, I. S. Cenzer, J. Boscardin, J. Fisher, and K. Covinsky. 2012. Half of older Americans seen in emergency department in last month of life; most admitted to hospital, and many die there. *Health Affairs* 31(6):1277-1285.

Smith, S., A. Brick, S. O'Hara, and C. Normand. 2014. Evidence on the cost and cost-effectiveness of palliative care: A literature review. *Palliative Medicine* 28(2):130-150.

Spettell, C. M., W. S. Rawlins, R. Krakauer, J. Fernandes, M. E. S. Breton, W. Gowdy, S. Brodeur, M. MacCoy, and T. A. Brennan. 2009. A comprehensive case management program to improve palliative care. *Journal of Palliative Medicine* 12(9):827-832.

Spillman, B. 2012. Financial preparedness for long-term care needs in old age. In *Consumer knowledge and financial decisions: Lifespan perspectives*, edited by D. J. Lamdin. New York: Springer. Pp. 239-253.

Starks, H., S. Wang, S. Farber, D. A. Owens, and J. R. Curtis. 2013. Cost savings vary by length of stay for inpatients receiving palliative care consultation services. *Journal of Palliative Medicine* 16(10):1215-1220.

Steuerle, C. E., and C. Quakenbush. 2012. *Social Security and Medicare taxes and benefits over a lifetime: 2012 update*. Washington, DC: Urban Institute. http://www.urban.org/UploadedPDF/412660-Social-Security-and-Medicare-Taxes-and-Benefits-Over-a-Lifetime.pdf (accessed August 15, 2014).

Stukel, T. A., E. S. Fisher, D. E. Wennberg, D. A. Alter, D. J. Gottlieb, and M. J. Vermeulen. 2007. Analysis of observational studies in the presence of treatment selection bias: Effects of invasive cardiac management on AMI survival using propensity score and instrumental variable methods. *Journal of the American Medical Association* 297(3):278-285.

Temel, J. S., J. A. Greer, A. Muzikansky, E. R. Gallagher, S. Admane, V. A. Jackson, C. M. Dahlin, C. D. Blinderman, J. Jacobsen, W. F. Pirl, J. A. Billings, and T. J. Lynch. 2010. Early palliative care for patients with metastatic non small-cell lung cancer. *New England Journal of Medicine* 363(8):733-742.

Teno, J. M., P. L. Gozalo, J. P. Bynum, N. E. Leland, S. C. Miller, N. E. Morden, T. Scupp, D. C. Goodman, and V. Mor. 2013. Change in end-of-life care for Medicare beneficiaries: Site of death, place of care, and health care transitions in 2000, 2005, and 2009. *Journal of the American Medical Association* 309(5):470-477.

Thomas, K. S., and V. Mor. 2013. Providing more home-delivered meals is one way to keep older adults with low care needs out of nursing homes. *Health Affairs* 32(10):1796-1802.

Tilson, S., and G. J. Hoffman. 2012. *Addressing Medicare hospital readmissions* (R42546). Washington, DC: Congressional Research Service.

Topf, L., C. A. Robinson, and J. L. Bottorff. 2013. When a desired home death does not occur: The consequences of broken promises. *Journal of Palliative Medicine* 16(8):875-880.

Ubel, P. A., S. R. Berry, E. Nadler, C. M. Bell, M. A. Kozminski, J. A. Palmer, W. K. Evans, E. L. Strevel, and P. J. Neumann. 2012. In a survey, marked inconsistency in how oncologists judged value of high-cost cancer drugs in relation to gains in survival. *Health Affairs* 31(4):709-717.

Unroe, K. T., and D. E. Meier. 2013. Quality of hospice care for individuals with dementia. *Journal of the American Geriatrics Society* 61:1212-1214.

U.S. Burden of Disease Collaborators. 2013. The state of U.S. health, 1990-2010: Burden of diseases, injuries, and risk factors. *Journal of the American Medical Association* 310(6):591-608.

U.S. Department of Justice. 2013. *Hospice of Arizona and related entities pay $12 million to resolve False Claims Act allegations*. News release. March 20. http://www.justice.gov/opa/pr/2013/March/13-civ-326.html (accessed July 25, 2013).

Verdier, J. M., M. Au, and J. Gillooly. 2011. *Managing the care of dual eligible beneficiaries: A review of selected state programs and special needs plans*. Washington, DC: MedPAC.

Walke, L. M., A. L. Byers, R. McCorkle, T. R. Fried. 2006. Symptom assessment in community-dwelling older adults with advanced chronic disease. *Journal of Pain and Symptom Management* 31(1):31-37.

Weeks, W. B., S. S. Rauh, E. B. Wadsworth, and J. N. Weinstein. 2013. The unintended consequences of bundled payments. *Annals of Internal Medicine* 158(1):62-64.

Weiner, J. S., and S. A. Cole. 2004. Three principles to improve clinician communication for advance care planning: Overcoming emotional, cognitive, and skill barriers. *Journal of Palliative Medicine* 7(6):817-829.

Wennberg, J. E., E. S. Fisher, D. C. Goodman, and J. S. Skinner. 2008. *Tracking the care of patients with severe chronic illness: The Dartmouth Atlas of Health Care 2008.* Lebanon, NH: Dartmouth Medical School. http://www.dartmouth.edu/~jskinner/documents/2008_Chronic_Care_Atlas.pdf (accessed February 22, 2014).

Wiener, J. M., W. Anderson, G. Khatutsky, Y. Kaganova, J. O'Keeffe. 2013. *Medicaid spend down: New estimates and implications for long-term services and supports financing reform.* Final report. http://www.rti.org/pubs/rti_medicaid-spend-down_3-20-13_1.pdf (accessed February 1, 2014).

Wilensky, G. 2014. Developing a viable alternative to Medicare's physician payment strategy. *Health Affairs* 33(1):153-160.

Wright, A. A., and I. T. Katz. 2007. Letting go of the rope: Aggressive treatment, hospice care, and open access. *New England Journal of Medicine* 357(4):324-327. http://www.nejm.org/doi/full/10.1056/NEJMp078074 (accessed February 22, 2014).

Yabroff, K. R., J. S. Mandelblatt, and J. Ingham. 2004. The quality of medical care at the end-of-life in the USA: Existing barriers and examples of process and outcome measures. *Palliative Medicine* 18(3):202-216.

Yang, Y. T., and M. M. Mahon. 2011. Considerations of quality-adjusted life-year in palliative care for the terminally ill. Letter. *Journal of Palliative Medicine* 14(11):1197.

Yoon, J., M. E. Domino, E. C. Norton, G. S. Cuddeback, J. P. Morrissey. 2013. The impact of changes in psychiatric bed supply on jail use by persons with severe mental illness. *Journal of Mental Health Policy and Economics* 16(2):81-92.

Young, K., R. Garfield, M. Musumeci, L. Clemans-Cope, and E. Lawton. 2013. *Medicaid's role for dual eligible beneficiaries.* Menlo Park, CA: KFF, Kaiser Commission on Medicaid and the Uninsured. http://kaiserfamilyfoundation.files.wordpress.com/2013/08/7846-04-medicaids-role-for-dual-eligible-beneficiaries.pdf (accessed February 22, 2013).

6

Public Education and Engagement

The Institute of Medicine (IOM) report *Approaching Death* (IOM, 1997) suggests that "a continuing public discussion is essential to develop a better understanding of the modern experience of dying, the options available to dying patients and families, and the obligations of communities to those approaching death" (IOM, 1997, p. 270). The rationale for this conclusion is that creation of a more supportive environment for people near the end of life and their caregivers and families—one that would ensure that people die free of avoidable distress and "find the peace or meaning that is significant to them"—requires attitudes and actions that can be motivated, strengthened, and sustained through continued public discussion. The committee responsible for that report believed that public officials, professional organizations, religious leaders, and community groups should bear the greatest responsibility for encouraging this discussion and for providing the specific information needed by patients and families faced with advancing illness. The "whole-community model for care at the end of life" presented in the report elaborates on this idea, describing potential public education programs "that aim to improve general awareness, to encourage advance care planning, and to provide specific information at the time of need about resources for physical, emotional, spiritual, and practical caring at the end of life" (IOM, 1997, p. 117).

Likewise, the IOM report *When Children Die* (IOM, 2003) includes several recommendations concerning better communication about end-of-life issues in ways that encompass but are somewhat broader than the activities of advance care planning. The report calls for information programs and resources to help families advocate for appropriate care for

345

their children and themselves, and cites as a priority research on methods for improving communication and decision making.

In the years since these reports were issued, the need for culturally appropriate public education and engagement about end-of-life care continues, and it is manifest at several levels. The committee responsible for the present report perceives several fundamental needs:

- at the societal level, to build support for constructive public policy related to the organization and financing of end-of-life care and for institutional and provider practices that promote high-quality, compassionate, sustainable care;
- at the community/family level, to raise public awareness and elevate expectations about care options in the final phase of life, the needs of caregivers, and the hallmarks of high-quality culturally relevant and appropriate care; and
- at the individual level, to motivate and facilitate advance care planning and meaningful conversations with family, other caregivers, and clinicians about values, goals, and preferences for care.

The nation has a long way to go to meet these needs. Not only do most Americans lack knowledge about end-of-life care choices, which they will at some point so urgently need, but also the health community and other leaders have not fully and productively utilized public education and engagement strategies to make that knowledge available in ways that are meaningful and relevant to diverse population groups. Worse, statements of some leaders have misled the public on these issues (see the discussion of "death panels" later in this chapter).

The proportion of the U.S. population that is aged 65 and older has more than tripled over the past century, from 4 percent in 1900 to 14 percent in 2012 (Hobbs and Stoops, 2002; U.S. Census Bureau, 2013). Yet despite this aging of America, many have not thought about the kinds of health care decisions they will face as they age or develop serious chronic conditions. As time and technology progress, those decisions will become increasingly complicated.

In this chapter, the terms "public education" and "public engagement" have slightly different meanings. "Public education" generally refers to one-way communication with audiences through media, print, and online channels, while "public engagement" refers to efforts to involve audience members and may include two-way communication and interactivity. The former is passive; the latter is active and may merge into advocacy.

This chapter begins by providing an overview of the current state of public awareness about end-of-life care. Next is a description of events and activities that have led to a changing climate for discussion of death and dying and encouraged advance care planning. The chapter then explores considerations relevant to developing public education and engagement campaigns on end-of-life topics. This is followed by discussion of several controversial issues that have dominated recent public dialogue on death and dying. The chapter ends with the committee's recommendation on public education and engagement.

THE STATE OF PUBLIC KNOWLEDGE ABOUT END-OF-LIFE CARE

In describing a "learning health system," the IOM suggests that "the success of and innovations in healthcare delivery should depend on direct consumer engagement in the design of healthcare models and their aims" and that "citizen and patient engagement is central to taking advantage of advances in the personalization of care based on genetics, preferences, and circumstances" (IOM, 2011, p. 33). But what is known on consumer thinking on the delivery of care near the end of life and the readiness to engage around this topic? Recent polls provide an overall impression, and the views of individuals who addressed the committee in its three public sessions and the 578 people who submitted comments to the study's website provide some deeper perspectives (see Appendix C), although the full range of sociocultural perspectives may not be completely represented in public polls or public comments to the committee.

Trends in Fundamental Attitudes

In the 2011 Living Well at the End of Life poll of a national sample of U.S. adults, 86 percent of respondents said they thought end-of-life care should be "a top priority for the health care system in this country" (Regence Foundation and National Journal, 2011a, p. 2). More than 90 percent said hospice care should be a top priority, and once the term "palliative care" was explained, 96 percent said it should be a top priority as well.

A Pew Research Center (2013) survey of a nationally representative sample of nearly 2,000 adults provides recent information about Americans' attitudes regarding a number of aspects of end-of-life care, updating information from similar surveys conducted in 1990 and 2005. Since 1990, the proportion of adults who believe that "medical staff should do everything possible to save the life of a patient in all circumstances" has doubled. In part, this increase is due to a much smaller percentage who replied "don't know" to the same question in 2013. However, the percentage who believe "there are at least some circumstances where a patient should be allowed to die" also fell over the period, from 73 to 66 percent.

Nevertheless, many Americans say they would tell their own doctors to stop treatment so they could die:

- if they had an incurable disease and were suffering a great deal of pain (57 percent),
- if they had an incurable disease and were totally dependent on another for care (52 percent), or
- if they had an incurable disease and it were difficult to function in day-to-day life (46 percent).

These percentages have remained about the same since 1990, although at the same time, a growing number of people—35 percent, compared with 28 percent in 1990—say they would tell their doctor to do everything possible to keep them alive even if they were suffering a great deal of pain and there were no possibility of recovery. Again, much of this shift is due to people previously unsure.

On the other hand, 62 percent of those surveyed believe individuals have a moral right to end their own lives if they are suffering great pain with no hope of improvement—a 7 percent increase from 1990. Substantial numbers also believe people have the right to commit suicide if they have an incurable disease (56 percent), when they are ready to die and living has become a burden (38 percent), or when their care is an extremely heavy burden on the family (32 percent). In this survey, the public was equally divided on the question of whether physicians should be allowed to prescribe a lethal drug to assist a person seeking suicide.

Although the majority of black Protestants (61 percent) and Hispanic Catholics (57 percent) would ask their doctors to "do everything possible" to keep them alive even if they were suffering great pain and had no hope of improvement, large numbers of both groups (39 percent and 43 percent, respectively) feel differently or have not decided. This finding underscores the point made in Chapter 3 that clinicians cannot make assumptions about patients' beliefs and preferences based on race, ethnicity, religion, or culture. They must ask.

Understanding of Care Choices

Basic Terminology

Expecting people to understand what they are reading and hearing about end-of-life care or to have meaningful conversations about the subject presumes a common vocabulary. This report emphasizes the importance of high-quality palliative care, but 78 percent of Americans responding to a 2011 survey did not know what palliative care is (CAPC, 2011), and in a more recent survey, 83 percent said they had not heard of it (CHCF, 2012).

Even medical professionals conflate "palliative care" with "end-of-life care," when in fact palliative care can be appropriate at any stage of a serious illness when active steps are needed to reduce pain and symptoms and improve quality of life (CAPC, 2011). Nor do clinicians always correctly distinguish between "palliative care" and "hospice," the latter being a model for delivering palliative services.

In this report, the committee also repeatedly refers to the importance of family caregivers. When people were asked what term they would use to describe "loved ones who care for [people] at the end of their lives," however, nearly half of respondents did not have a term for that role, one-quarter said "family," and one-quarter responded "caregiver" or "caretaker" (Calabrese-Eck, 2013).

In Chapter 3, the committee strongly endorses the need for people to name a health care agent. Because this role has numerous titles in state law and in practice—including, for example, "agent," "surrogate," and "health care power of attorney"—confusion is inevitable. When people were asked what term they would use to refer to the "person they designate to make healthcare decisions on their behalf," 30 percent of respondents did not know what to call such a person, 32 percent said "family," 15 percent "power of attorney," 11 percent "beneficiary/executor" (perhaps recognizing this person has legal authority), and 10 percent "caregiver" (Calabrese-Eck, 2013).

Terminology matters when it comes to controversial end-of-life issues as well. While a Gallup survey conducted in May 2013 found that only 51 percent of respondents supported doctors' helping a terminally ill patient "commit suicide" if requested by the patient, 70 percent supported such a policy—a percentage similar to that found in 1990—when the practice was described as allowing doctors to "end a (terminally ill) patient's life by some painless means" if requested. Recognizing that the term "assisted suicide" is problematic, advocates for this policy often term it "physician aid in dying"; in Oregon, which was the first state to allow the practice through a 1994 ballot initiative,[1] and elsewhere, it is sometimes called "death with dignity" (Levine, 2014). Gallup's question using the "painless means" wording also specified that both patient and family requested it, whereas the "assisted suicide" question specified only the patient's requesting it (Saad, 2013).

In short, the foundation for effective communication is not laid, and "the terminology that the health care system uses and the way information is presented is often not aligned with what consumers use and seek" (C-TAC, 2014, p. 2).

---

[1] Oregon Death with Dignity Act, OR. REV. STAT. §§ 127.800-127.995 (2006).

Concerns About Care

Americans have two consistent concerns about care near the end of life that are reflected in a number of recent polls—the cost of care and being a burden on their families:

- Asked what would concern them if they or a family member became seriously ill, Americans ranked the potential cost of treatment as their highest concern (overall ranking 8.1 on a 10-point scale) (Regence Foundation and National Journal, 2011a).
- In a 2011 poll, Californians were asked about important concerns at the end of life, and the top concern was making sure the family was not burdened financially by care (67 percent) (CHCF, 2012).
- In the same survey, 60 percent of respondents (68 percent of African American respondents) said it was extremely important to them to make sure their family is not burdened by difficult decisions about their care.

The public's concerns about costs and impacts on the family are well founded, as discussed in other chapters of this report.

Expression of Individual Preferences

The 2013 Pew survey referenced above found that 37 percent of Americans say they have given a great deal of thought and 35 percent say they have given some thought to their preferences regarding medical treatment near the end of life; among those aged 75 and older, one-quarter have given the issue little or no thought. Among people who say they have given the issue considerable thought, most (88 percent) have captured their preferences either in writing or in conversation with others. Americans who are older, white, and have more education or higher incomes are more likely to have put their wishes in writing. (Chapter 3 reviews this literature in more detail.)

Nevertheless, among Americans aged 65 and older, more report talking with their children about what to do with family belongings (76 percent) than about how to handle their medical care if they can no longer make their own decisions (63 percent) or can no longer live independently (55 percent). Even fewer adult children of older parents say the discussion about medical care decision making has occurred (57 percent) (Pew Research Center, 2009).

If people find the topic of care preferences difficult to discuss with family members, discussion with their health care providers appears to be no easier. Research conducted in the U.S. population in general (not specifically among those with serious advanced illnesses) has found that most (8 in 10) want their clinician to listen to them and to have the full truth about their diagnosis; yet only 6 in 10 say that their provider listens to them, and fewer than half say their provider asks about their goals and concerns for their health and health care (Alston et al., 2012). And although the cost of health care is of concern to patients with serious illnesses, few physicians (16 percent) report having any education or training regarding financial issues and how to discuss them (Regence Foundation and National Journal, 2011b).

According to Alston and colleagues (2012, p. 7), "Unsurprisingly, 30 percent of people said they 'very often' get health information from a source other than their health care provider. The most common sources were their spouse or partner (15 percent), the Internet (9 percent), and a friend or family member who works in health care (6 percent)." Likewise, with respect to palliative and end-of-life care in particular, people said they received most of their information from family members and friends (49 percent) (Regence Foundation and National Journal, 2011a). In this study, only about one-third of respondents said they received such information most often from their doctor or health care provider or the news media, and 45 percent said they received very little or no such information from their physician. When asked how much they trusted the information they received, respondents gave high ratings to information that came from doctors or other health care providers (76 percent) and from family and friends (69 percent). The information that came from the news media received high trust ratings from only 17 percent of respondents.

Surveys indicate that most people (70-80 percent) want a patient experience that includes deep engagement in shared decision making; however, a substantial gap exists between what people want and what they receive. Those who do become more engaged report a better experience (Alston et al., 2012). Written public testimony gathered for this study through an on-line questionnaire (see Appendix C) indicates the often poor communication patients and families have with clinicians. People feel that explanations are rushed, issues are not explained, choices are not understood, and clinicians do not listen. Good communication, by contrast, is greatly appreciated. The way to establish good communication, one caregiver said, is to "ask patients and families what *they* want," which is a message of Chapter 3.

Experts in health care communication believe a combination of three elements—clinician expertise, patient and family goals and concerns, and medical evidence[2]—is necessary for truly informed health care decisions, and in general, Americans strongly value all three (Alston et al., 2012). What is needed is to mobilize that general support in the specific context

---

[2]Shortcomings in the U.S. population with respect to literacy and health literacy, which are essential to the interpretation of medical evidence, are discussed in Chapter 3.

of advanced illness. Death and dying can be a difficult, emotional issue for both public engagement and private discussion. For most people, until a family member is actually facing a serious illness, interest is just too low, the psychological barriers are too high, and preoccupation with the demands of daily life is a ready excuse not to engage. At least in the short term, that reluctance must be acknowledged and societal means found to help people understand that, in most instances, good information is available when they want it.

Public education and engagement efforts should aim to normalize difficult conversations and help people from diverse communities acquire the information and skills needed to participate meaningfully in those conversations. As a result, more people might obtain the care they want and need as they near the end of life.

THE CHANGING CLIMATE FOR DISCUSSION OF DEATH AND DYING

Events and activities since 1997 have changed the climate for discussions of death and dying, and the topic is not the taboo it was a few decades ago. As more people in the baby boom generation reach age 65—some 10,000 a day until 2030 (Pew Research Center, 2010)—public interest in and acceptance of information on death and dying will likely increase. As previously noted, the Pew Research Center (2013) found that the proportion of surveyed Americans indicating that they have given a great deal of thought to their end-of-life wishes was 37 percent in 2013, up from 28 percent in 1990. This rising interest presents opportunities for reaching people more effectively with tailored information directed at those who access different media (or no media at all), those who rely on languages other than English, and those for whom lay educators (for example, *promotoras*) may be the most effective and culturally appropriate educational approach, as well as other means to reach those currently underserved.

A number of significant national efforts have encouraged more effective advance care planning and "having the conversation" and sought to improve end-of-life care more generally. National organizations, including the National Hospice and Palliative Care Organization, the Center to Advance Palliative Care, several insurers, private foundations, and others, have attempted to raise public awareness about what constitutes good end-of-life care and how people can go about obtaining it.

In recent years, end-of-life experiences have been the subject of numerous family memoirs. Mitch Albom's 1997 book *Tuesdays with Morrie* has sold more than 14 million copies. Websites have been created to facilitate care planning conversations (for example, The Conversation Project, DeathWise, Aging with Dignity and *Five Wishes*, and Engage with Grace), organize discussions on end-of-life topics (for example, Death Cafe, Death over Dinner),[3] and support community-level advocacy (for example, Project Compassion). Some focus on medical decisions, some discuss relationships, and some also cover financial issues. Major movies, television series such as Showtime's 2013 *Time of Death*, and individual episodes of dramatic programs have shown greater realism with respect to death and dying. Local and national documentaries (notably Bill Moyers' PBS series *On Our Own Terms*) have covered the topic extensively, providing tools for individual action and community engagement and serving as the impetus for activities in hundreds of communities nationwide (RWJF, 2004a). Box 6-1 lists these and other examples of recent efforts to bring attention to end-of-life issues.

The written public testimony gathered for this study supports public education initiatives that would help normalize discussions of death and dying (see Appendix C). Comments encourage both television advertising campaigns and improvements in the relevant content of entertainment programming (such as more realistic portrayals of the likely outcome of resuscitation). Projects such as Hollywood Health and Society at the University of Southern California's Annenberg School for Communication and Journalism advise on a range of health topics. The Writers Project of the Robert Wood Johnson Foundation's Last Acts initiative worked with television writers and producers specifically on death and dying issues, with the goal of increasing the realism of depictions of end-of-life decision making and promoting understanding of palliative care (Hollywood Health and Society, 2014; RWJF, 2004b).

The idea that American society can have a national conversation about death and dying is supported by the confluence of several social forces (Novelli, 2013):

- Many Americans have seen how the current health care system has treated their parents and other family members and do not want that for themselves. This activated consumer generation is likely to be less passive about accepting care that violates their own wishes.
- Many people have stories about a death gone wrong, and increasingly, people are sharing those stories. This shared yet intensely private experience is common to people of all racial, ethnic, religious, social, political, educational, and occupational groups.

---

[3] "Discussing end-of-life issues over dinner" coverage at http://www.aarp.org/money/investing/info-10-2013/death-dinner-parties-discuss-end-of-life.html?sf19245178=1 (accessed December 17, 2014).

BOX 6-1
Examples of Recent Efforts to Bring Attention
to End-of-Life Dilemmas and Approaches

General Awareness Movements and Advance Care Planning
   The Conversation Project: http://theconversationproject.org
   DeathWise: https://www.deathwise.org
   Engage with Grace: http://www.engagewithgrace.org
   Death Cafe: http://www.deathcafe.com
   Death over Dinner: http://www.deathoverdinner.org;
      http://blog.tedmed.com/?tag=death-over-dinner
   Project Compassion: http://project-compassion.org
   Aging with Dignity and *Five Wishes*: http://agingwithdignity.org;
      http://www.agingwithdignity.org/five-wishes.php
   Community Conversations on Compassionate Care (Compassion and
      Support): https://www.compassionandsupport.org
   National Healthcare Decisions Day: http://www.nhdd.org
   Life Before Death: The Lien Foundation: http://www.lifebeforedeath.com/
      index.shtml
   Before I Die: http://beforeidie.cc
   Death Clock: http://www.deathclock.com

Films and Television Series
   Time of Death: http://www.sho.com/sho/time-of-death/home
   On Our Own Terms: http://www.pbs.org/wnet/onourownterms
   Honoring Choices Minnesota: http://www.honoringchoices.org
   A Good Day to Die: http://thediemovie.wordpress.com
   Ways to Live Forever: http://trailers.apple.com/trailers/independent/
      waystoliveforever
   How to Die in Oregon: http://www.howtodieinoregon.com/trailer.html
   Amour (Academy Award Winner, Best Foreign Language Film):
      http://www.sonyclassics.com/amour

- Leadership in public education is emerging at the local level in communities around the country and nationally through coalitions and
  collaborations.[4]

Features of several continuing public education efforts focused on the
issue of advance care planning are provided in Table 6-1.

---

[4]Coalitions and organizations currently participating in public education efforts include
National Healthcare Decisions Day and the National Alliance for Caregiving, plus numerous
independent organizations, such as the Caregiver Action Network, Compassionate Friends,
and the Informed Medical Decisions Foundation.

CONSIDERATIONS FOR PUBLIC EDUCATION AND ENGAGEMENT CAMPAIGNS

Several recommendations presented in this report might be considered for inclusion in public education and engagement initiatives. Such efforts are likely to be more successful if the end-of-life care topic pursued is highly relevant to an organization's mission and reflects the interests of the audiences that organization serves. For example, libraries might create reading lists or host book discussion groups on end-of-life topics, employers might review financial and end-of-life planning with employees nearing retirement, and senior centers might be concerned with raising awareness of caregiver issues. Coalitions of organizations might manage a broader set of topics and recruit members well positioned to address them.

The following subsections provide a brief review of major considerations entailed in developing a public education and engagement campaign. These considerations—sponsorship, audiences, messages, channels, and evaluation—are adaptable to a variety of organizations and themes. They can be understood in terms of either communications or social marketing[5] (audience versus target market, for example).

Sponsorship

Especially with topics as sensitive as advance care planning and end-of-life care, the choice of a credible and trustworthy entity to sponsor a public education and engagement effort is critical. In many communities, coalitions of organizations have come together to sponsor a project, bringing in more people and providing assurance that the effort is broad based.

As reviewed in Chapter 1, a great many stakeholder groups have a professional or civic interest in end-of-life issues. They include health and social services professionals, clergy, volunteers, and others who provide direct care and counseling; those who manage health care institutions and programs, run public and private insurance programs, and advocate for better care; state and federal policy makers; and business executives and union leaders. Health care systems and voluntary health organizations may be able to deliver credible messages, but sponsorship and participation in coalitions are often broader than that. Other organizations—such as labor unions, religious organizations, public health agencies, and insurers—interested in the health and welfare of their members or the community also may become interested. A sponsor or coalition partner can be as large as a

---

[5]Social marketing is the application of marketing principles to issues and causes involving personal behavior (antismoking campaigns, for example) or community betterment (promoting HIV/AIDS awareness, for example) (Grier and Bryant, 2005; Walsh et al., 1993).

TABLE 6-1 Features of Selected Organizations' Public Awareness and Engagement Activities Related to Advance Care Planning

Feature	Honoring Choices Minnesota[a]	Aging with Dignity and Five Wishes[b]	The Conversation Project[c]	Community Conversations on Compassionate Care (CCCC)[d]	National Healthcare Decisions Day Initiative (NHDD)[e]
Purpose	Encourage discussions of end-of-life care preferences	Improve how people talk about and plan for end-of-life care	Ensure that end-of-life care wishes are expressed and respected	Motivate advance care planning discussions and completion of advance directives	Inspire, educate and empower the public and providers about the importance of advance care planning
Target audience	Anyone over age 18	All adults, especially those who would be "champions" of the message		Anyone over age 18	General public and health care providers
Time frame	2008-present	1997-present	2012-present	2002-present	2008-present
Outreach methods	Volunteers; media; partnerships with the faith community, multicultural groups, health and human services providers	Mass media, word of mouth, professional associations, champions, translation of the Five Wishes advance directive into 27 languages	National media campaign, website, social media, traditional media, entertainment industry, employers, faith community	Volunteer coalition; employer outreach; dissemination of educational tools through workshops, print, video, Internet, and broadcast and social media	Public events, website, email, social media

Selected progress measures	Six documentaries broadcast 28 times to 163,833 households; nearly 50,000 page views of Honoring Choices website; project conducts awareness surveys, tracks completion of advance directives	More than 20 million *Five Wishes* documents distributed; 30,000 organizations help distribute	More than 50,000 downloads of materials, which include a Conversation Starter Kit and a guide on how to talk to one's doctor	One million printed advance care planning booklets, active website; 40-60 percent of target populations have health care proxies	Participation by more than 110 national organizations, 1,200 state and local organizations, and 1.7 million members of the general public; 37 states with dedicated state liaisons; more than 29,000 advance directives completed on NHDDs (April 16) between 2008 and 2013
Budget	First 3 years: $1.8 million (including documentary production); core: $350,000/year	First 5 years: $1 million; subsequently self-sustaining			

SOURCES:

*a*Personal communication, S. Schettle, Twin Cities Medical Society and Honoring Choices Minnesota, December 5, 2013.
*b*Personal communication, P. Malley, Aging With Dignity, December 6, 2013.
*c*Personal communication, H. Warshaw, The Conversation Project, December 7, 2013.
*d*CCCC, 2008, 2014; Personal communication, P. Bomba, Community Conversations on Compassionate Care, February 2, 2014.
*e*Personal communication, N. A. Kottkamp, National Healthcare Decisions Day, December 3, 2013.

national mental health organization or as small as one of its local chapters, a national religious body or an individual congregation.

Excellus BlueCross BlueShield, serving Upstate New York, has supported a Community-Wide End-of-Life/Palliative Care Initiative since 2001 that engages a broad array of professionals, consumers, and other collaborators from diverse backgrounds. This collaboration has achieved heightened awareness of the value of advance care planning and greatly increased the percentage of people who have completed health care proxies (through its Community Conversations on Compassionate Care Program); has implemented Medical Orders for Life-Sustaining Treatment (MOLST) (New York's Physician Orders for Life-Sustaining Treatment [POLST] paradigm initiative) and eMOLST programs, described in Chapter 3; has led regional and statewide discussions and encouraged improved policies related to high-quality palliative and end-of-life care, including pain management and use of feeding tubes; has engaged in additional community-wide education efforts; and has conducted a number of surveys to establish baseline data and determine progress toward measurable goals (CCCC, 2014).

Audiences

Different end-of-life messages are relevant to different audiences, and there are various ways to segment audiences for the purpose of crafting messages with maximum appeal. The general rule of thumb in audience segmentation is to have relevant sameness within groups and relevant differences between groups (Andreason, 1995; Noar, 2006). Policy makers and health care leaders might respond to one message, whereas members of racial and ethnic minority groups might be interested in another; likewise, older and younger adults would likely respond to different messages.

Clinician audiences are a vital complement to public audiences. Opportunities for engagement exist within the clinical community. For example, clinicians who believe health professions schools should do a better job of teaching about palliative care might work through a professional group—and possibly even attempt to engage segments of the public—to advocate for increased palliative care training. Likewise, senior centers, employer groups, and other entities might want to tie messages for caregivers to programs aimed at healthy living, retiree benefits, and so on.

Audiences defined as the "general public" or "all Americans 65 and older" are usually too diffuse to be maximally useful in campaign planning. The more carefully a market can be segmented into different groups, with different messages and appropriate media for each, the more likely the members of those groups are to respond as desired (Andreasen, 1995;

Grier and Bryant, 2005; Walsh et al., 1993). Given the usual limited funding for educational and engagement efforts, audience segments can be prioritized by importance or likelihood of response. Thus, "segmentation can help managers achieve both efficiency and effectiveness" (Andreasen, 1995, p. 177).

Audiences can be segmented by socioeconomic strata, by role (e.g., caregivers, clergy), by their involvement with the issue, and in many other ways. For example, research has shown that people who have had a recent hospitalization or who have been a caregiver for someone who recently died are particularly receptive to engaging in advance care planning (Carr and Khodyakov, 2007). They would be a natural audience for messages on that topic.

Timing may be important in identifying a target audience. The point at which a serious illness is diagnosed may be the most critical period of attention and focus for individuals who are ill and their families, and the time when they are most in need of useful information. People in this audience may be seeking relatively in-depth information about what to expect as their illness progresses and how to respond to increasing care requirements.

An additional consideration is whether and how to target by behavior. People who actively seek out health information—for example, on the Internet—might constitute a discrete audience segment. Or people may reach a stage of behavior change that prompts them to seek information (the "stages of change" decision-making model is described in Chapter 3). Even within audience groups, there may be significant subaudiences. Online information seekers may be inclined to view their doctors as collaborators to whom they can bring relevant health care information for review and follow-up, or they may make use of the information independently. Making good use of online information sources requires that people "have skills to effectively seek out the desired information, evaluate it, and then apply the information they find toward solving their health problems" (IOM, 2009, p. 10). Almost 60 percent of the very large number of Internet users who seek out online health information say they have used it in making health decisions, and almost 40 percent say they have used it to change the way they manage a chronic condition or pain (Fox, 2006). Nevertheless, information provided in Chapter 3 about the low level of health literacy raises some question as to whether people can use the information they find in a way most useful to them. By contrast, people who have difficulty finding answers to their health questions or understanding complex issues may prefer to rely on their physicians to provide them with information. Although both groups are active information seekers, they differ in where they look for information, the way they relate to physicians, and their demographic characteristics.[6]

Messages

Not until the target audiences have been chosen and some research on their current views on relevant themes has been conducted can the work of crafting specific messages begin. A number of past public engagement campaigns around end-of-life issues have focused on the concept of consumer/patient "control of your destiny" and the ability to "make your own decisions on your own terms" (for example, the public engagement campaign that accompanied Bill Moyers' public television series *On Our Own Terms* in 2000). Research on the efficacy and outcomes of this messaging has been insufficient to allow assessment of audience response to this specific approach. Message development often proceeds in stages, beginning with in-depth personal interviews or focus groups, to gain a deeper understanding of the views held on a subject by members of a target audience. Those insights can be part of the basis for survey questionnaires administered to larger groups to learn what aspects of an issue are most meaningful. Survey responses can be either programmed (forced choice) or open-ended. Open-ended comments are another rich source of opinion data.

Several recent end-of-life campaigns—aided by the ability to make resources available via the Web—are providing much more in the way of supporting materials to back up their basic messages (see Box 6-1 and Table 6-1). An example is The Conversation Project, discussed in Chapter 3, whose basic theme is that people need to talk about the important but difficult topic of end-of-life care. Its message is the provocative "Have you had the conversation?" It supports that message by providing a Conversation Starter Kit and personal stories that can help normalize the discussion of the topic (Bisognano and Goodman, 2013). Lately, The Conversation Project has extended its message to emphasize the importance of conversations with clinicians as well.

Channels

Healthy People 2020, the federal government's initiative to promote disease prevention and health promotion goals for the nation, acknowl-

---

[6]From Porter Novelli's 2013 ConsumerStyles survey. 2013 ConsumerStyles is an online survey (administered through GfK's KnowledgePanel®) among a representative sample of 6,717 U.S. adults, fielded March 29 to April 16, 2013. ConsumerStyles is Porter Novelli's tri-annual survey that tracks Americans' attitudes, lifestyle values, purchasing behaviors, technology use, and traditional and social media habits.

edges the important role of communications media in forming public views on health and disease. According to the U.S. Department of Health and Human Services (HHS, 2013), "Health communication and health information technology (IT) are central to health care, public health, and the way our society views health." Information on health and medical care is widely available through traditional print and broadcast outlets, as well as through the Internet and social media, with more than 70 percent of Americans using the Internet to acquire health information (Fox and Duggan, 2013). Typical mass media campaigns are only one way to reach and influence key target audiences on end-of-life topics. Communicating through intermediaries, such as faith communities, health care providers, and consumer affinity groups, is another approach. The Robert Wood Johnson Foundation's 10-year Last Acts campaign was built on a model of involving trusted organizations as "message carriers," and by its close, organizations of all sizes were participating and sharing information with their constituents (Patrizi et al., 2011). Social media can be useful channels as well, especially when they engage people who feel connected to the message source. Offering high-quality websites at moments of readiness is another potentially useful strategy.

Entertainment television has not been overlooked as a vehicle for carrying health-related messages (Singhal and Rogers, 2004), including messages about death and dying. Both long story arcs—such as the illness and death of Dr. Mark Greene at the end of *E.R.*'s eighth season—and specific episodes of a program (e.g., *N.Y.P.D. Blue*, *Gideon's Crossing*) have portrayed dilemmas and decisions that arise at the end of life. Some audience members who would never watch a documentary or attend a lecture on the topic are thereby exposed to valuable information (and sometimes misinformation). Social modeling theories suggest that audiences learn from fictional characters with whom they identify, making them more likely to emulate behavior that has positive outcomes and avoid behavior that has negative outcomes (Singhal and Rogers, 2004).

Evaluation

Evaluation is essential for campaigns to assess progress, make course corrections, and achieve meaningful results. Finding campaigns that have been well evaluated is difficult, however, and many of those that have been evaluated tackle topics that are so different from end-of-life care that comparisons may be elusive. The 2013 Pew Research Center survey cited earlier provides baseline data on consumer awareness, attitudes, and behavior regarding a number of issues related to advanced illness and end of life. Such national baseline information is a good starting point and with some refinement could be used to gauge the effectiveness of public awareness and engagement initiatives at the state or local level. Organizations that sponsor end-of-life public education and engagement initiatives might be able to adopt at least some of these tracking survey questions for their projects for both program improvement and accountability purposes, as well as the ability to compare their project's results with national trends. See Annex 6-1 at the end of this chapter for brief descriptions of selected health-related public information and engagement campaigns and their results.

CONTROVERSIAL ISSUES

Widely publicized controversies related to end-of-life care and dying are nothing new. These topics are perennial flashpoints for conflicts of values, particularly in a heterogeneous nation such as the United States. People's views on serious illness and the end of life, bereavement and loss, and the duties of caregivers are deeply held and vary across many societal dimensions (see Chapter 3), as well as individuals of similar backgrounds. These are vital public issues as well, and while people may differ in their opinions about them, dissemination of relevant facts and evidence will enable those opinions to be based, insofar as possible, on the facts as they are known and a candid assessment of their limits.

This section examines several contentious issues related to end of life that are certain to recur. Because their recurrence can be foreseen, stakeholders should be prepared and should work with like-minded individuals and groups to coordinate their messages and campaign aggressively and effectively to promote an evidence-based and factual approach to these topics. Moreover, concern about spurious attacks should not deter advocates of person-centered, family-oriented care from responsible public engagement, from making policy recommendations, or from advocacy.

Physician-Assisted Suicide

Supporters refer to the ethical principle of autonomy in advocating state laws and policies to allow physician-assisted suicide. However, many clinicians and others believe the practice violates a different fundamental principle: "Do no harm."

Opposition to public policy support for physician-assisted suicide goes beyond religious objections. Allowing people "a choice" of whether to end their lives may be fraught with opportunities for coercion and disruption of patients' trust absent vigorous attempts to ensure that all Americans have access to high-quality care that would meet complex needs near the end of life, as well as systemic changes that would lessen burdens (financial and otherwise) on family members. As the American Geriatrics Society (AGS) stated in its 1996 Supreme Court *amicus* brief in the case of *Vacco v. Quill*,

"The health care available to the terminally ill may be the most important factor influencing the care provided and may result in requests for
[physician-assisted suicide] that could be avoided if appropriate care were
available. . . . The AGS has been opposed to legalizing [physician-assisted
suicide] or physician involvement in euthanasia, primarily on the grounds
that our frail elderly patients are especially vulnerable to social coercion
and that the well-being of those who are old and sick is not being carefully
considered" (Lynn et al., 1997, pp. 497-499).

In 1997, the U.S. Supreme Court ruled that assisted suicide is not a
constitutionally protected right, although it did not bar states from formulating their own statutes to address it, and five now allow it under state law
or court authorization.[7] Legislatures in Oregon, Vermont, and Washington
have enacted laws that permit state residents to end their lives voluntarily
with a lethal dose of medication prescribed by a physician if they are "terminally ill" (Oregon), have a "terminal condition" (Vermont), or have a
life expectancy of less than 6 months (Washington).[8] During 2013, similar
legislation was introduced in at least six states, and proposals to specifically
outlaw the practice were introduced in two states. In Montana, legislation
was proposed on both sides of the question, and the state Supreme Court
ruled that physicians who help a person end his or her own life voluntarily
will not be subject to trial for homicide.[9] In early 2014, a New Mexico
judge ruled that terminally ill, mentally competent patients have the right
to "aid in dying" under the state constitution.[10] If upheld, that decision
may apply statewide. Continuing efforts to revise state laws guarantee that
this controversial issue will be recurrent, at least locally if not nationally
(Eckholm, 2014).

Withholding and Withdrawal of Life Support

Over the years, the issue of withholding and withdrawal (especially) of
life support has stimulated contentious public debates and led to numerous changes in law and policy. These debates have frequently focused on
women or minorities (Holloway, 2011). Many of their cases have prompted
unprecedented public intervention in what would ordinarily be considered
private family decisions.

The most widely publicized, and protracted, legal cases centered around
three young women who left no advance directives—Karen Ann Quinlan,

---

[7]*Washington v. Glucksberg*, 521 U.S. 702 (1997); *Vacco v. Quill*, 521 U.S. 793 (1997).

[8]Oregon Death with Dignity Act, OR. REV. STAT §§ 127.800-995, 1997; Washington
Death with Dignity Act, R.C.W. 70.245, 2009; Vermont Patient Choice and Control at the
End of Life Act, Act 39, 18 V.S.A. Chapter 113 (2013).

[9]*Baxter v. Montana*, 224 P.3d 1211 (Mont. 2009).

[10]*Morris v. Brandenberg*, D-202-CV-2012-02909 (N.M. 2d Jud. Dist., Jan. 13, 2014).

Nancy Beth Cruzan, and Teresa Marie Schiavo. Their sudden, unexpected, and permanent unconsciousness (from different causes) ignited strident public debates.[11] In each instance, the courts eventually decided that treatment could be withdrawn, but years of legal wrangling devastated family members and health care team members. According to Holloway (2011, p. 147), "When the body belongs to a woman or a member of a racial or ethnic minority, the privacy [that legal] protections ordinarily grant is already at risk." The notoriety of such cases may prompt people to consider their own end-of-life preferences.[12]

As of early 2014, two cases involving clashes over cessation of treatment of individuals declared brain dead again received considerable media attention. One in California involved an African American child whose family wanted her to continue receiving treatment (Debolt, 2014). The other was a Latino woman whose family and husband wanted life support withdrawn, but because she was pregnant, Texas state law was believed to prohibit it (Hellerman et al., 2014). In the latter case, after 2 months of public discussion, a judge ruled the Texas law was being misapplied and ordered an end to treatment. As of June 2014, the child in California had been kept alive on life support for 6 months after being declared brain dead (Debolt, 2014). As technology improves the ability to keep body systems functioning even without mental function, more such cases can be expected.

Distributive Justice and Futile Care

As discussed in previous chapters, when patients and families have a clear understanding of the course of a terminal illness, the consequences and experience of cure-oriented versus palliative care, and the quality of life each produces, most choose the palliative approach. A minority of patients nevertheless do want aggressive care, and at present, they usually receive it. As a result, some question whether patients should be entitled to medical interventions that hold no realistic promise of extending life or improving or maintaining quality of life. Because many critical care services are expensive, is this the best way to spend health care dollars?

The principle of autonomy would suggest that individuals should receive whatever services they want. However, the amount of money society

---

[11]For a fuller legal and historical review of these cases, see Fine (2005) and Johnson (2009).

[12]An assessment of 117 individuals aged 50 and older enrolled in an ongoing advance directive study during the period of the Schiavo controversy found that 92 percent had heard about the case and had taken one or more actions as a result: had become more certain about their choices (61 percent), talked to their family or friends about what they would want in a similar situation (66 percent), decided to complete an advance directive (37 percent), discussed advance care planning with their physician (8 percent), and/or completed an advance directive (3 percent) (Sudore et al., 2008).

has available to spend on health care is not infinite. There are trade-offs and opportunity costs, as spending on truly futile health care services may deprive other people of important benefits, and services that provide the patient no benefit may be thought of as too expensive regardless of their cost (Meisel, 2008).

Other countries have faced this issue and come to different conclusions, while U.S. policy makers have strictly avoided any measures—such as basing reimbursement policy on comparative effectiveness assessments—that might have the effect of limiting care (Satvat and Leight, 2011). Ironically, economists and policy analysts readily acknowledge that allocation decisions are actually common in the United States, based mainly on ability to pay; they are merely implicit and hidden, rather than explicit, transparent, and potentially more fair (Lauridsen et al., 2007; Swanson, 2009).

Tensions surrounding this issue might be alleviated if research continued to show that receiving more medical interventions near the end of life does not produce better outcomes in terms of longevity or quality of life, as other chapters of this report have documented. The nation can no longer pretend that there is no upper limit on what it can afford, and the debate will continue to be divisive if concern about health care costs results in some version of a cap on spending.

Making Dying Visible

Given Americans' acknowledged reluctance to discuss dying, an unlikely controversy arose in early 2014 about the use of social media to discuss the consequences of a serious illness. Lisa Bonchek Adams is an active user of social media—Facebook, Twitter, and her blog[13]—which she uses to talk about her metastatic breast cancer and coping with illness and grief and to urge her online followers to have cancer screenings. Although her illness is advanced and likely will eventually be the cause of her death, she was not dying at the time the controversy erupted.

Adams' use of social media to discuss her disease was questioned in separate opinion pieces in both *The Guardian* and *The New York Times* by writers who found that her public discussion of her illness was unseemly ("dying out loud") and who appeared to counsel passive acceptance as a more humane (and cheaper) alternative (Keller, 2014). People who follow Adams' posts, and Adams herself, were quick to point out the many inaccuracies and misinterpretations of her intent and her own personal choices (Elliott, 2014; Tufekci, 2014), and a widely publicized backlash ensued that resulted in useful media soul searching, namely around using "one woman's story as an occasion for debate about what might be wrong with broader

---

[13]See http://lisabadams.com (accessed December 17, 2014).

approaches to dying" (O'Rourke, 2014). Following this public outcry, *The Guardian* removed the controversial article from its website (Elliott, 2014)

The controversy highlights Americans' ambivalence about talking about dying, the sensitivity with which social justice principles need to be applied, and the dangers of making facile judgments about the care and treatment choices made by others. From a media analysis point of view, it shows evidence of the ability of story and of social media to engage people in a meaningful way if trust and respect are built over time, as Adams had done over a period of years.

The 2009 Controversy Over "Death Panels"

A significant setback to more effective advance care planning occurred when Section 1233 of a House bill (HR 3200, 111th Cong.) that led to the Patient Protection and Affordable Care Act of 2010 was withdrawn after false and misleading statements that it would establish "death panels." The provision would have reimbursed clinicians for the time spent in advance care planning with patients. Such conversations would have included discussion of the documents that can help ensure that patients' wishes regarding care are followed in the event they become unable to express them.[14]

Too often, clinicians, patients, and families embark on a treatment journey for a serious disease without important information and understanding

---

[14]Specifically, Section 1233 of HR 3200, 111th Cong., titled "Advance Care Planning Consultation," would have allowed "(A) An explanation by the practitioner of advance care planning, including key questions and considerations, important steps, and suggested people to talk to; (B) An explanation by the practitioner of advance directives, including living wills and durable powers of attorney, and their uses; (C) An explanation by the practitioner of the role and responsibilities of a health care proxy; (D) The provision by the practitioner of a list of national and State-specific resources to assist consumers and their families with advance care planning, including the national toll-free hotline, the advance care planning clearinghouses, and State legal service organizations (including those funded through the Older Americans Act of 1965): (E) An explanation by the practitioner of the continuum of end-of-life services and supports available, including palliative care and hospice, and benefits for such services and supports that are available under this title; and (F) . . . An explanation of orders regarding life sustaining treatment or similar orders, which shall include—(I) the reasons why the development of such an order is beneficial to the individual and the individual's family and the reasons why such an order should be updated periodically as the health of the individual changes; (II) the information needed for an individual or legal surrogate to make informed decisions regarding the completion of such an order; and (III) the identification of resources that an individual may use to determine the requirements of the State in which such individual resides so that the treatment wishes of that individual will be carried out if the individual is unable to communicate those wishes, including requirements regarding the designation of a surrogate decision-maker (also known as a health care proxy)" (America's Affordable Health Choices Act of 2009, HR 3200.IH, 111th Congress, 1st sess. http://www.gpo.gov/fdsys/pkg/BILLS-111hr3200ih/pdf/BILLS-111hr3200ih.pdf [accessed August 22, 2013]).

of the illness and its likely course, and at times with a conscious effort to protect another from the truth about these matters (Kumar and Temel, 2013; Piemonte and Hermer, 2013). Without understanding the likely course of illness and the risks and benefits of treatment choices, patients (and families) cannot make informed decisions about care (Hajizadeh et al., 2013; Weeks et al., 2012). By contrast, a good advance care planning process gives people "a way to think about death and dying"; for some people, that discussion can allow them to confront dying directly instead of its being a "vague, unmanageable concept" (Martin et al., 1999, p. 88).

At least an hour is usually needed to explore such topics thoroughly (Briggs et al., 2004; Detering et al., 2010). According to the National Center for Health Statistics (undated), in 2010, the average U.S. physician visit lasted only 21 minutes, and more than half of visits lasted 15 minutes or less. Lack of time and lack of payment make clinicians even less likely to have difficult conversations they may be reluctant to have in the first place.

The allegation of "death panels" was first made in 2009. Although no aspect of Section 1233 bore any resemblance to the accusation, it was repeated so often that many people came to regard it as truth. Public education efforts by medical and public health authorities were ineffective in countering this misinformation. The Kaiser Family Foundation's Health Tracking Poll of March 2012—2 years after passage of the Affordable Care Act—revealed that 36 percent of Americans erroneously believed the law actually contains a provision to "allow a government panel to make decisions about end-of-life care for people on Medicare," and 20 percent responded "don't know" (KFF, 2012). When that polling question was repeated in 2013, 40 percent said they believed the law contains this provision, and 21 percent did not know (KFF, 2013). Thus, 3 years after the act's passage, 60 percent of Americans either believed or were unsure whether "death panels" are law.

The politicization of discussion of end-of-life care has definitely had an impact on public perceptions of these issues. *

---

*Quotation from a response submitted through the online public testimony questionnaire for this study. See Appendix C.

Section 1233 of HR 3200 (111th Cong.) was strongly opposed by conservative protestors. House Minority Leader John Boehner and Representative Thaddeus McCotten (R-MI) said the legislation "may start us down a treacherous path toward government-encouraged euthanasia" (Boehner and McCotter, 2009; Pear and Herszenhorn, 2009)—opposition that was "startling because the need for such legislation had been recognized by both political parties for some time" (Altman and Shachtman, 2011, p. 282). In the months before the introduction of HR 3200 with Section 1233, two bills were introduced in the House and one in the Senate relating to orders for life-sustaining treatment and advance care planning, two with bipartisan support.[15]

Recent polls conducted with the American public also reveal strong support for advance care planning. In one 2011 poll,

- 97 percent agreed or strongly agreed that "it is important that patients and their families be educated about palliative care and end-of-life care options available to them along with curative treatment";
- 86 percent thought these discussions should be fully covered by health insurance; and
- 81 percent thought they should be fully covered by Medicare (Regence Foundation and National Journal, 2011a).

Similarly, when the California HealthCare Foundation polled 1,669 adult Californians (including 393 people who had lost a loved one in the previous year) about their attitudes toward end-of-life topics, respondents were asked, "One idea is to have insurance plans cover a doctor's time to talk with patients about treatment options towards the end of life. Do you think this is a good idea or a bad idea?" Eighty-one percent of respondents thought it was a "very good" or "somewhat good" idea (CHCF, 2012).[16] Although the question was worded neutrally, this level of support was significant—especially because public opinion research indicates that 43 percent of American consumers do not trust their health insurance plan (PRG, 2012).

So why did the important effort represented by Section 1233 fail? Leaving aside the fear that underlies many Americans' unwillingness to contemplate mortality, concerns about paying for advance care planning were exacerbated by opposition to comparative effectiveness research. Opponents claim that such research will prevent Americans from obtaining treatments they want and lead to rationing based on an external view of

---

[15]Advance Planning and Compassionate Care Act of 2009, HR 2911, 111th Cong.; Life Sustaining Treatment and Medical Preferences Act of 2009, HR 1898, 111th Cong.; and Advance Planning and Compassionate Care Act of 2009, S 1150, 111th Cong. HR 1898 and S 1150 had bipartisan support. Furthermore, previous versions of S 1150 had been introduced in 2007 (S 464, 110th Cong.), 2002 (S 2857, 107th Cong.), 1999 (S 628, 106th Cong.), and 1997 (S 1345, 105th Cong.), all with bipartisan support.

[16]The group most likely to say it was a bad idea were men aged 65 and older; 30 percent of this group thought it was a "somewhat bad" or "very bad" idea.

their likely effectiveness or excessive expense. While other countries do factor cost comparisons into decisions on which services to reimburse with public monies (Satvat and Leight, 2011), the U.S. approach explicitly prohibits any consideration of treatment costs (Altman and Shachtman, 2011).

The objections to facilitating advance care planning may be misplaced when, as discussed in Chapter 3, some evidence suggests that people who do plan for their care most often choose less aggressive care. This choice has been associated with increased survival, better quality of life, and decreased stress and psychological impacts on family members (Mack et al., 2010; Temel et al., 2010; Wright et al., 2008). No association has been found between having an advance directive discussion or document and earlier death (Fischer et al., 2010). Indeed, according to Winter and Parks (2012, p. 741), "Ironically, we found that those who avoid living wills and end-of-life conversations are the least likely to have treatment wishes respected, because their proxies are unlikely to know their wishes."

Improving the care people receive at the end of life by giving them the care they actually want while saving money by avoiding costly and futile interventions people do not want could have been a strategy with multiple benefits for the health system. But the discussion of these two goals—individual care and collective savings—in the same public conversation may help explain why the proposed provision "became the lightning rod it did" (Kaebnick, 2013, p. 2). Accordingly, some commentators would keep the financial argument completely out of the advance care planning discussion (Fried and Drickamer, 2010). As a *Washington Post* opinion piece said, because health care reform was promoted in large part on the grounds that it would control rising and unsustainable health care costs (Antos et al., 2009), in that context, "citizens are not delusional to conclude that the goal [of Section 1233] is to reduce end-of-life spending" (Robinson, 2009).

In early January 2011, the Centers for Medicare & Medicaid Services (CMS) withdrew "voluntary advance care planning" as a specified element of the Medicare annual wellness visit (HHS, 2011). This decision was due to the discordant views of stakeholders, "including those who disagreed when the idea of voluntary advance care planning was first proposed under the Patient Protection and Affordable Care Act" (Holley, 2011). The CMS final rule acknowledged as much:

> It has since become apparent that we did not have an opportunity to consider prior to the issuance of the final rule the wide range of views on this subject held by a broad range of stakeholders (including members of Congress and those who were involved with this provision during the debate on the Affordable Care Act). Therefore, we are rescinding the provision of the final rule that includes voluntary advance care planning as a specified element of the annual wellness visits providing personalized prevention

plan services, and returning to the policy that was proposed, which was limited to the elements specified in the Act. (HHS, 2011)

In August 2013, the bipartisan team of Senators Mark Warner of Virginia and Johnny Isakson of Georgia again pursued the goal of reimbursement for advance care planning discussions by introducing the Care Planning Act of 2013.[17] According to Warner, the bill "is about honoring a patient's choice, not making it for them" (Mundy, 2013). Nevertheless, the staying power of the distortions around "death panels" may have doomed the senators' initiative.

As Piemonte and Hermer (2013, p. 24) advise, "If we are ever to make progress toward creating policy that incentivizes physicians to engage in constructive end of life conversations, we need to do so in a way that appeals to the shared values of those across the political spectrum." Recent public opinion research suggests there is ample support for advance care planning and insurance that covers it. Targeted public education and engagement efforts may move the needle on these policy initiatives.

RECOMMENDATION

Recommendation 5. Civic leaders, public health and other governmental agencies, community-based organizations, faith-based organizations, consumer groups, health care delivery organizations, payers, employers, and professional societies should engage their constituents and provide fact-based information about care of people with advanced serious illness to encourage advance care planning and informed choice based on the needs and values of individuals.

Specifically, these organizations and groups should

- use appropriate media and other channels to reach their audiences, including underserved populations;
- provide evidence-based information about care options and informed decision making regarding treatment and care;
- encourage meaningful dialogue among individuals and their families and caregivers, clergy, and clinicians about values, care goals, and preferences related to advanced serious illness; and
- dispel misinformation that may impede informed decision making and public support for health system and policy reform regarding care near the end of life.

---

[17]Care Planning Act of 2013 (S 1439, 113th Cong., 1st sess.).

In addition,

- health care delivery organizations should provide information and materials about care near the end of life as part of their practices to facilitate clinicians' ongoing dialogue with patients, families, and caregivers;
- government agencies and payers should undertake, support, and share communication and behavioral research aimed at assessing public perceptions and actions with respect to end-of-life care, developing and testing effective messages and tailoring them to appropriate audience segments, and measuring progress and results; and
- health care professional societies should prepare educational materials and encourage their members to engage patients and their caregivers and families in advance care planning, including end-of-life discussions and decisions.

All of the above groups should work collaboratively, sharing successful strategies and promising practices across organizations.

REFERENCES

ALF (American Legacy Foundation). 2012. *truth®*. http://legacyforhealth.org/content/download/621/7337/file/truth_fact_sheet_January_2012.pdf (accessed May 2, 2014).

ALF. 2014. *National education campaigns: Keeping young people from using tobacco.* http://legacyforhealth.org/what-we-do/national-education-campaigns/keeping-young-people-from-using-tobacco (accessed May 2, 2014).

Alston, C., L. Paget, G. Halvorson, B. Novelli, J. Guest, P. McCabe, K. Hoffman, C. Koepke, M. Simon, S. Sutton, S. Okun, P. Wicks, T. Undem, V. Rohrbach, and I. Von Kohorn. 2012. *Communicating with patients on health care evidence.* Discussion paper. Washington, DC: IOM. http://www.iom.edu/~/media/Files/Perspectives-Files/2012/Discussion-Papers/VSRT-Evidence.pdf (accessed January 22, 2014).

Altman, S., and D. Shactman. 2011. *Power, politics, and universal health care.* Amherst, NY: Prometheus Books.

Andreasen, A. R. 1995. *Marketing social change: Changing behavior to promote health, social development, and the environment.* San Francisco, CA: Jossey-Bass.

Antos, J., J. Bertko, M. Chernew, D. Cutler, D. Goldman, M. McClellan, E. McGlynn, M. Pauly, L. Schaeffer, and S. Shortell. 2009. *Effective steps to address long-term health care spending growth.* Washington, DC: Engelberg Center for Health Care Reform at The Brookings Institution. http://www.brookings.edu/~/media/research/files/reports/2009/9/01%20btc/0826_btc_fullreport.pdf (accessed August 30, 2013).

Asbury, L. D., F. L. Wong, S. M. Price, and M. J. Nolin. 2008. The VERB™ campaign: Applying a branding strategy in public health. *American Journal of Preventive Medicine* 34(Suppl. 6):S183-S187.

Berkowitz, J. M., M. Huhman, C. D. Heitzler, L. D. Potter. M. J. Nolin, and S. W. Banspach. 2008. Overview of formative, process, and outcome evaluation methods used in the VERB™ campaign. *American Journal of Preventive Medicine* 34(Suppl. 6):S222-S229.

Bisognano, M., and E. Goodman. 2013. Engaging patients and their loved ones in the ultimate conversation. *Health Affairs* 32(2):203-206.

Boehner, J., and T. McCotter. 2009. *Statement by House GOP leaders Boehner and McCotter on end-of-life treatment counseling in Democrats' health care legislation.* http://www.speaker.gov/press-release/statement-house-gop-leaders-boehner-and-mccotter-end-life-treatment-counseling (accessed April 22, 2014).

Briggs, L. A., K. T. Kirchhoff, B. J. Hammes, M. K. Song, and E. R. Colvin. 2004. Patient-centered advance care planning in special patient populations: A pilot study. *Journal of Professional Nursing* 20(1):47-58.

Calabrese-Eck, L. 2013. *Understanding consumer attitudes, barriers, and word-strings around advanced care.* Presented at the Consumer Research Symposium, sponsored by the Coalition to Transform Advanced Care, Washington, DC, June 27. http://www.slideshare.net/bsinatro/leigh-calabrese-eck (accessed February 8, 2014).

CAPC (Center to Advance Palliative Care). 2011. *2011 public opinion research on palliative care.* http://www.capc.org/tools-for-palliative-care-programs/marketing/public-opinion-research/2011-public-opinion-research-on-palliative-care.pdf (accessed February 8, 2014).

Carr, D., and D. Khodyakov. 2007. Health care proxies: Whom do young old adults choose and why? *Journal of Health and Social Behavior* 48(2):180-194.

Carroll, T. E., and L. Van Veen. 2002. Public health social marketing: The Immunise Australia program. *Social Marketing Quarterly* 8(1):55-61.

CCCC (Community Conversations on Compassionate Care). 2008. *An advance care planning program: A community-wide end-of-life/palliative care initiative project.* Post presented at the Blue Cross Blue Shield Association Conference. http://www.compassionandsupport.org/pdfs/CCCC-poster.pdf (accessed May 14, 2014).

CCCC. 2014. *Community Conversations on Compassionate Care.* https://www.compassionandsupport.org/index.php/for_patients_families/advance_care_planning/community_conversations (accessed May 14, 2014).

CHCF (California HealthCare Foundation). 2012. *Final chapter: Californians' attitudes and experiences with death and dying.* http://www.chcf.org/publications/2012/02/final-chapter-death-dying (accessed February 8, 2014).

C-TAC (Coalition to Transform Advanced Care). 2014. *Consumer perceptions and needs regarding advanced illness care: Are we listening?* Washington, DC: C-TAC.

Debolt, D. 2014. Brain-dead finding for California girl may test unique N.J. law. *The Seattle Times*, June 21. http://seattletimes.com/html/nationworld/2023899650_njjahixml.html (accessed June 24, 2014).

Detering, K. M., A. D. Hancock, M. C. Reade, and W. Silvester. 2010. The impact of advance care planning on end of life care in elderly patients: Randomised controlled trial. *British Medical Journal* 340:c1345.

Eckholm, E. 2014. "Aid in dying" movement takes hold in some states. *The New York Times*, February 7. http://nyti.ms/1g3sOPV (accessed February 8, 2014).

El-Guebaly, N. 2005. Don't drink and drive: The successful message of Mothers Against Drunk Driving (MADD). *World Psychiatry* 4(1):35-36.

Elliott, C. 2014. Why an article on Lisa Boncheck Adams was removed from the Guardian site. *The Guardian*, January 16. http://gu.com/p/3mv4g (accessed April 30, 2014).

Emery, S. Y. Kim, Y. K. Choi, G. Szczpka, M. Wakefield, and F. J. Chaloupka. 2012. The effects of smoking-related television advertising on smoking and intentions to quit among adults in the United States: 1999-2007. *American Journal of Public Health* 102:751-757.

Evans, W. D., J. Wasserman, E. Bertolotti, and S. Martino. 2002. Branding behavior: The strategy behind the truthSM campaign. *Social Marketing Quarterly* 8:17-29.

Farrelly, M. C., C. G. Healton, K. C. Davis, P. Messeri, J. C. Hersey, and M. L. Haviland. 2002. Getting to the truth: Evaluating national tobacco countermarketing campaigns. *American Journal of Public Health* 92:901-907.

Farrelly, M. C., K. C. Davis, M. L. Haviland, P. Messeri, and C. G. Healton. 2005. Evidence of a dose-response relationship between "truth" antismoking ads and youth smoking prevalence. *American Journal of Public Health* 95:425-431.

Farrelly, M. C., K. C. Davis, J. Duke, and P. Messeri. 2009a. Sustaining "truth": Changes in youth tobacco attitudes and smoking intentions after 3 years of a national antismoking campaign. *Health Education Research* 24(1):42-48.

Farrelly, M. C., J. Nonnemaker, K. C. Davis, and A. Hussin. 2009b. The influence of the national truth® campaign on smoking initiation. *American Journal of Preventive Medicine* 36(5):379-384.

FDA (U.S. Food and Drug Administration). 2014a. *The Real Cost Campaign.* http://www. fda.gov/AboutFDA/CentersOffices/OfficeofMedicalProductsandTobacco/AbouttheCenter forTobaccoProducts/PublicEducationCampaigns/TheRealCostCampaign/default.htm (accessed May 2, 2014).

FDA. 2014b. *The Real Cost: Campaign overview.* http://www.fda.gov/downloads/AboutFDA/ CentersOffices/OfficeofMedicalProductsandTobacco/AbouttheCenterforTobacco Products/PublicEducationCampaigns/TheRealCostCampaign/UCM384307.pdf (accessed May 2, 2014).

Fell, J. C., and R. B. Voas. 2006. Mothers Against Drunk Driving (MADD): The first 25 years. *Traffic Injury Prevention* 7:195-212.

Fine, R. L. 2005. From Quinlan to Schiavo: Medical, ethical, and legal issues in severe brain injury. *Baylor University Medical Center Proceedings* 18:303-310.

Fischer, S. M., S-J. Min, and J. S. Kutner. 2010. Advance directive discussions do not lead to death. *Journal of the American Geriatrics Society* 58(2):400-401.

Fox, S. 2006. *Online health search 2006.* Washington, DC: Pew Internet & American Life Project. http://www.pewinternet.org/files/old-media//Files/Reports/2006/PIP_Online_ Health_2006.pdf.pdf (accessed April 23, 2014).

Fox, S., and M. Duggan. 2013. *The diagnosis difference. Part two: Sources of health information. Pew Research Internet Project.* http://www.pewinternet.org/2013/11/26/part-two-sources-of-health-information (accessed May 13, 2014).

Fried, T. R., and M. Drickamer. 2010. Garnering support for advanced [*sic*] care planning. *Journal of the American Medical Association* 303(3):269-270.

Grier, S., and C. A. Bryant. 2005. Social marketing in public health. *Annual Review of Public Health* 26:319-339.

Hajizadeh, N., K. Crothers, and R. S. Braithwaite. 2013. Using modeling to inform patient-centered care choices at the end of life. *Journal of Comparative Effectiveness Research* 2(5):497-508.

Hellerman, C., J. Morris, and M. Smith. 2014. Brain-dead Texas woman taken off ventilator. *CNN.* http://www.cnn.com/2014/01/26/health/texas-pregnant-brain-dead-woman (accessed June 24, 2014).

HHS (U.S. Department of Health and Human Services). 2011. Medicare program; amendment to payment policies under the physician fee schedule and other revisions to part B for CY2011. *Federal Register* 76(6):1366-1367. http://www.gpo.gov/fdsys/pkg/FR-2011-01-10/pdf/2011-164.pdf (accessed August 5, 2014).

HHS. 2013. *Health communication and health information technology.* http://www.healthy people.gov/2020/topicsobjectives2020/overview.aspx?topicid=18 (accessed December 11, 2013).

Hobbs, F., and N. Stoops. 2002. *Demographic trends in the 20th century: Census 2000 special reports.* Washington, DC: U.S. Census Bureau. http://www.census.gov/prod/2002pubs/censr-4.pdf (accessed April 22, 2014).

Holley, D. 2011. CMS rule reversal: Understanding the impact on advance care planning. *ABA Health eSource* 7(7). http://www.americanbar.org/newsletter/publications/aba_health_esource_home/aba_health_law_esource_1103_holley.html (accessed February 10, 2014).

Holloway, K. F. C. 2011. *Private bodies, public texts: Race, gender, and a cultural bioethics.* Durham, NC: Duke University Press.

Hollywood Health and Society. 2014. *USC Annenberg School for Communication and Journalism, Hollywood Health & Society.* http://hollywoodhealthandsociety.org (accessed June 24, 2014).

Holtgrave, D. R., K. A. Wunderink, D. M. Vallone, and C. G. Healton. 2009. Cost-utility analysis of the national truth® campaign to prevent youth smoking. *American Journal of Preventive Medicine* 36(5):385-388.

Huhman, M., C. Heitzler, and F. Wong. 2004. The VERB campaign logic mode: A tool for planning and evaluation. *Preventing Chronic Disease* 1(3):1-6. http://www.cdc.gov/pcd/issues/2004/jul/pdf/04_0033.pdf (accessed January 27, 2014).

Huhman, M. E., L. D. Potter, M. J. Nolin, A. Piesse, D. R. Judkins, S. W. Banspach, and F. L. Wong. 2010. The influence of the VERB campaign on children's physical activity in 2002 to 2006. *American Journal of Public Health* 100(4):638-645.

IOM (Institute of Medicine). 1997. *Approaching death: Improving care at the end of life.* Washington, DC: National Academy Press.

IOM. 2003. *When children die: Improving palliative and end-of-life care for children and their families.* Washington, DC: The National Academies Press.

IOM. 2009. *Health literacy, eHealth, and communication: Putting the consumer first.* Washington, DC: The National Academies Press.

IOM. 2011. *Patients charting the course: Citizen engagement and the learning health system.* Washington, DC: The National Academies Press.

Johnson, S. H. 2009. Quinlan and Cruzan: Beyond the symbols. In *Health law & bioethics*, edited by S. H. Johnson, J. H. Krause, R. S. Saver, and R. F. Wilson. Frederick, MD: Aspen Publishers. Pp. 53-75.

Kaebnick, G. E. 2013. A win-win? Editorial. *The Hastings Center Report* 43(4):2.

Keller, B. 2014. Heroic measures. *The New York Times*, January 12. http://nyti.ms/JTkpDa (accessed January 21, 2014).

KFF (The Henry J. Kaiser Family Foundation). 2012. *Kaiser health tracking poll—March 2012.* http://kaiserfamilyfoundation.files.wordpress.com/2013/01/8285-f.pdf (accessed July 26, 2013).

KFF. 2013. *Kaiser health tracking poll—March 2013.* Figure 11. http://kff.org/health-reform/poll-finding/march-2013-tracking-poll (accessed July 26, 2013).

Kumar, P., and J. S. Temel. 2013. End-of-life care discussions in patients with advanced cancer. *Journal of Clinical Oncology* 31(27):3315-3319.

Lauridsen, S. M. R., M. S. Norup, P. J. H. Rossel. 2007. The secret art of managing healthcare expenses: Investigating implicit rationing and autonomy in public healthcare systems. *Journal of Medical Ethics* 33:704-707.

Levine, D. 2014. "Death with dignity" or "assisted suicide"? *Governing.* http://www.governing.com/topics/health-human-services/gov-death-with-dignity-rhetoric.html (accessed March 12, 2014).

Lynn, J., F. Cohn, J. H. Pickering, J. Smith, and A. M. Stoeppelwerth. 1997. American Geriatrics Society on physician-assisted suicide: Brief to the United States Supreme Court. *Journal of the American Geriatrics Society* 45(4):489-499.

Mack, J. W., J. C. Weeks, A. A. Wright, S. D. Block, and H. G. Prigerson. 2010. End-of-life discussions, goal attainment, and distress at the end of life: Predictors and outcomes of receipt of care consistent with preferences. *Journal of Clinical Oncology* 28(7):1203-1208.

MADD (Mothers Against Drunk Driving). 2014. *Mission and history*. http://www.madd.org/about-us/mission (accessed May 2, 2014).

Martin, D. K., E. C. Thiel, and P. A. Singer. 1999. A new model of advance care planning: Observations from people with HIV. *Archives of Internal Medicine* 159(1):86-92.

McCarthy, J. D., and M. Wolfson. 1996. Resource mobilization by local social movement organizations: Agency, strategy, and organization in the movement against drinking and driving. *American Sociological Review* 61(6):1070-1088.

Meisel, A. 2008. End-of-life care. In *From birth to death and bench to clinic: The Hastings Center bioethics briefing book for journalists, policymakers, and campaigns*, edited by M. Crowley. Garrison, NY: The Hastings Center. Pp. 51-54. http://www.thehastingscenter.org/Publications/BriefingBook/Detail.aspx?id=2270 (accessed July 10, 2013).

Mundy, A. 2013. Senators revive push for end-of-life-care planning. *The Wall Street Journal*, August 1. http://blogs.wsj.com/washwire/2013/08/01/senators-try-to-revive-bill-for-end-of-life-planning (accessed August 1, 2013).

National Center for Health Statistics. undated. *National Ambulatory Medical Care Survey: 2010 summary tables*. Tables 27 and 28. http://www.cdc.gov/nchs/data/ahcd/namcs_summary/2010_namcs_web_tables.pdf (accessed August 29, 2013).

Noar, S. M. 2006. A 10-year retrospective of research in health mass media campaigns: Where do we go from here? *Journal of Health Communication* 11:21-42.

Novelli, B. 2013. *Dying better in America*. Presented at TEDxGeorgetown, Washington, DC. http://www.youtube.com/watch?v=Q-DbcF5gIh0 (accessed February 13, 2014).

O'Rourke, M. 2014. Tweeting cancer. *The New Yorker*. http://www.newyorker.com/online/blogs/culture/2014/01/tweeting-cancer.html (accessed January 24, 2014).

Patrizi, P., E. Thompson, and A. Spector. 2011. *Improving care at the end of life: How the Robert Wood Johnson Foundation and its grantees built the field*. Princeton, NJ: RWJF. http://www.rwjf.org/content/dam/farm/reports/reports/2011/rwjf69582 (accessed May 20, 2014).

Pear, R., and D. Herszenhorn. 2009. Democrats push health care plan while issuing assurances on Medicare. *New York Times*, July 28. http://www.nytimes.com/2009/07/29/health/policy/29health.html (accessed January 22, 2014).

Pew Research Center. 2009. *Growing old in America: Expectations vs. reality*. http://www.pewsocialtrends.org/files/2010/10/Getting-Old-in-America.pdf (accessed January 21, 2014).

Pew Research Center. 2010. *Baby boomers retire*. http://www.pewresearch.org/daily-number/baby-boomers-retire (accessed January 24, 2014).

Pew Research Center. 2013. *Views on end-of-life medical treatments*. http://www.pewforum.org/files/2013/11/end-of-life-survey-report-full-pdf.pdf (accessed November 25, 2013).

Piemonte, N. M., and L. Hermer. 2013. Avoiding a "death panel" redux. *Hastings Center Report* 43(4):20-28.

PRG (Peppers & Rogers Group). 2012. *Measuring the value of trust in healthcare*. http://www.peppersandrogersgroup.com/view.aspx?docId=33579 (accessed August 15, 2013).

Regence Foundation and National Journal. 2011a. *Living well at the end of life: Research findings from 2011 public opinion research*. http://syndication.nationaljournal.com/communications/NationalJournalRegenceToplines.pdf (accessed January 22, 2014).

Regence Foundation and National Journal. 2011b. *Living well at the end of life: Research findings from 2011 public opinion research*. http://syndication.nationaljournal.com/communications/NationalJournalRegenceDoctorsToplines.pdf (accessed January 22, 2014).

Richardson, A. K., M. Green, H. Xiao, N. Sokol, and D. Vallone. 2010. Evidence for truth®: The young adult response to a youth-focused anti-smoking media campaign. *American Journal of Preventive Medicine* 39(6):500-506.

Robinson, E. 2009. Behind the rage, a cold reality. *The Washington Post*, August 11. http://articles.washingtonpost.com/2009-08-11/opinions/36799409_1_health-insurance-health-care-health-care-costs (accessed August 22, 2013).

RWJF (Robert Wood Johnson Foundation). 2004a. *Moyers' prime time PBS program on dying in America generates large audience, boosts awareness of end-of-life issues.* http://www.rwjf.org/reports/grr/038858.htm (accessed January 22, 2014).

RWJF. 2004b. *End-of-life issues get an airing on prime-time tv.* http://www.rwjf.org/content/dam/farm/reports/program_results_reports/2004/rwjf63987 (accessed June 24, 2014).

Saad, L. 2013. U.S. support for euthanasia hinges on how it's described: Support is at low ebb on the basis of wording that mentions "suicide." *Gallup Politics.* http://www.gallup.com/poll/162815/support-euthanasia-hinges-described.aspx (accessed March 18, 2014).

Satvat, A., and J. Leight. 2011. Comparative effectiveness. In *Health care delivery in the United States*, 10th ed., edited by A. R. Kovner and J. R. Knickman. New York: Springer. Pp. 277-295.

Singhal, A., and E. M. Rogers. 2004. The status of entertainment-education worldwide. In *Entertainment-education and social change: History, research, and practice*, edited by A. Singhal, M. J. Cody, E. M. Rogers, and M. Sabido. Mahwah, NJ: Lawrence Erlbaum Associates. Pp. 3-20.

Sudore, R. L., C. S. Landefeld, S. Z. Pantilat, K. M. Noyes, and D. Schillinger. 2008. Reach and impact of a mass media event among vulnerable patients: The Terri Schiavo Story. *Journal of General Internal Medicine* 23(11):1854-1857.

Swanson, A. 2009. Rational as a necessity. *Annals of Health Law: Advance Directive* 19(1):1-11. http://www.luc.edu/media/lucedu/law/centers/healthlaw/pdfs/advancedirective/pdfs/issue3/swanson.pdf (accessed May 16, 2014).

Temel, J. S., J. A. Greer, A. Muzikansky, E. R. Gallagher, S. Admane, J. A. Jackson, C. M. Dahlin, C. D. Blinderman, J. Jacobsen, W. F. Pirl, J. A. Billinbs, and T. J. Lynch. 2010. Early palliative care for patients with metastatic non-small-cell lung cancer. *New England Journal of Medicine* 363(8):733-742.

Tufekci, Z. 2014. Social media is a conversation, not a press release. *Medium.* https://medium.com/technology-and-society/4d811b45840d (accessed January 21, 2014).

U.S. Census Bureau. 2013. *Annual estimates of the resident population for selected age groups by sex for the United States, states, counties, and Puerto Rico Commonwealth and Municiios: April 1, 2010 to July 1, 2012.* http://factfinder2.census.gov/bkmk/table/1.0/en/PEP/2012/PEPAGESEX (accessed April 22, 2014).

Walsh, D. C., R. E. Rudd, B. A. Moeykens, and T. W. Moloney. 1993. Social marketing for public health. *Health Affairs* 12(2):104-119.

Weeks, J. C., P. J. Catalano, A. Cronin, M. D. Finkelman, J. W. Mack, N. L. Keating, and D. Schrag. 2012. Patients' expectations about effects of chemotherapy for advanced cancer. *New England Journal of Medicine* 367(17):1616-1625.

Winter, L., and S. M. Parks. 2012. Acceptors and rejecters of life-sustaining treatment: Differences in advance care planning characteristics. *Journal of Applied Gerontology* 31(6):734-742.

Wong, F., M. Huhman, C. Heitzler, L. Asbury, R. Bretthauer-Mueller, S. McCarthy, and P. Londe. 2004. VERB™—a social marketing campaign to increase physical activity among youth. *Preventing Chronic Disease* 1(3):1-7. http://www.cdc.gov/pcd/issues/2004/jul/pdf/04_0043.pdf (accessed January 27, 2014).

Wong, F. L., M. Greenwall, S. Gates, and J. Berkowtiz. 2008. It's what you do!: Reflections on the VERB™ campaign. *American Journal of Preventive Medicine* 34(Suppl. 6):S175-S182.

Wright, A. A., B. Zhang, A. Ray, J. W. Mack, E. Trice, T. Balboni, S. L. Mitchell, V. A. Jackson, S. D. Block, P. K. Maciejewski, and H. G. Prigerson. 2008. Associations between end-of-life discussions, patient mental health, medical care near death, and caregiver bereavement adjustment. *Journal of the American Medical Association* 300(14):1665-1673.

ANNEX 6-1:
SELECTED PUBLIC ENGAGEMENT CAMPAIGNS
ON HEALTH-RELATED TOPICS

Campaign	Goals	Target Populations
VERB™*a* Launched June 2002	Increase and maintain physical activity among tweens (children ages 9 to 13)	Primary audience: tweens (children 9 to 13) Secondary audience: Parents and other adult influencers of tweens

Methodology	Evidence of Impact or Future Directions
Campaign messages were developed that spoke directly to tweens, in their language, and through their trusted channels. Outreach to parents and other adults lagged, but when implemented, focused on gaining their buy-in to the campaign in order to garner support for the initiative. Multimedia campaign included paid television, radio, print, Internet, and out-of-home advertising; unpaid added-value public service announcements; community-based promotions ("Longest Day of Play" and "Extra Hour for Extra Action"), events, and street marketing; community, corporate, and media partnerships; and online presence.	In 2006, 75 percent of surveyed tweens had awareness of the VERB campaign (prompted and unprompted), an increase from 67 percent in 2003, the first year of data collection. Campaign exposure was found to have a dose-response effect on previous-day physical activity during data collection in 2004, 2005, and 2006. This association was statistically significant in 2004 and 2005. A dose-response effect of campaign exposure on attitudes and beliefs relating to physical activity, including outcome expectations, self-efficacy, and social influences, was also found in 2006.

continued

Campaign	Goals	Target Populations
Mothers Against Drunk Driving (MADD)[b] Launched September 1980	Prevent underage drinking; stop drunk driving; reduce the number of accidents, injuries, and deaths from drunk driving and support victims of drunk driving	Youth, victims and families of victims of drunk driving, policy makers
"The Real Cost" AntiTobacco Campaign[c] Announced February 2014	Reduce the number of youth cigarette smokers; prevent teenagers from trying cigarettes, or if they have already done so, get them to quit	Teens aged 12-17 who are at risk for using or have experimented with cigarettes

Methodology	Evidence of Impact or Future Directions
The Campaign to Eliminate Drunk Driving advocates for strategies and technologies that reduce the likelihood of drunk driving, including law enforcement, ignition interlock devices, and other technologies that can determine alcohol impairment. A PowerTalk21 national day encourages parents to talk with their children about alcohol. A legislative agenda includes advocacy for and measurement of enactment of new local and national laws relating to the minimum drinking age, server liability, and sobriety checkpoints. Services for victims include participation in victim impact panels, emotional support, assistance, and court accompaniment. Personalization of traffic crash victims so they were not just numbers helped people acknowledge not only the statistics but also the actual lives cut short. MADD leaned heavily on the National Highway Traffic Safety Administration's research and program staff to meet the need for coordinating policy changes with science.	MADD played major roles in the passage of laws relating to the minimum legal drinking age, youth zero tolerance, and lower blood alcohol limits. MADD estimates that it has saved more than 27,000 young lives through the implementation of minimum drinking age laws alone. Alcohol-related traffic deaths in the United States decreased from an estimated 30,000 in 1980, when MADD was founded, to 16,694 in 2004, although complex factors likely contributed to this reduction, and it is unknown how much of this reduction can be attributed to MADD.
A multimedia education campaign educates at-risk teenagers by spotlighting the health hazards of smoking in advertisements and on social media. Television, radio, web, cinema, print, and out-of-home advertising shows the costs of smoking, including skin damage, gum disease, tooth loss, and loss of control due to addiction. Ads are compelling, provocative, graphic, and attention grabbing.	The U.S. Food and Drug Administration will evaluate the campaign through a multiyear, nationwide, longitudinal study to assess changes in tobacco-related knowledge, attitudes, and behaviors.

continued

Campaign	Goals	Target Populations
"Truth" AntiTobacco Campaign[d] Launched February 2000	Prevent teens from ever trying a cigarette and reduce youth smoking	Primary audience: teenagers aged 12-17 Secondary audience: young adults aged 18-24
"Immunise Australia" Program Social Marketing Campaign[e] Launched February 1997	Increase the number of children up to age 6 who have been fully immunized	Mothers with children up to age 5 Secondary audience included family, friends, and health care providers

SOURCES:
   [a]Asbury et al., 2008; Berkowitz et al., 2008; Huhman et al., 2004, 2010; Wong et al., 2004, 2008.
   [b]El-Guebaly, 2005; Fell and Voas, 2006; MADD, 2014; McCarthy and Wolfson, 1996.
   [c]FDA, 2014a,b.

Methodology	Evidence of Impact or Future Directions
A countermarketing campaign includes • television advertisements exposing big tobacco's marketing and manufacturing practices and the health effects, social costs, and addictiveness of tobacco use; • media and corporate partnerships with MTV, BET, G4, Fuse, and Virgin Mobile; • a website and social media, which include facts, games, and contests; and • a grassroots *truth* tour that travels the country to connect with youth and engage them on a peer-to-peer level at concerts, sporting events, and other venues, encouraging them to rebel by *not* smoking, typically stopping in more than 50 cities per tour.	Exposure to the campaign is associated with changes in tobacco-related attitudes, beliefs, and behaviors among teens and young adults. Exposure to *truth* advertisements was associated with higher odds of intention to quit smoking and of having made a quit attempt in the past 12 months. From 2000 to 2004, it is estimated that *truth* was significantly associated with reduced youth smoking prevalence and prevented more than 450,000 teens and young adults from using tobacco. From 2000 to 2002, *truth* saved $1.9-$5.4 billion in medical care costs to society. The Office of Juvenile Justice and Delinquency Prevention included *truth* in its portfolio of effective programs. *Truth* has also been lauded by the Centers for Disease Control and Prevention (CDC), the U.S. Department of Health and Human Services (HHS), and President George W. Bush.
Health care provider education and engagement included distribution of more than 60,000 *Australian Immunisation Handbooks*, a column in a provider publication, and an interactive satellite program. Community education and engagement included television commercials, print advertisements in magazines and posters in health care facilities, three Immunisation Awareness Days, a national immunization hotline, and distribution of information materials.	Recognition of the television advertisement was very high (80 percent), as was message recall (97 percent of those who recognized the ad). There was an increase of knowledge and behaviors relating to vaccination of young children. After the campaign, 45 percent of parents reported that they had checked their child's immunization status, compared with 36 percent before the campaign; 33 percent reported that they had taken their children to be immunized during the campaign, compared with 22 percent before the campaign. Prior to the campaign launch, 76 percent of children 12 months of age were fully vaccinated. This proportion increased to 85 percent in the year after the campaign, 88 percent 3 years later, and 91 percent 4 years later.

[d]ALF, 2012, 2014; Emery et al., 2012; Evans et al., 2002; Farrelly et al., 2002, 2005, 2009a,b; Holtgrave et al., 2009; Richardson et al., 2010.

[e]Carroll and Van Veen, 2002.

Glossary[1]

Advance care planning: The whole process of discussion of end-of-life care, clarification of related values and goals, and embodiment of preferences through written documents and medical orders. This process can start at any time and be revisited periodically, but it becomes more focused as health status changes. Ideally, these conversations (1) occur with a person's health care agent and primary clinician, along with other members of the clinical team; (2) are recorded and updated as needed; and (3) allow for flexible decision making in the context of the patient's current medical situation.

Advance directive: A broad term encompassing several types of patient-initiated documents, especially living wills and documents that name a health care agent. People can complete these forms at any time and in any state of health that allows them to do so.

Basic palliative care: Palliative care that is delivered by health care professionals who are not palliative care specialists, such as primary care clinicians, physicians who are disease-oriented specialists (such as oncologists and cardiologists), and nurses, social workers, pharmacists, chaplains, and others who care for this population but are not certified in palliative care.

Chronic pain: Ongoing or recurrent pain lasting beyond the usual course of acute illness or injury or, generally, more than 3 to 6 months and adversely

---

[1]Glossary terms without a citation are definitions created and derived by the committee.

affecting the individual's well-being. A simpler definition for chronic or persistent pain is pain that continues when it should not (American Chronic Pain Association, 2013).

Comparative effectiveness research: The generation and synthesis of evidence to compare the benefits and harms of alternative methods for preventing, diagnosing, treating, and monitoring a clinical condition or improving the delivery of care (IOM, 2009).

Direct care worker: Nursing assistants, home health and home care aides, personal care workers and personal care attendants who provide hands-on care, supervision, and emotional support to people with chronic illnesses and disabilities. These individuals work in a variety of settings, including nursing homes, assisted living and other residential care settings, adult day care, and private homes (Kiefer et al., 2005).

Dual eligibles: Individuals who are jointly enrolled in Medicare and Medicaid, and who are eligible to receive benefits from both programs. All dual-eligible beneficiaries qualify for full Medicare benefits, which cover their acute and postacute care. Dual-eligible beneficiaries vary in the amount of Medicaid benefits for which they qualify (CBO, 2013).

Durable power of attorney for health care: Identifies the person (the health care agent) who should make medical decisions in case of a patient's incapacity.

End-of-life care: Refers generally to the processes of addressing the medical, social, emotional, and spiritual needs of people who are nearing the end of life. It may include a range of medical and social services, including disease specific interventions as well as palliative and hospice care for those with advanced serious conditions who are near the end of life.

Family: Not only people related by blood or marriage, but also close friends, partners, companions, and others whom patients would want as part of their care team.

Fee-for-service: A payment system in which a health care program or plan pays providers a fee for each covered service performed for its enrollees (CBO, 2013).

Frailty: A clinically recognizable state of increased vulnerability resulting from aging-associated decline in reserve and function across multiple physiologic systems such that the ability to cope with everyday or acute stressors is compromised (Xue, 2011).

Health care agent: An individual designated in an advance directive who should make medical decisions in case of a patient's incapacity.

HITECH Act: The Health Information Technology for Economic and Clinical Health (HITECH) Act was enacted under Title XIII of the American Recovery and Reinvestment Act of 2009 and officially established the Office of the National Coordinator for Health Information Technology at the U.S. Department of Health and Human Services. The act includes incentives designed to accelerate the adoption of health information technology by the health care industry, health care providers, consumers, and patients, largely through the promotion of electronic health records and secure electronic health information exchange.[2]

Hospice: A service delivery system that provides palliative care for patients who have a limited life expectancy and require comprehensive biomedical, psychosocial, and spiritual support as they enter the terminal stage of an illness or condition. It also supports family members coping with the complex consequences of illness, disability, and aging as death nears (NQF, 2006).

Learning health care system: A health care system in which science, informatics, incentives, and culture are aligned for continuous improvement and innovation, with best practices being seamlessly embedded in the care process, patients and families being active participants in all elements of care, and new knowledge being captured as an integral by-product of the care experience (IOM, 2012).

Life-sustaining treatment: Medical procedures that replace or support an essential bodily function. Life-sustaining treatments include cardiopulmonary resuscitation (CPR), mechanical ventilation, artificial nutrition and hydration, dialysis, and certain other treatments (HHS, 2008).

Living will: A written or video statement about the kind of medical care a person does or does not want under certain specific conditions if no longer able to express those wishes.

---

[2]Health Information Technology for Economic and Clinical Health (HITECH) Act, Title XIII of Division A and Title IV of Division B of the American Recovery and Reinvestment Act of 2009 (ARRA), Public Law 111-5, 111th Cong., 1st sess. (February 17, 2009).

Long-term care: An array of health care, personal care, and social services generally provided over a sustained period of time to people of all ages with chronic conditions and with functional limitations. Their needs are met in a variety of care settings such as nursing homes, residential care facilities, and individual homes (IOM, 2001a).

Meaningful use: The use of certified electronic health record technology in a purposeful manner (such as electronic medication prescribing), ensuring that the technology is connected in a manner that provides for the electronic exchange of health information to improve the quality of care (CDC, 2012).

Medicare hospice benefit: A benefit available under Medicare Part A that allows Medicare beneficiaries who choose hospice care to receive non-curative medical and support services for their terminal illness. To be eligible, beneficiaries must be certified by a physician to be terminally ill with a life expectancy of 6 months or less. Hospice care under Medicare includes both home care and inpatient care, when needed, and a variety of services not otherwise covered by Medicare (CMS, 2013).

Medicare Part A: Also known as the Hospital Insurance program, covers inpatient hospital services and skilled nursing facility, home health, and hospice care (IOM, 2013).

Medicare Part B: Also known as the Supplementary Medical Insurance program, helps pay for physician, outpatient, home health, and preventive services (IOM, 2013).

Medicare Part C (Medicare Advantage Plan): Allows beneficiaries to enroll in a private plan, such as a health maintenance organization, preferred provider organization, or private fee-for-service plan, as an alternative to the traditional fee-for service program. These plans receive payments from Medicare to provide Medicare-covered benefits, including hospital and physician services—and in most cases, prescription drug benefits (IOM, 2013).

Medicare Part D: The outpatient prescription drug benefit, established by the Medicare Modernization Act of 2003 and launched in 2006. The benefit is delivered through private plans that contract with Medicare—either stand-alone prescription drug plans or Medicare Advantage prescription drug plans (IOM, 2013).

Palliative care: Care that provides relief from pain and other symptoms, supports quality of life, and is focused on patients with serious advanced illness and their families. Palliative care may begin early in the course of treatment for a serious illness and may be delivered in a number of ways across the continuum of health care settings, including in the home, nursing homes, long-term acute care facilities, acute care hospitals, and outpatient clinics.

Patient-centered care: Health care that establishes a partnership among practitioners, patients, and their families (when appropriate) to ensure that decisions respect patients' wants, needs, and preferences and that patients have the education and support they need to make decisions and participate in their own care (IOM, 2001b).

POLST: Physician Orders for Life-Sustaining Treatment, created with and signed by a health professional, usually a physician (in some states a nurse practitioner or physician assistant), for someone who is seriously ill. Because they are actual doctor's orders, other health professionals, including emergency personnel, are required to follow them. POLST involves a clinical process designed to facilitate communication between health care professionals and patients, their families, their health care agents, or their designated surrogates. The POLST medical orders (forms) cover a range of topics likely to emerge in care of a patient near the end of life relating to that patient's goals of care and treatment preferences.

Specialty palliative care: Palliative care that is delivered by health care professionals who are palliative care specialists, such as physicians who are board certified in this specialty, palliative-certified nurses, and palliative care–certified social workers, pharmacists, and chaplains.

Spirituality: Refers to the way individuals seek and express meaning and purpose and the way they experience their connectedness to the moment, to self, to others, to nature, and to the significant or sacred (Pulchalski et al., 2009).

Surrogate: A person who, by default, becomes the substitute decision maker for an individual who has no appointed agent (HHS, 2008).

Systems-based approach: An organized, deliberate approach to the identification, assessment, and management of a complex clinical problem; may include checklists, treatment algorithms, provider education, quality improvement initiatives, and changes in delivery and payment models (Weissman and Meier, 2011).

Vulnerable populations: People from ethnic, cultural, and racial minorities, people with low educational attainment or low health literacy, and those in prisons or having limited access to care for geographic or financial reasons. Also included are people with serious illnesses, multiple chronic diseases, and disabilities (physical, mental, or cognitive); the frail elderly; those without accesses to needed health services; as well as nearly all people nearing the end of life.

REFERENCES

American Chronic Pain Association. 2013. *Glossary.* http://www.theacpa.org/Glossary (accessed November 1, 2013).

CBO (Congressional Budget Office). 2013. *Dual-eligible beneficiaries of Medicare and Medicaid: Characteristics, health care spending, and evolving policies.* CBO publication no. 4374. Washington, DC: U.S. Government Printing Office.

CDC (Centers for Disease Control and Prevention). 2012. *Meaningful use: Introduction.* http://www.cdc.gov/ehrmeaningfuluse/introduction.html (accessed August 5, 2014).

CMS (Centers for Medicare & Medicaid Services). 2013. *Medicare hospice benefits.* Baltimore, MD: CMS. http://www.medicare.gov/Pubs/pdf/02154.pdf (accessed August 5, 2014).

HHS (U.S. Department of Health and Human Services). 2008. *Advance directives and advance care planning: Report to Congress.* http://aspe.hhs.gov/daltcp/reports/2008/adcongrpt.htm (accessed August 7, 2013).

IOM (Institute of Medicine). 2001a. *Improving the quality of long-term care.* Washington, DC: National Academy Press.

IOM. 2001b. *Envisioning the national health care quality report.* Washington, DC: National Academy Press.

IOM. 2009. *Initial national priorities for comparative effectiveness research.* Washington, DC: The National Academies Press.

IOM. 2012. *Best care at lower cost: The path to continuously learning health care in America.* Washington, DC: The National Academies Press.

IOM. 2013. *Variation in health care spending: Target decision making, not geography.* Washington, DC: The National Academies Press.

Kiefer, K., L. Harris-Kojetin, D. Brannon, T. Barry, J. Vasey, and M. Lepore. 2005. *Measuring long-term care work: A guide to selected instruments to examine direct care worker experiences and outcomes.* Washington, DC: Institute for the Future of Aging Services.

NQF (National Quality Forum). 2006. *A national framework and preferred practices for palliative and hospice care quality: A consensus report.* Washington, DC: NQF.

Puchalski, C., B. Ferrell, R. Virani, S. Otis-Green, P. Baird, J. Bull, H. Chochinov, G. Handzo, H. Nelson-Becker, M. Prince-Paul, K. Pugliese, and D. Sulmasy. 2009. Improving the quality of spiritual care as a dimension of palliative care: The report of the consensus conference. *Journal of Palliative Medicine* 12(10):885-904.

Weissman, D. E., and D. E. Meier. 2011. Identifying patients in need of a palliative care assessment in the hospital setting: A consensus report from the center to advance palliative care. *Journal of Palliative Medicine* 14(1):17-23.

Xue, Q. L. 2011. The frailty syndrome: Definition and natural history. *Clinics in Geriatric Medicine* 27(1):1-15.

Appendix A

Data Sources and Methods

The Committee on Approaching Death: Addressing Key End-of-Life Issues was asked to assess the current state of health care for persons of all ages with a serious illness or medical condition who are likely approaching death and who require coordinated care, appropriate personal communication, and individual and family support. The purpose of this study was to assess the delivery of health care, social, and other supports to both the person approaching death and the family; person-family-provider communication of values, preferences, and beliefs; advance care planning; health care costs, financing, and reimbursement related to end-of-life care; and salient education of health professionals, patients, families, employers, and the public at large. To respond comprehensively to its charge, the committee examined data from a variety of sources. These sources included a review of the literature since the release of the 1997 Institute of Medicine (IOM) report *Approaching Death: Improving Care at the End of Life* and the 2003 report *When Children Die: Improving Palliative and End-of-Life Care for Children and Their Families*, public input obtained through a series of workshops and meetings, three commissioned papers, a public questionnaire soliciting experiences with end-of-life care, and written public comments on aspects of the study charge. The study was conducted over a 18-month period.

DESCRIPTION OF THE STUDY COMMITTEE

The study committee comprised 21 individuals with expertise in aging, palliative care, hospice, pediatrics, mental health, spirituality, caregiving, finance, health administration, public engagement, legal studies, health disparities, ethics, and health systems research. See Appendix G for biographical sketches of the committee members. The committee convened for six 2-day meetings in February 2013, May 2013, July 2013, September 2013, December 2013, and February 2014.

LITERATURE REVIEW

Several strategies were used to identify literature relevant to the committee's charge. First, a search of bibliographic databases, including MEDLINE, EMBASE, and SCOPUS, was conducted to obtain articles from peer-reviewed journals. The keywords used in searches included *advance directives, aging, bereavement, caregivers, chaplains, chronic disease, clinical and supportive care, communication, community engagement, continuing medical education, cultural barriers, death and dying, decision making, demographic shifts, disparities, epidemiology, ethics, ethnic groups, financing, fiscal realities, graduate medical education, health care delivery, health care quality, hospice, nursing, nursing home care, pain management, palliative care, patients, payment systems, pediatrics, pharmacy, professional education, professional standards, psychosocial care, public health, public-private partnerships, racial and ethnic differences, religion, social work, spirituality, team-based care, technology, vulnerable populations,* and *workforce development.*

Staff sorted through approximately 4,500 articles to identify those that were relevant to the committee's charge and created an EndNote database. In addition, committee members, meeting participants, and members of the public submitted articles and reports on these topics. The committee's database included more than 1,500 relevant articles and reports.

PUBLIC MEETINGS

The committee hosted three public meetings to obtain additional information on specific aspects of the study charge. These meetings were held in conjunction with the committee's February, May, and July 2013 meetings. Subject-matter experts were invited to the public meetings to present information and recommendations for the committee's consideration. The committee also held open forums at each public meeting at which members of the public were encouraged to provide testimony on any topics related to the study charge.

The first public meeting was intended to focus on a discussion of the committee's task, as well as provide a summary of the IOM's two most recent studies in the topic area, which generated the two reports cited above—*Approaching Death: Improving Care at the End of Life* and *When Children Die: Improving Palliative and End-of-Life Care for Children and Their Families*. The second meeting focused on family caregiver experiences and needs, as well as national and state policies impacting caregivers. The meeting also featured representatives of community organizations focused on end-of-life care, as well as a detailed summary of state-specific programs and policies for individuals approaching death. The third meeting featured speakers who discussed clinical ethics, spiritual and religious needs of individuals near the end of life, and empirical and legal issues regarding advance directives.

At each public meeting, the committee heard testimony and comments from a broad range of stakeholders, including individuals living with chronic disease, family members of people approaching death, health care providers, and individuals representing national and regional advocacy groups. The committee found this input to be highly informative for its deliberations. Agendas for the three public meetings are presented in Boxes A-1 through A-3.

ADDITIONAL ACTIVITIES

After the committee's third meeting in Houston, Texas, some members participated in mobile rounds. This activity was sponsored by the MD Anderson Cancer Center's Texas Community Bus Rounds program. Committee members had the opportunity to visit patients enrolled in home hospice care and to observe the delivery of care provided by members of the palliative care team at the MD Anderson Cancer Center.

The committee also hosted a theatrical performance in August 2013 at the Chautauqua Institution in New York. The performance by Outside the Wire included a reading of the ancient Greek play *Women of Trachis* by Sophocles as a catalyst for a town hall discussion about death and end-of-life care as it touches patients, families, and health professionals. The event was facilitated by Bryan Doerries, artistic director for Outside the Wire, with performances by T. Ryder Smith (as Heracles), Alex Morf (as Hyllus), and Bryan Doerries (as the Chorus). The panel comprised Patricia Bomba, M.D., FACP, vice president and medical director of geriatrics at Excellus BlueCross BlueShield; Christine Cassel, M.D., president and CEO of the National Quality Forum; Harvey Fineberg, M.D., Ph.D., then-president of the IOM; and Philip Pizzo, M.D., professor and former dean at the Stanford University School of Medicine. The event included a discussion with the more than 500 attendees about their reactions to the reading and experiences and thoughts related to serious illness, aging, and end-of-life issues.

In addition to testimony at these meetings, the committee solicited public input on topics relevant to its charge through its website. More than

500 individuals provided written testimony. A summary of these comments can be found in Appendix C.

COMMISSIONED PAPERS

The committee commissioned three papers from experts in subject-matter areas relevant to the study charge. These papers were intended to provide greater analysis and in-depth information on selected topics of interest to the committee:

- A paper written by Haiden Huskamp of Harvard Medical School and David Stevenson of the Vanderbilt University School of Medicine provides a detailed analysis of financing and payment methods in end-of-life care, as well as possible reforms to federal eligibility and payment policies (see Appendix D).
- A paper written by Melissa Aldridge and Amy Kelley of the Mount Sinai Icahn School of Medicine reviews the epidemiology of individuals approaching death, including demographics, clinical characteristics, and patterns of health care utilization. It also reviews current programs and models of care aimed at high-cost populations and suggests future research opportunities for evaluating this part of the population (see Appendix E).
- A paper written by Chris Feudtner, Wenjun Zhong, Jen Faerber, and Dingwei Dai of The Children's Hospital of Pennsylvania and James Feinstein of the Ann & Robert H. Lurie Children's Hospital of Chicago reviews the challenges and opportunities of delivering pediatric end-of-life care and palliative care. The paper provides analysis on the epidemiology of children approaching death, in addition to potential implications for utilizing those data to make changes in pediatric end-of-life care (see Appendix F).

BOX A-1
PUBLIC SESSION AGENDA

Wednesday, February 20, 2013

National Academy of Sciences
2101 Constitution Avenue NW, Lecture Room
Washington, DC 20418

1:00 p.m. WELCOME AND INTRODUCTIONS

Judith A. Salerno, M.D., M.S.
Leonard D. Schaeffer Executive Officer
Institute of Medicine

David M. Walker and Philip A. Pizzo, M.D.
Co-Chairs
Committee on Approaching Death: Addressing Key End-of-Life
Issues

1:15 p.m. COMMITTEE PERSPECTIVES ON STUDY CHARGE

Committee members will discuss areas that should be considered
during the course of the study.

2:15 p.m. STAKEHOLDER PERSPECTIVES ON STUDY CHARGE

Members of the public will have an opportunity to provide 3 minutes
of comments/testimony in any area related to the study charge.

Susan Friedman
Deputy Director of Government Relations
American Osteopathic Association

Nneka Mokwunye, Ph.D.
Director
Center for Ethics, Washington Hospital Center

Evan DeRenzo, Ph.D.
Senior Clinical Ethicist
Center for Ethics, Washington Hospital Center

William Benson
Principal
Health Benefits ABCs and International Association for Indigenous
Aging

continued

BOX A-1 Continued

Mickey MacIntyre
Chief Program Officer
Compassion & Choices

Rosalind Kipping
President
Compassion & Choices National Capital Area Chapter

Lisa Culver, M.B.A.
Senior Specialist, Clinical Practice
American Physical Therapy Association

Barry Passett, M.D.
Physician

Joan Harrold, M.D.
Medical Director & Vice President of Medical Services
Hospice & Community Care

Kristen Santiago, M.S.
Manager, Strategic Initiatives
C-Change

David Longnecker, M.D.
Director
Association of American Medical Colleges

Sally Welsh, M.S.N., R.N.
CEO
Hospice and Palliative Nurses Association

Marie Delvalle-Mahoney, M.D.
Physician
Canon Hospice and North Shore Hospitalists, LLC

Mollie Gurian, J.D., M.P.H.

Cameron Muir, M.D.
Executive Vice President, Quality & Access
Capital Caring/The Innovations Group

3:15 p.m. BREAK

3:25 p.m OVERVIEW OF 1997 IOM REPORT
APPROACHING DEATH: IMPROVING CARE AT THE END OF LIFE

Christine K. Cassel, M.D.
Former Chair of the Committee on Care at the End of Life

OVERVIEW OF 2003 IOM REPORT
WHEN CHILDREN DIE: IMPROVING PALLIATIVE AND END-OF-LIFE CARE FOR CHILDREN AND THEIR FAMILIES

Pamela S. Hinds, Ph.D., R.N., FAAN
Former Member of the Committee on Palliative and End-of-Life Care for Children and Their Families

DISCUSSION

5:00 p.m. ADJOURN and RECEPTION

BOX A-2
PUBLIC SESSION AGENDA

Wednesday, May 29, 2013

Stanford University School of Medicine
300 Pasteur Drive, Always Building
Stanford, CA 94305

8:30 a.m. **WELCOME AND INTRODUCTIONS**

David M. Walker and Philip A. Pizzo, M.D.
Co-Chairs
Committee on Approaching Death: Addressing Key End-of-Life
Issues

8:45 a.m. **POLICIES AND CAREGIVING AT THE END OF LIFE**

Lynn Friss Feinberg, M.S.W.
Senior Strategic Policy Advisor
Independent Living/Long-Term Care
AARP Public Policy Institute

Ms. Feinberg will provide an overview of policies that support family
caregivers, including future policy needs at the end of life.

9:15 a.m. **FAMILY CAREGIVER EXPERIENCES AND NEEDS**

Barbara Sourkes, Ph.D.
Kriewall-Haehl Director, Palliative Care Program
Lucile Packard Children's Hospital
Stanford University School of Medicine

Dr. Sourkes will provide an overview of critical issues that families
face, both the universal themes that cross the life span and those
that are specific to either adult or pediatric care at the end of life.
She will moderate a panel of family caregivers who will provide their
perspectives on challenges in communication, decision making, and
obtaining optimal care for themselves as well as their loved ones.

Panelists:
Joanne Barr
Carla Reeves
Jim Santucci
Alyson Yisrael

10:30 a.m.   BREAK

**10:45 a.m.   COMMUNITY ORGANIZATIONS FOCUSED ON END-OF-LIFE
                CARE**

VJ Periyakoil, M.D.
Director
Palliative Care Education and Training
Stanford University School of Medicine

Dr. Periyakoil will provide an overview of the opportunities
and challenges related to providing culturally effective care
for multicultural Americans. She will moderate a panel of
representatives from community-based organizations effectively
meeting the end-of-life needs of diverse populations. Panelists will
describe the services they provide, the varied populations they
serve, and lessons learned about effective strategies for facilitating
access to quality end-of-life care.

Panelists:
Alex Briscoe
Director
Alameda County Health Care Services Agency

Marilyn Ababio
Hospice Systems Coordinator
Alameda County Health Services Agency

Sandy Chen Stokes, R.N., M.S.N.
Founder
Chinese American Coalition for Compassionate Care

Jean Yih
Board Chair
Chinese American Coalition for Compassionate Care

Barbara Beach, M.D.
Co-founder and Medical Director
George Mark Children's House

12:00 p.m.   LUNCH

continued

BOX A-2 Continued

12:45 p.m.   STATE-LEVEL PROGRAMS AND POLICIES

Panelists will provide an overview of programs, policies, and
legislation pertaining to care at the end of life.

Susan Tolle, M.D.
Director
Center for Ethics in Health Care
Oregon Health and Science University

Myra Christopher
Kathleen M. Foley Chair for Pain and Palliative Care
Center for Practical Bioethics

Margaret Metzger, J.D.
Health Care Consultant
Wellesley, Massachusetts

2:00 p.m.   PUBLIC COMMENT

Members of the public who register will have 3 minutes to comment
on any topic related to the study charge.

Marilyn Golden
Senior Policy Analyst
Disability Rights Education & Defense Fund

Jeffrey Kaufhold, M.D.
Chair, Ethics Committee
Greater Dayton Area Hospital Association

Renée Berry
Chief Executive Officer
BeMoRe

Amy Vandenbroucke, J.D.
Executive Director
National POLST Paradigm Task Force

Pat Dodson, M.A.
Advisory Board Member
Compassion & Choices

Paula Taubman
Northern California Executive Director
Compassion & Choices

Thomas White, Ph.D.
Member, Board of Directors
Compassion & Choices

Stephanie Harman, M.D.
Clinical Assistant Professor
Stanford School of Medicine

Devon Dabbs
Executive Director and Co-Founder
Children's Hospice and Palliative Care Coalition

Heidi Engel, D.P.T.
Physical Therapist and Clinical Instructor
University of California, San Francisco Medical Center

L. Alberto Molina
Assistant Director of Interpreter Services
Stanford Hospital & Clinics

Angelica Villagran
VMI Coordinator
Stanford Hospital & Clinics

Johanna Parker
Lead Interpreter for Education and Training
Stanford Hospital & Clinics

3:00 p.m.   **ADJOURN**

BOX A-3
PUBLIC SESSION AGENDA

Monday, July 22, 2013

Baylor College of Medicine
One Baylor Plaza
Board Room, Room M-100
Houston, TX

1:00 p.m.   WELCOME AND COMMITTEE INTRODUCTIONS

David M. Walker and Philip A. Pizzo, M.D.
Co-Chairs
Committee on Approaching Death: Addressing Key End-of-Life
Issues

Paul Klotman, M.D.
President and CEO
Baylor College of Medicine

1:15 p.m.   CLINICAL ETHICS

Jeremy Sugarman, M.D., M.P.H.
Harvey M. Meyerhoff Professor of Bioethics and Medicine
Johns Hopkins Berman Institute of Bioethics

Dr. Sugarman will present an overview of end-of-life decision-making
principles, including respect for patients' values, goals, choices, and
dignity; advance care planning; surrogate decision making; the role
of current best interests of the incompetent patient; conscientious
objections by health care workers and institutions; justice; and
allocation of limited resources.

Rebecca Dresser, J.D.
Daniel Noyes Kirby Professor of Law
Professor of Ethics in Medicine
Washington University in St. Louis
Former Member, President's Council on Bioethics

Ms. Dresser will provide an overview of the President's Council on
Bioethics 2005 report *Taking Care: Ethical Caregiving in Our Aging
Society.* She will focus on the importance of respect for human life
and dignity and caring for persons who are disabled or enfeebled.

2:00 p.m.	**DISCUSSION**
2:30 p.m.	**BREAK**
2:45 p.m.	**ADDRESSING SPIRITUAL AND RELIGIOUS NEEDS**

Farr A. Curlin, M.D.
Associate Professor of Medicine
Co-Director, Program on Medicine and Religion
Faculty, MacLean Center for Clinical Medical Ethics
The University of Chicago

Dr. Curlin will examine the importance of spiritual needs and concerns for patients near the end of life and the value of religion as a source of support for many patients. He will consider the value of health care professionals inquiring about those needs and concerns; the benefits (in terms of patient outcomes) of addressing those needs as part of high-quality palliative care; the importance of the conscience and integrity of physicians and health care workers in end-of-life care; and ethical dilemmas that arise in a diverse, pluralistic society when the health care professional holds strong religious beliefs that differ sharply from the religious beliefs of the patient.

The Rev. Charles R. Millikan, D.Min.
Vice-President for Spiritual Care and Values Integration
The Methodist Hospital System
Houston, Texas

Rev. Millikan will discuss how in a multidisciplinary health care team in end-of-life care, the patient's spiritual needs and concerns can be addressed in a respectful way. He will consider the role of hospital chaplains in helping patients address these issues in a nondenominational way, as well as the role of the patient's own religious advisors.

| 3:25 p.m. | **DISCUSSION** |
| 4:00 p.m. | **ADJOURN DAY #1 PUBLIC SESSION** |

continued

BOX A-3 Continued

Tuesday, July 23, 2013

Texas Children's Cancer Center
6701 Fannin Street
Auditorium
Houston, TX

9:00 a.m.   **WELCOME AND COMMITTEE INTRODUCTIONS**

David M. Walker and Philip A. Pizzo, M.D.
Co-Chairs
Committee on Approaching Death: Addressing Key End-of-Life
Issues

9:15 a.m.   **EMPIRICAL AND LEGAL ISSUES REGARDING POLST**

Susan E. Hickman, Ph.D.
Associate Professor, Indiana University School of Nursing
Co-Director, Research in Palliative and End-of-Life Communication
and Training (RESPECT) Center, Indiana University-Purdue
University Indianapolis (IUPUI)
Senior Affiliate, IU Health Fairbanks Center for Medical Ethics

Dr. Hickman will present a critical overview of empirical evidence
regarding the impact of Physician Orders for Life-Sustaining
Treatment (POLST) on clinical care and outcomes. Does POLST
lead to fewer days in the intensive care unit in the last week of
life, CPR before death, etc.? Do states that have robust POLST
programs have different levels of specific medical interventions in
end-of-life care? Does POLST reduce disputes regarding end-of-life
decisions? Does POLST prevent complicated grieving by survivors
or decision regret?

Rebecca Sudore, M.D.
Associate Professor of Medicine
University of California, San Francisco

Dr. Sudore will review challenges and limitations in advance care
planning and POLST, with particular attention to vulnerable patients.
She will consider the importance of conversations in advance care
planning, as well as documentation of orders and the challenges
entailed in improving these conversations.

Alan Meisel, J.D.
Director, Center for Bioethics and Health Law
Dickie, McCamey and Chilcote Professor of Bioethics, and Professor of Law and Psychiatry
University of Pittsburgh

Mr. Meisel will discuss legal issues that might present challenges to a patient and family who wish to use the POLST form or other types of advance care planning. May a surrogate complete a POLST for a patient who has already lost decision-making capacity? Are there restrictions on using POLST to decline feeding tubes in patients with severe dementia or stroke? Are these limitations communicated effectively to patients and families using POLST? Have there been cases involving POLST in the courts? What other legal approaches to advance care planning have states implemented, such as default priority for surrogates and oral appointment of health care proxies, and how have they worked in practice?

10:00 a.m. DISCUSSION

10:45 a.m. BREAK

11:00 a.m. PUBLIC COMMENT

Members of the public who register will have 5 minutes to comment on any topic related to the study charge.

Diane Coleman
President and CEO
Not Dead Yet

Cynthia Taniguchi
Project Manager, Provider Implementation
McKesson Specialty Health

Donald Molony, M.D.
Professor of Medicine
University of Texas Houston Medical School

Robert J. Hesse, Ph.D.
Vice Chairman, Institute for Spirituality and Health
The Texas Medical Center

12:00 p.m. ADJOURN

Appendix B

Recommendations of the Institute of Medicine's Reports *Approaching Death* (1997) and *When Children Die* (2003): Progress and Significant Remaining Gaps

Significant progress has been made in improving the care of people near the end of life since the publication of the Institute of Medicine (IOM) reports *Approaching Death: Improving Care at the End of Life* (IOM, 1997) and *When Children Die: Improving Palliative and End-of-Life Care for Children and Their Families* (IOM, 2003), yet gaps still remain. This appendix highlights just some of the advances that have been made, as well as a selection of the areas in which efforts are still needed.

APPROACHING DEATH

1997 Recommendation 1: People with advanced, potentially fatal illnesses and those close to them should be able to expect and receive reliable, skillful, and supportive care.

- As of 2009, 63 percent of U.S. hospitals with at least 50 beds, 85 percent of hospitals with more than 300 beds, and all Veterans Administration hospitals reported having a palliative care team—an increase of 138 percent from 2000 (CAPC, 2011; Edes et al., 2007; Morrison et al., 2011). In 2011, an estimated 1.65 million patients received hospice services; a million of them died under hospice care during that year (NHPCO, 2012a). In comparison, *Approaching Death* (IOM, 1997) notes that 390,000 patients were served by hospice in 1995, representing just 17 percent of all deaths that year.

- In 2001, 19 percent of all Medicare decedents accessed hospice for 3 or more days. By 2007, this proportion had increased to 30 percent (NHPCO, 2012a).
- A number of demonstration projects related to end-of-life care, including those of the Sutter Medical Network, Kaiser Permanente, and Aetna's Compassionate Care Program, have been completed, creating potential new care delivery models (Brumley and Hillary, 2002; Brumley et al., 2007; Krakauer et al., 2009; Labson et al., 2013; Meyer, 2011; Spettell et al., 2009).
- Additional pilot efforts have taken place in difficult-to-serve rural areas.
  - A National Rural Health Association Technical Assistance Project, funded by the Health Resources and Services Administration, Office of Rural Health Policy (HRSA-ORHP), provided assistance in "Community Oriented Planning for Palliative Care" to three rural communities. One of these efforts focused on linkages among service agencies and developed a volunteer program to support patients with complex care issues (Stratis Health, 2009).
  - A separate rural pilot program involved 10 rural Minnesota communities that established or strengthened local palliative care programs through the Minnesota Rural Palliative Care Initiative (October 2008 to April 2010). As of April 2011, 6 of the 10 were enrolling patients and providing interdisciplinary palliative care services, while the other 4 had developed and/or improved processes to enhance palliative care services (Stratis Health, 2011).
- The Center to Advance Palliative Care,[1] established at Mount Sinai School of Medicine in New York City with funding from the Robert Wood Johnson Foundation (RWJF) in 1999, is a national resource providing health care professionals with tools, training, and technical assistance to increase access to quality palliative care services in hospitals and other health settings. It also works to improve relevant payment and regulatory policies.

Remaining gaps:

- Only about two-thirds of hospitals nationwide offer some type of palliative care program, and the lessons learned in centers of palliative care excellence are not available to everyone (NHPCO, 2012a).

---

[1] See http://www.capc.org (accessed December 17, 2014).

- Patients in small hospitals (those with fewer than 50 beds, which represent about one in five U.S. hospitals), public hospitals (54 percent), and sole community provider hospitals (40 percent)[2] have much less access to palliative medicine. These institutions also typically serve uninsured and rural Americans (NHPCO, 2012a).
- Accreditation standards for hospitals and nursing homes do not currently require that hospitals offer a quality palliative care program; however, the Joint Commission has established a voluntary advanced certification program for palliative care programs (Joint Commission, 2014).
- The rate of health care transitions among fee-for-service Medicare beneficiaries increased between 2000 and 2009, including the rate of transitions both in the last 90 days of life and in the last 3 days of life (Teno et al., 2013).
- Caregiving takes an enormous emotional, physical, and financial toll on individuals, and this role could be better supported by health care providers and employers and through public policy (Abernethy et al., 2008; Coalition to Transform Advanced Care, 2013; DOL, 2013; Kilbourn et al., 2011; Payne et al., 1999; Reinhard et al., 2012).
- Despite some positive trends in integrating palliative and disease-specific treatment, greater efforts are needed (Matlock et al., 2010). As long as palliative care is considered "separate from" the main business of health care, it is vulnerable to being omitted or ignored.

1997 Recommendation 2: Physicians, nurses, social workers, and other health professionals must commit themselves to improving care for dying patients and to using existing knowledge effectively to prevent and relieve pain and other symptoms.

- The number of palliative care teams within hospital settings has increased by approximately 148 percent, from more than 600 in 2000 to more than 1,600 in 2012 (CAPC, 2012).

Remaining gaps:

- Studies of pain management and symptom burden have shown undertreatment by health care providers (Kutner et al., 2001; Swetz et al., 2012; Wilkie and Ezenwa, 2012).
- A 2011 IOM report also notes persistent undertreatment of pain near the end of life (IOM, 2011).

---

[2] Totals add to more than 100 percent because some hospitals are in more than one category.

- There is little objective information about the knowledge and attitudes of health professionals regarding care of patients near the end of life.
- A greater emphasis is needed on team care and coordinated services across care settings.

1997 Recommendation 3: Because many problems in care stem from system problems, policy makers, consumer groups, and purchasers of health care should work with health care practitioners, organizations, and researchers to

(a) *strengthen methods for measuring the quality of life and other outcomes of care for dying patients and those close to them;*

- The National Consensus Project for Quality Palliative Care (NCP), launched in 2002, represents the nation's major hospice and palliative care organizations and has developed and disseminated three versions of its *Clinical Practice Guidelines for Quality Palliative Care* (2004, 2009, and 2013) (Dahlin, 2009, 2013; NCP, 2004).
- The National Quality Forum (NQF) used these guidelines to develop its report *A National Framework and Preferred Practices for Palliative and Hospice Care Quality,* published in 2006 (NQF, 2006).
- With the Assessing Care of Vulnerable Elders (ACOVE) initiative, RAND Corporation developed a large set of quality indicators, including indicators relevant or specific to care near the end of life (Walling et al., 2010; Wenger et al., 2007).
- The PEACE Project (Prepare, Embrace, Attend, Communicate, Empower) reviewed 174 potential measures of quality for hospice and palliative care, and gave 34 high ratings (Hanson et al., 2010; Schenck et al., 2010).
- The Measuring What Matters initiative, an effort by the American Academy of Hospice and Palliative Medicine (AAHPM) Quality and Practice Standards Task Force and the Hospice and Palliative Nurses Association (HPNA) Research Advisory Group, seeks to identify a set of basic, advanced, and aspirational evidence-based performance measures that are relevant to all hospice and palliative care programs (American Academy of Hospice and Palliative Medicine, undated-a,b,c).
- A Toolkit of Instruments to Measure End-of-Life Care was developed[3] and is accepted and widely used in the field (Mularski et al., 2007).

---

[3]See http://www.chcr.brown.edu/pcoc/toolkit.htm (accessed December 17, 2014); http://www.chcr.brown.edu/pcoc/resourceguide/resourceguide.pdf (accessed December 17, 2014).

- as the "family interview" quality assessment tool by almost 900 National Hospice and Palliative Care Organization (NHPCO) hospice member organizations, which have created a database of several hundred thousand family surveys that are a rich resource for new research, including studies of the quality of care and outcomes for patients with dementia and cancer;
- in informing the development of national, state, and local indicators of end-of-life care quality; and
- in a range of other research.

(b) *develop better tools and strategies for improving the quality of care and holding health care organizations accountable for care at the end of life;*

- NHPCO now reports data related to patient outcomes and measures; family evaluation of hospice care, palliative care, and bereavement services; and team attitudes and relationships (NHPCO, undated-a).
- Medicare's Hospice Quality Reporting Program (HQRP), established under the Patient Protection and Affordable Care Act (ACA), requires hospice programs to report quality data publicly (CMS, undated; HHS, 2013).[4]
  - Hospices were initially required by the Centers for Medicare & Medicaid Services (CMS) to report on two measures: first reports on Quality Assessment and Performance Improvement programs were due in January 2013, and those on pain control performance, using NQF's pain measure (#0209), by April 2013.
  - Beginning in 2014, however, these previously used measures will be discontinued, and the hospices will be required under the HQRP to complete and submit to CMS the Hospice Item Set (HIS), which collects data on seven NQF-endorsed measures.
  - In addition to the HIS quality reporting requirements, CMS will require that hospices, starting in 2015, complete the Hospice Experience of Care Survey, which will gather information from caregivers of deceased hospice patients about patient and family experiences with hospice care.
- NHPCO has developed a Quality Partners performance improvement program and additional quality resources for hospices (NHPCO, undated-b).

---

[4]Patient Protection and Affordable Care Act of 2010, Public Law 111-148, 111th Cong., 2d sess. (March 23, 2010), § 3004(c).

(c) *revise mechanisms for financing care so that they encourage rather than impede good end-of-life care and sustain rather than frustrate coordinated systems of excellent care;*

- The Medicare Hospice Benefit covered hospice services for more than 1.1 million beneficiaries in 2010 (MedPAC, 2012). To elect the Medicare Hospice Benefit, patients must forgo all curative treatments and opt solely for comfort care. Eligibility is based on a life expectancy of 6 months or less (CMS, 2013a).
- Demonstration projects at Sutter Medical Network, Kaiser Permanente, and Aetna, noted above, have successfully tested an expanded version of hospice that uses the concept of "concurrent care," which does not require patients to give up curative treatments, a major barrier to hospice enrollment (Brumley and Hillary, 2002; Brumley et al., 2007; Krakauer et al., 2009; Labson et al., 2013; Meyer, 2011; Spettell et al., 2009).
- The ACA amends current law regarding pediatric hospice care to eliminate the requirement for electing either curative or hospice care when it is paid for through Medicaid and state Children's Health Insurance Programs (CHIPs).[5]
- The ACA further calls for a concurrent care demonstration program to test whether concurrent care would save money while improving Medicare patients' quality of life.[6] In March 2014, CMS launched the Medicare Care Choices Model, which will allow selected Medicare-certified hospices to provide palliative care services to patients with certain serious advanced illnesses who meet the Medicare Hospice Benefit eligibility criteria but are still receiving curative care (CMS, 2014).
- A new Medicare-Medicaid Coordination Office is established under the ACA, and is charged with facilitating the integration and alignment of federal Medicare and state Medicaid funding into a single source of financial support (CMS, 2013b).
- Models of managed care for the dually eligible have shown promise among certain populations, including individuals in nursing homes and those with advanced dementia (Brown and Mann, 2012; Goldfeld et al., 2013; Kane et al., 2002).

---

[5]Patient Protection and Affordable Care Act of 2010, Public Law 111-148, 111th Cong., 2d sess. (March 23, 2010), Section 2302 Concurrent Care for Children.

[6]Patient Protection and Affordable Care Act of 2010, Public Law 111-148, 111th Cong., 2d sess. (March 23, 2010), Section 3140 Medicare Hospice Concurrent Care Demonstration Program.

Remaining gaps:

- The hospice care payment methodology and the base rates have not been recalibrated since the benefit was established in 1983 (MedPAC, 2012).
- In 2009, the Medicare Payment Advisory Commission (MedPAC) made recommendations to reform the hospice payment system so it would provide relatively higher payments at the beginning and end of the hospice stay (U-shaped payment curve), rather than the current equal daily payment (MedPAC, 2009).
- Under a 2009 CMS rule, the Budget Neutrality Adjustment Factor (BNAF)—a key factor in calculating the Medicare hospice wage index—will be phased out over 7 years, resulting in a permanent reduction in hospice reimbursement rates of approximately 4.2 percent (CMS, 2009a; Hospice Action Network, 2013).
- The ACA alters the Medicare hospice rate formula, wage index, and payment rate through
  - introduction of a productivity adjustment factor, which will lower annual hospice payments by an additional 11.8 percent over the next decade (CMS, 2013c; Hospice Action Network, 2013); and
  - reduction of the hospice market basket update by 0.3 percentage points (CMS, 2013c).
- CMS's Bundled Payments for Care Improvement Initiative specifically excludes hospice services (CMS, 2013d).
- Financial incentives still drive the volume of services delivered and lead to fragmentation of the health care system and high costs (Kamal et al., 2012; Kumetz and Goodson, 2013; MedPAC, 2011; Schroeder and Frist, 2013).

(d) *reform drug prescription laws, burdensome regulations, and state medical board policies and practices that impede effective use of opioids to relieve pain and suffering.*

- In 2004, the Federation of State Medical Boards of the United States, Inc., adopted new revised management guidelines as the "Model Policy for the Use of Controlled Substances for the Treatment of Pain," emphasizing the problem of undertreatment (FSMB, 2004).[7]

---

[7]State-by-state opioid prescribing policies can be found at http://www.medscape.com/resource/pain/opioid-policies (accessed December 17, 2014).

- As part of its End of Life initiatives, RWJF funded researchers at the University of Wisconsin to support their work in assessing laws, regulations, and guidelines relating to pain treatment (Patrizi et al., 2011; RWJF, 2008).
  - *Achieving Balance in Federal and State Pain Policy: A Guide to Evaluation*, published by the University of Wisconsin Pain & Policy Studies Group in 2000 and updated in 2003, presents findings of a systematic evaluation of pain-related policies of the federal government, the 50 states, and the District of Columbia. Subsequent versions of this guide have been supported by the American Cancer Society, the American Cancer Society Cancer Action Network, and the LIVESTRONG Foundation (Pain & Policy Studies Group, 2014a).
  - From 2000 to 2003, RWJF funded the development of *Achieving Balance in State Pain Policy: A Progress Report Card*, which graded all states based on their policy content. The report card is currently supported by the American Cancer Society, the American Cancer Society Cancer Action Network, and the LIVESTRONG Foundation (Pain & Policy Studies Group, 2014b). The most recent report card, for calendar year 2013, found that
    - 96 percent of states received a grade higher than C, an improvement from 88 percent in 2008;
    - 15 states received a grade of A, indicating state policies that best balance pain management and drug control, while only 8 states (Alaska, Illinois, Louisiana, Missouri, Nevada, Oklahoma, Tennessee, and Texas) received below a B, and no states received below a C; and
    - since 2006, no state has seen a reduction in its pain policy grade.

Remaining gaps:

- Physicians report persistent opinions—voiced by patients' families, other physicians, or other health care professionals—that common palliative practices, including palliative sedation and prescribing of pain medications for symptom management, are euthanasia or murder (Goldstein et al., 2012).
- A 2007 review of state pain policies notes that "potential barriers [to pain management] are restrictive drug control and health care policies governing the medical use of prescription medications for pain management, palliative care, or end-of-life care" (Gilson et al., 2007, p. 342).

- A 2011 IOM report also recognizes persistent undertreatment of pain near the end of life. The report acknowledges that restrictive regulatory and law enforcement policies negatively impact the appropriate use of opioid drugs for all patients experiencing pain, and that "frequently [hospice and palliative care programs] must rely on opiate medications at levels that would be inappropriate in other, nonterminal situations" (IOM, 2011, p. 85).

1997 Recommendation 4: Educators and other health professionals should initiate changes in undergraduate, graduate, and continuing education to ensure that practitioners have relevant attitudes, knowledge, and skills to care well for dying patients.

- AAHPM, which began with 250 founding member physicians in 1988, had nearly 5,000 members as of mid-2013 (American Academy of Hospice and Palliative Medicine, undated-d).
- As of the start of the 2014-2015 academic year, there were 107 accredited subspecialty training fellowship programs in the United States, collectively producing approximately 227 new palliative medicine physicians per year (ACGME, 2014).
- Accreditation standards for undergraduate baccalaureate nursing programs, adopted by the American Association of Colleges of Nursing in 2008, specify that all baccalaureate nursing graduates should be prepared to "implement patient and family care around resolution of end-of-life and palliative care issues, such as symptom management, support of rituals, and respect for patient and family preferences" (AACN, 2008, p. 31).
- The Education in Palliative and End-of-Life Care (EPEC) project began in 1999 as a train-the-trainer program for physicians and other health professionals, geared to teaching both its curriculum and educational approaches to improving palliative care. As of 2010, there were more than 2,000 EPEC trainers in the United States and 16 other countries (EPEC, 2012).
- In 2000, the End-of-Life Nursing Education Consortium (ELNEC) project began providing undergraduate and graduate nursing faculty, continuing education providers, staff development educators, specialty nurses, and others with training in palliative care so they could teach this essential information to nursing students and practicing nurses. As of April 2013, more than 15,400 nurses and other health care professionals had received ELNEC training, and in turn had returned to their institutions and communities to train more than 390,000 nurses and other health care providers (AACN, 2014a; ELNEC, 2013).

- Around this same time, the End-of-Life/Palliative Education Resource Center[8] was launched to share educational resource material among the community of health professional educators involved in palliative care education. It continues to be an authoritative source of information today.
- The Project on Death in America (PDIA) Faculty Scholars program (1995-2003) selected 87 scholars (from 740 applicants), 83 percent of whom were physicians and 13 percent nurses. An analysis of the scholars' subsequent careers found that the program was "successful in . . . developing a core group of clinical and academic leaders to advance the field of palliative care" (Sullivan et al., 2009, p. 157).
- PDIA's Social Work Leadership and Development Awards funded 42 social work leaders and led to the first Social Work Summit on End-of-Life and Palliative Care in 2002 (PDIA, 2004; SWHPN, undated). The work continues today under the auspices of the Social Work Hospice and Palliative Care Network, which has more than 500 members.[9]

Remaining gaps:

- The medical school curriculum is required to cover end-of-life care (Liaison Committee on Medical Education, 2013); education in palliative care is offered in 99 percent of U.S. medical schools, usually as part of another course; and all medical schools offer some type of instruction on death and dying, although the average total instruction is only 17 hours in the 4-year curriculum (Dickinson, 2011).
- While structured medical school curricula in hospice and palliative medicine, especially those that incorporate experiential and clinical aspects, have demonstrated effectiveness, they still are not widespread (Quill et al., 2003; Ross et al., 2001; von Gunten et al., 2012).
- Hospice and palliative medicine content is relatively lacking in many board certification examinations in specialties in which basic palliative care is especially relevant, accounting for only 2 percent of the board certification exam in oncology (ABIM, 2013a) and 3 percent in general internal medicine (ABIM, 2013b).
- In 2011-2013, only 3 of the 49 accredited U.S. schools of public health offered a course on end-of-life care policy. Another 6 public

---

[8] See http://www.eperc.mcw.edu/EPERC.htm?docid=67983 (accessed December 17, 2014).
[9] See http://www.swhpn.org (accessed December 17, 2014).

health schools offered some content on end-of-life concerns, but most of these offerings embedded this content in courses on aging policy and so did not consider the entire life span (Lupu et al., 2013).

1997 Recommendation 5: *Palliative care should become, if not a medical specialty, at least a defined area of expertise, education, and research.*

- In 2006, the American Board of Medical Specialties approved hospice and palliative medicine as a medical subspecialty of 10 participating boards, and the Accreditation Council for Graduate Medical Education voted to accredit fellowship training programs in this subspecialty. By 2009, CMS had approved palliative medicine as a subspecialty (CMS, 2009b).
- In the United States, there were 2,887 physicians certified by the American Board of Hospice and Palliative Medicine as of 2008, and there were 566 advanced practice nurses certified by the National Board for Certification of Hospice and Palliative Nurses (NBCHPN®) and almost 10,771 NBCHPN®-certified registered nurses as of March 2011 (CAPC, 2011). Between 2008 and 2012, 6,356 physicians across all 10 participating board specialties became board certified in hospice and palliative medicine (ABEM, 2013; ABFM, 2013; ABIM, 2013c; ABP, 2013; ABPMR, 2013; ABPN, 2013; ABS, 2013).[10]
- Approximately 4,400 physicians currently practice hospice and palliative medicine, as defined by board certification or membership in AAHPM (Lupu and AAHPM Workforce Task Force, 2010). Most practice this specialty part-time, yielding an estimated palliative physician workforce of 1,700-3,300 full-time equivalent (FTE) physicians.
- Since 2008, the National Association of Social Workers (NASW) has offered specialty certification in hospice and palliative care; as of 2014, there are 18 advanced practice specialty credentials offered by NASW (NASW, 2014).
- Concepts associated with pain management and palliative care are part of curriculum standards in pharmacotherapy (ACPE, 2011).
- A 2012 survey found that 82 percent of pharmacy schools offered some coursework on end-of-life care, typically as learning modules or lectures rather than devoted classes (Dickinson, 2013); on average, 6.2 hours was devoted to teaching students about death

---

[10]Personal communication, S. McGreal, ABMS, February 4, 2014.

and dying (Dickinson, 2013), an increase from 3.9 hours in 2001 (Herndon et al., 2003).

- Chaplains are certified by the Board of Chaplaincy Certification Inc., an affiliate of the 4,500-member Association of Professional Chaplains (BCCI, 2013). Specialty certification in palliative care (BCC-PCC) was introduced in 2013 as the first in an expected series of specialty chaplaincy certifications (APC, 2013).

Remaining gaps:

- An estimated 4,487 hospice and 10,810 palliative care physician FTEs are needed to staff the current number of hospice- and hospital-based palliative care programs at appropriate levels (Lupu and AAHPM Workforce Task Force, 2010).
- The Board of Pharmacy Specialties has considered adding pain and palliative medicine as a specialty, but it has yet to do so (BPS, 2011).

1997 Recommendation 6: The nation's research establishment should define and implement priorities for strengthening the knowledge base for end-of-life care.

- In 1997, the Director of the National Institutes of Health (NIH) designated the National Institute of Nursing Research (NINR) as NIH's lead institute for end-of-life research. In 2009, NINR established the Office of Research on End-of-Life Science and Palliative Care, Investigator Training, and Education (OEPC) (NINR, 2012).
- In 2013, NINR published *Building Momentum: The Science of End-of-Life and Palliative Care: A Review of Research Trends and Funding, 1997-2010*, which reviews the state of the research in end-of-life and palliative care since the 1997 IOM report *Approaching Death* was issued (NINR, 2013a). Among its findings are the following:
  - There was a tripling of publications on end-of-life and palliative care between 1997 and 2010.
  - Published studies focus primarily on advance care planning, pain and symptom management, and locations and types of care.
  - Research was supported by 37 federal organizations and more than 500 private nongovernmental organizations; an increase in funding from NIH has been seen since 1997, but so, too, has a reduction in private funding (from 48.5 percent of research support in 1997 to 24.8 percent in 2010).

- With support from a number of public and private funders, the National Palliative Care Research Center (NPCRC)[11] establishes priorities for palliative care research, works to develop a new generation of palliative care researchers, and coordinates and supports studies of ways to improve care for patients and families. The center's partner organization, the Center to Advance Palliative Care, enables rapid translation of these research findings into clinical practice.
- The Palliative Care Research Cooperative Group (PCRC), established in 2010, offers a mechanism for connecting researchers and clinicians across varied clinical settings; it facilitates timely completion of complex studies, including randomized controlled trials, by pooling resources and expertise across sites (Abernethy et al., 2010).
- The Patient-Centered Outcomes Research Institute (PCORI) was established under the ACA. Its research priorities and agenda are in line with many of the topics that require further study in the field of palliative care (PCORI, 2014).[12]

Remaining gaps:

- The 2013 NINR review mentioned above (NINR, 2013a) found a dearth of research on racial and ethnic populations; pediatric populations; caregiving; and ethical, cultural, and spiritual aspects of end-of-life care.
- A 2006 study found that more than 25 percent of published palliative medicine research was performed with no acknowledged extramural funding, and fewer than one-third of published studies were supported by NIH funding (Gelfman and Morrison, 2006).
- As of 2009, there were only 114 active NIH grants supporting palliative care research (CAPC, 2011).
- Palliative care accounted for only 0.2 percent of all NIH grants between 2006 and 2010 (Gelfman et al., 2010).
- The present report identifies a number of areas that warrant further research, including but not limited to
  - the development and application of evidence-based measures of quality of care near the end of life;
  - approaches to prognosis and the impact of more accurate prognosis on quality of care, quality of life, and other outcomes;

---

[11]See http://www.npcrc.org (accessed December 17, 2014).
[12]Patient Protection and Affordable Care Act of 2010, Public Law 111-148, 111th Cong., 2d Sess. (January 5, 2010), § 6301.

- diffusion of models of end-of-life care that have been found to be effective;
- the impact of the organization and financing of the health care system on the delivery, quality, and cost of care for patients near the end of life;
- financial, physical, and emotional impacts on caregivers;
- patient-provider communication and patient and family decision making near the end of life;
- pediatric advance care planning and involvement of pediatric patients in decision making about their care near the end of life; and
- the development of meaningful-use criteria relating to end-of-life care and advance care planning and the impact of these criteria on outcomes.

1997 Recommendation 7: A continuing public discussion is essential to develop a better understanding of the modern experience of dying, the options available to patients and families, and the obligations of communities to those approaching death.

- Since 1997, numerous public education efforts focused on issues of advance care planning and palliative care have been launched. These campaigns have had varying sponsorship, and some have been coalition efforts. Their goals have varied, but many have stressed
  - the importance of advance care planning ("having the conversation"),
  - what palliative care and hospice are, and
  - the right to good pain management.
- Numerous public education and engagement efforts and campaigns have begun and/or continue, including
  - The Conversation Project and the Institute for Healthcare Improvement's (IHI's) Conversation Ready Initiative (http://theconversationproject.org);
  - DeathWise (https://www.deathwise.org);
  - Engage with Grace (http://www.engagewithgrace.org);
  - Death Cafes (http://www.deathcafe.com);
  - Death over Dinner (http://www.deathoverdinner.org, http://blog.tedmed.com/?tag=death-over-dinner [accessed December 17, 2014]);
  - Project Compassion (http://project-compassion.org);

- Aging with Dignity and *Five Wishes* (http://agingwithdignity.org; http://www.agingwithdignity.org/five-wishes.php [accessed December 17, 2014]);
- Community Conversations on Compassionate Care (Compassion and Support) (https://www.compassionandsupport.org);
- National Healthcare Decisions Day (http://www.nhdd.org);
- It's About How You LIVE campaign (NHPCO Caring Connections) (http://www.caringinfo.org/i4a/pages/index.cfm?pageid= 3380 [accessed December 17, 2014]);
- Life Before Death (The Lien Foundation) (http://www.life beforedeath.com/index.shtml [accessed December 17, 2014]);
- Before I Die (http://beforeidie.cc);
- Death Clock (http://www.deathclock.com);
- Time of Death (http://www.sho.com/sho/time-of-death/home [accessed December 17, 2014]);
- PBS's "On Our Own Terms: Moyers on Dying" (http://www.pbs.org/wnet/onourownterms [accessed December 17, 2014]);
- Honoring Choices, the Minnesota/Twin Cities Public Television documentary series and related materials (http://www.honoringchoices.org);
- A Good Day to Die (http://thediemovie.wordpress.com);
- Ways to Live Forever (http://trailers.apple.com/trailers/independent/waystoliveforever [accessed December 17, 2014]);
- How to Die in Oregon (http://www.howtodieinoregon.com/trailer.html [accessed December 17, 2014]);
- Amour (http://www.sonyclassics.com/amour);
- PBS Frontline documentary "Facing Death" (http://www.pbs.org/wgbh/pages/frontline/facing-death [accessed December 17, 2014]); and
- Inside Out documentary "Quality of Death: End of Life Care in America" (http://insideout.wbur.org/documentaries/quality ofdeath [accessed December 17, 2014]).
- Two of the National Rural Health Association's three Technical Assistance Project community-based teams—in Franklin, North Carolina, and Ruleville, Mississippi—focused their efforts on developing provider and community education and outreach plans around advance directives (Stratis Health, 2009).

Remaining gaps:

- Misunderstandings persist among both the general public and health care providers about the differences in meaning of such terms as "palliative care," "end-of-life care," and "hospice," as well as "agent," "surrogate," "caregiver," and "family" (CAPC, 2011; CHCF, 2012).

- The persistent reluctance to talk about death—among clinicians, patients and families, and policy makers—remains a barrier to appropriate care at the individual level and to social policies that would improve the quality of life of dying people and their families (Pew Research Center, 2009, 2013; Walling et al., 2008).

WHEN CHILDREN DIE

2003 Recommendation 1: Pediatric professionals, children's hospitals, hospices, home health agencies, professional societies, family advocacy groups, government agencies, and others should work together to develop and implement clinical practice guidelines and institutional protocols and procedures for palliative, end-of-life, and bereavement care that meet the needs of children and families.

- NHPCO developed *Standards of Practice for Pediatric Palliative Care and Hospice* (NHPCO, 2009), which identifies four diagnostic categories of patients who should be offered palliative care and/ or hospice services. They are children with
  - "life-threatening conditions for which curative treatment may be feasible but can fail, where access to palliative care services may be beneficial alongside attempts at life-prolonging treatment and/or if treatment fails;
  - conditions where early death is inevitable and there may be long periods of intensive treatment aimed at prolonging life, allowing participation in normal activities, and maintaining quality of life (e.g., life-limiting conditions);
  - progressive conditions without curative treatment options, where treatment is exclusively palliative after diagnosis and may extend over many years; and
  - irreversible but nonprogressive conditions entailing complex health care needs leading to complications and the likelihood of premature death" (NHPCO, 2009, pp. 5-6).
- Children's Hospice International issued the *Children's Program of All-Inclusive Coordinated Care for Children and Their Families (ChiPACC) Standards of Care and Practice Guidelines* in September 2005. It covers 16 care components, including access to care, ethics, care teams, assessment processes, and bereavement services (Children's Hospice International, 2005).

- *The Hastings Center Guidelines for Decisions on Life-Sustaining Treatment and Care Near the End-of-Life, Second Edition*, released in 2013, includes guidelines on decision making about life-sustaining treatment for the continuum of pediatric populations, including nonviable and viable neonates, young children, older children, adolescents, and mature and emancipated minors (Hastings Center, 2013).
- In its *Report of the Children & Adolescents Task Force of the Ad Hoc Committee on End-of-Life Issues,* the American Psychological Association (APA) published information about the role of psychologists in providing psychosocial care and bereavement services to children near the end of life and their families. The report also covers issues related to research, education and training, and policy with respect to care for this population (APA, 2005).
- In 2010, the Association of Pediatric Hematology/Oncology Nurses, in partnership with the Children's Oncology Group Nursing Discipline, published *Pediatric Oncology Palliative and End-of-life Care Resource*, which provides information about palliative care to nurses caring for critically and terminally ill children with cancer (Ethier et al., 2010). It contains information on pain and symptom management, management of psychosocial issues, bereavement and grief, and other topics.
- The National Cancer Institute, through its Physician Data Query (PDQ®) database, has developed summaries on pediatric supportive care for both patients (NCI, 2013) and health professionals (NCI, 2014).
- From 2005 to 2010, Hospice of Michigan implemented its Pediatric Early Care (PEC) program, which is for families of children from birth to 21. PEC assists patients and families from the time of diagnosis, providing support in palliative care education; grief and loss; sibling support; memory-making activities; patient advocacy; insurance assistance; community resource access; and integration with service providers, medical staff, and those at other social and community locations, including schools, workplaces, and places of worship (Hospice of Michigan, undated).
- While not specific to pediatric populations, NQF put forth preferred practices for end-of-life care and bereavement care for all patients with serious and complex illness and their families (NQF, 2006).
- A number of children's hospitals, including St. Jude Children's Research Hospital and Boston Children's Hospital, have implemented institution-specific guidelines and procedures relating to the initiation of palliative care (Baker et al., 2008).

2003 Recommendation 2: Children's hospitals, hospices, home health agencies, and other organizations that care for seriously ill or injured children should collaborate to assign specific responsibilities for implementing clinical and administrative protocols and procedures for palliative, end-of-life, and bereavement care. In addition to supporting competent clinical services, protocols should promote the coordination and continuity of care and the timely flow of information among caregivers and within and among care sites including hospitals, family homes, residential care facilities, and injury scenes.

- In April 2006, Massachusetts' health care reform legislation resulted in the establishment of the statewide Pediatric Palliative Care Network (PPCN) program, administered by the Massachusetts Department of Public Health (Massachusetts Department of Public Health, 2014). In 2010, PPCN involved 11 hospice programs that provided services to 227 children with life-limiting illnesses. A 2011 assessment of the program found that implementing this model successfully is "highly feasible at relatively low cost" (Bona et al., 2011, p. 1217). In contrast with public benefit programs, such as Medicaid and CHIP, eligibility is not based on a family's income level, insurance type, or insured status. There is no life expectancy requirement for participation in the program, which provides services for pain and symptom management; case management; counseling and psychosocial support; respite care; complementary therapies; spiritual care; and bereavement services for family, caregivers, siblings, and others.
- NHPCO has developed a number of tools to support hospice and palliative medicine health care teams, although these resources do not include content specific to pediatric populations (NHPCO, undated-c). Topics include
  - interdisciplinary team competency;
  - cultural competency in grief and loss;
  - delivering bad news: helpful guidance that also helps the patient; and
  - talking about treatment options and palliative care.

2003 Recommendation 3: Children's hospitals, hospices with established pediatric programs, and other institutions that care for children with fatal or potentially fatal medical conditions should work with professional societies, state agencies, and other organizations to develop regional information programs and other resources to assist clinicians and families in local and outlying communities and rural areas.

- In 2007, NHPCO conducted its second member Survey on Pediatric Services, receiving 378 responses. Overall, 78 percent of responding hospices reported that they served pediatric patients, and 37 percent had a formal pediatric program in place. Of those without a dedicated pediatric team, 22 percent had specialized staff providing only pediatric services (Friebert, 2009).
- Two of the Center to Advance Palliative Care's (CAPC's) eight Palliative Care Leadership Centers (PCLCs) are based in children's hospitals and provide health professionals with close, hands-on experiences, as well as a 12-month mentoring follow-up to guide them through the challenges of program growth and sustainability. The PCLC pediatrics training is relevant to pediatric palliative care programs at every stage of development, whether involving teams from children's hospitals or pediatric programs within a general hospital, and tailored to the specific operational needs of each program (CAPC, 2014).
- Pilot programs and local/regional palliative care networks have been established in some rural communities.
  - The Rural Palliative Care Network at Vermont Children's Hospital expands Fletcher Allen Health Care's Palliative Medicine Service and allows the hospital's clinicians to share their palliative care expertise with the region's clinicians and community hospital staff. The network's services include telemedicine consultations, a palliative medicine hotline, a palliative medicine mentorship program, site visits, and weekly case conferences (Fletcher Allen Health Care, 2014).
  - The Massachusetts PPCN, mentioned above, is a statewide program with the participation of hospice and palliative care programs in metropolitan and rural areas (Bona et al., 2011; Massachusetts Department of Public Health, 2014).

2003 Recommendation 4: Children's hospitals, hospices, and other institutions that care for seriously ill or injured children should work with physicians, parents, child patients, psychologists, and other relevant experts to create policies and procedures for involving children in discussions and decisions about their medical condition and its treatment. These policies and procedures—and their application—should be sensitive to children's intellectual and emotional maturity and preferences and to families' cultural backgrounds and values.

- One of the preferred practices outlined in NQF's *A National Framework and Preferred Practices for Palliative and Hospice Care Quality* is "Decisionmaking of Minors," which states: "For minors with decisionmaking capacity, document the child's views and preferences for medical care, including asset for treatment, and give them appropriate weight in decisionmaking. Make appropriate staff members available to both the child and the adult decisionmaker for consultation and intervention when the child's wishes differ from those of the adult decisionmaker" (NQF, 2006, p. 45)

- Advance directive documents specifically geared to pediatric patients have been developed. For example, the creators of the *Five Wishes* living will (18 million of which are in circulation in the United States) have developed *My Wishes*, "a booklet written in everyday language that helps children express how they want to be cared for in case they become seriously ill," and *Voicing My Choices: A Planning Guide for Adolescents & Young Adults*, which "helps young people living with a serious illness to communicate their preferences to friends, family and caregivers" (Aging with Dignity, 2014; Lyon et al., 2013; Wiener et al., 2008, 2012).
- One recent study found that the implementation of advance directives for pediatric patients entails several particular barriers. For example, emergency department personnel are uncomfortable honoring them, schools may not accept them, and parents seeking to honor their children's wishes encounter negative reactions from others (Lotz et al., 2013).

2003 Recommendation 5: Children's hospitals and other hospitals that care for children who die should work with hospices and other relevant community organizations to develop and implement protocols and procedures [around bereavement services].

- A 2011 study found that 24 of 28 surveyed pediatric palliative care programs (86 percent) reported having a staff chaplain on their clinical team, although their roles varied widely (Fitchett et al., 2011).
- While not specific to pediatric populations, NQF recommends that all palliative care and hospice models include bereavement support for at least 13 months after the patient's death. This framework suggests preferred practices for the development and implementation of grief and bereavement care plans (NQF, 2006).

2003 Recommendation 6: Public and private insurers should restructure hospice benefits for children to (a) add hospice care to the services required by Congress in Medicaid and other public insurance programs for children and to the services covered for children under private health plans; (b) eliminate eligibility restrictions related to life expectancy, substitute criteria based on a child's diagnosis and severity of illness, and drop rules requiring children to forgo curative or life-prolonging care (possibly in a case management framework); and (c) include outlier payments for exceptionally costly hospice patients. (See bullets under Recommendation 7.)

2003 Recommendation 7: *In addition to modifying hospice benefits, Medicaid and private insurers should modify policies restricting benefits for other palliative services related to a child's life-threatening medical condition.*

- As noted earlier, the ACA removed the prohibition on receiving concurrent treatment (hospice and curative services) for children under Medicaid and CHIP. Children may be enrolled simultaneously in programs that provide supplemental services not covered by Medicaid and CHIP, such as specialized home health care, case management, respite care, and family support services (NHPCO, 2010).[13]
- A number of states have obtained waivers from CMS rules to establish or augment pediatric palliative services. In 2005, Florida became the first state to use a managed care waiver program to offer concurrent hospice and curative treatment for qualified children (Florida Agency for Health Care Administration, 2009, 2013). California, Colorado, and North Dakota use supplemental services waivers; New York and North Carolina use waivers for medically fragile children. A different model has been developed in Washington State under its Early and Periodic Screening, Diagnosis, and Treatment program (NHPCO, 2010, 2012b).
- State Medicaid programs must cover hospice services for children even if they do not include hospice services for adults (CMS, 2010).

Remaining gaps:

- To qualify for concurrent care, the child must be within the last 6 months of life if the disease runs its normal course, as certified by a physician (NHPCO, 2010).
- Under this benefit, children are limited to a state's existing Medicaid hospice and other services (NHPCO, 2010).

2003 Recommendation 8: *Federal and state Medicaid agencies, pediatric organizations, and private insurers should cooperate to (1) define diagnosis*

---

[13]Patient Protection and Affordable Care Act of 2010, Public Law 111-148, 111th Cong., 2d Sess. (January 5, 2010), § 2302 Concurrent Care for Children.

and, as appropriate, severity criteria for eligibility for expanded benefits for palliative, hospice, and bereavement services; (2) examine the appropriateness for reimbursing pediatric palliative and end-of-life care of diagnostic, procedure, and other classification systems that were developed for reimbursement of adult services; and (3) develop guidance for practitioners and administrative staff about accurate, consistent coding and documenting of palliative, end-of-life, and bereavement services.

- As previously mentioned, NHPCO developed *Standards of Practice for Pediatric Palliative Care and Hospice* (NHPCO, 2009), which identifies four diagnostic categories of patients, listed above, who should be offered palliative care and/or hospice services.

2003 Recommendation 9: Medical, nursing, and other health professions schools or programs should collaborate with professional societies to improve the care provided to seriously ill and injured children by creating and testing curricula and experiences [for health care professionals].

- At Children's Hospital Boston, physicians participated with nurses, social workers, psychologists, and chaplains involved in pediatric critical care in a day-long interprofessional communication program, the Program to Enhance Relational and Communication Skills, created by the Institute for Professionalism and Ethical Practice (Meyer et al., 2009).

2003 Recommendation 10: To provide instruction and experiences appropriate for all health care professionals who care for children, experts in general and specialty fields of pediatric health care and education should collaborate with experts in adult and pediatric palliative care and education to develop and implement [model curricula, residency program requirements, pediatric palliative care fellowships, introductory and advanced continuing education programs, and strategies to evaluate techniques and tools for educating health professionals in palliative care, end-of-life, and bereavement care].

- EPEC-Pediatrics has 23 core and two elective topics, taught through 20 distance learning modules and six 1-day, in-person conference sessions (EPEC, 2013). Since 2012, physicians and nurse practitioners have participated in "Become an EPEC-Pediatrics Trainer" workshops.[14]

---

[14]Personal communication, S. Friedrichsdorf, Children's Hospitals and Clinics of Minnesota, February 6, 2014.

- ELNEC developed an ELNEC-Pediatric Palliative Care curriculum in 2003, updated in 2009 with content about perinatal and neonatal issues (AACN, 2014b).
- As noted earlier, in September 2006, the American Board of Medical Specialties approved the creation of hospice and palliative medicine as a subspecialty of 10 participating boards, which include pediatrics (American Academy of Hospice and Palliative Medicine, undated-e). Between 2008 and 2012, 210 pediatricians became board certified in hospice and palliative medicine, accounting for 3 percent of all board-certified physicians in this subspecialty (ABP, 2013).
- NBCHPN® administers the following hospice and palliative pediatric nurse examinations accredited by the American Board of Nursing Specialties through 2015:
  - Advanced Certified Hospice and Palliative Nurse,
  - Certified Hospice and Palliative Nurse,
  - Certified Hospice and Palliative Licensed Nurse,
  - Certified Hospice and Palliative Nursing Assistant,
  - Certified Hospice and Palliative Care Administrator,
  - Nurse Certified in Perinatal Loss Care, and
  - Certified Hospice and Palliative Pediatric Nurse (NBCHPN®, 2014).
- The Accreditation Council for Graduate Medical Education requires that pediatric training programs include formal instruction related to the "impact of chronic diseases, terminal conditions, and death on patients and their families" (ACGME, undated).
- Other curricula and education programs have been developed by organizations including the following:
  - Children's International Project on Palliative/Hospice Services (ChiPPS)—developed a core curriculum for varied populations of health professionals that can be used to design, develop, and implement individualized education and training programs (NHPCO, undated-d).
  - Initiative for Pediatric Palliative Care (IPPC)—developed curriculum materials and conducted educational retreats throughout the United States and Canada for interdisciplinary teams, including clinicians from pediatric and neonatal intensive care units and parents of children with life-threatening conditions (Solomon et al., 2010).

Remaining gap:

- There is still a clear need for additional pediatric palliative care preparation during residency training. While no formal, standardized training of medical students and residents currently exists, a few programs and institutions are piloting or implementing such programs (Carter and Swan, 2012; Schiffman et al., 2008).

2003 Recommendation 11: *The National Center for Health Statistics, the National Institutes of Health, and other relevant public and private organizations, including philanthropic organizations, should collaborate to improve the collection of descriptive data—epidemiological, clinical, organizational, and financial—to guide the provision, funding, and evaluation of palliative, end-of-life, and bereavement care for children and families.*

- In 2009, NHPCO published *NHPCO Facts and Figures: Pediatric Palliative and Hospice Care in America*, which compiles data from various articles and reports (Friebert, 2009).
- NHPCO has been collecting data using the voluntary National Data Set (NDS) since 1999. The NDS provides a platform for data-driven evaluation of the performance of the hospice industry. While this tool is not specific to pediatric populations, it does collect information relevant to hospices that serve pediatric populations either exclusively or alongside adult hospice patients. NHPCO has added an annual national Palliative Care Supplement to the NDS (NHPCO, 2013). In 2007, NHPCO conducted a Survey on Pediatric Services and received 378 responses from member hospice providers offering information about their pediatric patient population and services (Friebert, 2009).

2003 Recommendation 12: *Units of the National Institutes of Health and other organizations that fund pediatric oncology, neonatal, and similar clinical and research centers or networks should define priorities for research in pediatric palliative, end-of-life, and bereavement care. Research should focus on infants, children, adolescents, and their families, including siblings, and should cover care from the time of diagnosis through death and bereavement. Priorities for research include but are not limited to the effectiveness of (a) clinical interventions, including symptom management; (b) methods for improving communication and decision making; (c) innovative arrangements for delivering, coordinating, and evaluating care, including interdisciplinary care teams and quality improvement strategies; and (d) different approaches to bereavement care.*

- Recent NIH grant programs supporting research on pediatric end-of-life care include
  - Advancing Palliative Care Research for Children Facing Life-Limiting Conditions, a $1.25 million NINR-sponsored program supporting biobehavioral research aimed at improving quality of life, including bereavement support, for children (NIH, 2010); and
  - Improving Care for Dying Children and Their Families (2004-2007), a program under the auspices of several institutes designed to support research that will improve the quality of life for children who are approaching the end of life; the quality of the dying process; and bereavement following the child's death among family members, friends, and care providers (NIH, 2004).
- NINR's *Palliative Care: Conversations Matter®* campaign focuses on improving communication about pediatric palliative care among patients, families, and health care providers (NINR, 2013b).
- NPCRC funds grants in the following areas of interest: pain and symptom management, communication, and models of health care delivery (NPCRC, undated-a). It offers funds through four different funding mechanisms: pilot and exploratory project support grants, junior faculty career development awards, infrastructure support for collaborative study, and research design/statistical support grants (NPCRC, undated-b).
  - Funding to date has supported projects aimed at elucidating, among other topics, communication and decision making, symptom burden, and quality of life among pediatric patient populations (NPCRC, 2010).
  - In 2013, NPCRC established the Lord Pediatric Palliative Care Career Development Awards with the support of the Lord Foundation (NPCRC, 2013).

Remaining gaps:

- The NINR-published review *Building Momentum: The Science of End-of-Life and Palliative Care: A Review of Research Trends and Funding, 1997-2010* reports that research involving pediatric populations increased between 1997 and 2010, but still accounted for a small proportion (less than 10 percent) of all end-of-life and palliative care research publications (NINR, 2013a).
  - Research among solely children (defined as newborn to age 17) increased from 2.5 percent in 2003 to 6.3 percent in 2010.

- Research among combined populations of children and adults increased from 3.4 percent in 2003 to 5.4 percent in 2010.
- The present report identifies the need for further research among pediatric populations in a number of topic areas, including
  - approaches to symptom management and bereavement support;
  - the impact of palliative care on clinical outcomes and patient and family experience;
  - involvement of children in end-of-life decision making, approaches to decision support and communication, and the development of guidelines for pediatric and adolescent advance care planning;
  - care received in various settings, including outpatient settings, hospices, and emergency departments and through home health agencies; and
  - staffing, management, and financing of hospital-based pediatric palliative care and community-based pediatric hospice services.

REFERENCES

AACN (American Association of Colleges of Nursing). 2008. *The essentials of baccalaureate education for professional nursing practice.* Washington, DC: AACN. https://www.aacn.nche.edu/education-resources/BaccEssentials08.pdf (accessed February 10, 2014).

AACN. 2014a. *End-of-Life Nursing Education Consortium (ELNEC).* http://www.aacn.nche.edu/elnec (accessed February 11, 2013).

AACN. 2014b. *ELNEC-Pediatric Palliative Care.* http://www.aacn.nche.edu/elnec/about/pediatric-palliative-care (accessed July 30, 2014).

ABEM (American Board of Emergency Medicine). 2013. *Annual report, 2012-2013.* East Lansing, MI: ABEM. https://www.abem.org/public/docs/default-source/publication-documents/2012-13-annual-report.pdf?sfvrsn=8 (accessed January 31, 2014).

Abernethy, A. P., D. C. Currow, B. S. Fazekas, M. A. Luszcz, J. L. Wheeler, and M. Kuchibhatla. 2008. Specialized palliative care services are associated with improved short- and long-term caregiver outcomes. *Support Care Cancer* 16:585-597.

Abernethy, A. P., N. M. Aziz, E. Basch, J. Bull, C. S. Cleeland, D. C. Currow, D. Fairclough, L. Hanson, J. Hauser, D. Ko, L. Lloyd, R. S. Morrison, S. Otis-Green, S. Pantilat, R. K. Portenoy, C. Ritchie, G. Rocker, J. L. Wheeler, S. Y. Zafar, and J. S. Kutner. 2010. A strategy to advance the evidence base in palliative medicine: Formation of a palliative care research cooperative group. *Journal of Palliative Medicine* 13(12):407-413. http://www.ncbi.nlm.nih.gov/pubmed/21105763 (accessed September 20, 2013).

ABFM (American Board of Family Medicine). 2013. *Diplomate statistics.* Lexington, KY: ABFM. https://www.theabfm.org/about/stats.aspx (accessed December 4, 2013).

ABIM (American Board of Internal Medicine). 2013a. *Medical oncology: Certification examination blueprint.* Philadelphia, PA: ABIM. http://www.abim.org/pdf/blueprint/medon_cert.pdf (accessed November 29, 2013).

ABIM. 2013b. *Internal medicine: Certification examination blueprint.* Philadelphia, PA: ABIM. http://www.abim.org/pdf/blueprint/im_cert.pdf (accessed November 29, 2013).

ABIM. 2013c. *Number of certificates issued—all candidates.* Philadelphia, PA: ABIM. http:// www.abim.org/pdf/data-candidates-certified/all-candidates.pdf (accessed December 3, 2013).

ABP (American Board of Pediatrics). 2013. *Number of diplomate certificates granted through December 2012.* Chapel Hill, NC: ABP. https://www.abp.org/ABPWebStatic/?anticache= 0.1225979424765275#murl%3D%2FABPWebStatic%2FaboutPed.html%26surl%3D% 2Fabpwebsite%2Fstats%2Fnumdips.htm (accessed December 3, 2013).

ABPMR (American Board of Physical Medicine and Rehabilitation). 2013. *Examination statistics.* Rochester, MN: ABPMR. https://www.abpmr.org/candidates/exam_statistics. html (accessed December 3, 2013).

ABPN (American Board of Psychiatry and Neurology, Inc.). 2013. *Initial certification statistics.* Buffalo Grove, IL: ABPN. http://www.abpn.com/cert_statistics.html (accessed December 4, 2013).

ABS (American Board of Surgery). 2013. *Diplomate totals.* Philadelphia, PA: ABS. http://www. absurgery.org/default.jsp?statsummary (accessed December 3, 2013).

ACGME (Accreditation Council for Graduate Medical Education). 2014. *Number of accredited programs for the current academic year (2013-2014), United States.* Chicago, IL: ACGME. https://www.acgme.org/ads/Public/Reports/Report/3 (accessed April 14, 2014).

ACGME. undated. *ACGME program requirements for graduate medical education in pediatrics.* http://www.acgme-i.org/web/requirements/Pediatrics.pdf (accessed February 15, 2013).

ACPE (Accreditation Council for Pharmacy Education). 2011. *Accreditation standards and guidelines for the professional program in pharmacy leading to the doctor of pharmacy degree.* Chicago, IL: ACPE. https://www.acpe-accredit.org/pdf/FinalS2007Guidelines2.0.pdf (accessed January 27, 2014).

Aging with Dignity. 2014. *Five Wishes resources.* https://www.agingwithdignity.org/five-wishes-resources.php (accessed July 28, 2014).

American Academy of Hospice and Palliative Medicine. undated-a. *Measuring what matters.* http://aahpm.org/quality/measuring-what-matters (accessed March 4, 2014).

American Academy of Hospice and Palliative Medicine. undated-b. *Top twelve measures— background information, evidence, and clinical user panel (CUP) comments.* http:// aahpm.org/uploads/education/MWM%20Top%2012%20Measure%20Information%20 and%20Comments.pdf (accessed July 23, 2014).

American Academy of Hospice and Palliative Medicine. undated-c. *Frequently asked questions (FAQs) about Measuring What Matters.* http://aahpm.org/uploads/education/MWM%20 FAQ%20List.pdf (accessed July 23, 2014).

American Academy of Hospice and Palliative Medicine. undated-d. *History of AAHPM.* http:// aahpm.org/about/history (accessed July 15, 2014).

American Academy of Hospice and Palliative Medicine. undated-e. *ABMS certification.* http://184.106.197.112/certification/default/abms.html (accessed July 15, 2014).

APA (American Psychological Association). 2005. *Report of the Children & Adolescent Task Force of the Ad Hoc Committee on End-of-Life Issues.* Washington, DC: APA. http:// www.apa.org/pi/aids/programs/eol/end-of-life-report.pdf (accessed August 6, 2014).

APC (Association of Professional Chaplains). 2013. *The Association of Professional Chaplains introduces palliative care specialty certification.* News release. May 1. Schaumburg, IL: APC. http://www.professionalchaplains.org/Files/news/pr_palliative_care_specialty_ certification.pdf (accessed August 6, 2014).

Baker, J. N., P. S. Hinds, S. L. Spunt, R. C. Barfield, C. Allen, B. C. Powell, L. H. Anderson, and J. R. Kane. 2008. Integration of palliative care principles into the ongoing care of children with cancer: Individualized care planning and coordination. *Pediatric Clinics of North America* 55(1):223-250.

BCCI (Board of Chaplaincy Certification Inc.). 2013. *BCCI certification*. Schaumburg, IL: APC. http://bcci.professionalchaplains.org/content.asp?pl=25&contentid=25 (accessed December 3, 2013).

Bona, K., J. Bates, and J. Wolfe. 2011. Massachusetts' Pediatric Palliative Care Network: Successful implementation of a novel state-funded pediatric palliative care program. *Journal of Palliative Medicine* 14(11):1217-1223.

BPS (Board of Pharmacy Specialties). 2011. *BPS approves ambulatory care designation; explores new specialties in pain and palliative care, critical care and pediatrics*. Washington, DC: BPS. http://www.bpsweb.org/news/pr_041911.cfm (accessed January 24, 2014).

Brown, R., and D. R. Mann. 2012. *Best bets for reducing Medicare costs for dual eligible beneficiaries: Assessing the evidence*. Issue Brief. Menlo Park, CA: The Henry J. Kaiser Family Foundation.

Brumley, R. D., and K. Hillary. 2002. *The TriCentral Palliative Care Program toolkit*. Oakland, CA: Kaiser Permanente.

Brumley, R. D., S. Enquidanos, P. Jamison, R. Seitz, N. Morgenstern, S. Saito, J. McIlwane, K. Hillary, and J. Gonzales. 2007. Increased satisfaction with care and lower costs: Results of a randomized trial of in-home palliative care. *Journal of the American Geriatric Society* 55(7):993-1000.

CAPC (Center to Advance Palliative Care). 2011. *America's care of serious illness: A state-by-state report card on access to palliative care in our nation's hospitals*. New York: CAPC. http://reportcard.capc.org/pdf/state-by-state-report-card.pdf (accessed July 15, 2014).

CAPC. 2012. *Growth of palliative care in U.S. hospitals: 2012 snapshot*. http://www.capc.org/capc-growth-analysis-snapshot-2011.pdf (accessed February 18, 2013).

CAPC. 2014. *PCLC overview*. http://www.capc.org/palliative-care-leadership-initiative/overview (accessed February 17, 2013).

Carter, B. S., and R. Swan. 2012. Pediatric palliative care instruction for residents: An introduction to IPPC. *American Journal of Hospice and Palliative Care* 29(5):375-378.

CHCF (California HealthCare Foundation). 2012. *Final chapter: Californians' attitudes and experiences with death and dying*. http://www.chcf.org/~/media/MEDIA%20LIBRARY%20Files/PDF/F/PDF%20FinalChapterDeathDying.pdf (accessed August 7, 2013).

Children's Hospice International. 2005. *Children's Program of All-Inclusive Coordinated Care for Children and Their Families (ChiPACC) standards of care and practice guidelines*. http://www.chionline.org/standards-of-care-and-practice-guidelines (accessed August 6, 2014).

CMS (Centers for Medicare & Medicaid Services). 2009a. Medicare program; hospice wage index for fiscal year 2010, final rule. *Federal Register* 74(150):39384-39433. http://www.gpo.gov/fdsys/pkg/FR-2009-08-06/pdf/E9-18553.pdf (accessed July 18, 2014).

CMS. 2009b. *New physician specialty code for hospice and palliative care*. http://www.cms.gov/Regulations-and-Guidance/Guidance/Transmittals/downloads/R1715CP.pdf (accessed July 29, 2014).

CMS. 2010. *State Medicaid directors' letter re: hospice care for children in Medicaid and CHIP*. http://downloads.cms.gov/cmsgov/archived-downloads/SMDL/downloads/SMD10018.pdf (accessed February 16, 2013).

CMS. 2013a. *Medicare hospice benefits*. http://www.medicare.gov/Pubs/pdf/02154.pdf (accessed February 18, 2013).

CMS. 2013b. *About the Medicare-Medicaid Coordination Office*. http://www.cms.gov/Medicare-Medicaid-Coordination/Medicare-and-Medicaid-Coordination/Medicare-Medicaid-Coordination-Office (accessed December 2, 2013).

CMS. 2013c. Medicare program; FY 2014 hospice wage index and payment rate update; hospice quality reporting requirements; and updates on payment reform; final rule. *Federal Register* 78:152. http://www.gpo.gov/fdsys/pkg/FR-2013-08-07/pdf/2013-18838.pdf (accessed July 25, 2014).

CMS. 2013d. *Bundled payments for care improvement initiative: General information.* http://innovation.cms.gov/initiatives/Bundled-Payments (accessed January 30, 2014).

CMS. 2014. *Fact sheets: Medicare Care Choices Model.* http://www.cms.gov/Newsroom/MediaReleaseDatabase/Fact-sheets/2014-Fact-sheets-items/2014-03-18.html (accessed July 18, 2014).

CMS. undated. *User guide for hospice quality reporting data collection.* http://www.cms.gov/Medicare/Quality-Initiatives-Patient-Assessment-Instruments/Hospice-Quality-Reporting/Downloads/UserGuideforDataCollection-.pdf (accessed June 18, 2014).

Coalition to Transform Advanced Care. 2013. *Summary Report of National Summit on Advanced Illness Care. January 29-30, 2013.* http://advancedcarecoalition.org/wp-content/uploads/2012/11/2013-Summit-Summary-.pdf (accessed January 14, 2014).

Dahlin, C., ed. 2009. *Clinical practice guidelines for quality palliative care.* 2nd ed. Pittsburgh, PA: National Consensus Project for Quality Palliative Care. http://www.nationalconsensusproject.org/guideline.pdf (accessed July 17, 2014).

Dahlin, C., ed. 2013. *Clinical practice guidelines for quality palliative care.* 3rd ed. Pittsburgh, PA: National Consensus Project for Quality Palliative Care. http://www.nationalconsensusproject.org/NCP_Clinical_Practice_Guidelines_3rd_Edition.pdf (accessed July 17, 2014).

Dickinson, G. E. 2011. Thirty-five years of end-of-life issues in U.S. medical schools. *American Journal of Hospice and Palliative Care* 28(6):412-417.

Dickinson, G. E. 2013. End-of-life and palliative care education in U.S. pharmacy schools. *American Journal of Hospice and Palliative Medicine* 30(6):532-535.

DOL (U.S. Department of Labor). 2013. *Wage and hour division: Family and Medical Leave Act.* http://www.dol.gov/whd/fmla (accessed August 27, 2013).

Edes, T., S. Shreve, and D. Casarett. 2007. Increasing access and quality in Department of Veterans Affairs care at the end of life: A lesson in change. *Journal of the American Geriatrics Society* 55(10):1645-1649.

ELNEC (End-of-Life Nursing Education Consortium). 2013. *End-of-life Nursing Education Consortium (ELNEC) fact sheet.* Washington, DC: AACN.

EPEC (Education in Palliative and End-of-life Care). 2012. *EPEC history.* http://www.epec.net/history.php (accessed August 5, 2014).

EPEC. 2013. *EPEC—pediatrics.* Chicago, IL: EPEC. http://epec.net/epec_pediatrics.php?curid=6 (accessed November 25, 2013).

Ethier, A. M., J. Rollins, and J. Stewart. 2010. *Pediatric oncology palliative and end-of-life care resource.* Chicago, IL: Association of Pediatric Hematology/Oncology Nurses.

Fitchett, G., K. A. Kyndes, W. Cadge, N. Berlinger, E. Flanagan, and J. Misasi. 2011. The role of professional chaplains on pediatric palliative care teams: Perspectives from physicians and chaplains. *Journal of Palliative Medicine* 14(6):704-707.

Fletcher Allen Health Care. 2014. *Rural Palliative Care Network.* http://www.fletcherallen.org/services/other_services/specialties/palliative_care/for_providers (accessed February 11, 2013).

Florida Agency for Health Care Administration. 2009. *Children's Medical Service Network partners in care: Together for kids.* http://ahca.myflorida.com/medicaid/quality_management/mrp/contracts/med052/final_annual_pic_report_february_2009.pdf (accessed February 11, 2013).

Florida Agency for Health Care Administration. 2013. *Florida Medicaid summary of services fiscal year 12/13.* http://ahca.myflorida.com/Medicaid/pdffiles/2012-2013_Summary_of_Services_Final_121031.pdf (accessed February 16, 2013).

Friebert, S. 2009. *NHPCO facts and figures: Pediatric palliative and hospice care in America.* http://www.nhpco.org/sites/default/files/public/quality/Pediatric_Facts-Figures.pdf (accessed April 2009).

FSMB (Federation of State Medical Boards). 2004. *Model policy for the use of controlled substances for the treatment of pain.* http://www.fsmb.org/pdf/2004_grpol_Controlled_Substances.pdf (accessed July 15, 2014).

Gelfman, L. P., and R. S. Morrison. 2006. Research funding for palliative medicine. *Journal of Palliative Medicine* 11(1):36-43.

Gelfman, L. P., Q. Du, and R. S. Morrison. 2010. An update: NIH research funding for palliative medicine 2006-2010. *Journal of Palliative Medicine* 16(2):125-129.

Gilson, A. M., D. E. Joranson, and M. A. Maurer. 2007. Improving state pain policies: Recent progress and continuing opportunities. *CA: A Cancer Journal for Clinicians* 57:341-353.

Goldfeld, K. S., D. C. Grabowski, D. J. Caudry, and S. L. Mitchell. 2013. Health insurance status and the care of nursing home residents with advanced dementia. *JAMA Internal Medicine* 173(22):2047-2053.

Goldstein, N. E., L. M. Cohen, R. M. Arnold, E. Goy, S. Arons, and L. Ganzini. 2012. Prevalence of formal accusations of murder and euthanasia against physicians. *Journal of Palliative Medicine* 15(3):334-339.

Hanson, L. C., L. P. Scheunemann, S. Zimmerman, F. S. Rokoske, and A. P. Schenck. 2010. The PEACE project review of clinical instruments for hospice and palliative care. *Journal of Palliative Medicine* 13(10):1253-1260.

Hastings Center. 2013. *The Hastings Center guidelines for decisions on life-sustaining treatment and care near the end of life.* Washington, DC: Hastings Center.

Herndon, C. M., K. Jackson, D. S. Fike, and T. Woods. 2003. End-of-life care education in United States pharmacy schools. *American Journal of Hospice and Palliative Care* 20(5):340-344.

HHS (U.S. Department of Health and Human Services). 2013. Medicare program; FY2014 hospice wage index and payment rate update; hospice quality reporting requirements; and updates on payment reform. *Federal Register* 78(152):48234-48281. http://www.gpo.gov/fdsys/pkg/FR-2013-08-07/pdf/2013-18838.pdf (accessed June 18, 2014).

Hospice Action Network. 2013. *The Medicare hospice benefit & recent changes impacting the hospice community.* http://hospiceactionnetwork.org/linked_documents/get_informed/policy_resources/RecentChangesMHB.pdf (accessed February 18, 2013).

Hospice of Michigan. undated. *Pediatric early care.* http://www.hom.org/?page_id=49 (accessed February 11, 2013).

IOM (Institute of Medicine). 1997. *Approaching death: Improving care at the end of life.* Washington, DC: National Academy Press.

IOM. 2003. *When children die: Improving palliative and end-of-life care for children and their families.* Washington, DC: The National Academies Press.

IOM. 2011. *Relieving pain in America: A blueprint for transforming prevention, care, education, and research.* Washington, DC: The National Academies Press.

Joint Commission. 2014. *Facts about the advanced certification program for palliative care.* http://www.jointcommission.org/certification/palliative_care.aspx (accessed June 2, 2014).

Kamal, A. H., D. C. Currow, C. S. Ritchie, J. Bull, and A. P. Abernethy. 2012. Community-based palliative care: The natural evolution for palliative care delivery in the U.S. *Journal of Pain and Symptom Management* 46(2):254-264.

Kane, R. L., G. Keckhafer, and J. Robst. 2002. *Evaluation of the Evercare Demonstration Program: Final report.* http://www.cms.gov/Medicare/Demonstration-Projects/Demo ProjectsEvalRpts/downloads/Evercare_Final_Report.pdf (accessed February 22, 2014).

Kilbourn, K., A. Costenaro, S. Madore, K. DeRoche, D. Anderson, T. Keech, and J. S. Kutner. 2011. Feasibility of a telephone-based counseling program for informal caregivers of hospice patients. *Journal of Palliative Medicine* 14(11):1200-1205.

Krakauer, R., C. M. Spettell, L. Reisman, and M. J. Wade. 2009. Opportunities to improve the quality of care for advanced illness. *Health Affairs* 28(5):1357-1359.

Kumetz, E. A., and J. D. Goodson. 2013. The undervaluation of evaluation and management professional services: The lasting impact of current procedural terminology code deficiencies on physician payment. *Chest* 144(3):740-745.

Kutner, J. S., C. T. Kassner, and D. E. Nowels. 2001. Symptom burden at the end of life: Hospice providers' perceptions. *Journal of Pain and Symptom Management* 21(6):473-480.

Labson, M. C., M. M. Sacco, D. E. Weissman, and B. Gornet. 2013. Innovative models of home-based palliative care. *Cleveland Clinic Journal of Medicine* 80(Suppl. 1):e530-e535.

Liaison Committee on Medical Education. 2013. *Functions and structure of a medical school: Standards for accreditation of medical education programs leading to the M.D. degree.* Chicago, IL: American Medical Association, and Washington, DC: Association of American Medical Colleges. https://www.lcme.org/publications/functions2013june.pdf (accessed November 26, 2013).

Lotz, J. D., R. J. Jox, G. D. Borasio, M. Führer. 2013. Pediatric advance care planning: A systematic review. *Pediatrics* 131(3):e873-e880.

Lupu, D., and AAHPM Workforce Task Force. 2010. Estimate of current hospice and palliative medicine physician workforce shortage. *Journal of Pain and Symptom Management* 40(6):899-911.

Lupu, D., C. Deneszczuk, T. Leystra, R. McKinnon, and V. Seng. 2013. Few U.S. public health schools offer courses on palliative and end-of-life care policy. *Journal of Palliative Medicine* 16(12):1582-1587.

Lyon, M. E., S. Jacobs, L. Briggs, Y. I. Cheng, and J. Wang. 2013. Family-centered advance care planning for teens with cancer. *JAMA Pediatrics* 167(5):460-467.

Massachusetts Department of Public Health. 2014. *Pediatric palliative care network.* http://www.mass.gov/ppcn (accessed July 25, 2014).

Matlock, D. D., P. N. Peterson, B. E. Sirovich, D. E. Wennberg, P. M. Gallagher, and F. L. Lucas. 2010. Regional variations in palliative care: Do cardiologists follow guidelines? *Journal of Palliative Medicine* 13(11):1315-1319.

MedPAC (Medicare Payment Advisory Commission). 2009. *Report to Congress: Medicare payment policy—Chapter 6: Reforming Medicare's hospice benefit.* http://www.medpac.gov/chapters/Mar09_ch06.pdf (accessed August 28, 2014).

MedPAC. 2011. *The sustainable growth rate system: Policy considerations for adjustments and alternatives.* http://www.medpac.gov/chapters/jun11_ch01.pdf (accessed May 15, 2014).

MedPAC. 2012. *Report to Congress: Medicare payment policy—Chapter 11: Hospice services.* http://www.medpac.gov/chapters/Mar12_Ch11.pdf (accessed March 2012).

Meyer, E. C., D. E. Sellers, D. M. Browning, K. McGuffie, M. Z. Solomon, and R. D. Truog. 2009. Difficult conversations: Improving communication skills and relational abilities in health care. *Pediatric Critical Care Medicine* 10(3):352-359.

Meyer, H. 2011. Changing the conversation in California about care near the end of life. *Health Affairs* 30(3):390-393.

Morrison, R. S., R. Augustin, P. Souvanna, and D. E. Meier. 2011. America's care of serious illness: A state-by-state report card on access to palliative care in our nation's hospitals. *Journal of Palliative Medicine* 14(10):1094-1096.

Mularski, R. A., S. M. Dy, L. R. Shugarman, L.R., A. M. Wilkinson, J. Lynn, P. G. Shekelle, S. C. Morton, V. C. Sun, R. G. Hughes, L. K. Hilton, M. Maglione, S. L. Rhodes, C. Rolon, and K. A. Lorenz. 2007. A systematic review of measures of end-of-life care and its outcomes. *Health Services Research* 42(5):1848-1870.

NASW (National Association of Social Workers). 2014. *NASW professional social work credentials and advanced practice specialty credentials.* Washington, DC: NASW. https://www.socialworkers.org/credentials/list.asp (accessed January 8, 2014).

NBCHPN® (National Board for Certification of Hospice and Palliative Nurses). 2014. *NBCHPN certifications offered.* http://www.nbchpn.org/DisplayPage.aspx?Title=Certifications%20 Offered (accessed July 30, 2014).

NCI (National Cancer Institute). 2013. *Pediatric supportive care (PDQ®), patient version.* http://www.cancer.gov/cancertopics/pdq/supportivecare/pediatric/Patient (accessed July 30, 2014).

NCI. 2014. *Pediatric supportive care (PDQ®), health professional version.* http://www.cancer.gov/cancertopics/pdq/supportivecare/pediatric/healthprofessional (accessed July 30, 2014).

NCP (National Consensus Project for Quality Palliative Care). 2004. National Consensus Project for Quality Palliative Care: Clinical practice guidelines for quality palliative care, executive summary. *Journal of Palliative Medicine* 7(5):611-627.

NHPCO (National Hospice and Palliative Care Organization). 2009. *Standards of practice for pediatric palliative care and hospice.* Alexandria, VA: NHPCO. http://www.nhpco.org/sites/default/files/public/quality/Ped_Pall_Care%20_Standard.pdf.pdf (accessed July 15, 2014).

NHPCO. 2010. *Concurrent care for children implementation toolkit.* Alexandria, VA: NHPCO. http://www.nhpco.org/sites/default/files/public/ChiPPS/CCCR_Toolkit.pdf (accessed February 13, 2013).

NHPCO. 2012a. *NHPCO facts and figures: Hospice care in America.* http://www.nhpco.org/sites/default/files/public/Statistics_Research/2012_Facts_Figures.pdf (accessed February 10, 2013).

NHPCO. 2012b. *Pediatric concurrent care.* Alexandria, VA: NHPCO Mary J. Labyak Institute for Innovation. http://www.nhpco.org/sites/default/files/public/ChiPPS/Continuum_Briefing.pdf (accessed July 28, 2014).

NHPCO. 2013. *National Data Set (NDS).* http://www.nhpco.org/performance-measures/national-data-set-nds (accessed February 15, 2013).

NHPCO. undated-a. *Performance measures.* http://www.nhpco.org/performancemeasures (accessed February 10, 2013).

NHPCO. undated-b. *Quality partners.* http://www.nhpco.org/qualitypartners (accessed July 15, 2014).

NHPCO. undated-c. *Tools and resources.* http://www.nhpco.org/tools-and-resources (accessed February 18, 2013).

NHPCO. undated-d. *Pediatric hospice.* http://www.nhpco.org/pediatric-hospice (accessed July 30, 2014).

NIH (National Institutes of Health). 2004. *PA-04-057: Improving care for dying children and their families.* http://grants2.nih.gov/grants/guide/pa-files/PA-04-057.html (accessed February 15, 2013).

NIH. 2010. *RFA-NR-10-006: Advancing palliative care research for children facing life-limiting conditions.* http://grants.nih.gov/grants/guide/rfa-files/RFA-NR-10-006.html (accessed February 15, 2013).

NINR (National Institute of Nursing Research). 2012. *Spotlight on end-of-life research.* https://www.ninr.nih.gov/researchandfunding/spotlight-on-end-of-life-research (accessed February 11, 2013).

NINR. 2013a. *Building momentum: The science of end-of-life and palliative care. A review of research trends and funding, 1997-2010.* Bethesda, MD: NINR. http://www.ninr.nih. gov/sites/www.ninr.nih.gov/files/NINR-Building-Momentum-508.pdf (accessed July 20, 2014).

NINR. 2013b. *Palliative Care: Conversations Matter®.* http://www.ninr.nih.gov/newsand information/conversationsmatter?utm_source=NINR%20News%20and%20Notes&utm_ medium=Newsletter&utm_content=NINR%27s%20Pediatric%20Palliative%20Care%20 Campaign&utm_campaign=Palliative%20Care%3A%20Conversations%20Matter#. U-J6nWNCx2B (accessed August 6, 2014).

NPCRC (National Palliative Care Research Center). 2010. *$1.8 million awarded for palliative care research.* http://www.npcrc.org/news-detail.aspx?id=108 (accessed July 30, 2014).

NPCRC. 2013. *NPCRC announces new opportunities for pediatric and geriatric palliative care research applications.* http://www.npcrc.org/news-detail.aspx?id=127 (accessed July 30, 2014).

NPCRC. undated-a. *Grants Program: Areas of interest.* http://www.npcrc.org/content/33/ Areas-of-Interest.aspx (accessed February 15, 2013).

NPCRC. undated-b. *Grants Program: Funding opportunities.* http://www.npcrc.org/ content/19/Funding-Opportunities.aspx (accessed February 15, 2013).

NQF (National Quality Forum). 2006. *A national framework and preferred practices for palliative and hospice care quality: A consensus report.* Washington, DC: NQF.

Pain & Policy Studies Group. 2014a. *Achieving balance in federal and state pain policy: A guide to evaluation (CY2013).* Madison: Pain & Policy Studies Group, University of Wisconsin Carbone Cancer Center. http://www.painpolicy.wisc.edu/sites/www.painpolicy. wisc.edu/files/evalguide2013.pdf (accessed July 14, 2014).

Pain & Policy Studies Group. 2014b. *Achieving balance in state pain policy: A progress report card (CY2013).* Madison: Pain & Policy Studies Group, University of Wisconsin Carbone Cancer Center. http://www.painpolicy.wisc.edu/sites/www.painpolicy.wisc.edu/ files/prc2013.pdf (accessed July 14, 2014).

Patrizi, P., Thompson, E., and Spector, A. 2011. *Improving care at the end of life: How the Robert Wood Johnson Foundation and its grantees built the field.* RWJF retrospective series. http://www.rwjf.org/content/dam/farm/reports/reports/2011/rwjf69582 (accessed March 2011).

Payne, S., P. Smith, and S. Dean. 1999. Identifying the concerns of informal carers in palliative care. *Palliative Medicine* 13:37-44.

PCORI (Patient-Centered Outcomes Research Institute). 2014. *About us.* http://www.pcori. org/about-us/landing (accessed July 24, 2014).

PDIA (Project on Death in America). 2004. *Shaping the future of social work in palliative & end-of-life care.* New York: PDIA. http://www.swhpn.org/swlda/archive/Downloads/ January-March%2004%20Newsletter.pdf (accessed July 15, 2014).

Pew Research Center. 2009. *Growing old in America: Expectations vs. reality.* http://www. pewsocialtrends.org/files/2010/10/Getting-Old-in-America.pdf (accessed January 21, 2014).

Pew Research Center. 2013. *Views on end-of-life medical treatments.* http://www.pewforum. org/files/2013/11/end-of-life-survey-report-full-pdf.pdf (accessed November 25, 2013).

Quill, T. E., E. Dannefer, K. Markaki, R. Epstein, J. Greenlaw, K. McGrail, and M. Milella. 2003. An integrated biopsychosocial approach to palliative care training of medical students. *Journal of Palliative Medicine* 6(3):365-380.

Reinhard, S. C., C. Levine, and S. Samis. 2012. *Home alone: Family caregivers providing complex chronic care.* Washington, DC: AARP, Public Policy Institute.

Ross, D. D., H. C. Fraser, and J. S. Kutner. 2001. Institutionalization of a palliative and end-of-life education program in a medical school curriculum. *Journal of Palliative Medicine* 4(4):512-518.

RWJF (Robert Wood Johnson Foundation). 2008. *State policies design to curb misuse of controlled substances restrict legit pain treatment: Reform needed.* Analysis of state policies on pain management (program results). Princeton, NJ: RWJF. http://www.rwjf.org/content/dam/farm/reports/program_results_reports/2008/rwjf64200 (accessed July 15, 2014).

Schenck, A. P., F. S. Rokoske, D. D. Durham, J. G. Cagle, and L. C. Hanson, 2010. The PEACE project: Identification of quality measures for hospice and palliative care. *Journal of Palliative Medicine* 13(12):1451-1459.

Schiffman, J. D., L. J. Chamberlain, L. Palmer, N. Contro, B. Sourkes, and T. C. Sectish. 2008. Introduction of a pediatric palliative care curriculum for pediatric residents. *Journal of Palliative Medicine* 11(2):164-170.

Schroeder, S. A., and W. Frist. 2013. Phasing out fee-for-service payment. *New England Journal of Medicine* 368(21):2029-2031.

Solomon, M. Z., D. M. Browning, D. L. Dokken, M. P. Merriman, and C. H. Rushton. 2010. Learning that leads to action: Impact and characteristics of a professional education approach to improve the care of critically ill children and their families. *Archives of Pediatrics and Adolescent Medicine* 164(4):315-322.

Spettell, C. M., W. S. Rawlins, R. Krakauer, J. Fernandes, M. E. S. Breton, W. Gowdy, S. Brodeur, M. MacCoy, and T. A. Brennan. 2009. A comprehensive case management program to improve palliative care. *Journal of Palliative Medicine* 12(9):827-832.

Stratis Health. 2009. *National Rural Health Association Technical Assistance Project final report.* http://www.stratishealth.org/documents/NRHA_PC_Report_09-09.pdf (accessed February 18, 2013).

Stratis Health. 2011. *Minnesota Rural Palliative Care Initiative: Learning Collaborative Project brief.* http://www.stratishealth.org/documents/PC_Stratis_Health_MRPCI_project_brief_2011.pdf (accessed February 18, 2013).

Sullivan, A. M., N. M. Gadmer, and S. D. Block. 2009. The Project on Death in America faculty scholars program: A report on scholars' progress. *Journal of Palliative Medicine* 12(2):155-159.

Swetz, K. M., T. D. Shanafelt, L. B. Drozdowicz, J. A. Sloan, P. J. Novotny, L. A. Durst, R. P. Frantz, and M. D. McGoon. 2012. Symptom burden, quality of life, and attitudes toward palliative care in patients with pulmonary arterial hypertension: Results from a cross-sectional patient survey. *The Journal of Heart and Lung Transplantation* 31(10):1102-1108.

SWHPN (The Social Work in Hospice and Palliative Care Network). undated. *Charting the course for the future of social work in end-of-life and palliative care: A report of the 2nd Social Work Summit on End-of-Life and Palliative Care.* http://www.swhpn.org/monograph.pdf (accessed July 15, 2014).

Teno, J. M., P. L. Gozalo, J. P. Bynum, N. E. Leland, S. C. Miller, N. E. Morden, T. Scupp, D. C. Goodman, and V. Mor. 2013. Change in end-of-life care for Medicare beneficiaries: Site of death, place of care, and health care transitions in 2000, 2005, and 2009. *Journal of the American Medical Association* 309(5):470-477.

von Gunten, C. F., P. Mullan, R. A. Nelesen, M. Soskins, M. Savoia, G. Buckholz, and D. E. Weissman. 2012. Development and evaluation of a palliative medicine curriculum for third-year medical students. *Journal of Palliative Medicine* 15(11):1198-1217.

Walling, A., K. A. Lorenz, S. M. Dy, A. Naeim, H. Sanati, S. M. Asch, and N. S. Wenger. 2008. Evidence-based recommendations for information and care planning in cancer care. *Journal of Clinical Oncology* 26(23):3896-3902.

Walling, A., S. M. Asch, K. Lorenz, C. P. Roth, T. Barry, K. L. Kahn, and N. S. Wenger. 2010. The quality of care provided to hospitalized patients at the end of life. *Archives of Internal Medicine* 170(12):1057-1063.

Wenger, N. S., Roth, C. P., Shekelle, P., and the ACOVE Investigators. 2007. Introduction to the Assessing Care of Vulnerable Elders-3 quality indicator measurement set. *Journal of the American Geriatrics Society* 55:S247-S252.

Wiener, L., E. Ballard, T. Brennan, H. Battles, P. Martinez, and M. Pao. 2008. How I wish to be remembered: The use of an advance care planning document in adolescent and young adult populations. *Journal of Palliative Medicine* 11(10):1309-1313.

Wiener, L., S. Zadeh, H. Battles, K. Baird, E. Ballard, J. Osherow, and M. Pao. 2012. Allowing adolescents and young adults to plan their end-of-life care. *Pediatrics* 130(5):897-905.

Wilkie, D. J., and M. O. Ezenwa. 2012. Pain and symptom management in palliative care at the end of life. *Nursing Outlook* 60(6):357-364.

Appendix C

Summary of Written Public Testimony

The committee solicited written testimony about care for individuals who are likely approaching death. In addition to testimony provided at the committee's public meetings (see Appendix A), comments were received through an online survey[1] (see Box C-1). The committee asked for thoughts, stories, and comments from individuals who have a serious and progressive illness or condition and their families, caregivers, and care providers, as well as others who are interested in end-of-life care. The committee was particularly interested in testimony about barriers to care, opportunities for improving care, patient and family experiences with care, and experiences of health care providers. The committee received 578 responses. These comments, along with the in-person testimony described in Appendix A, provided rich context for the committee's work. This appendix provides highlights and a brief summary of the experiences and opinions of those who provided this testimony. Box C-1 provides an overview of the survey used to solicit this testimony.

Responses were received from a wide range of individuals. Caregivers who provided compelling testimony included husbands, wives, sisters, brothers, sons, daughters, nieces, godchildren, parents, cousins, in-laws, friends, and neighbors. The majority of those cared for were elderly, but

---

[1] Respondents were informed that the Institute of Medicine would not record identifying information such as individuals' names, email addresses, or IP addresses. Only aggregated responses without personally identifying information were presented to the committee and placed in the public access file for this project. Respondents were also told that their responses might be referenced or quoted in this report.

BOX C-1
Survey Overview and Testimony Questions

The Institute of Medicine is undertaking a project that will examine care for individuals approaching death. The committee will assess the delivery of health care, social, and other supports to both the person approaching death and the family; person-family-provider communication of values, preferences, and beliefs; advance care planning; health care costs, financing, and reimbursement; and education of health professionals, patients, families, employers, and the public at large.

You may submit comments in any or all of the following areas.

Experiences Receiving Care

Question 1: If you are an individual living with a serious progressive illness or condition, or a loved one of an individual please describe your experiences receiving care. Your stories may include how you have talked with health care providers, your family, and friends; how you have discussed and reviewed your spiritual or religious needs, your finances, or any other issues. Your stories may also include what you liked and did not like about communication with your providers and others who gave you support, treatment approaches, or any other aspects of care.

Question 2: If you are a family member or friend of an individual who has died, what care or supports did you need and/or receive while your family member or friend was in the advanced stages of their condition. What care or supports did you need and/or receive after they died? What care or support did you NOT receive and wish you had received during the illness, at the time of death, or afterwards.

many were in midlife, and some were adolescents and young adults. Some individuals who were themselves living with serious illness and/or likely approaching death also provided their own perspectives. The illnesses and conditions described included Alzheimer's disease, various types of cancer, heart failure, dementia, kidney failure, liver failure, Parkinson's disease, AIDS, and bone fractures.

An array of health care professionals also provided compelling testimony. Many wrote about their experiences both as professionals and as caregivers for loved ones. Testimony was received from ethicists, social workers, chaplains, priests, pastors, and health care administrators, as well as dieticians, oncologists, nephrologists, nurses, cardiologists, neurologists, pediatricians, psychologists, and intensive care unit (ICU) physicians. Many

Experiences Providing Care

Question 3: If you are a health care professional, please tell us about your experiences in providing care to individuals with a serious progressive illness or condition and their families. What are the problems, opportunities, challenges, and successes you encounter? Does the term "end of life" impact the willingness of the individuals you work with to engage in the provision of care or the willingness to receive it? Please indicate what type of professional you are (discipline/specialty).

Barriers to Care

Question 4: What do you see as the biggest barriers to care (for individuals with serious progressive illness or condition) that is appropriate and easy to access?

Improving Care

Question 5: What three changes in the U.S. health care system could improve care of individuals with serious progressive illness?

Additional Comments

Question 6: If you have additional thoughts about improving research, care, and education for or about individuals with a serious illness or medical condition who are likely approaching death, or if you would like to share information related to the committee's work, please use the space provided below to do so. You may also email documents or articles to support your testimony to eol@nas.edu.

of these professionals experienced similar challenges and frustrations, in their roles as both caregivers and health care professionals.

PERCEPTIONS OF DEATH

Many respondents, including caregivers and health care professionals, commented on the ways in which the topic of death is perceived by some health professions and among some patients and families. The perceptions were predominantly ones of fear. One caregiver commented, "Americans don't see death as a part of life." Another added that we are "too afraid to talk about death." Health care professionals also commented about such fears among some of the patients and families they cared for but also among their colleagues. One said, "Physicians are not comfortable discussing EOL [end-of-life] choices."

Health care providers and nonproviders alike commented on the barrier presented by the "healing culture" of medicine and the belief by providers that death means failure. Said a critical care physician, "One of the biggest challenges I face in taking care of patients with advanced progressive illness is the unwillingness of some (not all, probably not even many) to face death and accept it as a part of life just like birth, marriage, etc. We are plagued by a complete lack of understanding and acceptance that we are going to die—our entire medical system is oriented to staving off death. As a clinician, I often feel a failure when someone dies under my care, even though in retrospect (and in the now) the course was laid out long ago by the disease process. Opportunities lie in educating the populace as a whole about death and its inevitability."

Respondents also commented on perceptions of death within American culture. For example, one person remarked, "people in our culture are terrified of death and dying. It has been institutionalized and privatized to the point people are terrified of one of the few experiences we all have in common." A provider, a chaplain, commented on the reasons for these perceptions by saying that "the politicization of discussion of end-of-life care (death panels associating the discussion of end-of-life choice with euthanasia) has definitely had an impact on public perception of these issues." Caregivers and providers alike noted that a fear of death and dying is reflected in legal and legislative systems. Said a caregiver who cared for a dying spouse, "The matter of choice in the time and place of dying is a personal one, and the political and legal system should have NOTHING to say in the matter." A palliative care nurse practitioner noted, "Politicians are afraid to discuss end of life care for fear of hearing the words 'rationing' or 'death panels.'" An emergency medicine physician, who is currently caring for a family member, stated, "I think many physicians fear being sued because the most advanced treatment is not implemented."

"Like most Americans I never thought of death or end-of-life issues until I was forced to. I had no idea how unprepared I was emotionally, mentally, financially, and spiritually to face my grandmother and mother's terminal illnesses," wrote another caregiver.

COMMUNICATION

Importance of Conversation

An important theme that emerged from the testimony was the importance of clear and honest communication between providers and patients and their families. Many stories relayed the impact of not having sufficient information, not understanding choices, and not feeling heard. For example, one caregiver said, "But, perhaps medical professionals could try to explain earlier and more clearly what is really going on. It's dizzying, confusing, and emotionally difficult to navigate the medical establishment and to almost literally translate what they are telling patients and families." One respondent with a serious illness described his/her perception that providers were not willing to talk about what will happen. Another wrote, "I have not seen lack of willingness to provide great end of life care, but rather the failure to point out that the end of life is approaching." Another important issue raised by one caregiver was the problem of ageism and stereotyping of the elderly and its effect on care, including the "tendency of medical providers to talk with loved ones rather than respecting the patient and keeping the patient at the center of the conversation."

However, there were also stories that relayed the impact of positive communication. A caregiver wrote: "When my dad passed just a few years ago, I was most grateful for medical personnel who took the time to listen sympathetically to my anxieties, fears, and questions. My most troubling question was, 'Am I doing enough? Am I doing the right thing?' They kindly offered options for care and counseled me as to what seemed reasonable, given his deteriorating condition."

Many health care providers of all types acknowledged that there is fear and reluctance to provide honest and clear information, and that professionals need to talk more openly about options near the end of life. A provider noted, "Most patients and families are not afraid of having an honest discussion about serious illnesses or 'end of life' if it's done well and professionally."

There were several comments by providers about the terminology used by providers when talking with patients and families. Some believed that the term "end of life" should not be used. One person stated that it was not compatible with the medical profession's philosophy of saving lives. Another commented that the term was important to use because it is unambiguous and helps patients and families hear the truth. Other providers suggested that terms such as "serious illness" and "end-stage illness" were more appropriate to use.

With regard to suggestions for improving communication, one caregiver simply stated, "Ask patients what they want." Many others, including patients themselves, indicated that just having conversations was important. Said one caregiver, "What I appreciate most is honesty, accurate information, and empathy from health care providers."

Advance Care Planning and Advance Directives

Another facet of communication reflected in the testimony was the use and honoring of advance directives. Some caregivers relayed stories of how care preferences were not assessed, and advance directives were not honored. Said one: "My mother has multiple sclerosis and is receiving excellent care from one of the top medical centers for MS [multiple sclerosis] in the nation. Despite the level of medical treatment, not one person has ever discussed her goals for treatment, her values and preferences, or what she would want doctors to do if something happened to her and she couldn't communicate." Another caregiver described the following situation: "My aunt had a DNR [do not resuscitate] on file when she was in the skilled nursing facility following a fall and fractured hip. She was moved to a new room the day after she got there and that evening was dying of aspiration. They tried to resuscitate her for ONE HOUR before giving up and thankfully, she was released from this torture and died. She was 90 years old. The reason they did this was that they had failed to move her DNR from one room to another, and yet, they somehow managed to move her azalea plant that I brought to her that day to her new room. Words cannot express how heartbreaking and infuriating this is to me."

Other caregivers submitted comments expressing frustration about the inability to have conversations about advance directives. A caregiver stated, "Not sure how to get doctors to talk about advance directives, i.e., MOLST [Medical Orders for Life-Sustaining Treatment]. My dad's doctor signed it—no discussion, etc., and told me (I'm a nurse) to go over the information and fill it out with my dad."

Some caregivers commented that people need not only to have directives, but also the cooperation of family and providers. Many stories revealed the emotional impact that resulted when family members and physicians disagreed with the stated wishes of a patient. Among those living with serious illness, comments on this topic conveyed the importance of having advance directives, and it was suggested that digital advance directives be made standard practice to help ensure that they will be known and honored.

PROVISION OF CARE:
DELIVERY, QUALITY, COORDINATION, AND TIMING

Individuals living with serious illness, caregivers, providers, and others wrote many compelling stories about how care was received and provided. Testimony revealed challenges with the coordination and continuity of care and with receiving the care individuals wanted (including limited interventions) when they wanted it.

One issue raised frequently by caregivers was a feeling that too many procedures and unnecessary surgeries occurred in the care of their loved one. A wife wrote, "When my late husband was battling a brain tumor in the last months of his life, the doctors wanted him to undergo another surgery. We knew enough to ask: what will this add to my quality of life and life span? The answer was: 'well, the surgery, as you know is difficult, but it can add a few weeks to your life.'" Another caregiver commented that more treatment may be too much for some, but helpful to others: "I have seen many patients get chemotherapy treatment long after they have lost their quality of life and think that a little honesty may have given them more quality in the time they had left. I have also seen many patients live a high quality of life while receiving chemotherapy, which I think should be a determining factor when deciding treatment options." A person living with a serious and chronic condition commented: "I have made it clear that I will be fighting until the end. I have said so through my advance directive."

Other concerns expressed by caregivers included the fragmentation of care and lack of care coordination. These problems were also reported by providers. One provider, a primary care internist, said, "Tear down the barriers between acute hospital, home, nursing home, assisted living, hospice. Transitions among these are not easy, and any one doctor has a great deal of trouble navigating and coordinating them all." Another person said regarding the care of his/her father: "The doctors that I have encountered in his care don't want to talk about palliative care, advance directives, and any kind of general plan of care for him. Each specialist works in a silo, rather than a collaboration of care. We will bring tests results with us, so that one physician is aware of what others are doing."

Another major concern expressed by respondents related to the adequacy of pain relief in individuals with serious illness. A provider believed that there was too much fear of addiction to pain medication, which prevents adequate pain control in patients. Still another provider reported that there was fear of hastening death by providing adequate pain relief.

Many caregivers relayed wonderfully positive experiences with hospice and palliative care, which benefited both the patient and family. One husband wrote: "The most important help we got was from hospice. They provided pain control, help for me as a care giver, unstinting nursing care for my wife, and the option of palliative sedation if she needed it. After she died they provided the grief support I so desperately needed." Other caregivers noted that while their experience with hospice was good overall, there were challenges, such as the level and timeliness of assistance and assistance provided when a regular nurse is off duty, as well as obtaining adequate pain control. Once caregiver wrote: "My mother died 3 years ago in the aftermath of a heart attack. She fortunately received hospice care in an excellent hospital setting. The disturbing thing about her last hours was that the hospital nurses would not administer enough pain medication to moderate her suffering. The hospice nurses checked in on her only once a day—we had been assured that she would be kept 'completely comfortable' but that was not the case, since the hospital staff insisted they did not want to medicate her to a level of unresponsiveness." There were additional comments about hospice being a misunderstood service. For example, one provider said: "One of the biggest barriers to care regarding hospice services is the misunderstanding of patients that if you sign up for hospice you are giving up on living. The misconstrued notion that everyone has given up hope if you sign up for hospice. This could not be further from the truth." While there were reports from providers that palliative care has become increasingly medicalized and less holistic, many providers and caregivers expressed that it was a very helpful service, one that was not offered soon enough.

Other topics mentioned as barriers to care included difficulty finding care for those with behavioral issues, the use of technology that makes the end of life more difficult to determine, and a lack of training about disability culture and lifestyle. In addition, policies and procedures were mentioned as preventing patient-centered care. One patient remarked, "Policies and procedures take center stage and the patient is a 'bit player' in the drama that unfolds." There were also numerous comments that expressed support for or opposition to physician aid in dying.

A wide range of respondents offered suggestions for reducing barriers to good care. Providers called for increased coordination of care, more patient-centered care, earlier access to hospice (including an extension of the benefit to a 1-year prognosis rather than 6 months) and palliative care, and better access to home care.

Like providers, caregivers suggested that better coordination of care should be provided, even mandated, and that hospice should be offered early. Other suggestions from caregivers and those living with serious illness related to social supports and assistance in coping, such as the need for skilled advocates, social workers, better grief support, respite care, home visits, and pain control. Some stories relayed the extent of depression in loved ones who were dying and some who died by suicide. Some caregivers stated that more attention should be paid to the mental and cognitive health of people during the course of their illness. In addition, a multitude of stories spoke to the benefit and necessity of spiritual care. One person, the adult child of a dying man, wrote that the chaplain was able to explore some of his/her father's questions that he did not want to discuss with his children. Another respondent commented, "I needed a chaplain's care, and did not receive it, while she was dying, and afterwards. I get support from the congregation of which I am a part, but that is different, more diffuse care. I wanted to be able to talk about my friend, the courageous decision she made, the quality of her dying, and how my world changed with her death."

NEED FOR EDUCATION

Many of the topics raised in the sections above led to suggestions for education—for patients, family, providers, and the public at large. Testimony included ideas for ways to help change perceptions of death. A number of respondents suggested that public education initiatives are needed, such as television commercials to help normalize discussions of death and dying. One respondent recommended that providers work with producers in Hollywood to paint a more realistic picture of illness, codes, and other events surrounding the end of life.

To help patients and families, the use of technology was encouraged. One provider suggested that "improving the availability of communication with a cell phone, texting system that insures 24-hour care would be a great improvement. Access to videos online to discuss some of the issues related to terminal care, medications used by families to comfort patients, discussions to have with the patient to comfort and encourage, and a host of other needed information topics would be very helpful." Other providers thought that patients and families should receive more education on the benefits of hospice and palliative care. Interestingly, many caregivers (and some providers) made the same recommendation for providers.

Additional suggestions were made regarding education for providers. These suggestions included formal curriculum requirements on or exposure to end-of-life care, humanities requirements for medical students, and training in effective communication. Training was also recommended for direct care workers and religious leaders.

COST OF CARE AND REIMBURSEMENT POLICIES

The cost of care was a serious concern expressed by caregivers. One commented, "Individuals with long term illness should not impoverish their families through medical costs. We need SERIOUS change to funding." Another caregiver remarked that "the emotional cost is great, the financial cost is astronomical."

Providers expressed frustration that the fee-for service model poses a problem for providing care for the ill and those near the end of life, that Medicare regulations drive care, and that there are financial incentives to treat patients aggressively. One provider commented, "I wish doctors were given more support to be there." A nurse wrote, after reflecting on the death of a loved one, "We must look at restructure of reimbursement, so providers have incentives to spend the time that is needed, rather than getting paid fee for services and losing sight of what is most important."

Health care professionals recommended many changes in reimbursement policies. Providers suggested payment for communication about treatment choices and goals of care, increased coverage for palliative care and hospice, and funding for coordination of care and other ancillary services (such as nursing time to address symptoms, health care navigators). Some providers also thought that compensation should be provided for transitional care. One palliative care nurse wrote about the need for "financial incentives that focus on quality of life, symptom management and caregiver burdens." Caregivers noted that they experienced challenges when dealing with insurance companies. One respondent stated, "The challenges come with insurance companies and what they think is necessary or not necessary. The insurance companies may take their time to respond to our requests and frequently need more documentation. Their rules may change and what was acceptable 1 month may need clarification for the prescription to be filled by the pharmacy." Caregivers also called for an easier process for filing claims and reimbursement for home health palliative care, and supported payment for discussions with providers about goals of care.

STRESS ON CAREGIVERS

Caregivers expressed a range of additional concerns that reflect issues related to stress on caregivers and other barriers to care. There were numerous reflections on the emotional and logistical difficulties faced by caregivers. One noted, "Caregivers are the backbone of care for this population. We are unpaid and under tremendous emotional distress." Another commented, "Health care providers ought to take the time to consider the spouse or caregiver of a disabled or elderly person who is brought to them for treatment. Sometimes, the 'bringer' may be the person who needs the most care." One caregiver mentioned the difficulties posed by sibling ineligibility for the Family and Medical Leave Act. In describing caring for a sick spouse, one respondent wrote, "There are days when it's hard for me not to laugh when well-meaning people advise me to take care of myself. . . . My husband's illness is my illness. I belong to a caregivers group, which is supportive. People who are not caregivers do not understand the continuous burden of the role and seem to think it can be walked away from or put aside forever or for a while. Not so. The stress feels as if I'm constantly holding my breath."

Respondents also reported difficulties related to transportation and hospital parking. One provider wrote, "Issues my patients have, who is going to do the food shopping, how is my spouse going to cope, how does my spouse get a respite from caring for me." Many caregivers described the amount and types and difficulty of care they were required to offer. A chaplain who is also a caregiver for a spouse wrote about his/her experience: "The biggest shock for me has been how much our current system requires the patient in this situation to have a relative looking out for them. Some people are alone." Another caregiver, reflecting on caring for his/her father during the end of his life, wrote, "His disease progressed rapidly and we were struggling with his daily care. We did hire a nurse for the last days of our father's life as my sister and I felt unable to carry out some of the medical procedures that we felt required more skill than we were able to handle (catheterization). I am astounded that it would be expected of any caregiver, especially an elderly spouse." Describing the burden seen on families caring for loved ones, one provider wrote, "The idea that families are often forced to make great personal and financial sacrifices to do what is best for their loved one is inexcusable for a country such as ours."

While many caregivers and loved ones remarked that they received support during their grief and bereavement from health care providers, hospice companies, loved ones, and faith communities, others noted that these services and supports were inadequate or nonexistent. Reflecting on the passing of her mother-in-law, one respondent wrote, "Following her death, other than mailed pamphlets we received no bereavement care. My husband and sister-in-law, in particular, could have used this after losing both parents in less than 2 years." While most providers and caregivers told of their experiences caring for adult parents, siblings, family members, and friends, some described the experience of caring for or losing a child. One respondent wrote, "I was transported to the emergency department during a miscarriage, and once the team determined that my life was not in danger from the blood loss, I was dismissed. There was no screening or assessment or offer of support—no recognition that this 'loss' was potentially traumatic—no moment of compassionate connection for what to me was the loss of a child."

Another respondent talked about the passing of a parent: "Afterwards, I was so tired and often felt others did not appreciate the grief I experienced. Grief is a real issue that ultimately everyone if [they live] long enough, will pass through."

CONCLUSION

The committee is grateful to the hundreds of individuals who shared their experiences and perspectives on care for individuals with serious illness and for those who are likely approaching death. Their responses shed light on the challenges faced and on supports that helped ease burdens. The following reflection from a caregiver perhaps summarizes some of the important messages from the many submissions received: "The success is that for the most part, when you take the time to find out what's most important to patients and families, they make very reasonable choices. The challenge is that our health care system does not encourage these conversations, our professional providers frequently do not have the time or training, and treatment measures default to those that are not patient-centered."

Appendix D

Financing Care at the End of Life and the Implications of Potential Reforms

Haiden A. Huskamp, Ph.D.[1]

David G. Stevenson, Ph.D.[2]

As with other health care services, the manner in which end-of-life care is financed in the United States has a substantial impact on the care that is delivered. In the following paper, we examine the implications of financing and payment methods for end-of-life care for utilization, quality, and expenditures of individuals with advanced illness. After presenting context about service utilization, expenditures, and insurance coverage at the end of life, we highlight key limitations of current financing approaches, including incentives for overutilization, fragmentation, and inattention to quality of care. We discuss possible reforms to end-of-life care financing and the potential trade-offs involved, paying particular attention to bundled payment approaches and targeted changes to eligibility and payment policies. We conclude with broad guidance about factors to consider in advancing public policy in this important area.

FINANCING CARE AT THE END OF LIFE AND THE IMPLICATIONS OF POTENTIAL REFORMS

Introduction

As with other health care services, the manner in which end-of-life care is financed in the United States has a substantial impact on the care that is

[1]Department of Health Care Policy, Harvard Medical School, 180 Longwood Avenue, Boston, MA 02115, huskamp@hcp.med.harvard.edu, 617-432-0838.

[2]Department of Health Policy, Vanderbilt University School of Medicine, 2525 West End Avenue, Suite 1200, Nashville, TN 37203, David.Stevenson@vanderbilt.edu, 615-322-2658.

delivered. Not only does coverage in public and private insurance programs shape the services for which individuals are eligible, but also the interaction between coverage and approaches to payment exerts a strong influence on the intensity, setting, and quality of care that is provided. In this appendix, we examine the implications of financing and payment of end-of-life care in the United States and discuss potential reforms and their possible impacts. We focus primarily on the Medicare program, given its prominent role in paying for and shaping end-of-life care. We detail relevant research findings where possible, while also identifying gaps in the knowledge base. We conclude with broad guidance about factors to consider in advancing public policy in this important area.

UTILIZATION AND EXPENDITURES FOR INDIVIDUALS AT THE END OF LIFE

Approximately 2.5 million individuals die each year from a variety of causes, including sudden acute illness, accident, suicide, homicide, and long-term chronic conditions (Minino, 2013). Approximately three-quarters (74 percent) of deaths occur among persons aged 65 and older (Minino, 2013). In contrast to nonelderly decedents, death among the elderly is most likely to occur after a diagnosis of advanced chronic illness as opposed to a sudden, unexpected death. Of all deaths in 2011 among persons aged 65 and older, 26 percent were due to heart disease, 22 percent to cancer, 7 percent to chronic lower respiratory diseases, 6 percent to stroke, and 5 percent to Alzheimer's disease (Minino, 2013). For the one-quarter of all deaths among the nonelderly, a much larger proportion is due to accidents, homicide, suicide, or acute episodes of illness. For example, 38 percent of all 2011 deaths among those aged 1-24, 26 percent among those aged 25-44, and 7 percent among those aged 45-64 were due to accidents (Minino, 2013).

Services Used at the End of Life

Individuals suffering from advanced illness may use a variety of life-prolonging and palliative services after their diagnosis. While the inpatient share of Medicare expenditures for decedents aged 65 and older in a given year has dropped dramatically over the past 30 years, inpatient care still accounted for half of all Medicare spending—50.2 percent—among elderly decedents in 2006 (see Table D-1) (Riley and Lubitz, 2010). Physician services accounted for 18.8 percent, skilled nursing facility (SNF) care for 10.4 percent, hospice for 9.7 percent, other outpatient services for 6.8 percent, and home health care for 4.1 percent (Riley and Lubitz, 2010). Although inpatient spending as a proportion of total spending at the end of life has

TABLE D-1 Percent of Medicare Payments by Service Type for Medicare Decedents Aged 65 and Older

Services	1978	2006
Inpatient Hospital	76.3	50.2
Physician and Other Medical	17.3	18.8
Outpatient	2.6	6.8
Hospice	0.0	9.7
Skilled Nursing Facility (SNF)	1.9	10.4
Home Health	1.8	4.1

SOURCE: Riley and Lubitz, 2010.

declined substantially along with an increased role for hospice care, it is important to note that many Medicare beneficiaries still have intensive service use at the end of life (Barnato et al., 2004; Riley and Lubitz, 2010). In fact, many Medicare beneficiaries access the hospice benefit only after spending time in the hospital and the intensive care unit (ICU), and then do so only for short periods of time (Teno et al., 2013).

Approximately one-quarter of Medicare spending is incurred by individuals in their last year of life, a proportion that has remained virtually unchanged since the late 1970s (Riley and Lubitz, 2010). Focusing only on Medicare expenditures provides a narrow picture of health care spending at the end of life, particularly for nursing home residents, approximately two-thirds of whom are dually eligible for Medicare and Medicaid and receive Medicaid-financed long-term services and supports. While some have pointed to the relatively large share of Medicare spending devoted to care in the final year of life to support an argument that growth in health care spending is driven largely by the increased use of high-cost aggressive treatment for individuals near death, Scitovsky (1984) argued that changes in technology and intensity of treatment had not disproportionately affected utilization and spending for patients at the end of life relative to other elderly Medicare patients who are ill, and thus that spending should not be a disproportionate target of cost containment efforts. Lubitz also concluded that Medicare beneficiaries in their final year of life did not account for a larger share of Medicare expenditures after the emergence of new medical technologies, demonstrating that the dying were utilizing care in ways similar to those of other patients (Lubitz and Riley, 1993). It is also important to note that calculations of spending in the last year of life can be made only by looking backward from the decedent's date of death. These calculations do not necessarily reflect "real-time" decision making by patients and families about care in the final year of life, as 1-year survival is extremely difficult to predict.

Elderly individuals with advanced illness and their families face considerable financial risk from out-of-pocket health care expenditures in the final years of life (Kelley et al., 2013b). Studying elderly Medicare beneficiaries who died between 2002 and 2008, Kelley and colleagues found that average out-of-pocket spending in the 5 years before death was $38,688 (in 2008 dollars). Expenditures were highly skewed, however, with a 90th percentile of $89,106. For one-quarter of decedents, out-of-pocket expenditures exceeded the household's baseline total assets. Reaffirming the importance of including long-term services and supports in calculations of spending at the end of life as mentioned above, nursing home costs accounted for half of the expenses for those in the top quartile of spending (Kelley et al., 2013b).

Variation in Utilization and Spending at the End of Life

Although spending on end-of-life care is uniformly high, the Dartmouth Atlas documented substantial geographic variation in use of end-of-life care services and spending by hospital referral region (HRR) over time, which researchers and policy makers viewed as evidence of wide regional differences in physician practice patterns (Goodman et al., 2011). For example, in 2007, the average number of days spent in an ICU for chronically ill Medicare beneficiaries in the last 6 months of life varied from 0.7 in Minot, North Dakota, to 10.7 in Miami, Florida (Goodman et al., 2011). In this same population, the percentage dying in a hospital varied from 12.0 percent in Minot, North Dakota, to 45.8 percent in Manhattan, New York, and the average number of days spent enrolled in hospice varied from a low of 6.1 in Elmira, New York, to a high of 39.5 in Odgen, Utah (Goodman et al., 2011).

A July 2013 report by the Institute of Medicine's Committee on Geographic Variation in Health Care Spending sheds new light on the literature on variations in health care spending and utilization at the end of life (IOM, 2013). First, the report documents large variation in health care spending at all levels of geography studied, including HRRs; hospital service areas; core-based statistical areas (CBSAs); physician practices; and even the level of an individual physician after controlling for demographic characteristics, insurance plan factors, and market-level characteristics. Importantly, the variation in total Medicare spending was driven largely by the utilization of post-acute services, including SNF services, home health care, hospice, inpatient rehabilitation, and long-term acute care; if there were no variation in post-acute care expenditures, then variation in total Medicare spending would decrease by 73 percent (IOM, 2013). One potential implication of these findings is that the integrated payment and bundled payment demonstrations we describe below (e.g., where acute, post-acute, and other health care services are more integrated in their financing and delivery) could have greater relevance than simple geographic adjustments to administered payments alone in introducing efficiencies into the health care system.

WHO PAYS FOR CARE AT THE END OF LIFE?

As of 2011, the majority of the U.S. population (54 percent) had private health insurance coverage either through an employer (49 percent) or an individual/nongroup policy (5 percent) (KFF, 2011). Sixteen percent were covered by the Medicaid program, 13 percent by Medicare, and 1 percent by other public programs, with approximately 16 percent being uninsured (KFF, 2011). Although the Patient Protection and Affordable Care Act (ACA) will likely decrease the number of uninsured individuals and increase the proportion who have Medicaid and private coverage beginning in January 2014, the Medicare program is—and will remain—the predominant payer for end-of-life care in the United States, primarily because of the older ages at which most Americans die. Moreover, Medicare's role in shaping end-of-life care in the United States likely goes beyond the proportion of Americans who die as Medicare beneficiaries, given that older individuals are disproportionately likely to die from advanced illness as opposed to an accident or sudden acute event.

With some exceptions, such as the Medicare hospice benefit (described later in this appendix), insurance coverage for individuals with advanced and terminal illnesses reflects coverage that is available to enrollees more generally. The traditional Medicare program covers a broad range of preventive, acute, and post-acute care services for approximately 49 million beneficiaries (KFF, 2012d). Medicare Parts A and B cover hospital services; post-acute SNF care, home health, and rehabilitative services; physician services; durable medical equipment; and ambulance services. For those who elect to join a Part D plan, outpatient prescription drugs are also covered. Medicare's biggest coverage gap relates to the lack of coverage for long-term services and supports. In addition, cost-sharing requirements can be substantial for patients with high levels of service use. Approximately 12 million of the 49 million Medicare beneficiaries are enrolled in Medicare Advantage plans, which receive a capitated payment to cover all Part A and B services in addition to any supplemental services that the plan chooses (e.g., dental, vision) (KFF, 2012c). Of particular relevance to care at the end of life, Part A has covered hospice since 1983 for individuals with terminal illnesses who have an expected prognosis of 6 months or less and who agree to forgo curative treatment for the terminal condition.

Both Medicaid and private insurance plans typically cover a set of services similar to those covered by Medicare, although there is some variation. All state Medicaid programs are required to cover a set of mandated services, including hospital services (both inpatient and outpatient), physician services, home health services, and (unlike Medicare) long-term services and supports. State Medicaid programs are permitted—but not required—to cover prescription drugs, hospice, and personal care services. While an optional benefit, all 50 states and the District of Columbia cover prescription drugs, and all but one—Oklahoma—include hospice care as a covered benefit for adults. In early 2013, the Louisiana Department of Health and Hospitals announced plans to discontinue Medicaid coverage of hospice services as part of a broad set of budget cuts intended to balance the state's budget (Adelson, 2012). After opposition was raised, these plans were dropped (Adelson, 2013).

Private insurance coverage, including both covered benefits and cost-sharing requirements, varies greatly by plan, with some policies offering generous coverage and others offering more limited benefits. Private plans that will be offered through the ACA-created health insurance exchanges must cover services in 10 broad categories of "essential health benefits" (EHBs), using the state's specified "benchmark" plan (a private plan marketed in the state) as the guide for the generosity of coverage of these 10 types of services. States may also choose to mandate that exchange plans marketed in the state cover additional services. Hospice does not fall under one of the broad categories of EHBs that must be covered by all plans offered on the exchanges, so states are not required to insist that exchange plans cover it. Although hospice is currently covered by the benchmark plans for all 50 states and the District of Columbia, only 11 of the 50 states and the District of Columbia require hospice as a covered benefit for all plans offered through the exchanges.

KEY LIMITATIONS OF CURRENT FINANCING APPROACHES

The payment approaches used most commonly by Medicare, Medicaid, and commercial payers have a number of limitations that can contribute to suboptimal care at the end of life. Given its prominence in financing end-of-life care in the United States, we focus primarily on the role of Medicare, including the Medicare hospice benefit.

The Traditional Medicare Program

As noted above, Medicare finances health care for around 70 percent of the individuals who die each year in the United States. The program does not finance all services used at the end of life (as noted, for example, it does not cover long-term supportive services), but it pays for the vast majority of acute medical care and hospice that beneficiaries receive and thus plays a substantial role in shaping how health care providers deliver care for those who die. Although it can be difficult to discern the extent to which financing and payment alone lead to shortcomings in the provision of end-of-life care, researchers and other stakeholders often point to systemic incentives of the traditional Medicare program when discussing challenges such as burdensome, high-intensity treatments delivered at the end of life; fragmentation across payers and settings, which often leads to poor coordination of care; and benefit design features that inhibit delivering care that is in the best interest of patients.

Issues with the General Financing Approach

Excessive health care utilization at the end of life can be burdensome for patients and offers little clinical value. Previous studies of the Medicare population have shown high rates of hospitalization and use of intensive procedures at the end of life (Hogan et al., 2001; Kwok et al., 2011; Lubitz and Riley, 1993; Teno et al., 2013). In addition to the cultural and professional norms that shape physician behavior, a key determinant of older patients' end-of-life care may relate to the fee-for-service (FFS) payment system that is the foundation of reimbursement for services used by the nearly three-quarters of Medicare beneficiaries enrolled in the traditional Medicare program (IOM, 1997). FFS payment provides incentives to deliver more—and often more aggressive—care, and can lead to fragmentation in financing and delivery. More generally, the predominance of FFS payment in U.S. health care financing is often identified as a key impediment to addressing problems of low-value, poor-quality care, as well as rapidly growing health care expenditures (Schroeder and Frist, 2013).

Beyond incentivizing the delivery of more services and procedures, the traditional Medicare program historically has done little to encourage coordination across settings or benefit categories. Medicare generally uses a "silo" approach to reimbursement, employing a separate payment approach for a given provider type for a specific type of service. This approach ignores interrelationships between providers and the care they deliver and can distort clinical decision making. For example, hospitals and post-acute care providers are paid prospectively established rates for inpatient, SNF, and home health care. Hospitals receive a fixed payment for an inpatient hospital stay based on the diagnosis-related group (DRG) methodology, regardless of length of stay or costs incurred. The DRG payment system encourages hospitals to discharge patients as early as possible; in fact, implementation of the DRG system was associated with a decline in hospital lengths of stay and more frequent rehospitalizations (Lave, 1989). In contrast, nursing homes receive a fixed per diem amount for SNF, based on residents' resource utilization groups (RUGs) acuity score, an approach that incentivizes providers to capture fully residents' acuity and therapy needs but not necessarily to limit their lengths of stay. In somewhat of a hybrid of these two approaches, home health agencies are paid a prospectively determined rate for 60-day episodes of care. Importantly, none of these payment approaches gives providers any incentive or mechanism to coordinate the services individuals receive, despite the interrelated trajectories of patients between these settings.

The Medicare program's fragmented approach to payment interacts in negative ways with its largely disjointed approach to determining eligibility across service categories (e.g., eligibility and payment are defined separately for post-acute care services such as SNF care and home health care, despite overlap in populations served and services offered). This fragmented dynamic is confounded further when individuals are dually eligible for Medicare and Medicaid. The classic example of this disjuncture and its potential negative impact on beneficiaries is the perverse incentive that nursing homes have to hospitalize dually eligible residents who, in some instances, could be treated more successfully and efficiently in the nursing home. The financial incentive to shift residents onto the Medicare SNF benefit where possible is created by the disparity between Medicare SNF payments and the generally much lower Medicaid nursing home room and board payments. This challenge has received increasing attention in recent years as the financial and health costs of avoidable hospitalizations and rehospitalizations have become better understood, and interventions and strategies to address them have become more widespread (Lipsitz, 2013; Segal, 2011; Teno et al., 2013).

A related dynamic of particular importance to end-of-life care is the potential barrier the SNF benefit can present for nursing home residents' enrollment in hospice (residents may not enroll in hospice while receiving Medicare-financed post-acute care, unless the two services are treating distinct conditions). In particular, nursing homes and beneficiaries face financial disincentives to enrollment in Medicare hospice instead of Medicare-financed SNF care when both are an option. For individuals being discharged from the hospital who are eligible for either the hospice or SNF benefit, the nursing home generally receives much lower reimbursement for hospice-enrolled residents (whose nursing home care is typically paid for by Medicaid) relative to residents who are utilizing the Medicare SNF benefit. Moreover, residents not Medicaid eligible are liable for paying room and board costs if they choose hospice instead of SNF care (dually eligible residents are not subject to cost sharing for nursing home care during a hospice/long-term care stay or SNF stay). Calculating precise numbers of residents enrolled in SNF care who could benefit from earlier admission to hospice is difficult; however, previous research has identified a sizable minority of individuals who transition from SNF care to hospice within 1 day of SNF discharge, possibly suggesting that financial factors influence the timing of referral (Aragon et al., 2012; Hoffmann and Tarzian, 2005; Miller et al., 2012; Zerzan et al., 2000). The clinical implications of these incentives for residents and the nature of the transition from skilled-rehabilitative care to hospice care are unclear.

The Hospice Benefit as the Primary Financing Mechanism for Palliative Care

The primary mechanism for financing palliative services in the Medicare program (and, for that matter, in most state Medicaid programs and commercial insurance plans) is the hospice benefit. As discussed above, a beneficiary is eligible for the Medicare hospice benefit only if two physicians (one of whom can be the hospice physician) certify that the individual has a prognosis of 6 months or less should the illness run its natural course and if the beneficiary agrees to forego treatments intended to cure the illness or prolong life. These two requirements often limit timely enrollment in the hospice benefit, especially in the context of how the benefit is currently used. Defining hospice eligibility relative to the 6-month prognosis mark can be quite difficult, especially for individuals with noncancer diagnoses (Christakis and Lamont, 2000; Sachs et al., 2004). Moreover, limiting hospice to individuals who agree to forego curative therapies creates an artificial distinction between potentially life-prolonging and palliative therapies and could impede both enrollment and quality of care (Meier, 2013; Temel et al., 2010).

Together these eligibility requirements can serve to delay or prevent enrollment in the Medicare hospice benefit for some beneficiaries, effectively denying them access to palliative care services. Of the almost half (45.2 percent in 2011) of Medicare decedents who use the hospice benefit before their death, approximately one-quarter enroll 5 or fewer days before death (MedPAC, 2013), a period that most agree does not allow the individual or his/her caregivers to obtain the full benefits of hospice services (Bradley et al., 2004; Iwashyna and Christakis, 1998; Kelley et al., 2012; Taylor et al., 2007). Equally troubling is that many short-stay hospice users enroll in the benefit only after a hospitalization, and often after a hospitalization that includes an ICU stay. For example, one study estimates that 40 percent of individuals who used hospice for 3 or fewer days in 2009 had a hospitalization with an ICU stay prior to hospice admission (Teno et al., 2013). In other words, even though an increasing number of Medicare beneficiaries are using the hospice benefit, many do so only after exhausting high-intensity services.

Although palliative care can be introduced at any point in a person's illness to manage symptoms and maximize quality of life, Medicare offers little explicit coverage of palliative care outside of hospice. The Medicare Prescription Drug Improvement and Modernization Act of 2003 (the MMA) authorized a one-time payment to a hospice for evaluation and counseling services provided by a hospice physician for a beneficiary who has not elected the hospice benefit and has a prognosis of 6 months or less (fiscal year [FY] 2005 payment rate = $54.57). In addition, physicians may provide some palliative care consultation in the context of physician services financed by Medicare Part B. While these options provide some financing for physician discussions with patients about end-of-life care preferences and planning, the often time-intensive discussions are poorly reimbursed, in part because of lower value units assigned to the provision of evaluation and management services relative to the provision of procedures under the Resource Based Relative Value Scale (RBRVS) used to determine Medicare physician reimbursement rates for different types of services. Outside of the hospice benefit and these narrow provisions for physician consultation, there is no direct financing stream for palliative care services under the Medicare program (CAPC, 2009). Yet despite the lack of direct financing, many U.S. hospitals currently offer palliative care consultation services. Researchers report that the number of such programs in hospitals with 50 or more beds increased from 658 (24.5 percent) to 1,486 (58.5 percent)—a 125.8 percent increase—from 2000 to 2008 (CAPC, 2010).

Legislation has recently been introduced in both houses of Congress that would provide Medicare and Medicaid reimbursement for advance care planning. In March 2013, Congressman Earl Blumenauer introduced the Personalize Your Care Act (HR 5795), which would provide Medicare and Medicaid coverage for voluntary consultations with health care professionals about advance care planning every 5 years or after a change in health status. In August 2013, Senators Mark Warner and Johnny Isakson introduced the Care Planning Act (S 1439), which would provide Medicare and Medicaid coverage for voluntary discussions about treatment goals and options for patients with advanced illness that result in a documented care plan. The prospects for passage of these two bills are unclear.

Specific Concerns About the Current Hospice per Diem Payment Approach

Currently, for 97 percent of Medicare-financed hospice days, Medicare pays the hospice agencies an all-inclusive per diem payment (i.e., the FY 2014 routine home care rate of $156.26 per day, which is adjusted for differences in local wage rates) to provide all care related to the terminal condition; the other 3 percent of days are billed under one of three other allowable categories (continuous home care, general inpatient care, or inpatient respite) (MedPAC, 2013). In contrast to Medicare reimbursement for other providers, hospice payments are not adjusted for case mix or setting of care, and there is no provision for additional reimbursement for particularly high-cost cases (i.e., outlier payments) (Huskamp et al., 2010).

While this approach to payment may have been appropriate when hospice was used almost exclusively by cancer patients living at home (i.e., when the benefit was first implemented in the 1980s), it is less sufficient in the context of the much greater diversity in the diagnoses and settings of current hospice users, and of hospice providers as well.

The Medicare Payment Advisory Commission (MedPAC) and others have raised a number of concerns about the current payment approach for the Medicare hospice benefit. First, while hospice costs are generally higher for the first and last days of a hospice stay, the routine home care per diem payment is uniform throughout the stay, making longer stays more profitable (Huskamp et al., 2001, 2008, 2010). MedPAC has documented dramatic increases in mean length of stay over the past decade, driven largely by increases in duration of very long hospice stays (MedPAC, 2012). Importantly, these increases are not just a result of the greater portion of hospice users with noncancer diagnoses, as increased lengths of stay extend across diagnosis categories (MedPAC, 2012). In 2009, MedPAC recommended that the payment system be changed such that per diem payments are higher for days at the beginning and end of a hospice stay and lower for the middle days as length of stay increases (MedPAC, 2009). Second, the structure of the hospice benefit—with no adjustments for particularly high-cost stays—limits access for individuals with high-cost palliative care needs (Huskamp et al., 2001; Lorenz et al., 2004). A national survey of hospices found that 78 percent had at least one enrollment policy that could restrict access for individuals with high-cost palliative care needs (Carlson et al., 2011). Third, 18 percent of Medicare hospice stays in 2010 ended in live discharge from hospice, raising concerns about the quality of care received by these beneficiaries and questions about whether hospices are following the eligibility criteria for the benefit (MedPAC, 2013). Fourth, increasing numbers of hospice recipients are using the much more expensive general inpatient (GIP) care category of hospice services, raising questions about the appropriateness of such use (HHS OIG, 2013). Finally, hospice costs are lower on average for hospice users living in nursing homes than for those in the community, suggesting potential efficiencies in joint management of care by the hospice and nursing home (HHS OIG, 1997, 2013; Huskamp et al., 2010; MedPAC, 2013). In addition, hospice staff members provide more aide visits but fewer nurse visits to nursing home residents than to community-based residents, raising questions of duplicative payments because room and board fees paid by Medicaid or by patients themselves are intended to cover aide services needed by residents (Miller, 2004).

Researchers have argued that the current structure of the Medicare hospice benefit may be a particularly poor fit in the nursing home setting. Beyond the barrier that the SNF benefit can create for nursing home residents' enrollment in hospice and the need to pay appropriately for services that can overlap with nursing home care discussed above, several features of the nursing home population pose challenges vis-à-vis the hospice benefit: diagnoses of noncancer terminal conditions (for which, as noted, prognostication can be even more difficult than for cancer patients) are typically more common than in the community; levels of cognitive impairment are often high, and many residents do not have family members involved in their care to assist with the hospice election process; and physicians are often based off site, making it more difficult to discuss hospice with patients and family members (Huskamp et al., 2010).

Medicare Managed Care

Relative to the traditional Medicare (TM) program described above, providers serving the nearly 30 percent of beneficiaries enrolled in the Medicare Advantage (MA) program may be better positioned to promote the use of recommended services at the end of life while discouraging the use of unnecessary invasive procedures (Stevenson et al., 2013). MA plans generally are paid on a per-person—rather than per-service—basis, thereby rewarding plan efforts to manage chronic disease and to minimize unnecessary treatment intensity at the end of life. Importantly, hospice is one of the few benefits "carved out" of Medicare's managed care program. When managed care enrollees enter hospice, FFS Medicare becomes the payer for both hospice care and care unrelated to the terminal condition; health plans remain liable only for any supplemental benefits they provide beyond those in TM, such as vision or dental care. This policy creates a strong financial incentive for plans to promote hospice enrollment among their more expensive terminally ill enrollees, while also diminishing—at least somewhat—incentives to develop integrated, high-quality palliative care networks for people with advanced illness. MedPAC voted in January 2014 to end this hospice carve-out policy, recommending that MA plans begin to cover hospice services for the first time. The likelihood that this recommendation, to be released in the March 2014 report, will be implemented remains unclear.

Previous studies using data from the 1990s confirmed higher rates of Medicare hospice enrollment in managed care versus TM while concluding that this elevated use did not appear inappropriate (McCarthy et al., 2003; Riley and Herboldsheimer, 2001; Virnig et al., 2001). Yet these data are now almost two decades old and preceded passage of the MMA, which has led to markedly increased enrollment of Medicare beneficiaries in managed care plans (Afendulis et al., 2012). Outside of comparing hospice enrollment between MA and TM enrollees, few studies have characterized the intensity or quality of end-of-life care in the MA program. One recent study analyzed end-of-life care for MA and TM decedents matched on age, sex, race/ethnicity, and geography (Stevenson et al., 2013). Although the study could not assess the appropriateness of service use or the quality of end-of-life care delivered, its findings suggest that MA plans may do a better job of minimizing high-intensity procedures at the end of life. MA enrollees used hospice more frequently at the end of life than those being cared for in traditional Medicare, although this difference narrowed over the 2003-2009 study period. After accounting for differential enrollment in hospice, MA enrollees also used fewer inpatient services overall and had markedly lower emergency department use at the end of life compared with matched TM enrollees.

Other Integrated Financing Models

In addition to the MA program, other approaches to integrated financing and delivery have relevance for Medicare beneficiaries with advanced illness and offer potential advantages over Medicare's traditional FFS program. For instance, the Program of All-Inclusive Care for the Elderly (PACE) is an integrated model of financing and delivery for dually eligible older people who have nursing home–level clinical needs while also having the potential to be cared for in the community with adequate supports. Providers receive capitated payments from Medicare and Medicaid and offer enrollees comprehensive, interdisciplinary care across the health care continuum. A number of evaluations have assessed the potential of PACE to keep enrollees out of nursing homes and hospitals and to generate savings (Mukamel et al., 2007); however, few have focused specifically on the potential of such models to improve care at the end of life. Although studies have noted some benefits to PACE enrollment with respect to end-of-life care (e.g., reduced hospitalizations, improved end-of-life care planning, patient-centered care) (Famakinwa, 2010; Mukamel et al., 2002), wide variation also has been observed across PACE sites. Other integrated models of financing—including MA Special Needs Plans, focused on specific, high-risk populations, and more recent state integrated care demonstrations—have similar potential to improve the coordination of care. However, little solid evidence has documented the fulfillment of this potential in these types of models to date (Grabowski, 2007, 2009).

General Lack of Focus on Quality of Care in Current Financing and Regulatory Approaches

Whether in the TM or MA context, an important impediment to improving the financing and delivery of end-of-life care for beneficiaries is the lack of established quality measures. It has become increasingly common for both public and private payers to include in provider contracts financial incentives for providers to meet specified performance standards in an effort to improve the quality of care delivered to a population. However, existing contracts that include performance standards rarely include standards relevant to the provision of high-quality end-of-life care. For example, the Medicare accountable care organization (ACO) Shared Savings Program (MSSP) and Pioneer ACO demonstrations (discussed later) include 33 performance metrics in contracts with ACOs, not one of which is related to the provision of high-quality end-of-life care (Architecture for Humanity, 2012). Similarly, Blue Cross Blue Shield of Massachusetts' (BCBSMA's) Alternative Quality Contract, an innovative model that gives large provider organizations a global payment that covers all care plus bonuses of up to 10 percent of the global payment for meeting specified performance standards, includes a total of 64 performance standards (32 related to ambulatory care and 32 to hospital care), none of which focuses on end-of-life care (BCBSMA, 2010).

One sees a similar lack of focus on palliative and end-of-life care in public reporting systems that are intended to assist patients in selecting high-quality providers while also encouraging providers to improve quality of care. For instance, although the National Quality Forum (NQF) recently endorsed a set of quality measures with relevance to palliative and end-of-life care (NQF, 2012), the Healthcare Effectiveness Data and Information Set (HEDIS) measures that are used to assess and monitor MA plans historically have not included such measures. Although nearly 28 percent of Americans die in a nursing home (Teno et al., 2013), the Nursing Home Compare website reports information on few clinical or other measures relevant for assessing the quality of end-of-life care (it does report the percentage of long- and short-stay residents who self-report moderate to severe pain), instead focusing on measures of functional outcomes (Huskamp et al., 2012). The lack of measures appropriate to end-of-life care on the Nursing Home Compare website may not be surprising given the deemphasis on such measures in nursing home inspection surveys, which focus more on measures related to restoration and maintenance of function for residents. Yet the almost exclusive focus on the latter types of measures has the potential to impede appropriate end-of-life care for residents, because some measures that may address natural symptoms experienced in the dying process (e.g., functional decline, weight loss, dehydration) could be interpreted as implying poor-quality nursing home care (Huskamp et al., 2012). Perhaps as a further indication of this focus, the most recent version of the nursing home resident assessment form (the Minimum Data Set, Version 3.0) drops any reference to advance care planning, something that was included in the previous iteration.

Although progress has been made in developing quality measures for end-of-life care, as evidenced most prominently by the recent NQF endorsement (NQF, 2012), incorporating these measures into provider payment and oversight will be essential as health care is shaped increasingly by more integrated financing and delivery systems such as MA plans and newer innovations such as ACOs and patient-centered medical homes. Policy development in this area needs to ensure adequate provider networks for patients (e.g., including access to palliative care specialists), suitable quality measurement for oversight, and sufficiently flexible financial incentives to foster coordination of care and mitigate incentives for selection or for stinting on needed care.

As required by Section 3004 of the ACA, all Medicare-certified hospice agencies must report a set of hospice quality measures starting in FY 2014 or face payment reductions (a 2 percentage point decrease in the market basket update for that year). These measures include information about pain screening and assessment, dyspnea screening and assessment, the percentage of opioid users who are offered or prescribed a bowel regimen, and documented discussions about treatment preferences and patients' beliefs and values. The ACA also stipulates that hospice quality measures ultimately will be publicly reported (the timetable has yet to be announced), as the Centers for Medicare & Medicaid Services (CMS) already does with quality measures for other types of Medicare providers.

POSSIBLE FINANCING REFORMS AND POTENTIAL IMPLICATIONS FOR END-OF-LIFE CARE

A number of payment and delivery reforms that are planned or currently under way would impact the utilization, cost, and quality of services for patients with advanced illnesses, perhaps addressing some of the problems described above, but also possibly introducing other concerns. Some of these reforms are being implemented as Medicare demonstration programs authorized under the ACA; others are being considered or adopted more broadly in the Medicare program, the commercial market, and/or state Medicaid programs.

Bundling of Payments to Providers

There is now broad national interest on the part of payers, including private insurers, Medicare, and Medicaid, in identifying alternatives to FFS payment (Kirwan and Iselin, 2009; Schroeder and Frist, 2013). Growing attention is focusing on bundled payment models as an alternative that could lead to lower expenditures and increased efficiency (Cutler and Ghosh, 2012). Instead of reimbursing each provider individually for every service delivered to a patient, bundled payment models entail payments for bundles of related services. The bundle of services can be defined relatively narrowly (e.g., to include both physician and nonphysician services delivered during an acute inpatient stay) or more broadly (e.g., to include all acute inpatient care and post-acute care related to an index hospitalization), with the broadest bundle including all services provided to an individual over the course of 1 year (i.e., a global budget).

Depending on how they are structured, models that bundle payments across types of providers have the potential to remove some existing incentives related to setting of care that result from a "silo-based" payment system (e.g., a nursing home's incentive to hospitalize residents to receive higher payments upon discharge). Bundled payments can also give providers greater flexibility to tailor service delivery, as well as incentives for improved coordination of care (Hackbarth et al., 2008). However, these arrangements also raise some concerns. Paying health care providers a fixed fee to cover a bundle of services provides strong incentives for the efficient delivery of services within the bundle. However, this arrangement also creates incentives for providers to increase the volume of bundles delivered as a way to increase revenue, and encourages them to direct care to services not included in the bundle where possible, limiting the potential for savings (Weeks et al., 2013). More important, relative to an FFS system, paying providers a fixed rate that covers a bundle of services can create incentives for them to stint on care or attempt to select patients who have lower-than-average expected costs, creating potential access problems for relatively sicker patients—something that is seen currently in the Medicare hospice benefit (Aldridge et al., 2012). Even with risk adjustment methods to adjust the bundled rate for observable characteristics related to a patient's expected costs, variation in expected spending across individuals within a bundle that is not accounted for by risk adjustment methods will remain, creating incentives for selection. Also, bundling payment for services delivered by different types of providers conceivably could restrict the patient's choice of provider (Sood et al., 2011). For example, if Medicare began paying hospitals a bundled rate for acute and related post-acute care, hospitals might limit their network of post-acute providers in order to negotiate favorable rates (in exchange for volume of patient referrals) with a subset. As discussed in more detail below, a more recent emphasis of bundled payment approaches is the incorporation of quality metrics to incentivize providers to balance quality and efficiency concerns in their provision of care.

In response to the strong incentives that would be created by a pure bundled payment approach for these services, Feder has called for caution in implementation, suggesting a hybrid payment approach that involves the sharing of both risk and savings on the part of providers (Feder, 2013). This type of mixed payment method, which has been proposed for use in health care reimbursement for decades (Newhouse, 1994), could help temper incentives for selection and stinting while still creating an incentive for increased efficiency (in a sense, splitting the difference between the positive and negative incentives created). Others have called for an outlier payment system, as is used in the Medicare reimbursement system for acute inpatient care (Carter et al., 2012). In addition, most agree that performance measures with financial incentives for achieving high-quality care should be included in efforts to bundle payments (see the discussion below) (Schroeder and Frist, 2013; Sood et al., 2011).

Medicare demonstrations of two important models that involve the bundling of payments have recently been undertaken: (1) the Medicare Bundled Payments for Care Improvement Initiative (BPCII) and (2) the MSSP and the Pioneer ACO Program.

In January 2013, CMS announced the provider organizations that will participate in the BPCII, a demonstration that will test several models for bundling provider payments. These models include one that bundles all post-acute services delivered after hospital discharge, one that bundles an acute inpatient admission with post-acute care delivered within 180 days of discharge, and one that bundles an acute inpatient admission with any related readmissions within 30 days of discharge (CMS, 2013a).

The BPCII is not Medicare's first effort at bundling payments. In the 1990s, Medicare conducted the Heart Bypass Center Demonstration, which paid seven hospitals an all-inclusive, per-discharge, bundled rate covering all hospital and physician services provided during the inpatient stay for coronary artery bypass graft (CABG) surgery. Over the 5-year demonstration period (1991-1996), Medicare saved approximately 10 percent on in-hospital spending for CABG surgery recipients, with no evidence of a worsening in health outcomes (Health Care Financing Administration, 1998). In January 2011, CMS implemented a change in the prospective payment system for end-stage renal disease (ESRD), which involved expanding the bundle of services for which dialysis providers are paid to include dialysis-related lab tests and injectable medications such as relatively high-cost erythropoiesis-stimulating agents (ESAs, which some argued were being overused), iron, and vitamin D analogs (Chambers et al., 2013). In addition to the expansion of the bundle, Congress required a Quality Incentive Program (QIP), which reduced payments to providers that failed to meet certain performance standards. Preliminary analyses of the impact of the changes suggest that ESA use dropped by approximately 15-20 percent immediately after implementation, while use of home-based therapies such as peritoneal dialysis increased (Collins, 2012; Fuller et al., 2013; Gilbertson et al., 2012). These data are preliminary and do not elucidate the impact on health outcomes; a longer-term, more detailed study is needed. Nevertheless, these early findings suggest that a change in the bundle of services could have important implications for both spending and quality of care.

While the experience of these previous demonstrations is informative, it does not necessarily generalize to the likely impacts of many of the bundling models being implemented or discussed today. Both the CABG and ESRD bundling demonstrations focused on relatively narrow bundles of services delivered by a single provider organization, while many of the current bundling models would involve bundling services across multiple types of providers.

The MSSP and the Pioneer ACO Program, both implemented in 2012, define a broad service bundle—all services financed by Medicare Parts A and B—in setting spending targets for participating organizations. Under the MSSP, implemented in 2012, participating ACOs are put at risk in one of two ways: (1) use of a "one-sided" approach to risk, whereby the ACO shares in any savings achieved relative to the benchmark spending level (calculated using Medicare Part A and B spending data from the previous 3 years, inflated to the performance year for beneficiaries assigned to the ACO) but is not subject to risk if expenditures exceed the benchmark; or (2) use of a "two-sided" approach to risk, whereby the ACO shares in any savings achieved while also sharing responsibility for spending that exceeds the benchmark (Cao et al., 2013). For the one-sided model, ACOs share in up to 50 percent of any savings, depending on their performance with respect to the 33 performance measures related to quality that are used by the program. ACOs that accept the two-sided model can share in up to 60 percent of savings, again depending on the achievement of performance standards. To date, only a small number of MSSP ACOs have opted for two-sided risk sharing, although current regulations state that all will be required to accept downside risk in the second contract period.

The Pioneer ACO model is an alternative to the MSSP that CMS is testing in 32 "advanced" organizations with experience operating under ACO-type risk-sharing arrangements (CMS, 2012). With the Pioneer model, ACOs can achieve higher levels of rewards and are subject to higher levels of risk than is the case under the MSSP during years 1 and 2 of the demonstration. Starting in year 3, ACOs are eligible to receive a prospective, per-beneficiary per-month payment instead of some or all FFS payments received under the current system (CMS, 2012).

In some respects, ACOs have a strong incentive to adopt care management practices that optimize palliative care and hospice use for individuals with advanced illness, provided these individuals remain assigned to the ACO (i.e., by using sufficient services with an ACO-contracted primary care physician). More specifically, previous studies have shown that early integration of palliative care for individuals with advanced illness has the potential to reduce health care costs overall (Morrison et al., 2008). At the same time, this incentive is tempered by the ability of ACOs to refer individuals outside of the ACO, for example, to a hospice agency or a primary care provider who does not contract with the organization. One key indicator of how ACOs respond to these incentives will be determined by the adequacy of the provider networks available for patients within the ACO with advanced illnesses (e.g., including access to palliative care specialists). A related indicator is the timing of palliative care and hospice utilization for individuals at the end of life. For instance, relative to trends currently seen in the Medicare program (described earlier in this appendix), will ACOs achieve hospice lengths of stay that allow individuals to realize the strengths of the benefit more fully, and will individuals access these services before they enter the hospital and ICU?

Early results from the first year of the MSSP show that nearly half (54 of 114) of the MSSP ACOs that began operation in 2012 had lower spending than projected, and 29 produced savings relative to the target that were large enough to allow them to share savings with Medicare (CMS, 2014c). Early results from the first year of the Pioneer ACO model suggest that Medicare spending per beneficiary for individuals enrolled in these organizations grew at a slower rate overall than spending for beneficiaries enrolled in the FFS program in their area, although results differed across Pioneer ACOs (L&M Policy Research, 2014). Relative to FFS beneficiaries in the same area, 8 Pioneer ACOs had significantly lower Medicare spending growth per beneficiary, 1 had significantly higher Medicare spending growth per beneficiary, and 23 had no statistically significant difference (L&M Policy Research, 2014). Pioneer ACOs performed better than FFS Medicare on 15 quality measures for which published data on FFS beneficiaries were available, and 25 of the 32 had lower risk-adjusted readmission rates relative to the benchmark rate for FFS beneficiaries (CMS, 2013e; Toussaint et al., 2013). However, none of the 33 quality performance standards relates specifically to end-of-life care.

In the commercial market, some payers have also begun experimenting with bundled payment models similar in many ways to the Medicare ACO demonstration programs. In 2009, BCBSMA adopted its Alternative Quality Contract (AQC), which gives provider organizations a risk-adjusted prospective payment for all primary and specialty care provided to a fixed population (the global budget) for a 5-year period. As noted above, AQC organizations are eligible for bonuses of up to 10 percent of their budget based on their performance on 64 outpatient and hospital measures, again none of which is particularly relevant or meaningful for end-of-life care.

AQC implementation was associated with a modest slowing of total spending growth, particularly among organizations that had previously been paid under FFS by BCBSMA, over the first 2 years of the contract (Song et al., 2011, 2012). The savings were driven primarily by a shift of outpatient care to providers with lower fees. However, effects appeared to differ based on prior risk contracting experience with BCBSMA; lower use explained about half of savings for enrollees of providers without prior BCBSMA risk contracting experience. AQC implementation was also associated with some improvements in the contract's performance standards, which were larger in year 2 than in year 1. The AQC evaluation was unable to assess the impact on care at the end of life because of relatively small numbers of decedents each year in this nonelderly commercial population.

If a key goal of bundled payment models (regardless of how broad the bundle) is to maintain or improve quality while increasing provider efficiency—something that was not a primary focus of many previous models intended to increase efficiency—then the success of these efforts will depend on the ability to measure and monitor quality of care for patients with advanced illness. As noted above, none of the new models being implemented or debated includes performance measures appropriate to measuring quality of care for patients with advanced illness.

As policy makers seek to incorporate quality measures into bundled payment and other coordinated care efforts, the role of such measures can be viewed as twofold. First, by integrating quality metrics into the financial incentives for providers, policy makers can help ensure that providers are delivering care that is aligned with expected standards. It should be noted, however, that while the literature on pay-for-performance (P4P) strategies suggests that P4P often does result in improved quality as measured by the metrics used in the P4P systems, the improvements are often relatively small in magnitude and may be somewhat narrowly focused on the clinical areas that are targeted through the measures (Colla et al., 2012; Mullen et al., 2010; Werner et al., 2013; Wilensky, 2011). Even if good measures of end-of-life care quality were to be incorporated in these arrangements, the extent to which overall quality of end-of-life care would improve in response to the incentives is unclear. A perhaps even more important role for quality measures in the context of financing reforms will be as part of a broad effort of oversight and monitoring of organizations responsible for providing end-of-life care. If policy makers detect important quality deficiencies that result from reforms to the financing of care, modifications can be made to such financing arrangements or to the oversight and compliance requirements for providers.

Another new initiative that is related conceptually to the idea of better integrating care individuals receive through the Medicare program involves integrating Medicare and Medicaid financing for individuals who are dually eligible for both programs. Also created by the ACA, the State Integrated Care and Financial Alignment Demonstrations for Dual Eligible Beneficiaries allow states to use one of two models to coordinate services for dually eligible individuals, something that has been challenging historically. Although few states have begun to implement their programs, 26 states have submitted applications to CMS for approval (CMS, 2013c). These programs have the potential to improve the coordination of medical and supportive services for dual eligibles at the end of life, but several caveats should be kept in mind when considering their possible future impact. First, although many states have expressed interest in developing these demonstrations, few programs are under way, and not all states will ultimately move forward with the initiative. Second, previous research has shown that achieving savings in the context of these programs is difficult, in part because states and provider organizations have relatively little experience in coordinating acute and supportive services for a frail population. Finally, and more specific to the context of end of life care, it appears that the state demonstration proposals either carve out Medicare-financed hospice care or explicitly exclude hospice enrollees from the demonstration (i.e., if individuals elect hospice, they are no longer enrolled in the demonstration) (CMS, 2013b; Grabowski, 2007; KFF, 2012a,b). Although palliative care is listed as an included benefit in some state proposals, most fail to mention palliative care services explicitly. One notable exception is South Carolina's proposal and memorandum of understanding with CMS, which details a new palliative care benefit for enrollees who may not meet hospice eligibility criteria (CMS, 2013d). The benefit is designed to provide care earlier in the continuum of illness or disease process, and the care can be provided in conjunction with potentially life-prolonging therapies.

In the context of discussing the potential value of coordinating long-term services and supports with other acute and post-acute care services, it is important to note that current provisions of the ACA do little to address the financing and delivery of long-term services and supports for non-Medicaid-eligible individuals, let alone how these services relate to the broader health care system. The Community Living Assistance Service and Supports (CLASS) Act (Title VIII of the ACA) could have bolstered the financial protection of individuals from long-term care costs, but it was repealed as part of the "fiscal cliff" deal in January 2013 (i.e., The American Taxpayer Relief Act of 2012). Although the Commission on Long-Term Care, which was created through the same legislation, was unable to reach consensus on any alternative approaches to financing of long-term services and supports, it did highlight the need to identify approaches that could better integrate these services and supports with other acute and post-acute services, including through bundled payment and interdisciplinary workforce development initiatives (U.S. Senate Commission on Long-Term Care, 2013).

Concurrent Care Models

The ACA calls on the Secretary of Health and Human Services to create a Medicare Hospice Concurrent Care demonstration program under which beneficiaries will no longer be required to forego curative therapies if they meet other eligibility criteria for the hospice benefit. Budget neutrality is required during the 3-year demonstration period, meaning that total Medicare expenditures under the demonstration must not exceed what Medicare spending would have been in the absence of the demonstration.

In March 2014, CMS released a request for applications for this demonstration program, called the Medicare Care Choices Model (CMS, 2014b), with applications due no later than June 2014. CMS plans to select at least 30 Medicare-certified hospice programs, including hospices that serve rural areas and those that serve urban areas, for participation in the demonstration. Beneficiaries who meet Medicare hospice eligibility criteria and have advanced cancers, chronic obstructive pulmonary disease (COPD), congestive heart failure (CHF), or HIV/AIDS are eligible for enrollment in the new model (CMS, 2014b). Participating hospices will provide services available under the Medicare hospice benefit for routine home care and inpatient respite levels of care (CMS, 2014a). CMS will pay participating hospices $400 per beneficiary per month for these services and for related care coordination activities (CMS, 2014a). Providers that deliver curative services to beneficiaries enrolled in the demonstration will be allowed to bill Medicare for the reasonable and necessary services they deliver (CMS, 2014a).

For a subset of its commercial clients, Aetna has used a concurrent care model for almost a decade. In 2004, Aetna expanded its hospice and palliative care benefits in two key ways: (1) by allowing members to receive curative therapies while enrolled in hospice (i.e., concurrent care) and (2) by requiring a prognosis of 12 or fewer months for hospice eligibility (as opposed to the 6-month prognosis requirement for the Medicare hospice benefit, which would still apply under the Medicare Concurrent Care demonstration) (Krakauer et al., 2009; Spettell et al., 2009). At the same time, Aetna implemented for all commercial and MA members a comprehensive case management program in which services are provided by a nurse care manager with extensive training in palliative care, using predictive modeling to identify potential enrollees for the program.

In a retrospective cohort study that matched current enrollees with historical controls, Spettell and colleagues (2009) compared expenditures, hospice use, and inpatient use for three groups of members who died in 2005, 2006, or 2007: (1) commercial enrollees who received the specialized case management and the traditional hospice benefit; (2) commercial enrollees who received both the case management and the expanded hospice benefit; and (3) MA enrollees who received the Medicare hospice benefit and case management. They found that hospice enrollment and mean number of hospice days for hospice users was substantially higher for all groups relative to the historical controls (who died in 2004). In contrast, the rate of inpatient stays was lower for the intervention groups relative to the controls: 17 percent of those receiving case management plus enhanced benefits had an inpatient stay versus 40 percent of their matched controls, and 23 percent of those receiving case management and traditional hospice benefits were hospitalized versus 43 percent of their controls. Commercial members with both case management and the expanded benefit had longer mean hospice stays than those who received case management and the traditional hospice benefit (37 versus 29 days, respectively), and both groups had longer mean stays than the historical controls.

Krakauer and colleagues (2009) estimate that the increase in hospice use and decrease in acute care service use resulted in a 22 percent decrease in spending compared with historical controls for the commercial member case management/traditional hospice benefit group (the authors provide no estimates for the other groups, nor do they discuss detailed methods). Given that hospice use was increasing during this period, the use of historical controls likely overstates the impact of the interventions. While the results of the Aetna experiment are informative, it is not possible to estimate accurately the potential impact of the Medicare concurrent care demonstration on expenditures using data from a program that offered both concurrent care and expanded hospice eligibility for a commercial under-65 population.

Outside of the Aetna program, no published studies shed light on the expected costs of concurrent care. Studies of cost savings associated with use of the Medicare hospice benefit document savings associated with stays of fewer than 30 days and stays lasting from 53 to approximately 105 days (Kelley et al., 2013a; Taylor et al., 2007). On the basis of these results, one might expect overall savings to the extent that concurrent care resulted in stays lasting fewer than 105 days. There are no data on the relationship between use of the Medicare hospice benefit and Medicare spending for longer stays because of smaller sample sizes in the upper tail of the distribution of stay duration. As a result, the extent to which demonstration sites might be able to meet the budget neutrality requirement could depend on who enrolls in the program and the duration of stays that result from the implementation of concurrent care.

While the Medicare Concurrent Care demonstration program was not implemented initially (with applications accepted starting only in spring 2014), a concurrent care requirement for children in Section 2302 of the ACA was implemented immediately after the act's passage. Effective March 2010, Medicaid and State Children's Health Insurance Programs (SCHIPs) may no longer require children up to age 21 to agree to forego curative therapies to be eligible for the hospice benefit. As noted above, although hospice is an optional benefit for Medicaid and SCHIP programs, the Early Periodic Screening, Diagnosis, and Treatment (EPSDT) provision requires that Medicaid and SCHIPs operating as Medicaid expansions cover hospice for children up to age 21 for whom a physician certifies a prognosis of 6 months or less, and the concurrent care requirement would apply to all of these children. Lindley and colleagues (2013) report that 31 of 50 states had implemented concurrent care for children by 2012, but there have been no published evaluations of the impact of the policy change on utilization of hospice services, spending, or quality of care.

If implemented broadly, concurrent care models should reduce barriers to accessing hospice. Existing concurrent care models would not, however, address any barriers to high-quality palliative care created by the 6-month prognosis requirement.

ACA-AUTHORIZED CHANGES TO MEDICARE HOSPICE REIMBURSEMENT

The ACA calls on the Secretary of Health and Human Services to implement revisions to the payment methodology for hospice services no earlier than October 1, 2013. The legislation requires that such changes be budget neutral in the fiscal year of their implementation. Medicare hospice payment changes could help reduce barriers to access and make payments more efficient, depending on the specific changes implemented by the secretary. For example, an outlier payment system for hospice care, whereby hospices would receive somewhat higher payments for particularly high-cost stays, could help increase access for patients with high-cost palliative care needs. Similarly, payments could be adjusted for case mix and/ or setting to ensure that they reflect the true cost of services delivered to hospice recipients. Of course, any reform of payment methodology could produce both intended and unintended consequences. Also, any given change implemented in isolation could produce very different outcomes than a package of individual changes combined to meet the budget neutrality provision of the law. Absent the more substantial reforms detailed above, it will be important to ensure that hospice payments are as fair and efficient as possible so as to facilitate both access to the benefit and its long-term sustainability.

CONCLUSION

Current approaches to financing services used by patients with advanced illness have a number of limitations that often lead to limited access to hospice and palliative care services and poor quality of care at the end of life. The ACA authorized a number of payment reforms, and payers are adopting or considering other changes as well. These reforms could address some—but likely not all—of the current limitations in financing (for example, in most cases they would not add the role of long-term services and supports for individuals at the end of life or at other points in their health trajectories). Policy makers should anticipate both the intended and unintended consequences of these reforms when structuring their design and implementation. To this end, we identify the following key elements as essential considerations for policy makers as they formulate and implement relevant reforms:

- As Medicare, Medicaid, and commercial payers move forward with efforts to bundle payment for groups of services, these models should incorporate performance metrics that are appropriate for patients with end-of-life care needs to ensure that the models do not result in lower quality of care for individuals with advanced illness. These measures would serve as the foundation for performance incentives in this area and should also be used in oversight and monitoring efforts to ensure high-quality care.
- In creating bundled payment systems, payers should consider mixed payment methods that involve providers sharing both risk and savings with the payer (as opposed to paying a fixed rate per bundle), especially while end-of-life care quality measures are in an early stage of development and use.
- Given the special concerns inherent in the financing of care for nursing home residents at the end of life, payment models that bundle acute, post-acute, and end-of-life care should be explored, again using mixed payment methods. Some package of hospice and palliative care services should be made available to nursing home residents while they are on the Medicare SNF post-acute care benefit.
- In the context of integrated care programs of all types, including MA programs, PACE, and ACO programs with risk-based payment such as the Medicare ACO demonstrations and the AQC, hospice and palliative care services should be included in the package of services for which these organizations are paid and held accountable.
  - Alternatives to carve-outs of hospice and palliative care services for individuals with advanced illness that ensure access to high-quality end-of-life and palliative care should be explored. Although prospects for implementation are unclear, MedPAC voted in January 2014 to recommend ending the hospice carve-out within the MA program.
  - Policy makers should ensure that these programs have adequate provider networks for patients (e.g., including access to palliative care specialists) and that they provide high-quality care to patients.

- Nursing homes should be held accountable for the quality of end-of-life care provided for all residents, including both those who do and do not use hospice. To support such expectations, nursing home survey processes, public reporting efforts such as Nursing Home Compare, and P4P efforts should incorporate performance measures appropriate for patients with advanced illness. In particular, the Nursing Home Compare tool could implement such improvements in the near term to ensure that its focus is not exclusively on restoration and maintenance of functioning.
- Changes in Medicare hospice benefit payment authorized by the ACA and implemented by the Secretary of Health and Human Services should attempt to match expected costs and payments for different types of hospice stays while ensuring access to high-quality end-of-life care for all beneficiaries with advanced illness, including those with high-cost palliative care needs. The impact of such changes on both expenditures and quality of care should be monitored on an ongoing basis.

REFERENCES

Adelson, J. 2012. Louisiana cuts health care, Medicaid and hospice programs to rebalance budget. *The Times-Picayune*, December 14, 2012. http://www.nola.com/politics/index.ssf/2012/12/louisiana_cuts_health_care_med.html (accessed December 18, 2014).

Adelson, J. 2013. Gov. Bobby Jindal backs down on Medicaid hospice elimination. *The Times-Picayune*, January 23, 2013. http://www.nola.com/politics/index.ssf/2013/01/gov_bobby_jindal_backs_down_on.html (accessed December 30, 2014).

Afendulis, C. C., M. B. Landrum, and M. E. Chernew. 2012. The impact of the Affordable Care Act on Medicare Advantage Plan availability and enrollment. *Health Services Research* 47(6):2339-2352.

Aldridge Carlson, M. D., C. L. Barry, E. J. Cherlin, R. McCorkle, and E. H. Bradley. 2012. Hospices' enrollment policies may contribute to underuse of hospice care in the United States. *Health Affairs (Millwood)* 31:2690-2698.

Aragon, K., K. Covinsky, Y. Miao, W. J. Boscardin, L. Flint, and A. K. Smith. 2012. Use of the Medicare posthospitalization skilled nursing benefit in the last 6 months of life. *Archives of Internal Medicine* 172:1573-1579.

Architecture for Humanity. 2012. *Design like you give a damn [2]: Building change from the ground up*. New York: Abrams Books.

Barnato, A. E., M. B. McClellan, C. R. Kagay, and A. M. Garber. 2004. Trends in inpatient treatment intensity among Medicare beneficiaries at the end of life. *Health Services Research* 39:363-375.

BCBSMA (Blue Cross Blue Shield of Massachusetts). 2010. *The Alternative Quality Contract*. http://www.bluecrossma.com/visitor/pdf/alternative-quality-contract.pdf (accessed July 28, 2014).

Bradley, E. H., H. Prigerson, M. D. Carlson, E. Cherlin, R. Johnson-Hurzeler, and S. V. Kasl. 2004. Depression among surviving caregivers: Does length of hospice enrollment matter? *American Journal of Psychiatry* 161:2257-2262.

Cao, X. Y., X. L. Jiang, X. L. Li, M. C. Hu Lo, and R. Li. 2013. Family functioning and its predictors among disaster bereaved individuals in China: Eighteen months after the Wenchuan earthquake. *PLoS ONE* 8(4):e60738.

CAPC (Center to Advance Palliative Care). 2009. *Making the case for hospital-based palliative care.* 2009. http://www.capc.org/building-a-hospital-based-palliative-care-program/case (accessed September 19, 2013).

CAPC. 2010. *Analysis of U.S. hospital palliative care programs: 2010 snapshot.* http://www.capc.org/news-and-events/releases/analysis-of-us-hospital-palliative-care-programs-2010-snapshot.pdf (accessed July 28, 2014).

Carlson, M. D., C. Barry, M. Schlesinger, R. McCorkle, R. S. Morrison, E. Cherlin, J. Herrin, J. Thompson, M. L. Twaddle, and E. H. Bradley. 2011. Quality of palliative care at US hospices: Results of a national survey. *Medical Care* 49:803-809.

Carter, C., A. B. Garrett, and D. Wissoker. 2012. Reforming Medicare payments to skilled nursing facilities to cut incentives for unneeded care and avoiding high-cost patients. *Health Affairs (Millwood)* 31:1303-1313.

Chambers, J. D., D. E. Weiner, S. K. Bliss, and P. J. Neumann. 2013. What can we learn from the U.S. expanded end-stage renal disease bundle? *Health Policy* 110:164-171.

Christakis, N. A., and E. B. Lamont. 2000. Extent and determinants of error in doctors' prognoses in terminally ill patients: Prospective cohort study. *British Medical Journal* 320:469-472.

CMS (Centers for Medicare & Medicaid Services). 2012. *Pioneer Accountable Care Organization Model: General fact sheet.* http://innovation.cms.gov/Files/fact-sheet/Pioneer-ACO-General-Fact-Sheet.pdf (accessed July 28, 2014).

CMS. 2013a. *Bundled Payments for Care Improvement (BPCI) initiative: General information.* http://innovation.cms.gov/initiatives/bundled-payments (accessed September 9, 2013).

CMS. 2013b. *Financial alignment initiative.* http://www.cms.gov/Medicare-Medicaid-Coordination/Medicare-and-Medicaid-Coordination/Medicare-Medicaid-Coordination-Office/FinancialModelstoSupportStatesEffortsinCareCoordination.html (accessed September 19, 2013).

CMS. 2013c. *Medicare-Medicaid enrollee state profiles.* http://www.cms.gov/Medicare-Medicaid-Coordination/Medicare-and-Medicaid-Coordination/Medicare-Medicaid-Coordination-Office/StateProfiles.html (accessed November 5, 2013).

CMS. 2013d. *Memorandum of understanding between the Centers for Medicare & Medicaid Services (CMS) and the state of South Carolina.* https://www.cms.gov/Medicare-Medicaid-Coordination/Medicare-and-Medicaid-Coordination/Medicare-Medicaid-Coordination-Office/Downloads/SCMOU.pdf (accessed July 25, 2014).

CMS. 2013e. *Pioneer Accountable Care Organizations succeed in improving care, lowering costs.* http://www.cms.gov/Newsroom/MediaReleaseDatabase/Press-Releases/2013-Press-Releases-Items/2013-07-16.html (accessed February 10, 2014).

CMS. 2014a. *Fact sheet: Medicare Care Choices Model.* http://www.cms.gov/Newsroom/MediaReleaseDatabase/Fact-sheets/2014-Fact-sheets-items/2014-03-18.html (accessed March 25, 2014).

CMS. 2014b. *Medicare Care Choices Model.* http://innovation.cms.gov/initiatives/Medicare-Care-Choices (accessed March 25, 2014).

CMS. 2014c. *Medicare's delivery system reform initiatives achieve significant savings and quality improvements—off to a strong start.* Press release. http://www.cms.gov/Newsroom/MediaReleaseDatabase/Press-Releases/2014-Press-releases-items/2014-01-30.html (accessed February 10, 2014).

Colla, C. H., D. E. Wennberg, E. Meara, J. S. Skinner, D. Gottlieb, V. A. Lewis, C. M. Snyder, and E. S. Fisher. 2012. Spending differences associated with the Medicare Physician Group Practice Demonstration. *Journal of the American Medical Association* 308:1015-1023.

Collins, A. J. 2012. *ESRD payment policy changes: The new "bundled" dialysis prospective payment system (PPS) in the United States.* National Kidney Foundation Spring Clinical Meeting, Washington, DC.

Cutler, D. M., and K. Ghosh. 2012. The potential for cost savings through bundled episode payments. *New England Journal of Medicine* 366:1075-1077.

Famakinwa, A. B. 2010. End-of-life care in a PACE program: Respecting the patient's wishes while supporting the caregiver. *Journal of the American Medical Directors Association* 11:528-530.

Feder, J. 2013. Bundle with care—rethinking Medicare incentives for post-acute care services. *New England Journal of Medicine* 369:400-401.

Fuller, D. S., R. L. Pisoni, B. A. Bieber, B. W. Gillespie, and B. M. Robinson. 2013. The DOPPS Practice Monitor for US dialysis care: Trends through December 2011. *American Journal of Kidney Diseases* 61:342-346.

Gilbertson, D., A. Collins, and R. Foley. 2012. *Transition in service utilization: Vascular access, injectables, hemoglobin levels, and transfusions.* Ann Arbor, MI: United States Renal Data System.

Goodman, D. C., A. R. Esty, E. S. Fisher, and C.-H. Chang. 2011. *Trends in variation in end-of-life care for Medicare beneficiaries with severe chronic illness.* Hanover, NH: The Dartmouth Institute for Health Policy and Clinical Practice.

Grabowski, D. C. 2007. Medicare and Medicaid: Conflicting incentives for long-term care. *Milbank Quarterly* 85:579-610.

Grabowski, D. C. 2009. Special needs plans and the coordination of benefits and services for dual eligibles. *Health Affairs (Millwood)* 28:136-146.

Hackbarth, G., R. Reischauer, and A. Mutti. 2008. Collective accountability for medical care—toward bundled Medicare payments. *New England Journal of Medicine* 359:3-5.

Health Care Financing Administration. 1998. *Medicare Participating Heart Bypass Center Demonstration.* https://www.cms.gov/Research-Statistics-Data-and-Systems/Statistics-Trends-and-Reports/Reports/downloads/oregon2_1998_3.pdf (accessed July 25, 2014).

HHS OIG (U.S. Department of Health and Human Services Office of Inspector General). 1997. *Hospice patients in nursing homes.* Washington, DC: HHS OIG.

HHS OIG. 2013. *Medicare hospice: Use of general inpatient care.* Washington, DC: HHS OIG.

Hoffmann, D. E., and A. J. Tarzian. 2005. Dying in America—an examination of policies that deter adequate end-of-life care in nursing homes. *The Journal of Law, Medicine & Ethics* 33:294-309.

Hogan, C., J. Lunney, J. Gabel, and J. Lynn. 2001. Medicare beneficiaries' costs of care in the last year of life. *Health Affairs (Millwood)* 20:188-195.

Huskamp, H. A., M. B. Buntin, V. Wang, and J. P. Newhouse. 2001. Providing care at the end of life: Do Medicare rules impede good care? *Health Affairs (Millwood)* 20:204-211.

Huskamp, H. A., J. P. Newhouse, J. C. Norcini, and N. L. Keating. 2008. Variation in patients' hospice costs. *Inquiry* 45:232-244.

Huskamp, H. A., D. G. Stevenson, M. E. Chernew, and J. P. Newhouse. 2010. A new Medicare end-of-life benefit for nursing home residents. *Health Affairs (Millwood)* 29:130-135.

Huskamp, H. A., C. Kaufmann, and D. G. Stevenson. 2012. The intersection of long-term care and end-of-life care. *Medical Care Research and Review* 69:3-44.

IOM (Institute of Medicine). 1997. *Approaching death: Improving care at the end of life.* Washington, DC: National Academy Press.

IOM. 2013. *Variation in health care spending: Target decision making, not geography.* Washington, DC: The National Academies Press.

Iwashyna, T. J., and N. A. Christakis. 1998. Attitude and self-reported practice regarding hospice referral in a national sample of internists. *Journal of Palliative Medicine* 1:241-248.

Kelley, A. S., S. L. Ettner, R. S. Morrison, Q. Du, and C. A. Sarkisian. 2012. Disability and decline in physical function associated with hospital use at end of life. *Journal of General Internal Medicine* 27:794-800.

Kelley, A. S., P. Deb, Q. Du, M. D. Aldridge Carlson, and R. S. Morrison. 2013a. Hospice enrollment saves money for Medicare and improves care quality across a number of different lengths-of-stay. *Health Affairs (Millwood)* 32:552-561.

Kelley, A. S., K. McGarry, S. Fahle, S. M. Marshall, Q. Du, and J. S. Skinner. 2013b. Out-of-pocket spending in the last five years of life. *Journal of General Internal Medicine* 28:304-309.

KFF (The Henry J. Kaiser Family Foundation). 2011. *Health insurance coverage of the total population.* http://kff.org/other/state-indicator/total-population (accessed July 25, 2014).

KFF. 2012a. *Explaining the state integrated care and financial alignment demonstrations for dual eligible beneficiaries.* Washington, DC: KFF.

KFF. 2012b. *State demonstrations to integrate care and align financing for dual eligible beneficiaries: A review of the 26 proposals submitted to CMS.* Washington, DC: KFF.

KFF. 2012c. *Total Medicare Advantage (MA) enrollment.* http://kff.org/other/state-indicator/ma-total-enrollment (accessed July 25, 2014).

KFF. 2012d. *Total number of Medicare beneficiaries.* http://kff.org/medicare/state-indicator/total-medicare-beneficiaries (accessed July 25, 2014).

Kirwan, L., and S. Iselin. 2009. *Recommendations of the Special Commission on the Health Care Payment System.* http://www.mass.gov/chia/docs/pc/final-report/final-report.pdf (accessed July 25, 2014).

Krakauer, R., C. M. Spettell, L. Reisman, and M. J. Wade. 2009. Opportunities to improve the quality of care for advanced illness. *Health Affairs (Millwood)* 28:1357-1359.

Kwok, A. C., M. E. Semel, S. R. Lipsitz, A. M Bader, A. E. Barnato, A. A. Gawande, and A. K. Jha. 2011. The intensity and variation of surgical care at the end of life: A retrospective cohort study. *Lancet* 378:1408-1413.

L&M Policy Research. 2014. *Effect of pioneer ACOs on Medicare spending in the first year.* Washington, DC: CMS.

Lave, J. R. 1989. The effect of the Medicare prospective payment system. *Annual Review of Public Health* 10:141-161.

Lindley, L. C., S. Edwards, and D. J. Bruce. 2013. Factors influencing the implementation of health care reform: An examination of the concurrent care for children provision. *American Journal of Hospice and Palliative Care* [epub ahead of print].

Lipsitz, L. A. 2013. The 3-night hospital stay and Medicare coverage for skilled nursing care. *Journal of the American Medical Association* 310(14):1441-1442.

Lorenz, K. A., S. M. Asch, K. E. Rosenfeld, H. Liu, and S. L. Ettner. 2004. Hospice admission practices: Where does hospice fit in the continuum of care? *Journal of the American Geriatrics Society* 52:725-730.

Lubitz, J. D., and G. F. Riley. 1993. Trends in Medicare payments in the last year of life. *New England Journal of Medicine* 328:1092-1096.

McCarthy, E. P., R. B. Burns, Q. Ngo-Metzger, R. B. Davis, and R. S. Phillips. 2003. Hospice use among Medicare managed care and fee-for-service patients dying with cancer. *Journal of the American Medical Association* 289:2238-2245.

MedPAC (Medicare Payment Advisory Commission). 2009. *Medicare payment policy.* Washington, DC: MedPAC.

MedPAC. 2012. *Report to the Congress: Medicare payment policy.* Washington, DC: MedPAC.

MedPAC. 2013. *Medicare payment policy.* Washington, DC: MedPAC.

Meier, D. E. 2013. *Palliative care and the health care crisis in the United States: A candid conversation with Dr. Diane Meier.* Syracuse, NY: Syracuse University Maxwell School of Citizenship and Public Affairs.

Miller, S. C. 2004. Hospice care in nursing homes: Is site of care associated with visit volume? *Journal of the American Geriatrics Society* 52:1331-1336.

Miller, S. C., J. C. Lima, and S. L. Mitchell. 2012. Influence of hospice on nursing home residents with advanced dementia who received Medicare-skilled nursing facility care near the end of life. *Journal of the American Geriatrics Society* 60:2035-2041.

Minino, A. M. 2013. *Death in the United States, 2011.* Washington, DC: Centers for Disease Control and Prevention.

Morrison, R. S., J. D. Penrod, J. B. Cassel, M. Caust-Ellenbogen, A. Litke, L. Spragens, and D. E. Meier. 2008. Cost savings associated with US hospital palliative care consultation programs. *Archives of Internal Medicine* 168:1783-1790.

Mukamel, D. B., A. Bajorska, and H. Temkin-Greener. 2002. Health care services utilization at the end of life in a managed care program integrating acute and long-term care. *Medical Care* 40:1136-1148.

Mukamel, D. B., D. R. Peterson, H. Temkin-Greener, R. Delavan, D. Gross, S. J. Kunitz, and T. F. Williams. 2007. Program characteristics and enrollees' outcomes in the Program of All-Inclusive Care for the Elderly (PACE). *Milbank Quarterly* 85:499-531.

Mullen, K. J., R. G. Frank, and M. B. Rosenthal. 2010. Can you get what you pay for? Pay-for-performance and the quality of healthcare providers. *The RAND Journal of Economics* 41:64-91.

Newhouse, J. P. 1994. Patients at risk: Health reform and risk adjustment. *Health Affairs (Millwood)* 13:132-146.

NQF (National Quality Forum). 2012. *NQF endorses palliative and end-of-life care measures.* http://www.qualityforum.org/News_And_Resources/Press_Releases/2012/NQF_Endorses_Palliative_and_End-of-Life_Care_Measures.aspx (accessed July 25, 2014).

Riley, G. F., and C. Herboldsheimer. 2001. Including hospice in Medicare capitation payments: Would it save money? *Health Care Financing Review* 23:137-147.

Riley, G. F., and J. D. Lubitz. 2010. Long-term trends in Medicare payments in the last year of life. *Health Services Research* 45:565-576.

Sachs, G. A., J. W. Shega, and D. Cox-Hayley. 2004. Barriers to excellent end-of-life care for patients with dementia. *Journal of General Internal Medicine* 19:1057-1063.

Schroeder, S. A., and Frist, W. 2013. Phasing out fee-for-service payment. *New England Journal of Medicine* 368:2029-2032.

Scitovsky, A. A. 1984. "The high cost of dying": What do the data show? *Milbank Memorial Fund Quarterly: Health and Society* 62:591-608.

Segal, M. 2011. *Dual eligible beneficiaries and potentially avoidable hospitalizations.* https://www.cms.gov/Research-Statistics-Data-and-Systems/Statistics-Trends-and-Reports/Insight-Briefs/downloads/PAHInsightBrief.pdf (accessed July 25, 2014).

Song, Z., D. G. Safran, B. E. Landon, Y. He, R. P. Ellis, R. E. Mechanic, M. P. Day, and M. E. Chernew. 2011. Health care spending and quality in year 1 of the alternative quality contract. *New England Journal of Medicine* 365:909-918.

Song, Z., D. G. Safran, B. E. Landon, M. B. Landrum, Y. He, R. E. Mechanic, M. P. Day, and M. E. Chernew. 2012. The "Alternative Quality Contract," based on a global budget, lowered medical spending and improved quality. *Health Affairs (Millwood)* 31:1885-1894.

Sood, N., P. J. Huckfeldt, J. J. Escarce, D. C. Grabowski, and J. P. Newhouse. 2011. Medicare's bundled payment pilot for acute and postacute care: Analysis and recommendations on where to begin. *Health Affairs (Millwood)* 30:1708-1717.

Spettell, C. M., W. S. Rawlins, R. Krakauer, J. Fernandes, M. E. Breton, W. Gowdy, S. Brodeur, M. MacCoy, and T. A. Brennan. 2009. A comprehensive case management program to improve palliative care. *Journal of Palliative Medicine* 12:827-832.

Stevenson, D. G., J. Z. Ayanian, A. M. Zaslavsky, J. P. Newhouse, and B. E. Landon. 2013. Service use at the end of life in Medicare advantage versus traditional Medicare. *Medical Care* 51(10):931-937.

Taylor, D. H., Jr., J. Ostermann, C. H. Van Houtven, J. A. Tulsky, and K. Steinhauser. 2007. What length of hospice use maximizes reduction in medical expenditures near death in the US Medicare program? *Social Science & Medicine* 65:1466-1478.

Temel, J. S., J. A. Greer, A. Muzikansky, E. R. Gallagher, S. Admane, V. A. Jackson, C. M. Dahlin, C. D. Blinderman, J. Jacobsen, W. F. Pirl, J. A. Billings, and T. J. Lynch. 2010. Early palliative care for patients with metastatic non-small-cell lung cancer. *New England Journal of Medicine* 363:733-742.

Teno, J. M., P. L. Gozalo, J. P. Bynum, N. E. Leland, S. C. Miller, N. E. Morden, T. Scupp, D. C. Goodman, and V. Mor. 2013. Change in end-of-life care for Medicare beneficiaries: Site of death, place of care, and health care transitions in 2000, 2005, and 2009. *Journal of the American Medical Association* 309:470-477.

Toussaint, J., A. Milstein, and S. Shortell. 2013. How the Pioneer ACO Model needs to change: Lessons from its best-performing ACO. *Journal of the American Medical Association* 310:1341-1342.

U.S. Senate Commission on Long-Term Care. 2013. *Commission on Long-Term Care: Report to the Congress*. Washington, DC: U.S. Senate Commission on Long-Term Care.

Virnig, B. A., E. S. Fisher, A. M. McBean, and S. Kind. 2001. Hospice use in Medicare managed care and fee-for-service systems. *American Journal of Managed Care* 7:777-786.

Weeks, W. B., S. S. Rauh, E. B. Wadsworth, and J. N. Weinstein. 2013. The unintended consequences of bundled payments. *Annals of Internal Medicine* 158:62-64.

Werner, R. M., R. T. Konetzka, and D. Polsky. 2013. The effect of pay-for-performance in nursing homes: Evidence from state Medicaid programs. *Health Services Research* 48:1393-1414.

Wilensky, G. R. 2011. Lessons from the Physician Group Practice Demonstration—a sobering reflection. *New England Journal of Medicine* 365:1659-1661.

Zerzan, J., S. Stearns, and L. Hanson. 2000. Access to palliative care and hospice in nursing homes. *Journal of the American Medical Association* 284:2489-2494.

Appendix E

Epidemiology of Serious Illness and High Utilization of Health Care

Melissa D. Aldridge, Ph.D., M.B.A.

Amy S. Kelley, M.D., M.S.H.S.

Prior to the adoption and implementation of programs aimed at reducing health care costs while providing high-quality care for patients, it is critical to have a comprehensive sense of the drivers of health care costs and the variability across different populations in annual health care spending. Health care reform debate in the United States is focused largely on the highly concentrated health care costs among a small proportion of the population and policy proposals to identify and target this "high-cost" group. The objective of this appendix is to characterize the population of individuals with the highest total health care costs using analyses of existing national datasets, peer-reviewed literature, and published reports. One of the greatest gaps in terms of the research we reviewed for this appendix is the lack of evidence regarding the impact of interventions or models of care on total health care costs. Most of the analyses we reviewed focused on only one payor—generally Medicare. Although such studies are informative, the focus on Medicare costs alone has led to the misperception that older adults and those at the end of life are the primary drivers of health care costs, and yet when one evaluates total health care costs, as we do in this appendix, that perception is not supported by the evidence.

We synthesize and augment existing evidence regarding individuals with high health care costs and describe this group in terms of demographics, clinical characteristics, and patterns of health care use. Based on existing evidence, we focus on individuals with chronic conditions and functional limitations. We then examine the costs and intensity of care for individuals at the end of life and present new findings regarding the overlap between the high-cost and end-of-life populations. We present results of our analyses identifying three patterns within the high-cost group: individuals who experience a discrete high-cost event in one year but who return to normal health and lower costs; individuals who persistently generate high annual health care costs due to chronic conditions, functional limitations, or other conditions; and individuals who have high health care costs because it is their last year of life. We conclude with a discussion of existing models of care that target high-cost populations and of future research to improve understanding of the population with highest health care costs. A critical next step in research is to evaluate the impact of various interventions on reducing total health care costs so that programs and policies implemented across the health care system truly reduce total costs rather than merely shifting costs from payor to payor.

CHARACTERIZING THE POPULATION WITH THE HIGHEST HEALTH CARE COSTS

Distribution and Trends in Total Health Care Costs

In 2011, the United States spent $2.7 trillion on health care, more than double what was spent in 2000 (CMS, 2014). It is projected that by 2040, 1 of every 3 dollars spent in the United States will be spent on health care (CBO, 2007; Emanuel, 2012). In evaluating these estimates and their relevance to health policy reform, however, it is important to understand the definition of health care costs that is used to calculate these estimates. The National Health Expenditure estimates (CMS, 2014) published annually by the Centers for Medicare & Medicaid Services (the source of the $2.7 trillion estimate for 2011) include a number of expenditure categories unrelated to direct patient care (see Figure E-1). Specifically, they include expenditures for government administration of health care programs; federal public health initiatives; investments in health care research, structures, and equipment; and non–patient care revenue, including revenue from gift shops and hospital cafeterias. Our analysis in this appendix focuses exclusively on the $1.6 trillion of patient care–related expenditures (shown in Figure E-1), with the goal of identifying policy solutions for addressing costs specifically related to patient care.

Health care reform debates that focus on health care costs generally fall into three major categories: (1) discussion of high total health care costs and reform proposals targeting how to decrease total costs, (2) discussion of the growth in health care costs over the past decade and reform proposals aimed at how to "bend" the cost curve, and (3) discussion of the highly concentrated health care costs among a small proportion of the population and policy proposals for identifying this "high-cost" group and significantly reducing their costs. The focus of this section of this appendix is on this

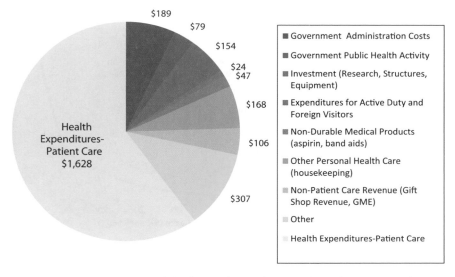

FIGURE E-1 Components of the $2.7 trillion of national health care expenditures, 2011.

NOTES: Expenditures are in billions of dollars; expenditure components were estimated based on the Centers for Medicare & Medicaid Services 2011 National Health Expenditure report (CMS, 2014), with adjustments based on estimates from Sing and colleagues (2006) and the 2011 Medical Expenditure Panel Survey data (AHRQ and HHS, 2011). GME = graduate medical education.

third category—characterizing the subpopulation with the highest health care costs.

The distribution of health care costs for the U.S. population consistently exhibits a significant "tail" segment of the population with extremely high costs. As of 2011, the top 5 percent of health care spenders (18.2 million people) accounted for an estimated 60 percent of all health care costs ($976 billion) (see Figure E-2). In this high-cost subgroup, total annual costs ranged from approximately $17,500 to more than $2,000,000 per person based on our analyses of the 2011 Medical Expenditure Panel Survey (MEPS) data (AHRQ and HHS, 2011), adjusted to include the nursing home population (National Center for Health Statistics, 2013).

Population with the Highest Health Care Costs

In an attempt to design policy solutions that target those individuals with exceptionally high health care costs, it is critical to understand the

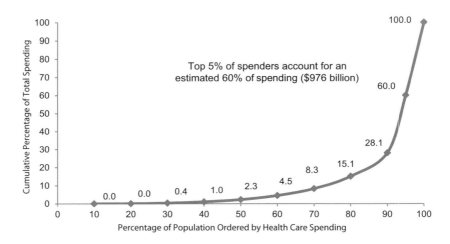

FIGURE E-2 Cumulative distribution of personal health care spending, 2011.
SOURCE: Total population and health care costs were obtained from the 2011 Medical Expenditure Panel Survey data (AHRQ and HHS, 2011), adjusted to include the nursing home population (National Center for Health Statistics, 2013). The entire nursing home population is estimated to be in the top 5 percent of total health care spending (see the section below on the nursing home population for details).

characteristics that define this population and thus potentially how and why they incur such high costs. Using our own analyses of the 2011 MEPS data combined with cost and population estimates for the nursing home population, we present findings regarding this high-cost population in terms of clinical characteristics and demographics.

The MEPS is a set of large-scale surveys of families and individuals, their medical providers (for example, doctors, hospitals, pharmacies), and employers across the United States (AHRQ and HHS, 2011). The households included in the survey are drawn from a nationally representative subsample of households. The MEPS collects data on the specific health services that Americans use, how frequently they use them, the cost of these services, and how they are paid for, as well as data on the cost, scope, and breadth of health insurance held by and available to U.S. workers.

The MEPS is considered the most complete source of data on the cost and use of health care and health insurance coverage for the U.S. population. The MEPS sample, however, does not include the population of individuals residing in nursing homes, and therefore we augmented our analyses of the MEPS data with estimates of the nursing home population sourced from the National Health Expenditure Accounts (CMS, 2014) and the Centers for Disease Control and Prevention (CDC) (Jones et al., 2009; National Center for Health Statistics, 2013; Sing et al., 2006).

To reiterate, unlike the National Health Expenditure estimate of $2.7 trillion of total costs—which includes expenditures for government administration of health care programs; federal public health initiatives; investments in health care research, structures, and equipment; and non–patient care revenue—our analyses in this section focus on the $1.6 trillion total costs for patient health care services.

Chronic Conditions and Functional Limitations

A substantial and growing body of work suggests that a key factor distinguishing individuals with the highest health care costs is the existence of both chronic conditions and functional limitations. Analyses of data on chronic conditions and health care costs have found that, of the population with the highest health care costs, greater than 75 percent have one or more of seven chronic conditions, including 42 percent with coronary artery disease, 30 percent with congestive heart failure, and 30 percent with diabetes (Emanuel, 2012). The U.S. Department of Health and Human Services (HHS) launched an initiative to both prevent and better manage care for multiple chronic conditions given their high prevalence and high associated health care costs. HHS reports that more than 25 percent of individuals in the United States have multiple chronic conditions, and the care of these individuals accounts for 66 percent of total health care spending (HHS, 2014). An analysis of U.S. health care spending recently reported in the *Journal of the American Medical Association* finds that chronic illnesses account for 84 percent of total health care costs (Moses et al., 2013).

A report to HHS by The Lewin Group (2010) takes this research a step further and evaluates the combination of chronic conditions and functional limitations as a way to identify the subgroup with the highest health care costs within the population with chronic conditions. This report concludes that the combination of chronic conditions and functional limitations is a better predictor of high health care costs than the number of chronic conditions alone. It finds that although nearly one-half of people living in the community have at least one chronic condition, fewer than one-third of those with chronic conditions have any functional limitation. Thus, the combination better pinpoints those with the greatest demand for health care and supportive services.

Throughout this analysis, we define a chronic condition as one that lasts or is expected to last 12 months or longer and either places limitations on normal function or requires ongoing care (The Lewin Group, 2010). A functional limitation is defined as having limitation in at least one of the following: physical activity (for example, walking, bending, stooping);

TABLE E-1 Population and Health Care Costs by Existence of Chronic Conditions and Functional Limitations

	No. of People	%	Health Care Costs	%
Total Population	312,514,999		$1,627,372,719,765	
No chronic conditions or functional limitations	149,340,364	48	186,301,532,393	11
Chronic conditions only	112,005,273	36	505,675,587,925	31
Functional limitations only	6,222,515	2	26,614,504,628	2
Chronic conditions and functional limitations	44,946,847	14	908,781,094,819	56

SOURCE: The percentage distribution of population and costs by chronic condition/functional limitation category was obtained from The Lewin Group (2010); total population and health care costs were obtained from the 2011 Medical Expenditure Panel Survey data (AHRQ and HHS, 2011), adjusted to include the nursing home population (CMS, 2014; National Center for Health Statistics, 2013; Sing et al., 2006).

normal life activity (for example, work, housework, school); an activity of daily living (ADL); or an instrumental activity of daily living (IADL) (The Lewin Group, 2010).

The impact of the combination of chronic conditions and functional limitations on health care costs is shown in Table E-1. Of the $1.6 trillion spent on health care in 2011, 56 percent ($909 billion) was for the 14 percent of the population who suffered from both chronic conditions and functional limitations. The second highest category of health care spenders was those with chronic conditions only. This population incurred 31 percent ($506 billion) of total costs and made up 36 percent of the population. *It is clear from these analyses that although the presence of chronic conditions is a key driver of health care costs, the addition of functional limitations appears to differentiate a high-cost group within those with chronic conditions.*

Consistent with the distribution of health care costs by chronic conditions and functional limitations shown in Table E-1, the population with both chronic conditions and functional limitations is disproportionately represented in the top 5 percent of health care spenders. Figure E-3 shows that those with both chronic conditions and functional limitations make up 72 percent of the top 5 percent of health care spenders while making up only 12 percent of the rest of the population. Not surprisingly, 50 percent of the lower-spending population has no chronic conditions or functional limitations, while only 5 percent of the high-cost population has neither of these characteristics.

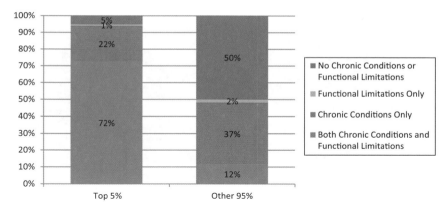

FIGURE E-3 Total health care costs for the top 5 percent and other 95 percent of spenders by existence of chronic conditions and functional limitations.
SOURCE: The percentage distribution of costs by chronic condition/functional limitation category and top 5%/other 95% categories was obtained from the National Institute for Health Care Management (NIHCM) Foundation (2012) analysis of 2009 Medical Expenditure Panel Survey data; these percentages were applied to health care costs from the 2011 Medical Expenditure Panel Survey data (AHRQ and HHS, 2011), adjusted to include the nursing home population (CMS, 2014; National Center for Health Statistics, 2013; Sing et al., 2006).

The combination of chronic conditions and functional limitations may be associated with higher health care costs for many reasons. The association may relate to the complexity of care coordination across multiple providers and settings, including duplication of test and procedures. It may also relate to increased use of specialists or increased likelihood of being hospitalized. A recent commentary in the *Journal of the American Medical Association* (Emanuel, 2012) suggests that an estimated 22 percent of health care expenditures are related to potentially avoidable complications, such as hospital admission for patients with diabetes with ketoacidosis or amputation of gangrenous limbs, or for patients with congestive heart failure for shortness of breath due to fluid overload (de Brantes et al., 2009; Emanuel, 2012). Reducing these potentially avoidable complications by only 10 percent would save more than $40 billion/year (Emanuel, 2012). Furthermore, the disproportionally higher costs for this group may reflect a lack of adequate community-based care and supportive services for those with functional limitations, which leaves patients with no alternative but to access the acute care hospital system by calling 911 or presenting to the emergency department.

Total Population, By Age

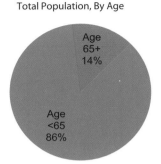

High-Cost Population, By Age

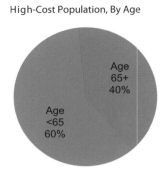

FIGURE E-4 Proportion of the total and high-cost populations by age.
SOURCE: 2011 Medical Expenditure Panel Survey data (AHRQ and HHS, 2011),
adjusted to include the nursing home population (CMS, 2012, 2014; National
Center for Health Statistics, 2013).

Age and Health Care Costs

Our analyses of the association between older age and higher health
care costs suggests that although individuals aged 65 and over are disproportionately in the top 5 percent of the population in terms of total health
care spending (see Figure E-4), almost two-thirds of the top 5 percent
spenders are younger than age 65. *Although older age may be a risk factor for higher health care costs, older adults make up the minority of the
high-cost spenders.* Furthermore, the proportion of total annual health care
spending for the population aged 65 or over (32 percent) has not changed
in a decade despite the growth in the size of that population (AHRQ and
HHS, 2011).

The pattern we have highlighted of individuals with both chronic
conditions and functional limitations generating disproportionately higher
health care costs is evident in both the population under age 65 and those
aged 65 and older (see Table E-2). *Specifically, those with chronic conditions and functional limitations in both groups incur more than 20 percent
of the nation's total annual health care expenditures (and together account
for more than half of total spending), yet each group makes up less than
10 percent of the total population.*

Race and Health Care Costs

The proportion of individuals who are nonwhite in the top 5 percent
of spenders compared with the bottom 95 percent is approximately the

TABLE E-2 Health Care Costs by Age, Chronic Conditions, and Functional Limitations

	Percentage of Population	Percentage of Health Care Costs
Age: Below 65		
No chronic conditions or functional limitations	46.2	11.5
Chronic conditions only	30.0	24.5
Functional limitations only	1.7	1.1
Chronic conditions and functional limitations	7.8	22.0
Age: 65 and Older		
No chronic conditions or functional limitations	1.1	0.4
Chronic conditions only	5.9	6.9
Functional limitations only	0.3	0.4
Chronic conditions and functional limitations	7.1	33.4

SOURCE: The percent distribution of population and costs by age and chronic condition/functional limitation category was obtained from The Lewin Group (2010); total population and health care costs were obtained from the 2011 Medical Expenditure Panel Survey data (AHRQ and HHS, 2011), adjusted to include the nursing home population (CMS, 2012, 2014; National Center for Health Statistics, 2013; Sing et al., 2006).

same (14.1 percent versus 20.5 percent) (see Figure E-5). The only notable difference is that the Asian population makes up only 2.0 percent of the top spenders and 5.2 percent of the lower spenders. Similarly, our analysis of the population with the top 5 percent of health care costs by both age and race (see Figure E-6) demonstrates that minority populations do not appear to account for a differential proportion of health care costs by age.

There is significant variation by race in terms of per person costs and payor (see Table E-3). The non-Hispanic white population has almost double the median per person cost of the non-Hispanic black population ($1,660 versus $878). For all races, private insurance is the largest payor. For the non-Hispanic white population, the proportion paid by private insurance is almost half, and the proportion paid by Medicaid is less than 10 percent. In contrast, for the non-Hispanic black and Hispanic populations, the proportion paid by private insurance is approximately one-third, and the proportion paid by Medicaid is roughly one-quarter.

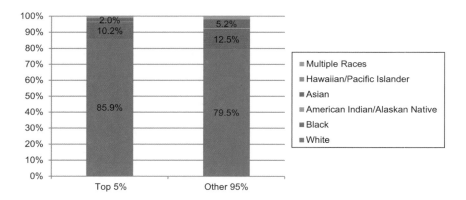

FIGURE E-5 Proportion of the top 5 percent and other 95 percent of spenders by race.
SOURCE: 2011 Medical Expenditure Panel Survey data (AHRQ and HHS, 2011), adjusted to include the nursing home population (CMS, 2014; Jones et al., 2009; National Center for Health Statistics, 2013; Sing et al., 2006).

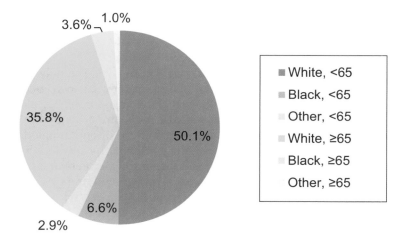

FIGURE E-6 Proportion of the high-cost population by age and race.
SOURCE: 2011 Medical Expenditure Panel Survey data (AHRQ and HHS, 2011), adjusted to include the nursing home population (CMS, 2014; Jones et al., 2009; National Center for Health Statistics, 2013; Sing et al., 2006).

TABLE E-3 Proportion of Health Care Costs by Race and Payor

Race/Ethnicity	Population (1,000s)	Per Person Cost		Total Cost (in millions)	Percentage by Payor				
		Median	Mean		OOP	Private	Medicare	Medicaid	Other
White, NH	198,127	1,660	5,604	991,244	14.9	46.7	25.9	6.0	6.5
Black, NH	37,322	878	4,677	138,138	8.8	31.2	23.6	24.6	11.8
Hispanic	52,717	637	3,289	126,189	13.0	34.5	19.1	23.1	10.3
Asian/ Hawaiian/PI, NH	16,814	792	4,355	56,675	11.2	37.8	14.1	31.0	6.0
AI/AK Native/ Multi, NH	6,146	1,157	3,430	18,479	15.1	36.1	15.4	18.1	15.4

NOTES: This table does not include the nursing home population. AI = American Indian; AK = Alaska; NH = non-Hispanic; OOP = out of pocket; PI = Pacific Islander.

SOURCE: 2011 Medical Expenditure Panel Survey data (AHRQ and HHS, 2011).

Health Care Costs by Payor

There has been very little change in the share of total health care costs paid by major payors in the past decade. In both 2000 and 2011, approximately 40 percent of all health care costs were paid by private insurance, followed by approximately 24 percent paid by Medicare (see Figure E-7). A slightly smaller share of health care costs was paid out of pocket by patients in 2011 (13.9 percent) compared with 2000 (19.4 percent). For the 5 percent of people with the highest health care costs in 2011, a similar proportion of their costs was paid by private insurance and Medicaid compared with the proportion of total costs for 2011, but a larger share (31.4 percent) of the costs of the high-cost population was paid for by Medicare, and a lower share (6.6 percent) was paid out of pocket by patients (see Figure E-7).

Not surprisingly, payor distribution differs by age because most people enroll in Medicare at age 65. The primary difference in payor by age group is a shift from private insurance as payor for those younger than 65 to Medicare as payor for those 65 and older (see Figure E-8).

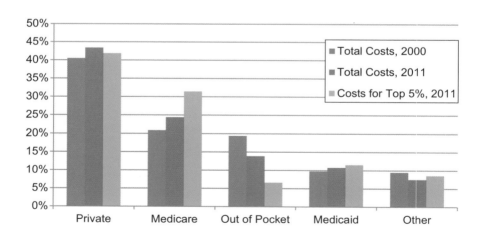

FIGURE E-7 Proportion of health care costs by payor, 2000 and 2011.
NOTE: This figure does not include the nursing home population because data on this population for 2000 were not available.
SOURCE: 2011 Medical Expenditure Panel Survey data (AHRQ and HHS, 2011).

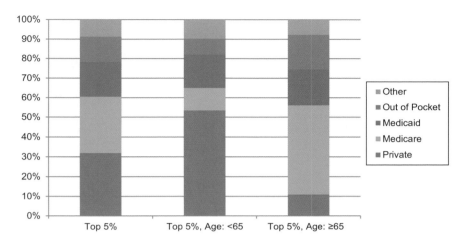

FIGURE E-8 Proportion of health care costs by payor for those younger than 65 and 65 and older.
SOURCE: 2011 Medical Expenditure Panel Survey data (AHRQ and HHS, 2011), adjusted to include the nursing home population (CMS, 2012, 2014; National Center for Health Statistics, 2013; Sing et al., 2006); payor data for the nursing home population were obtained from Moses et al. (2013) and assumed to be the same for the younger than 65 and 65 and older nursing home populations.

Epidemiology of Chronic Conditions

Overall, individuals aged 65 and older have a higher prevalence of chronic conditions and functional limitations (48 percent) compared with those younger than 65 (9 percent). Because of the large size of the population younger than 65, however, that population has a greater absolute number of individuals with chronic conditions and functional limitations (24 million, as compared with 22 million aged 65 or older).

For community-dwelling individuals with both chronic conditions and functional limitations, the most prevalent chronic conditions are hypertension, lipid metabolism disorder, arthritis disorders, and depressive disorders (The Lewin Group, 2010). The chronic conditions of allergies, chronic sinusitis, and asthma are more frequent among those with chronic conditions only than among those with both chronic conditions and functional limitations (The Lewin Group, 2010).

To best understand groups of chronic conditions, CDC has used the National Health Interview Survey to report the most common chronic condition triads among civilian, noninstitutionalized U.S. adults with at least three chronic conditions (Ward and Schiller, 2013) (see Table E-4).

TABLE E-4 Most Prevalent Chronic Condition Triads Among U.S. Adults, 2010

Sex, Age, and Triad	% (95% Confidence Interval)
Men	
Ages 18-44	
Arthritis/diabetes/hypertension	26.1 (16.70-38.45)
Asthma/diabetes/hypertension	15.5 (7.73-28.73)
Arthritis/asthma/hypertension	14.6 (7.17-27.31)
Arthritis/COPD/hypertension	12.2 (6.47-21.79)
Arthritis/CHD/hypertension	7.3 (3.23-15.83)
Ages 45-64	
Arthritis/diabetes/hypertension	28.3 (24.34-32.66)
Arthritis/CHD/hypertension	17.9 (14.52-21.86)
CHD/diabetes/hypertension	14.5 (11.37-18.22)
Arthritis/cancer/hypertension	11.2 (8.61-14.53)
Arthritis/asthma/hypertension	10.6 (8.03-13.91)
Ages ≥65	
Arthritis/diabetes/hypertension	28.2 (24.67-32.06)
Arthritis/cancer/hypertension	27.5 (23.97-31.31)
Arthritis/CHD/hypertension	27.2 (23.43-31.26)
CHD/diabetes/hypertension	17.8 (14.66-21.48)
Cancer/CHD/hypertension	14.6 (11.82-18.01)
Women	
Ages 18-44	
Arthritis/asthma/COPD	24.7 (17.68-33.50)
Arthritis/asthma/hypertension	21.3 (15.09-29.09)
Asthma/COPD/hypertension	19.8 (13.64-27.89)
Arthritis/COPD/hypertension	19.7 (13.82-27.32)
Arthritis/diabetes/hypertension	14.4 (9.65-21.03)
Ages 45-64	
Arthritis/diabetes/hypertension	30.5 (27.24-34.02)
Arthritis/asthma/hypertension	22.0 (19.00-25.35)
Arthritis/COPD/hypertension	18.4 (15.59-21.52)
Arthritis/cancer/hypertension	16.7 (13.80-20.09)
Arthritis/asthma/COPD	14.4 (12.08-17.16)
Ages ≥65	
Arthritis/diabetes/hypertension	32.6 (29.36-35.95)
Arthritis/cancer/hypertension	26.9 (23.95-30.13)
Arthritis/CHD/hypertension	19.3 (16.44-22.41)
Arthritis/COPD/hypertension	16.8 (14.19-19.84)
Arthritis/asthma/hypertension	16.5 (13.95-19.38)

NOTES: This table does not include the nursing home population. CHD = coronary heart disease; COPD = chronic obstructive pulmonary disease.
SOURCE: CDC, National Health Interview Survey, 2010 (Ward and Schiller, 2013).

The most prevalent triads of conditions were found to vary by both gender and age.

The Nursing Home Population

We estimate that in 2011, total health care costs related to residents of nursing facilities and continuing care retirement communities accounted for $296 billion, or 11 percent of the $2.7 trillion in total national health care expenditures and 18 percent of the $1.6 trillion in patient care–related expenditures analyzed in this report. This estimate is based on information from the National Health Expenditure Accounts (CMS, 2014), which report expenditures from nursing facilities for the care of their residents, in addition to estimates of the care of nursing home residents received outside of nursing facilities, such as during hospital stays (Sing et al., 2006). As of 2011, there were 1.4 million Americans residing in nursing facilities (National Center for Health Statistics, 2013). Thus, we estimate that the average annual health expenditure per nursing home resident is more than $200,000, which is significantly higher than the $17,500 minimum average annual health expenditure required to be in the top 5 percent of health care spenders based on MEPS data (AHRQ and HHS, 2011). Given that we do not have access to data on the distribution of health care expenditures for nursing home residents, we categorized the entire nursing home population as being in the top 5 percent of spenders in all analyses in this appendix. Further, given estimates that nearly all nursing home residents have at least one chronic condition and require assistance with one or more ADLs (Hing, 1989), we categorized the entire nursing home resident population as having both chronic conditions and functional limitations in this appendix.

In 2006, the most recent year for which data are available, 2.2 million (6 percent) of the Medicare population spent some portion of the year residing in a nursing home, and half of these individuals resided there for the full year. Nursing home residence is concentrated near the end of life and approaches 40 percent at the time of death (based on our analyses of the Health and Retirement Study [HRS] Medicare population). Much of this end-of-life nursing home care is provided under the skilled nursing facility (SNF) Medicare benefit, with nearly one in three Medicare beneficiaries using this benefit at some point during the last 6 months of life (Aragon et al., 2012). In addition, Medicare beneficiaries residing in nursing homes incur high costs related to hospitalizations (see Figure E-9). It is estimated that approximately 24 percent of these hospitalizations are related to ambulatory care–sensitive conditions and are therefore potentially preventable. This rate is even higher (30 percent) during a beneficiary's first 6 months following nursing home admission (Jacobson et al., 2010).

Hospitalizations account for the largest share of average Medicare spending per long-term care facility resident, 2006

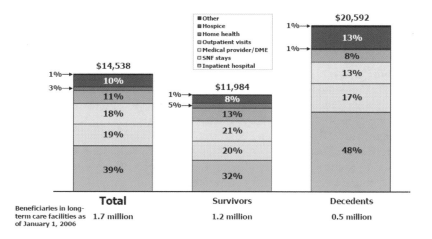

FIGURE E-9 Proportion of Medicare spending on hospital services among nursing home residents.

NOTE: Includes beneficiaries who were in long-term care facilities as of January 1, 2006, including those who died before the end of 2006. Excludes Medicare Advantage enrollees' spending. Excludes Medicare prescription of drug spending. DME = durable medical equipment; SNF = skilled nursing facility.

SOURCE: Jacobson et al., 2010. Reprinted with permission from The Henry J. Kaiser Family Foundation.

COST OF CARE AT THE END OF LIFE

Magnitude and Proportion of U.S. Health Care Spending on Decedents

We estimate that approximately 13 percent of the $1.6 trillion in health care costs is for the care of individuals in their last year of life (see Figure E-10). We computed this estimate using information from the HRS regarding the cost of care for individuals in the last year of life paid by Medicare, adjusted to account for the fact that 39 percent of costs in the last year of life are paid by sources other than Medicare, including Medicaid (10 percent), out of pocket (18 percent, primarily for nursing home care), and other sources (including private payers) (11 percent) (Hogan et

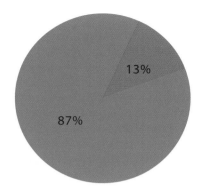

13%

87%

- Cost for Patients Not at the End of Life
- Cost for Patients at the End of Life

FIGURE E-10 Proportion of total health care costs for patients at the end of life. SOURCE: Numerator: Health and Retirement Study and linked Medicare data, decedents 2000-2008; adjusted to include non-Medicare payors (Hogan et al., 2001), and adjusted to 2011 dollars using the Bureau of Labor Statistics Consumer Price Index. Denominator: CMS 2011 National Health Expenditure report (CMS, 2014), with adjustments based on estimates from Sing and colleagues (2006) and the 2011 Medical Expenditure Panel Survey data (AHRQ and HHS, 2011) (see Figure E-1).

al., 2001), and adjusted to 2011 dollars using the Bureau of Labor Statistics Consumer Price Index. We then applied this estimated per person cost of care in the last year of life to the total number of deaths in 2011 to obtain the numerator of the 13 percent estimate shown in Figure E-10. As noted, the majority of costs in the last year of life (61 percent) are paid for by Medicare. Because of this, as well as the fact that Medicare is a readily available dataset for analysis, many analyses of the health care costs for decedents use estimates derived only from Medicare claims data. We consider this a limitation of the existing evidence regarding health care costs of decedents and have refined these analyses to estimate total health care costs in this appendix.

During 2012, enrollment in Medicare averaged about 50 million people. Net spending for the program was $466 billion. The Congressional Budget Office (CBO) expects Medicare spending to climb rapidly over the next decade, in part as a result of the retirement of the baby boomers (CBO, undated). This rate of spending is widely believed to be unsustainable, and the high rate of spending near the end of life is often cited as an area to examine for potential cost savings. Each year approximately 5 percent of fee-for-service (FFS) elderly Medicare beneficiaries die (Riley and Lubitz, 2010).

Change in Spending on Decedents Over Time

Medicare expenditures in the last year of life average 5 times greater than those in nonterminal years, and in recent years this end-of-life spending has accounted for approximately one-quarter of overall Medicare expenditures (see Figure E-11) (CMS, 2011; Hogan et al., 2001; Hoover et al., 2002; Lubitz and Riley, 1993; Riley and Lubitz, 2010). Over the past 30 years, overall health care costs have been climbing, but the proportion of spending by Medicare for decedents has been stable. The share of Medicare payments going to persons in their last year of life declined slightly from 28.3 percent in 1978 to 25.1 percent in 2006. After adjustment for age, sex, and death rates, however, there was no significant trend (see Figure E-12).

Variation in Spending Among Decedents

It is important to note that not all deaths result in high spending, and not all high spending occurs near death. For example, based upon data from the Medicare FFS population within the nationally representative HRS cohort adjusted to 2011 dollars, we find that while mean Medicare spending in the last year of life is $50,576 (median $37,152), 25 percent of beneficiaries incur $15,895 or less in Medicare spending in the final year of

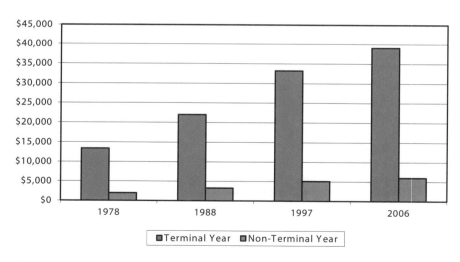

FIGURE E-11 Average per person spending on health care among decedents, 1978-2006.
SOURCE: Riley and Lubitz, 2010.

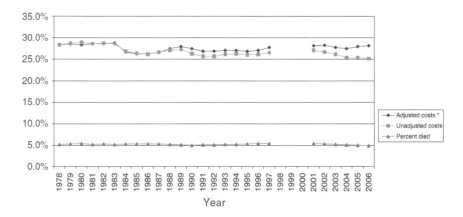

FIGURE E-12 Percentage dying and percentage of Medicare payments spent in the last 12 months of life among fee-for-service Medicare beneficiaries aged 65 and older, 1978-2006.
NOTES: Payment data not available for years 1998-2000.
*Costs adjusted for age, sex, and survival status of the 1978 sample.
SOURCE: Riley and Lubitz, 2010. Reprinted with permission from John Wiley and Sons. © Health Research and Educational Trust.

life. As Medicare spending accounts for approximately 60 percent of total health care spending (Hogan et al., 2001), we estimate that mean total health care spending in the last year of life is $82,911 (median $60,904), and 25 percent of beneficiaries incur $26,057 or less in spending in the final year of life (see Figure E-13).

Characteristics Associated with Increased Spending

Prior research has revealed significant variation in end-of-life health care spending across patient groups, hospitals, and geographic regions. The following subsections highlight several characteristics that have consistently been shown to be associated with variations in spending at the end of life. As previously mentioned, most existing analyses highlight only the characteristics of the Medicare population rather than the population of decedents as a whole.

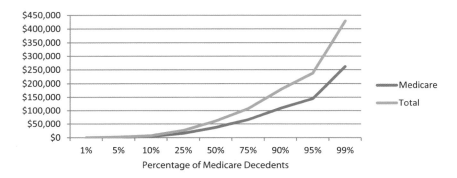

FIGURE E-13 Distribution of total health care and total Medicare spending in the last year of life among Medicare beneficiaries.
SOURCE: Health and Retirement Study and linked Medicare data, decedents 2000-2008, adjusted to 2011 dollar value using the Bureau of Labor Statistics Consumer Price Index.

Demographic Characteristics

Medicare expenditures in the last year of life decrease with age, especially for those aged 85 or older (see Figure E-14). This is in large part because the intensity of medical care in the last year of life decreases with increasing age (Levinsky et al., 2001; Kelley et al., 2011, 2012; Tschirhart et al., 2013). Race and ethnicity have also consistently demonstrated strong associations with costs of end-of-life health care. Hanchate and colleagues (2009), as one example, found that in the final 6 months of life, Medicare costs for non-Hispanic white patients averaged $20,166, while costs among black patients averaged $26,704 (32 percent higher) and among Hispanics, $31,702 (57 percent higher) (see Figure E-15) (Hanchate et al., 2009). The higher costs for Hispanics and blacks were attributed to greater use of hospital-based, life-sustaining interventions, including being more likely to be admitted to the intensive care unit (ICU) (39.6 for Hispanics, 32.5 percent for blacks, and 27.0 percent for whites); more intensive procedures, such as resuscitation and cardiac conversion (4.0 percent of Hispanics, 4.4 percent of blacks, and 2.7 percent of whites); mechanical ventilation (21.0 percent for Hispanics, 18.0 percent for blacks, and 11.6 percent for whites); and gastrostomy for artificial nutrition (9.1 percent for Hispanics, 10.5 percent for blacks, and 4.1 percent for whites) (Hanchate et al., 2009).

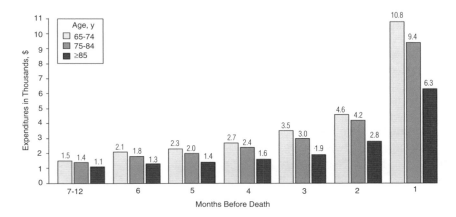

FIGURE E-14 Medicare spending in the last 12 months of life by age.

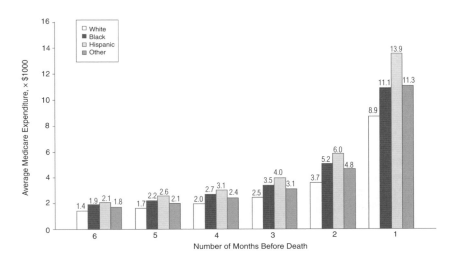

FIGURE E-15 Medicare spending in the last 6 months of life by race and ethnicity.

Health Characteristics: Medical Conditions,
Physical Function, and Debility

As described above, chronic conditions and functional limitations are associated with high health care spending. These relationships are also observed among decedents (see Table E-5).

In addition to chronic conditions and functional limitations, a few life-limiting conditions and catastrophic health events, such as advanced cancer or stroke, are also associated with higher costs at the end of life. Specific conditions and the different trajectories of functional decline seen with them are associated with different spending patterns prior to death. For example, functional decline may be due to progression of a chronic disease, such as chronic obstructive pulmonary disease (COPD), or the accumulation of multimorbidity or frailty, and in such cases this decline typically results in a steadily increasing pattern of health care spending (Chan et al., 2002; Lunney et al., 2002, 2003). Alternatively, people dying from single organ failure, such as congestive heart failure, may experience gradually diminishing physical function with periodic exacerbations of their illness, thus incurring very high episodic spending before death. Others who die suddenly, possibly from a stroke or motor vehicle accident, may incur little health care spending in their last year of life (Lunney et al., 2002, 2003). One recent study examined the impact of medical conditions and functional

TABLE E-5 Health Care Costs Among Medicare Fee-for-Service Beneficiaries by Chronic Conditions and by Functional Limitations in the Last Year of Life

	No. of People	%	Total Health Care Costs	%
Age: 65 or older, FFS Medicare beneficiaries				
No chronic conditions or functional limitations	15,484	1	$39,771,569	0
Chronic conditions only	411,774	28	28,271,965,777	23
Functional limitations only	20,323	1	613,233,917	0.5
Chronic conditions and functional limitations	1,037,419	70	94,197,646,891	77

NOTES: Functional limitation defined as needing help with any activities of daily living. Medicare costs represent on average 61 percent of total health care costs (Hogan et al., 2001). FFS = fee for service.
SOURCE: Health and Retirement Study and linked Medicare data, decedents 2000-2008, scaled to the full Medicare population and costs adjusted to 2011 dollars using the Bureau of Labor Statistics Consumer Price Index.

TABLE E-6 Association of Functional Status and Medical Conditions with Medicare Costs in the Last 6 Months of Life

Patient Characteristics	Adjusted Rate Ratio	95% Confidence Interval
Functional status (reference: independent in activities of daily living)		
Stable moderate impairment	1.12	0.92-1.36
Stable severe impairment	1.20	1.04-1.39
Decline from independent to moderate impairment	1.34	1.15-1.56
Decline from moderate to severe impairment	1.42	1.23-1.64
Decline from independent to severe impairment	1.64	1.46-1.84
Dementia/Alzheimer's disease	0.78	0.70-0.86
Diabetes	1.14	1.04-1.24
Chronic kidney disease	1.24	1.11-1.38
Stroke/transient ischemic attack	1.15	1.04-1.28
Congestive heart failure	1.08	0.98-1.18
Cancer	1.06	0.95-1.19
Chronic obstructive pulmonary disease	1.03	0.95-1.13
Depression	1.03	0.92-1.15

SOURCE: Health and Retirement Study and linked Medicare data, decedents 2000-2008. Adjusted for age, race, ethnicity, education, net worth, Medicaid, Medigap, nursing home residence, relative nearby, religiosity, Self Reported Health, three other chronic conditions, advance directive, regional hospital beds, and local pattern of end-of-life spending (Kelley et al., 2011).

decline simultaneously on end-of-life Medicare costs and demonstrated an independent and dose effect–like association between functional decline and increasing health care costs (Kelley et al., 2011). For example, a person experiencing a decline from functional independence to needing assistance with one ADL incurred 34 percent higher Medicare costs, all other factors being held equal, while a decline from independence to needing help with four or more ADLs was associated with 64 percent higher costs (see Table E-6).

Notably, this study found a negative association between dementia and total end-of-life Medicare costs, after adjusting for functional status, nursing home residence, and other characteristics. Patients suffering with dementia typically experience a long, slowly debilitating course of illness. A large portion of their health care expenses is focused on custodial and supportive care services, which are not covered by Medicare and therefore not represented in this study. A recent analysis of total health care costs associated with dementia found that the yearly costs per person attributable to dementia were approximately $50,000 (2010 U.S. dollars) (Hurd et al., 2013).

Advance Care Planning, Personal Preferences, and Goals of Care Discussions

Evidence is mixed regarding the impact of patient preferences on health care costs and treatment received. Many studies reveal a poor correlation. In the Study to Understand Prognoses and Preferences for Outcomes and Risks of Treatments (SUPPORT) trial, 35 percent of patients reported care conflicting with preferences, and such discord was associated with higher costs (Teno et al., 2002). In the same study, investigators found that the risk of in-hospital death, a marker of high end-of-life health care costs, was associated with greater hospital bed availability and not associated with patient preferences (Pritchard et al., 1998). Similarly, a prospective study of patient preferences for life-sustaining treatment found no relationship with treatment received (Danis et al., 1996).

However, conflicting evidence does exist. A study of the association between treatment-limiting advance directives and Medicare costs revealed a significant correlation with lower costs, but only within regions with patterns of high end-of-life health care spending (p = 0.04) (Nicholas et al., 2011). Zhang and colleagues (2009) found that among patients with advanced cancer, the cost of health care in the last week of life was 35.7 percent lower among patients who had reported discussions of end-of-life care preferences (p = 0.002).

Regional Variation

The wide variation in health care spending by geographic region has been the focus of extensive research and policy debate over the past three decades. The Dartmouth Atlas of Health Care, a leading contributor to this research, has focused primarily on Medicare spending, with particular interest in spending and patterns of utilization at the end of life. This work has highlighted a four-fold difference in Medicare end-of-life spending across geographic regions (see Figure E-16) (Fisher et al., 2003a).

Policy makers have seized upon these findings and suggested reform measures that would penalize high-spending and reward low-spending regions. An Institute of Medicine (2013) report, *Variation in Health Care Spending: Target Decision Making, Not Geography*, also notes wide regional variation in Medicare spending, but identifies the greatest variation in the use of post-acute services as opposed to hospital services. In addition,

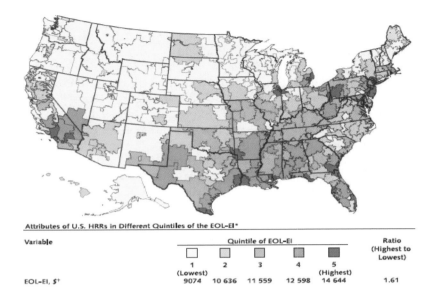

FIGURE E-16 Quintiles of Medicare spending in the last 2 years of life by region. SOURCE: Fisher et al., 2003a. Reprinted with permission from *Annals of Internal Medicine*.

the report cites wide regional variation in spending among private insurers; however, these patterns are not congruent with the patterns observed in Medicare and are more strongly related to differences in pricing. In sum, the report recommends against a geography-based value index or adjustment for Medicare services and instead suggests policies to promote high-value, patient-centered care.

Personal and Regional Factors Examined Simultaneously

A notable weakness in prior studies of regional variation is the inability to control adequately for severity of illness by studying claims or administrative data alone. This method also fails to assess and adjust for many of the other patient factors, such as function, that are known to be associated with spending. A recent examination of determinants of Medicare expenditures in the last 6 months of life aimed to consider simultaneously the influence of patients' social, medical, and functional characteristics while also adjusting for regional practice patterns and supply of medical resources, such as hospital beds and medical subspecialists. As hypothesized, this analysis revealed a strong, independent association of functional debility and decline with higher Medicare expenditures, and the same for selected medical conditions. In addition, after controlling for an extensive group of personal and health characteristics, regional factors continued to be significantly associated with Medicare costs. For example, a person in a region within the second quintile of practice pattern intensity, as measured by Dartmouth's End-of-Life Expenditure Index, incurs 10 percent more Medicare expenditures in the last 6 months of life than a person in a region within the lowest quintile, holding all other characteristics equal. Furthermore, each additional hospital bed per 10,000 residents was found to increase Medicare expenditures in the last 6 months of life by 1 percent if all other factors were held equal (Kelley et al., 2011). These findings support an independent effect of regional characteristics on health care spending, beyond the effect of patient-level factors.

Model or Settings of Care: Hospital Use

Hospital use accounts for the largest portion of Medicare expenditures near the end of life (CBO, undated; CMS, 2011). Over the past 30 years, overall use of hospital and ICU services has increased, while proportionally this use among decedents has remained stable (see Table E-7) (Riley and Lubitz, 2010). Wide variation in use of these services has also been noted

TABLE E-7 Measures of Inpatient Hospital Use Among Medicare Beneficiaries Aged 65 and Older by Survival Status, 1978-2006

Utilization Measure and Survival Status	1978	1988	1997	2002	2006
Percentage Hospitalized					
March decedents	64.5	63.7	62.6	62.8	62.5
Survivors	18.5	16.1	16.5	17.0	16.7
Percentage Undergoing Multiple Hospitalizations					
March decedents	20.3	22.2	24.5	25.6	27.0
Survivors	5.2	4.8	5.6	5.9	5.6
Percentage Using ICU/CCU Services					
March decedents	N/A	27.7	28.7	30.7	33.1
Survivors	N/A	4.6	5.6	6.1	6.3

NOTES: p <0.05 for positive linear trend in multiple hospitalizations for decedents and in ICU use for both decedents and survivors. Trends in multiple hospitalizations for survivors and percentage hospitalized for decedents and survivors were not statistically significant (Riley and Lubitz, 2010). CCU = critical care unit; ICU = intensive care unit.
SOURCE: Medicare Continuous History Sample, Fee-for-Service Medicare beneficiaries.

across beneficiaries and geographic regions. Among the decedent Medicare beneficiaries within the HRS cohort, one-quarter had no hospital days within the last 6 months of life, while 40 percent had 10 or more days. In an examination of the personal and regional factors associated with greater hospital use, one study found higher hospital use among all subjects with functional decline and those with stable severe functional disability compared with those functionally independent in their ADLs. For example, those declining from independence to severe debility experienced more than 9 additional hospital days in the last 6 months of life, other factors being held equal (Kelley et al., 2012). This study also revealed greater hospital use among blacks (6 more days on average) and Hispanics (5 more days).

PUTTING IT TOGETHER: THE INTERSECTION OF THE HIGH-COST AND END-OF-LIFE POPULATIONS

Estimating the Overlap in Population

Using our analyses of the population with the highest annual health care costs and the population at the end of life, we have generated an estimate of the overlap between these two groups. Specifically, of the estimated 18.2 million individuals annually who are in the 5 percent of the population with the highest health care costs, 11 percent (2.0 million) are in their last year of life (see Figure E-17). Further, of the 2.5 million annual deaths in the United States, 80 percent (2.0 million) were among individuals who incurred health care costs in their last year of life that place them in the top 5 percent of all spenders, while 20 percent (0.5 million) did not incur high health care costs in their last year of life.

Identifying Illness Trajectories

Given the relatively small proportion of the population with the highest health care costs who are at the end of life (11 percent), it is critical to gain a deeper understanding of the likely illness trajectories of the other 89 percent. We estimate that the population with the highest annual health care costs can be divided into three potential illness trajectories (see Figure E-18):

- individuals who have high health care costs because it is their last year of life (population at the end of life);
- individuals who persistently generate high annual health care costs due to chronic conditions, functional limitations, or other conditions who are not in their last year of life and who live for many

years, generating high health care expenses (population with persistently high costs); and

- individuals who experience a significant health event in one year but who return to normal health (population with a discrete high-cost event).

We estimate that the largest proportion of the population with the highest annual health care expenditures are individuals who experience a

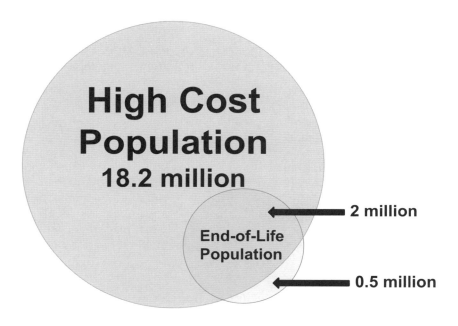

FIGURE E-17 Estimated overlap between the population with the highest health care costs and the population at the end of life.
NOTE: The entire nursing home population is estimated to be in the top 5 percent of total health care spending (see the earlier section on the nursing home population for details).
SOURCE: Total population and health care costs were obtained from the 2011 Medical Expenditure Panel Survey data (AHRQ and HHS, 2011), adjusted to include the nursing home population (National Center for Health Statistics, 2013). The distribution of total costs for the end-of-life population was estimated from the Health and Retirement Study and linked Medicare data, decedents 2000-2008, adjusted to include non-Medicare payors (Hogan et al., 2001) and adjusted to 2011 dollars using the Bureau of Labor Statistics Consumer Price Index.

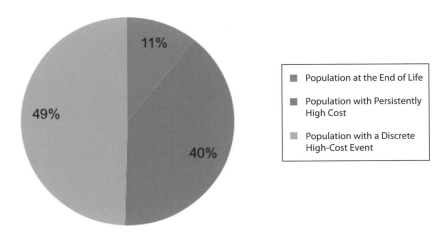

FIGURE E-18 Population with the highest health care costs (top 5 percent) by illness trajectory.
NOTES: The entire nursing home population is estimated to be in the top 5 percent of total health care spending (see the earlier section on the nursing home population for details). For a description of the calculation of illness trajectory groupings, see the discussion below.
SOURCE: 2011 Medical Expenditure Panel Survey data (AHRQ and HHS, 2011), adjusted to include the nursing home population (National Center for Health Statistics, 2013).

discrete event generating significant health care costs in a given year. We used evidence from a recent study (NIHCM Foundation, 2012) regarding the persistence of spending patterns over time. This study found that of individuals in the top 5 percent of health care spending in a given year, 62 percent were no longer in the top 5 percent of spending the next year. A portion of these individuals died; the rest transitioned to the bottom 95th percentile in health care spending the following year. Some examples of this illness trajectory might include people who have a myocardial infarction, undergo coronary bypass graft surgery, and return to stable good health after a period of rehabilitation; individuals who are diagnosed with early-stage cancer, complete surgical resection and other first-line therapies, and achieve complete remission; or people who are waiting for a kidney transplant on frequent hemodialysis and then receive a transplant and return to stable health. There may be relatively less opportunity for cost reductions in this population because many high-cost events may be unavoidable. Furthermore, given that most of these individuals return to better health (or at least return to the lower-cost population) within 1 year, health care dollars may already be well spent for them.

Population with Persistently High Costs (40 percent)

The second largest proportion of the high-cost population is those with persistently high health care costs. This subgroup is most likely characterized by the chronic conditions and functional limitations described earlier. Evidence suggests that this population tends to be older. A recent study (Cohen and Yu, 2012; NIHCM Foundation, 2012) revealed that among the population in the top 10 percent of health care spending persistently over a 2-year period, 42.9 percent were aged 65 or older, compared with only 19.2 percent of individuals who shifted from the top 10 percent to the bottom 75 percent in the following year. The existence of a subgroup of individuals with persistently high spending was also evident in an analysis of Medicare beneficiaries in which it was found that nearly half of beneficiaries who were high cost in 1997 were also high cost in 1996, and more than 25 percent were also high cost 4 years previously (CBO, 2005). Furthermore, 44 percent of those individuals remained high cost in 1998, and 25 percent were high cost in 2001 (see Figure E-19). This may be a key population for targeted interventions to reduce costs because such interventions may enable cost reductions across multiple years.

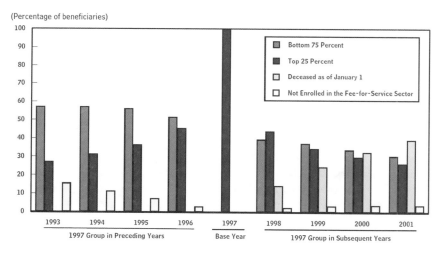

FIGURE E-19 Expenditure history of Medicare beneficiaries who constituted the top 25 percent of spending in 1997.
SOURCE: CBO, 2005.

Population at the End of Life (11 percent)

As described earlier, 80 percent of those in the last year of life are among the high-cost population. Functional debility and decline are strongly correlated with being among the highest spenders. In addition, some chronic illnesses, including diabetes, chronic kidney disease, dementia, and others, are associated with high health care costs, particularly in the setting of functional decline. Race and ethnicity are also noted to be consistent predictors of higher costs, although the reason for this association remains unclear, and it may be an artifact of poor-quality care or limited access to care over the life span (IOM, 2002). Finally, regional differences in spending and use of specific health care services, including hospital and ICU care, persist in studies controlling for patient factors.

Limitations and Gaps in the Evidence

Throughout this analysis, we have aggregated existing statistics and evidence and combined them with our own analyses and estimates. In a number of areas, the evidence presented here is limited by incomplete data. Studies of hospital and regional variation using only administrative claims do not adjust sufficiently for patient risk factors (i.e., health, function, and socioeconomic status) or patient preferences. Additionally, most prior studies have focused on single diseases or a single predictive factor in isolation, and thus are not generalizable to the broader population of seriously ill older adults with multiple chronic illnesses or advanced organ failure (Emanuel et al., 2003; Hamel et al., 1999; Shugarman et al., 2007; Zhang et al., 2003).

Additionally, measurement of diagnoses within administrative data does not adequately measure severity of illness. Variation exists in regional practice patterns in the use of diagnostic testing and billing codes, creating the potential for bias in analyses based on the measurement of chronic disease or total disease burden (Song et al., 2010; Welch et al., 2011). Many studies of the costs of care at the end of life have been retrospective mortality follow-back studies of decedents and are subject to selection bias because they cannot account for those who survived despite a high risk of death (Bach et al., 2004). These data, therefore, are particularly difficult to translate to policy or service design given the prognostic uncertainty associated with serious illness in real clinical settings.

Finally, as described earlier, we have made a number of assumptions regarding health care expenditures for nursing home residents given a lack of detailed data on this population. Further, our cost analyses do not include estimates for costs such as informal caregiving and lost wages. Consideration of these costs must be included in the context of any new or reformed design of health services because the economic implications of these costs for the aging population are potentially profound.

CONCLUSIONS AND RECOMMENDATIONS

Conclusions

Our analyses lead to the following conclusions:

- Although many proposals to reduce health care costs target the high cost of end-of-life care, on a population level, the cost of caring for individuals in their last year of life represents 13 percent of total annual health care spending, and these individuals make up just over 10 percent of the high-cost population.
- The population with both chronic conditions and functional limitations is a key driver of high health care costs. The addition of functional limitations appears to differentiate a high-cost group within those with chronic conditions and may characterize those who are persistently in the high-cost group.
- Instead of a focus on chronic conditions alone, a clinical indicator of one's potential to accrue high health care costs may be the onset of need for help with daily activities (functional limitations) in an individual with chronic conditions.
- Although older age may be a risk factor for higher health care costs, older adults make up the minority of the high-cost spenders. The proportion of total annual health care spending for the population aged 65 or older has not changed materially in a decade.
- Current data indicate that increased health care spending is not associated with higher-quality care, as measured by longevity, quality of life, and satisfaction (Fisher et al., 2003a,b; Mittler et al., 2010; Skinner et al., 2009; Wennberg et al., 2009; Yasaitis et al., 2009). Other studies of adults with serious illness suggest high-cost hospital-based treatment is often inconsistent with patient preferences and may contribute to patient suffering (Pritchard et al., 1998; Teno et al., 2002, 2007; Yasaitis et al., 2009; Zhang et al., 2009).

Maximizing value (i.e., increasing quality while reducing costs) in the care of the highest-cost, seriously ill individuals is a major challenge facing the nation's health care system and economy. The greatest strides in improving the quality and containing the costs of health care for the highest-cost population will be achieved by focusing research and clinical interventions on those with functional debility, chronic illnesses, and patterns of high health care utilization.

Recommendations

Our recommendations encompass expanding programs that already work to address high-cost populations; developing new programs or policies that better match patient needs with services; and considering the most appropriate target population for interventions based on population size, health care costs, and potential for health care savings.

Models That Currently Work to Align Patient
Goals with Treatment and Lower Costs

Palliative care A recent study examined the effect on hospital costs of palliative care team consultations for patients enrolled in Medicaid at four New York State hospitals and found that, on average, patients who received palliative care incurred $6,900 less in hospital costs during a given admission than a matched group of patients who received usual care. These reductions included $4,098 in hospital costs per admission for patients discharged alive and $7,563 for patients who died in the hospital. In addition, palliative care recipients spent less time in intensive care, were less likely to die in ICUs, and were more likely to receive hospice referrals than the matched usual care patients (Morrison et al., 2011). Similarly, a randomized controlled trial of palliative care in addition to usual care among patients newly diagnosed with stage IV non-small-cell lung cancer found that those in the intervention (palliative care) group had lower rates of emergency department visits and hospital admissions within the last 30 days of life, and they were less likely to receive chemotherapy within the last 14 days and more likely to be referred to hospice 4 days or longer prior to death. All measures are indicative of higher-quality and lower-cost end-of-life care (Temel et al., 2010).

Hospice Unlike palliative care, which is appropriate at any stage of serious illness, hospice is specific to care at the end of life. Hospice enrollment is restricted to patients with an estimated prognosis of 6 months or less and requires that patients forgo "curative" or disease-directed treatments. While extensive data support the high quality of hospice care, the impact of hospice enrollment on health care costs has been debated. A study (Kelley et al., 2013) using the HRS cohort decedent sample examined the impact on Medicare expenditures of hospice enrollment 1-7, 8-14, 15-30, and 53-105 days prior to death. Within all periods studied, hospice patients had significantly lower Medicare costs and lower rates of hospital and intensive care use, hospital readmission, and in-hospital death compared with propensity score-matched nonhospice controls. For example, patients being enrolled in hospice for 15-30 days resulted in $6,430 in savings to Medicare on average (see Figure E-20); patients enrolled in hospice for 53-105 days had 9 fewer hospital and 5 fewer ICU days compared with patients receiving usual care; and patients enrolled in hospice for 53-105 days had 15 percent fewer hospital readmissions and 40 percent fewer in-hospital deaths compared with patients receiving usual care.

Similarly, a study (Carlson et al., 2010) that followed more than 90,000 individuals with cancer found that total Medicare costs were significantly lower for those who remained continuously enrolled in hospice until death compared with those who disenrolled from hospice. The 11 percent of patients who disenrolled from hospice were more likely to be hospitalized (39.8 percent versus 1.6 percent), more likely to be admitted to the emergency department (33.9 percent versus 3.1 percent) or ICU (5.7 percent versus 0.1 percent), and more likely to die in the hospital (9.6 percent versus 0.2 percent). Patients who disenrolled from hospice died a median of 24 days following disenrollment, suggesting that the reason for hospice disenrollment was not improved health. Hospice disenrollees incurred higher

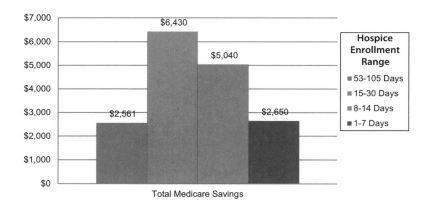

FIGURE E-20 Incremental effect of hospice enrollment on Medicare costs.
SOURCE: A version of this figure appears in Kelley et al., 2013. Reprinted with permission from Project HOPE/*Health Affairs*.

TABLE E-8 Hospice Enrollment Policies Potentially Restricting Access to Hospice Care, National Hospice Survey Data, 2008-2009

Policy	Percentage of Hospices (N = 591)
Patient cannot be receiving chemotherapy	61
Patient cannot be receiving total parenteral nutrition	55
Patient cannot be receiving transfusions	40
Patient cannot need an intrathecal catheter	32
Patient cannot continue to receive palliative radiation	30
Patient must have a caregiver at home	12
Patient cannot be receiving tube feeding	8
Hospice has all restrictive enrollment policies	0.8
Hospice has no restrictive enrollment policies	22

SOURCE: Aldridge et al., 2012.

per-day Medicare expenditures than patients who remained with hospice until death.

Despite the benefits of hospice for patients and families and the potential cost savings from greater hospice use, there are limitations in attempting to expand access to hospice care to a wider population. In addition to the eligibility criteria, which are considered a significant barrier to greater hospice use, hospices have been found to have varying enrollment policies aimed at restricting access to hospice care for potentially high-cost patients. A national survey of the enrollment policies of 591 U.S. hospices found that 78 percent of hospices had at least one enrollment policy that could restrict access to care for patients with potentially high-cost medical care needs, such as chemotherapy or total parenteral nutrition (see Table E-8) (Aldridge et al., 2012). This is particularly concerning given that the most complex patients and those with significant functional limitations may be those most in need of home-based palliative care, and yet hospices that could potentially provide such care may not be willing to take on such patients because of cost concerns. Smaller hospices, for-profit hospices, and hospices in certain regions of the country consistently reported more limited enrollment policies.

Programs aimed at improving health care services and reducing costs at the end of life will continue to be limited by physicians' inability to predict mortality accurately. In addition, interventions focused only on those near death will have limited opportunity to impact costs given the limited time span following intervention. Identifying patients with serious illness—that is, functional limitations and progressive chronic disease or organ failure—

is the first step in recognizing individuals who may be at risk of high-cost treatment. The additional factors noted above—race/ethnicity and regional patterns of care—require further study, but are clearly factors to consider in deploying limited resources and targeted efforts to improve the quality of communication and health care decision making.

Program of All-inclusive Care for the Elderly Those individuals eligible for both Medicare and Medicaid, the "dual-eligibles," are frequently among the highest-cost population. One program seeking to address both the care needs and the growing health care expenses of the dual-eligible population is the Program of All-inclusive Care for the Elderly (PACE). PACE is a long-term care delivery and financing program designed to provide comprehensive community-based care and prevent unnecessary use of hospital and nursing home care (Eng et al., 1997). Initial results from the PACE program in the 1990s demonstrated high-quality care with lower rates of hospitalization and lower costs. Yet expansion of the PACE model to other sites has been slow since 1997. Barriers cited include financial constraints, challenges with enrollment and referral sources, and model characteristics (Gross et al., 2004).

Open-access hospice programs Open-access hospice is an emerging model of care with the objective of providing hospice services to patients who need and want hospice care but may not be eligible under the Medicare eligibility criteria. Patients receive the medical symptom management and psychosocial support traditionally available through hospice while simultaneously retaining access to medical treatments designed to slow or halt their disease progression (Abelson, 2007). Although patients who receive care through open-access hospices may be covered by private insurance plans or may pay for their care out of pocket, initial reports (Abelson, 2007) indicate that the cost of caring for patients enrolled through open-access policies is generally absorbed by the hospice provider. Hospices may have financial incentives to provide care through open-access policies if these patients transition to hospice care earlier, which prolongs hospice length of stay and is therefore more profitable for the hospice provider.

The emergence of hospices with open-access policies signals the ability and willingness of some hospices to provide care outside of the Medicare hospice benefit and has the potential to improve access to hospice care. However, a recent study finds that only slightly more than one-quarter of hospices have such policies, and the majority of these hospice are nonprofit (Aldridge et al., 2012). This is concerning because it suggests that the open-access policy innovation may be unlikely to spread, given the substantial growth in the for-profit hospice sector during the past decade (Thompson et al., 2012). Between 2000 and 2009, four out of five hospice providers that entered the U.S. market were for-profit, and more than 40 percent of hospices operating in 2000 had changed ownership during that same decade (Thompson et al., 2012).

Hospital at Home® The Hospital at Home program was originally developed at Johns Hopkins to improve care for individuals with selected acute illnesses by providing acute hospital-level care in a patient's home instead of the hospital. Although the acute hospital is the standard venue for providing acute medical care for serious illness, it is expensive and may be hazardous for vulnerable older persons, who commonly experience functional decline, iatrogenic illness, and other adverse events during hospital admissions. Providing acute hospital-level care in a patient's home for carefully selected patients via Hospital at Home has been shown to improve patient safety, enhance quality, increase efficiency, reduce variations in practice, and reduce the costs of providing acute care for medical illness for Medicare beneficiaries (Frick et al., 2009; Leff et al., 2005, 2006). A 2012 meta-analysis of 61 randomized controlled trials found that Hospital at Home care led to a 19 percent reduction in costs with similar or improved clinical outcomes, including a 25 percent reduction in readmission rates, better patient satisfaction, and lower caregiver burden (Cryer et al., 2012).

Dissemination of the Hospital at Home program has been limited, however, by the lack of a feasible payment model in Medicare. There currently exists no mechanism in fee-for-service Medicare for reimbursing for these services; the services do not fit the statutory definition of acute hospital care because they are delivered to a patient outside the physical plant of the acute care hospital and therefore are not "at hospital" services. In fact, negative financial incentives exist in that the hospital would not receive reimbursement for the acute hospital admission. Further, there is no mechanism for receiving appropriate reimbursement for Hospital at Home services provided because these acute hospital-level services are well beyond the scope and intensity of reimbursable Medicare home health care services.

Identification of Target Population for Health Care Interventions to Reduce Costs

Our findings suggest that identification of the appropriate target population for cost-saving interventions is critical given the substantial variation in the size of different target populations, the costs generated by different populations, and the proportion of the target population likely to be impacted by an intervention. Using the statistics we have estimated for this report, Table E-9 compares three potential target populations and two hypothetical interventions to highlight the differences in potential cost savings. We assume that the percentage of the eligible population

TABLE E-9 Projected Cost Savings of Hypothetical Interventions by Target Population

Target Population*	Population Size	Total Costs ($bil)	Intervention	% of Population Impacted by Intervention	Potential Reduction in Health Care Costs (%)	Potential Reduction in Health Care Costs ($bil)
Age 65 or older with chronic conditions and functional limitations	22,092,740	$543	A	50	10	$27
			B	50	5	14
All individuals with chronic conditions and functional limitations	44,946,847	$909	A	50	10	45
			B	50	5	23
Individuals at the end of life	2,468,435	$200	A	50	10	10
			B	50	5	5

*Target populations are not mutually exclusive.

that will be impacted by each intervention is 50 percent in all cases and that the potential reduction in costs is either 10 percent or 5 percent. An intervention that targets all individuals with chronic conditions and functional limitations (45 million people), impacts half that population, and reduces costs by 10 percent will theoretically achieve double the reduction in health care costs compared with the same intervention that targets only older adults with chronic conditions and functional limitations ($45 billion versus $27 billion). Our estimates also highlight the fact that interventions aimed at individuals in their last year of life will generate smaller reductions in cost savings relative to interventions that target those with chronic conditions and functional limitations given the significantly smaller size of the end-of-life population and the limited time frame for cost reduction. In addition, given the complexity of identifying individuals in their last year of life relative to identifying individuals with chronic conditions and functional limitations, it is likely that an end-of-life intervention may have an even smaller effect on costs than shown in the table because it would likely impact less than 50 percent of the terminal population.

Standardized Identification of Seriously Ill
and Potentially High-Cost Patients

Add a flag to administrative data to identify functional debility Administrative datasets, including Medicare, Medicaid, and private insurer claims, are key sources of data for health services research and for identifying individuals who may benefit from tailored services. As described above, however, these data are lacking elements critical to the identification of serious illness. In particular, functional limitations and debility are major predictors of high total health care spending, yet are not available in the majority of claims data (Kelley et al., 2011). Therefore, the Centers for Medicare & Medicaid Services and other major payors should require the collection of functional status data with all inpatient, SNF, home health, and hospice claims. Functional status measures are already collected for clinical purposes in all of these settings, and a flag or indicator of functional limitation could be added as a modifier to claims in these settings. This single addition to standardized claims requirements would create an opportunity to study the costs and quality of care for patients with serious illness and to identify this high-cost and vulnerable population for interventions designed to improve care.

Use a trigger for screening based on utilization patterns Prospectively identifying those seriously ill, high-cost patients who do not have functional limitations is an additional challenge for the deployment of targeted interventions for this group. Therefore, we recommend using an algorithm based on the presence of selected chronic conditions and defined patterns of health care utilization to identify individuals for more thorough screening by a health care professional. For example, individuals with congestive heart failure who present to the emergency department two or more times within 1 year would be interviewed. Those with unmet need for health care and supportive services, uncontrolled symptoms, or excessive treatment or caregiver burden might qualify for an intervention program designed to improve care and avoid excessive or unnecessary costs.

Research Required

One of the greatest gaps in the research we have reviewed for this appendix is the lack of evidence regarding characteristics associated with high costs *in total* and the impact of interventions or models of care on *total* health care costs. Nearly all of the analyses we reviewed focused on only one payor—generally Medicare. Although such studies are informative, the focus on Medicare costs alone has led to the misperception that older adults and those at the end of life are the primary drivers of health care costs, and yet when one evaluates total health care costs, it is fairly clear that this is not the case. A critical next step in research is to evaluate the impact of various interventions on reducing total health care costs so that programs and policies implemented across the health care system truly reduce total costs rather than merely shift costs from payor to payor.

Second, comprehensive data for the study of high-cost, seriously ill patients are currently unavailable. The standardized collection of functional status measures and markers of high health care utilization recommended above would facilitate the study of "real-world" health care programs for this population. While this would be a critical step forward, rigorous, peer-reviewed research is also needed to promote high-value health care for this population. For example, a longitudinal prospective cohort study is needed to evaluate the current patterns of care for seriously ill and high-cost adults. Briefly, this study would recruit a large, diverse sample of adults with chronic illness, including those residing in nursing homes, from geographic regions that exhibit variability across a range of regional characteristics previously shown to be associated with treatment quality and intensity. Subjects would provide baseline data on a comprehensive range of demographic, psychosocial, functional, and medical characteristics, as well as pertinent measures of personal values and beliefs. They would also be asked to authorize access to their health care claims data from all relevant payors. The subjects would then be followed with brief yet frequent queries for signs of new serious illness or progressive debility. Those positively identified as possibly having serious illness would be interviewed regarding the period surrounding the onset of the illness and followed with serial interviews throughout the course of their illness. This study would address many of the current knowledge gaps by enrolling subjects prior to the onset of serious illness and measuring pertinent factors and potential confounders a priori. The sample selection would not be dependent upon time of death or even prognosis, and thereby would capture the full range of serious illness experiences. The step-wise prospective design would minimize sampling bias and allow for focused data collection among those with serious illness when and if it developed while minimizing the study's burden on subjects.

REFERENCES

Abelson, R. 2007. A chance to pick hospice. *New York Times*, February 10.

AHRQ (Agency for Healthcare Research and Quality) and HHS (U.S. Department of Health and Human Services). 2011. *Medical Expenditure Panel Survey*. http://meps.ahrq.gov/mepsweb (accessed September 2013).

Aldridge Carlson, M. D., C. L. Barry, E. J. Cherlin, R. McCorkle, and E. H. Bradley. 2012. Hospices' enrollment policies may contribute to underuse of hospice care in the United States. *Health Affairs (Millwood)* 31:2690-2698.

Aragon, K., K. Covinsky, Y. Miao, W. J. Boscardin, L. Flint, and A. K. Smith. 2012. Use of the Medicare posthospitalization skilled nursing benefit in the last 6 months of life. *Archives of Internal Medicine* 172:1573-1579.

Bach, P. B., D. Schrag, and C. B. Begg. 2004. Resurrecting treatment histories of dead patients: A study design that should be laid to rest. *Journal of the American Medical Association* 292:2765-2770.

Carlson, M. D., J. Herrin, Q. Du, A. J. Epstein, C. L. Barry, R. S. Morrison, A. L. Back, and E. H. Bradley. 2010. Impact of hospice disenrollment on health care use and medicare expenditures for patients with cancer. *Journal of Clinical Oncology* 28:4371-4375.

CBO (Congressional Budget Office). 2005. *High-cost Medicare beneficiaries*. http://www.cbo.gov/sites/default/files/cbofiles/ftpdocs/63xx/doc6332/05-03-medispending.pdf (accessed August 15, 2014).

CBO. 2007. *The long-term outlook for health care spending*. http://www.cbo.gov/ftpdocs/87xx/doc8758/MainText3.1.shtml (accessed September 2, 2013).

CBO. undated. *Medicare*. http://www.cbo.gov/topics/health-care/medicare (accessed September 6, 2013).

Chan, L., S. Beaver, R. F. Maclehose, A. Jha, M. Maciejewski, and J. N. Doctor. 2002. Disability and health care costs in the Medicare population. *Archives of Physical Medicine and Rehabilitation* 83:1196-1201.

CMS (Centers for Medicare & Medicaid Services). 2011. *Medicare trustees report*. https://www.cms.gov/Research-Statistics-Data-and-Systems/Statistics-Trends-and-Reports/ReportsTrustFunds/Downloads/TR2011.pdf (accessed September 6, 2013).

CMS. 2012. *Nursing home data compendium*. http://www.cms.gov/Medicare/Provider-Enrollment-and-Certification/CertificationandComplianc/downloads/nursinghomedatacompendium_508.pdf (accessed November 2013).

CMS. 2014. *National health expenditure data*. http://www.cms.gov/Research-Statistics-Data-and-Systems/Statistics-Trends-and-Reports/NationalHealthExpendData/index.html (accessed November 2013).

Cohen, S., and W. Yu. 2012. The concentration and persistence in the level of health expenditures over time: Estimates for the U.S. population, 2008-2009. AHRQ statistical brief #354. http://meps.ahrq.gov/mepsweb/data_files/publications/st354/stat354.pdf (accessed September 2013).

Cryer, L., S. B. Shannon, M. Van Amsterdam, and B. Leff. 2012. Costs for "hospital at home" patients were 19 percent lower, with equal or better outcomes compared to similar inpatients. *Health Affairs (Millwood)* 31:1237-1243.

Danis, M., E. Mutran, J. M. Garrett, S. C. Stearns, R. T. Slifkin, L. Hanson, J. F. Williams, and L. R. Churchill. 1996. A prospective study of the impact of patient preferences on life-sustaining treatment and hospital cost. *Critical Care Medicine* 24:1811-1817.

de Brantes, F., M. B. Rosenthal, and M. Painter. 2009. Building a bridge from fragmentation to accountability—the Prometheus Payment model. *New England Journal of Medicine* 361:1033-1036.

Emanuel, E. J. 2012. Where are the health care cost savings? *Journal of the American Medical Association* 307:39-40.

Emanuel, E. J., Y. Young-Xu, N. G. Levinsky, G. Gazelle, O. Saynina, and A. S. Ash. 2003. Chemotherapy use among Medicare beneficiaries at the end of life. *Annals of Internal Medicine* 138:639-643.

Eng, C., J. Pedulla, G. P. Eleazer, R. McCann, and N. Fox. 1997. Program of All-inclusive Care for the Elderly (PACE): An innovative model of integrated geriatric care and financing. *Journal of the American Geriatrics Society* 45:223-232.

Fisher, E. S., D. E. Wennberg, T. A. Stukel, D. J. Gottlieb, F. L. Lucas, and E. L. Pinder. 2003a. The implications of regional variations in Medicare spending. Part 1: The content, quality, and accessibility of care. *Annals of Internal Medicine* 138:273-287.

Fisher, E. S., D. E. Wennberg, T. A. Stukel, D. J. Gottlieb, F. L. Lucas, and E. L. Pinder. 2003b. The implications of regional variations in Medicare spending. Part 2: Health outcomes and satisfaction with care. *Annals of Internal Medicine* 138:288-298.

Frick, K. D., L. C. Burton, R. Clark, S. I. Mader, W. B. Naughton, J. B. Burl, W. B. Greenough, D. M. Steinwachs, and B. Leff. 2009. Substitutive Hospital at Home for older persons: Effects on costs. *American Journal of Managed Care* 15:49-56.

Gross, D. L., H. Temkin-Greener, S. Kunitz, and D. B. Mukamel. 2004. The growing pains of integrated health care for the elderly: Lessons from the expansion of PACE. *Milbank Quarterly* 82:257-282.

Hamel, M. B., R. B. Davis, J. M. Teno, W. A. Knaus, J. Lynn, F. Harrell, Jr., A. N. Galanos, A. W. Wu, and R. S. Phillips. 1999. Older age, aggressiveness of care, and survival for seriously ill, hospitalized adults. SUPPORT investigators. Study to understand prognoses and preferences for outcomes and risks of treatments. *Annals of Internal Medicine* 131:721-728.

Hanchate, A., A. C. Kronman, Y. Young-Xu, A. S. Ash, and E. Emanuel. 2009. Racial and ethnic differences in end-of-life costs: Why do minorities cost more than whites? *Archives of Internal Medicine* 169:493-501.

HHS (U.S. Department of Health and Human Services). 2014. *HHS initiative on multiple chronic conditions.* http://www.hhs.gov/ash/initiatives/mcc (accessed September 2013).

Hing, E. 1989. Nursing home utilization by current residents: United States, 1985. *Vital and Health Statistics* 13(102). http://www.cdc.gov/nchs/data/series/sr_13/sr13_102.pdf (accessed September 2013).

Hogan, C., J. Lunney, J. Gabel, and J. Lynn. 2001. Medicare beneficiaries' costs of care in the last year of life. *Health Affairs (Millwood)* 20:188-195.

Hoover, D. R., S. Crystal, R. Kumar, U. Sambamoorthi, and J. C. Cantor. 2002. Medical expenditures during the last year of life: Findings from the 1992-1996 Medicare current beneficiary survey. *Health Services Research* 37:1625-1642.

Hurd, M. D., P. Martorell, A. Delavande, K. J. Mullen, and K. M. Langa. 2013. Monetary costs of dementia in the United States. *New England Journal of Medicine* 368:1326-1334.

IOM (Institute of Medicine). 2002. *Unequal treatment: Confronting racial and ethnic disparities in health care*. Washington, DC: The National Academies Press.

IOM. 2013. *Variation in health care spending: Target decision making, not geography*. Washington, DC: The National Academies Press.

Jacobson, G., T. Neuman, and A. Damico. 2010. *Medicare spending and use of medical services for beneficiaries in nursing homes and other long-term care facilities: A potential for achieving medicare savings and improving the quality of care*. http://kaiserfamily foundation.files.wordpress.com/2013/01/8109.pdf (accessed October 2013).

Jones, A. L., L. L. Dwyer, A. R. Bercovitz, and G. W. Strahan. 2009. The National Nursing Home Survey: 2004 overview. *Vital Health Statistics* 13.

Kelley, A. S., S. L. Ettner, R. S. Morrison, Q. Du, N. S. Wenger, and C. A. Sarkisian. 2011. Determinants of medical expenditures in the last 6 months of life. *Annals of Internal Medicine* 154:235-242.

Kelley, A. S., S. L. Ettner, R. S. Morrison, Q. Du, and C. A. Sarkisian. 2012. Disability and decline in physical function associated with hospital use at end of life. *Journal of General Internal Medicine* 27:794-800.

Kelley, A. S., P. Deb, Q. Du, M. D. Aldridge Carlson, and R. S. Morrison. 2013. Hospice enrollment saves money for Medicare and improves care quality across a number of different lengths-of-stay. *Health Affairs (Millwood)* 32:552-561.

Leff, B., L. Burton, S. L. Mader, B. Naughton, J. Burl, S. K. Inouye, W. B. Greenough III, S. Guido, C. Langston, K. D. Frick, D. Steinwachs, and J. R. Burton. 2005. Hospital at Home: Feasibility and outcomes of a program to provide hospital-level care at home for acutely ill older patients. *Annals of Internal Medicine* 143:798-808.

Leff, B., L. Burton, S. Mader, B. Naughton, J. Burl, R. Clark, W. B. Greenough III, S. Guido, D. Steinwachs, and J. R. Burton. 2006. Satisfaction with Hospital at Home care. *Journal of the American Geriatrics Society* 54:1355-1363.

Levinsky, N. G., W. Yu, A. Ash, M. Moskowitz, G. Gazelle, O. Saynina, and E. J. Emanuel. 2001. Influence of age on Medicare expenditures and medical care in the last year of life. *Journal of the American Medical Association* 286:1349-1355.

The Lewin Group. 2010. *Individuals living in the community with chronic conditions and functional limitations: A closer look*. http://www.aspe.hhs.gov/daltcp/reports/2010/closerlook.pdf (accessed September 2013).

Lubitz, J. D., and G. F. Riley. 1993. Trends in Medicare payments in the last year of life. *New England Journal of Medicine* 328:1092-1096.

Lunney, J. R., J. Lynn, and C. Hogan. 2002. Profiles of older medicare decedents. *Journal of the American Geriatrics Society* 50:1108-1112.

Lunney, J. R., J. Lynn, D. J. Foley, S. Lipson, and J. M. Guralnik. 2003. Patterns of functional decline at the end of life. *Journal of the American Medical Association* 289:2387-2392.

Mittler, J. N., B. E. Landon, E. S. Fisher, P. D. Cleary, and A. M. Zaslavsky. 2010. Market variations in intensity of Medicare service use and beneficiary experiences with care. *Health Services Research* 45:647-669.

Morrison, R. S., J. Dietrich, S. Ladwig, T. Quill, J. Sacco, J. Tangeman, and D. E. Meier. 2011. Palliative care consultation teams cut hospital costs for Medicaid beneficiaries. *Health Affairs (Millwood)* 30:454-463.

Moses III, H., D. H. Matheson, E. R. Dorsey, B. P. George, D. Sadoff, and S. Yoshimura. 2013. The anatomy of health care in the United States. *Journal of the American Medical Association* 310:1947-1963.

National Center for Health Statistics. 2013. *Health, United States, 2012: With special feature on emergency care.* http://www.cdc.gov/nchs/data/hus/hus12.pdf#109 (accessed November 2013).

Nicholas, L. H., K. M. Langa, T. J. Iwashyna, and D. R. Weir. 2011. Regional variation in the association between advance directives and end-of-life Medicare expenditures. *Journal of the American Medical Association* 306:1447-1453.

NIHCM (National Institute for Health Care Management) Foundation. 2012, July. *The concentration of health care spending.* Data brief. http://www.nihcm.org/pdf/DataBrief3 %20Final.pdf (accessed September 2013).

Pritchard, R. S., E. S. Fisher, J. M. Teno, S. M. Sharp, D. J. Reding, W. A. Knaus, J. E. Wennberg, and J. Lynn J. 1998. Influence of patient preferences and local health system characteristics on the place of death. SUPPORT investigators. Study to understand prognoses and preferences for risks and outcomes of treatment. *Journal of the American Geriatrics Society* 46:1242-1250.

Riley, G. F., and J. D. Lubitz. 2010. Long-term trends in Medicare payments in the last year of life. *Health Services Research* 45:565-576.

Shugarman, L. R., C. E. Bird, C. R. Schuster, and J. Lynn. 2007. Age and gender differences in Medicare expenditures at the end of life for colorectal cancer decedents. *Journal of Women's Health* 16:214-227.

Sing, M., J. S. Banthin, T. M. Selden, C. A. Cowan, and S. P. Keehan. 2006. Reconciling medical expenditure estimates from the MEPS and NHEA, 2002. *Health Care Financing Review* 28:25-40.

Skinner, J., A. Chandra, D. Goodman, and E. S. Fisher. 2009. The elusive connection between health care spending and quality. *Health Affairs (Millwood)* 28:w119-w123.

Song, Y., J. Skinner, J. Bynum, J. Sutherland, J. E. Wennberg, and E. S. Fisher. 2010. Regional variations in diagnostic practices. *New England Journal of Medicine* 363:45-53.

Temel, J. S., J. A. Greer, A. Muzikansky, E. R. Gallagher, S. Admane, V. A. Jackson, C. M. Dahlin, C. D. Blinderman, J. Jacobsen, W. F. Pirl, J. A. Billings, and T. J. Lynch. 2010. Early palliative care for patients with metastatic non-small-cell lung cancer. *New England Journal of Medicine* 363:733-742.

Teno, J. M., E. S. Fisher, M. B. Hamel, K. Coppola, and N. V. Dawson. 2002. Medical care inconsistent with patients' treatment goals: Association with 1-year Medicare resource use and survival. *Journal of the American Geriatrics Society* 50:496-500.

Teno, J. M., A. Gruneir, Z. Schwartz, A. Nanda, and T. Wetle. 2007. Association between advance directives and quality of end-of-life care: A national study. *Journal of the American Geriatrics Society* 55:189-194.

Thompson, J. W., M. D. Carlson, and E. H. Bradley. 2012. US hospice industry experienced considerable turbulence from changes in ownership, growth, and shift to for-profit status. *Health Affairs (Millwood)* 31:1286-1293.

Tschirhart, E. C., Q. Du, and A. S. Kelley. In press. Factors influencing the use of intensive procedures in the last 6 months of life. *Journal of the American Geriatrics Society.*

Ward, B. W., and J. S. Schiller. 2013. Prevalence of multiple chronic conditions among US adults: Estimates from the National Health Interview Survey, 2010. *Preventing Chronic Disease* 10.

Welch, H. G., S. M. Sharp, D. J. Gottlieb, J. S. Skinner, and J. E. Wennberg. 2011. Geographic variation in diagnosis frequency and risk of death among Medicare beneficiaries. *Journal of the American Medical Association* 305:1113-1118.

Wennberg, J. E., K. Bronner, J. S. Skinner, E. S. Fisher, and D. C. Goodman. 2009. Inpatient care intensity and patients' ratings of their hospital experiences. *Health Affairs (Millwood)* 28:103-112.

Yasaitis, L., E. S. Fisher, J. S. Skinner, and A. Chandra. 2009. Hospital quality and intensity of spending: Is there an association? *Health Affairs (Millwood)* 28:w566-w572.

Zhang, B., A. A. Wright, H. A. Huskamp, M. E. Nilsson, M. L. Maciejewski, C. C. Earle, S. D. Block, P. K. Maciejewski, and H. G. Prigerson. 2009. Health care costs in the last week of life: Associations with end-of-life conversations. *Archives of Internal Medicine* 169:480-488.

Zhang, J. X., P. J. Rathouz, and M. H. Chin. 2003. Comorbidity and the concentration of health care expenditures in older patients with heart failure. *Journal of the American Geriatrics Society* 51:476-482.

Appendix F

Pediatric End-of-Life and Palliative Care: Epidemiology and Health Service Use

Chris Feudtner, M.D., Ph.D., M.P.H.[1,2]

Wenjun Zhong, Ph.D.[1]

Jen Faerber, Ph.D.[1]

Dingwei Dai, Ph.D.[1]

James Feinstein, M.D., M.P.H.[3]

Each year in the United States, just over 45,000 infants, children, and adolescents die, with another 18,500 deaths among young adults aged 20 to 24. These deaths, while representing only a small proportion of all deaths in America, are nevertheless vitally important when considering how the U.S. health care system can better meet the needs of patients approaching the end of life. Pediatric patients who die are widely acknowledged to present many challenges that distinguish them from adult patients: they live with and die from a wide array of often-rare diseases that require specialized care; the trajectory of their illness experiences is often either much shorter or far longer than that of adult patients; the child is always cared for in the context of a family, which also needs support and often care; the mechanism of financing health care in general and palliative care specifically is different for the young versus older adults; and serious pediatric illness and death during childhood present emotional and even spiritual challenges to those who love and care for these patients.

The past decade has witnessed remarkable changes in the care that can be provided to children with life-threatening conditions and their families. The field of interdisciplinary pediatric palliative care has become a well-recognized specialty, with an ever-increasing number of children's hospitals creating and developing interdisciplinary pediatric palliative care teams. Pediatric hospice has likewise advanced with the development and

---

[1]The Children's Hospital of Philadelphia.
[2]The Perelman School of Medicine at the University of Pennsylvania.
[3]The Children's Hospital of Colorado and the University of Colorado School of Medicine.

promulgation of practice standards, and with the increased possibility of pediatric patients with serious illness receiving hospice care concurrent with other modes of disease treatment. At the same time, all the challenges outlined above remain, and in certain ways as the opportunities to improve care for dying children have increased, the urgency of doing so has likewise increased. This appendix is intended to clarify the epidemiology and health service use of those receiving pediatric end-of-life and palliative care.

The analysis offered here is much more at the level of populations of patients as opposed to individual patients. Many of the most important aspects of pediatric end-of-life care can be understood only with what might be called the "3-foot view," obtained by sitting with patients and parents and care providers and listening to and learning from their experiences. This appendix, by contrast, is based on national mortality and health service data that offer a 3,000-foot view whereby general trends of disease and care can be seen, and on clinically detailed hospital data that allow a more specific 300-foot view of the ways in which groups of patients have received care.

DEFINITIONS

Before proceeding, we define and discuss key terms and concepts used throughout this appendix.

End of life: An ambiguous yet important period of time prior to death.

The end of life is perhaps best thought of as beginning when an illness, injury, or condition progresses to the point where the health status of the patient is diminished below a level that would make it possible to live in a way that is meaningful or acceptable to that individual and ends with the patient's death. This time period may represent the flash of a second (as is the case for patients who die instantly from trauma) or extend for several weeks or longer (as is the case for patients with progressive cancer who experience a mounting symptom burden).

The start of this time period, when the health status of the patient is judged to have descended below a threshold beyond which meaningful or acceptable quality of life is no longer possible, is subjective: seemingly similar patients and their families will make different judgments about what this threshold is, and thus when this time period starts. Because the start of this end-of-life period is a combination of both a biological process and value judgments, a change in either the patient's biology (such as physiologic organ failure) or a value judgment about the patient's health status (such as living with severe impairments that require technology support) can mark the beginning of the end of life.

Because this definition requires individual-level clarity about biology and value judgments, it cannot be applied in most large population datasets, which lack such data elements. As an approximation, then, epidemiologic and health services research can focus on a defined period of time prior to the day and time of death as the "end of life." This is a useful and often illuminating retrospective analytic strategy for population-level studies, but such uniform definitions should not be confused with the individual-level definition that is required for individual-level care and that is the required basis of any prospective study.

Care at the end of life: All forms of care—including medical, surgical, nursing, psychosocial, spiritual, and hospice—received by patients during the end-of-life period prior to death.

For the reasons discussed above, this period of time may vary substantially at the individual level across otherwise similar patients. During this period, moreover, the care received also can vary substantially depending upon the individual-level goals of care and available resources.

Palliative care: Care for patients with serious illness that is intended to palliate symptoms, enhance comfort, and improve quality of life.

Palliative care is compatible with other modes of care, such as disease-directed, cure-seeking, or life-prolonging care. Palliative care for patients with serious illness can begin long before they enter their end-of-life phase and can continue after they die, in the form of bereavement care for those who loved them. Palliative care is not synonymous with end-of-life care given the longer time frame in which it can be provided and the fact that the goals of end-of-life care often differ from those that guide palliative care, such as ongoing health maintenance interventions (for example, vaccinations), attendance at school, or involvement in other "normal" family and life activities.

Serious pediatric illness and life-threatening conditions: Illnesses and conditions that pose a significant risk of death and typically impose physical, emotional, and other forms of distressing symptoms upon patients at some point in the illness trajectory.

The distress caused by serious pediatric illness and life-threatening conditions can often be alleviated to varying degrees by the receipt of palliative care. Serious pediatric illness and life-threatening conditions are not prerequisites for the appropriate receipt of pediatric palliative care; patients with less severe forms of disease can also benefit from such care.

Pediatric age range: The range of ages at which patients with serious illness and life-threatening conditions are often treated by pediatric-oriented health care providers and hospitals.

The pediatric age range is not defined by a legal or administrative threshold (such as the 18th birthday, when individuals are granted some but not all rights and privileges of adulthood, or the 21st birthday, which is defined by the National Institutes of Health as the demarcation between children and adults). Rather, the pediatric age range is observed to extend from the prenatal period (when consultations about fetal health are provided by perinatologists) through young adulthood. At various points during the late teen years or early 20s, patients typically transition to adult-oriented health care providers (and indeed, for patients cared for by family physicians, the transition is one not of clinical provider but instead of the nature of the patient-clinician interaction). For pediatric patients with serious illness and life-threatening conditions, however, this transition is often delayed or avoided entirely because of concerns regarding continuity of care for very ill patients, or the need for specialized knowledge about disease processes or treatments that resides predominantly in pediatric clinicians and children's hospitals. While many of the studies and analyses discussed in this appendix are restricted to persons and patients below age 18 or 20, others extend the age range covered to 24 and even beyond, making it possible to see how the pediatric health care system is used to serve the needs of certain young adult patients.

DATA SOURCES

In addition to reviewing the published literature, we used the datasets described below in preparing this appendix.

Mortality Data

Centers for Disease Control and Prevention (CDC) mortality data (http://wonder.cdc.gov) are produced by the CDC's National Center for Health Statistics (NCHS). Currently, the dataset spans 1968 to 2010 and comprises a county-level national mortality file and a corresponding county-level national population file.

CDC mortality data based on the NCHS annual detailed mortality files include a record for every death of a U.S. resident recorded in the United States. The annual detailed mortality files contain an extensive set of variables derived from the death certificates. For the Compressed Mortality data, the source data records are condensed with only a subset of variables being retained: (1) state and county of residence; (2) year of death; (3) race; (4) sex; (5) for 1999-2010, Hispanic origin (not Hispanic or Latino, Hispanic or Latino); (6) age group at death (specific age recoded to 16 age groups); (7) underlying cause of death (1968-1978 with International Classification of Diseases [ICD]-8 codes, 1979-1998 with ICD-9 codes, and 1999-2010 with ICD-10 codes).

For the detailed mortality file or Multiple Cause of Death data, the data are based on death certificates for U.S. residents. Currently the data span the years 1999-2010. Each death certificate contains a single underlying cause of death, up to 20 additional multiple causes, and demographic data. The number of deaths, crude death rates or age-adjusted death rates, and 95 percent confidence intervals and standard errors for death rates can be obtained by place of residence (total United States, region, state, and county), age group (single year of age, 5-year age groups, 10-year age groups, and infant age groups), race, Hispanic ethnicity, gender, year, month and weekday of death, and cause of death (four-digit ICD-10 code or group of codes). Data are also available for injury intent and injury mechanism, drug/alcohol-induced causes, and urbanization categories, as well as place of death and whether an autopsy was performed.

The CDC mortality data are publicly available, and researchers need to agree to data use restrictions.

National Inpatient and Emergency Department Data

The Kids' Inpatient Dataset (KID, http://www.hcup-us.ahrq.gov/kidoverview.jsp) is part of the Healthcare Cost and Utilization Project (HCUP) sponsored by the Agency for Healthcare Research and Quality (AHRQ).

The KID, compiled every 3 years, is composed of hospitalization discharge data from approximately 3 million hospitalizations of patients under age 21. Versions exist for 1997, 2000, 2003, 2006, and 2009. Over the years, more states have been represented, with data from 44 states being included in 2009. The sample is constructed in a manner that allows weighted analyses to generate national estimates, equivalent in 2009 to approximately 7 million hospitalizations.

The KID contains more than 100 clinical and nonclinical variables for each hospital stay, including ICD-9, Clinical Modification (ICD-9-CM) diagnosis and external cause of injury codes; ICD-9-CM and Current Procedural Terminology, Fourth Edition (CPT®-4) procedure codes; admission and discharge status; patient demographic characteristics (e.g., sex, age, urban-rural designation of residence, national quartile of median household income for patient's zip code); expected payment source; total hospital charges; and hospital characteristics (e.g., region, trauma center indicator, urban-rural location, teaching status).

The Nationwide Emergency Department Sample (NEDS, http://www.hcup-us.ahrq.gov/nedsoverview.jsp) is also part of the HCUP. It is the largest all-payer emergency department (ED) database in the United States, yielding national estimates of hospital-based ED visits. In 2011, 28 HCUP states participated in the 2011 NEDS, providing data on 29 million ED visits at 951 hospitals.

The NEDS contains clinical and nonclinical variables regarding the ED encounter as well as linked data for any subsequent hospitalization, as described above for the KID. The dataset also identifies injury-related ED visits, including mechanism, intent, and severity of injury; total ED charges (for ED visits); and total hospital charges (for inpatient stays for ED visits that result in admission).

Both the KID and NEDS data are available for purchase through the HCUP Central Distributor. All users of the KID and NEDS must complete the online Data Use Agreement training, sign a Data Use Agreement, and send a copy to AHRQ.

Clinically Detailed Administrative Hospitalization Data

The Pediatric Health Information System (PHIS, http://www.chca.com/index_flash.html) is maintained by the Child Hospital Association (Kansas City, Kansas). It contains clinically detailed administrative discharge data on more than 18 million patient encounters from 43 not-for-profit, tertiary children's hospitals in the United States, representing most of the major metropolitan areas nationwide. The data are updated on a quarterly basis. The quality and reliability of the data are assured through a joint effort of the Child Hospital Association, the data manager (Thomson-Reuters, Durham, North Carolina), and participating hospitals. Data are accepted into the PHIS database only when classified errors occur in less than 2 percent of a hospital's quarterly data.

The Premier Perspective Database (PPD) is the product of a consortium of U.S. not-for-profit hospitals and health systems, maintained by Premier, Inc. (San Diego, California) (http://www.premierinc.com). It currently serves a broad array of academic medical centers, community-based hospitals, and other health care sites, distributed throughout the urban and rural United States. The PPD represents hospitals that admit both children and adults. It compiles hospital data from approximately one-sixth of all hospitalizations in the United States and contains information on more than 130 million patient discharges. About two-thirds of the member hospitals update their data monthly, and the rest update quarterly. Upon receiving data from participating hospitals, the PPD undertakes an extensive multi-phase data validation and correction process.

PHIS and PPD data elements are largely the same. They include patient characteristics (e.g., age, sex, admission and discharge dates, All Patient Refined-Diagnosis Related Groups [APR-DRGs]); diagnoses (e.g., discharge diagnosis based on ICD-9, order of diagnoses); pharmacy data (e.g., medications, route, date of administration, pharmacy charge); procedures (based on ICD-9 codes and date of procedure); supply (supply ordered, day supply delivered, and supply charge); laboratory tests (test ordered, date laboratory result delivered, but not actual results); radiologic imaging (imaging procedure, utilization of contrast media, date ordered, but not results);

and clinical services (including date provided and charge for the service). Researchers interested in using PHIS or PPD data should inquire with the respective data management organizations.

Other Data Sources and Data Needs

For the sake of thoroughness, we mention other large data sources not used in this appendix—in particular, Medicaid claims data and data from either health maintenance organizations (such as Kaiser Permanente and Group Health Cooperative) or commercial insurance plans. To date, only a limited number of epidemiologic and health services research studies regarding pediatric mortality and pediatric end-of-life and palliative care have used these data sources.

There is a compelling need for data that would provide a longitudinal "all services" perspective on the health care experience of pediatric patients with serious illness. By "all services," we mean to include hospital care; outpatient care; inpatient and outpatient pharmacy services; and home nursing, hospice, respite, and other services. Ideally, these data would be both "all payer" and "all services," providing a population-level perspective, so that any differences or confounding bias between patients covered, for example, by government versus commercial payers could be identified and accounted for. If not "all payer," a data source representing the various types of payers would be a major advance. Additionally, these data need to be organized such that individual patient experiences, while being appropriately deidentified, could be analyzed over time to discern patterns of care. Many data sources, such as the KID and NEDS, do not enable such longitudinal analyses. The development of a data source with these characteristics would represent a major advance for pediatric end-of-life and palliative care research.

Finally, a data source is needed that includes indicators of the goals of care, such as the occurrence of a "goals of care" discussion between the patient/parent and the medical team, or the initiation of "do not attempt resuscitation" orders, with timestamps regarding when such markers of goals of care occur. These data would enable analysis of how care changes in response to such occurrences and whether care provided is congruent with care goals. Because of practical considerations concerning how such data on goals of care would be obtained, these data sources would likely be much smaller than those outlined above.

FINDINGS AND INTERPRETATIONS

Annual Number of Deaths and Trends Over Time

In 2010, there were 45,068 deaths in the United States among persons aged 19 or younger and another 18,664 deaths among persons aged 20-24. Combining these groups, there were 63,732 deaths.

Historically, as depicted in Figure F-1a, the number of deaths has declined remarkably since 1968, especially among those in the infant age range. This decline in numbers is not due to a decline in the overall size of the population in this age range; in a corresponding manner, the rates of death (per person in each age range) have also plummeted (see Figure F-1b).

Age Distribution of Pediatric Deaths

The peak age of pediatric mortality, by far, is during the first year of life (see Figure F-2a). Accordingly, pediatric palliative care must be designed to address the needs of neonates and infants, as well as their parents and families.

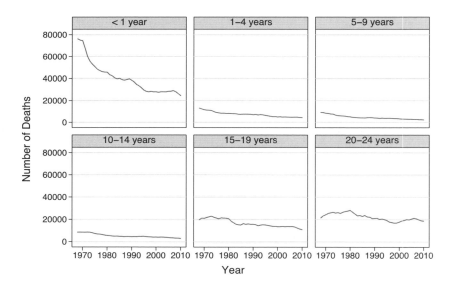

FIGURE F-1a Annual number of pediatric deaths in the United States, 1968-2010. SOURCE: Based on Multiple Cause of Death data 1968-2010 from CDC WONDER online database.

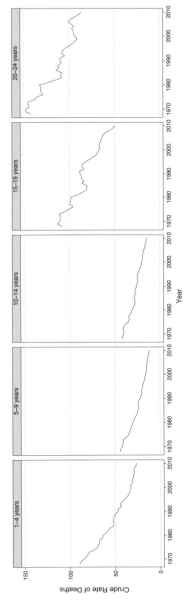

FIGURE F-1b Annual rates of pediatric deaths in the United States, 1968-2010.
NOTE: Omits infants, whose rate declined from 2,178 to 623 per 10,000 persons.
SOURCE: Based on Multiple Cause of Death data 1968-2010 from CDC WONDER online database.

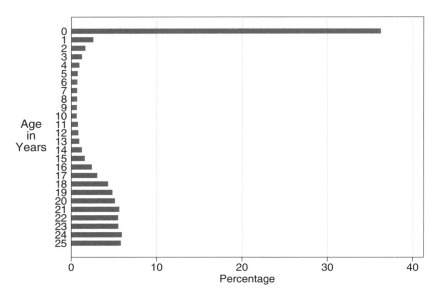

FIGURE F-2a Age distribution of pediatric deaths by year of age.
SOURCE: Based on Multiple Cause of Death data 2010 from CDC WONDER online database.

A closer look at the age distribution of pediatric deaths within the first year of life reveals the prominence of deaths within the first hours of life (see Figure F-2b). These rapid demises require that palliative care for these infants and their parents be close at hand, which is to say in places where infants are born (and antenatally as well, for prenatal visits and potentially the development of palliative care birth plans) and in newborn nurseries and neonatal intensive care units.

Causes of Pediatric Death

The single most important cause of pediatric and young adult deaths is trauma and other external causes, followed by conditions arising in the perinatal period (as underscored in the previous figures) and congenital malformations and chromosomal abnormalities (see Figure F-3).

Prevalence of Children with Conditions Warranting Palliative Care

Estimating the prevalence or number of children with conditions warranting palliative care is a difficult task for at least four reasons.

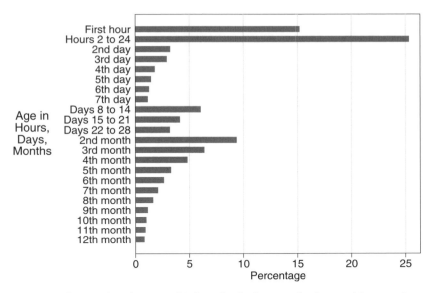

FIGURE F-2b Age distribution of infant deaths by month, day, and hours of age.
SOURCE: Based on Multiple Cause of Death data 2010 from CDC WONDER
online database.

First, the case definition of "children with conditions warranting palliative care" is not clear-cut and is based to some degree on perspectives and
values. At one end of a spectrum, case definition might be cases of children
who are actively dying and in pain or suffering because of a symptom other
than pain, and for whom palliative care is clearly needed and warranted
(as part of end-of-life care). Near the middle of the spectrum are cases of
children who are not actively dying but are likely to die in the ensuing
months or next few years as a result of either the progressive worsening of
their underlying condition or their medical fragility (what are termed here
"life-threatening conditions"), and these cases are also likely to benefit
from the receipt of palliative care. Toward the other end of the spectrum
are cases of children who are unlikely to live out a normal life span, can be
expected to live with significant impairments, and may or may not currently
have symptoms that could be ameliorated with palliative care interventions
(so-called life-limiting conditions).

Second, imbedded in the definitions of both life-threatening and life-
limiting conditions are probability statements regarding the prognosis for
how long the children will live and the likelihood that they have symptoms
that could be ameliorated (or more generally, that their quality of life

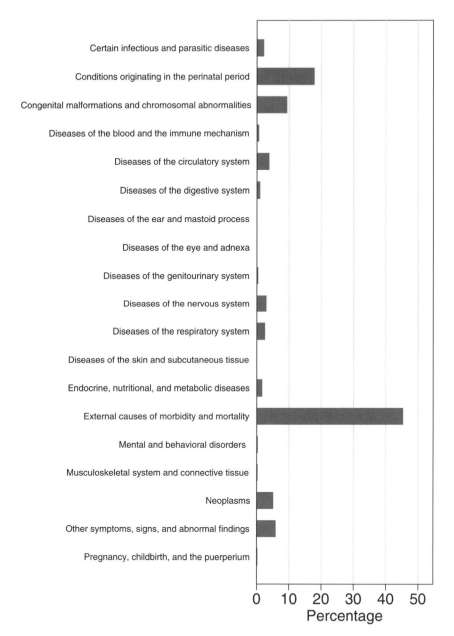

FIGURE F-3 Major causes of pediatric death.
SOURCE: Based on Multiple Cause of Death data 2010 from CDC WONDER online database.

or that of their parents or family could be improved). How large these probabilities need to be is largely a value-based decision. For example, would a patient with the following characteristics qualify as having a life-threatening condition that warrants palliative care: a combination of a 10 percent chance of dying in the next week, a 50 percent chance of dying sometime this coming year, and a 20 percent chance that symptom management could be improved with a palliative care approach?

Third, it is necessary to clarify the differences between point prevalence and period prevalence and their relevance for program development and policy considerations. Point prevalence refers to the number of cases at a given moment in time. Point prevalence is important for the design of clinical service programs, because it provides guidance on how much capacity these programs should have to take care of a specific number of patients. Period prevalence refers to the number of cases over a period of time, most often 1 year. For pediatric palliative care, period prevalence will be larger than point prevalence, because during the time period of 1 year, many cases will have both entered into the case definition (that is, developed the underlying condition) and died. Period prevalence is also relevant to program and policy development—not to understand the required daily capacity of palliative care teams but to understand the total palliative care workload of these teams. To clarify this distinction, consider two simplified scenarios. First, if the point prevalence were only 1 patient in a particular population but all the cases cared for by this team died within 1 day, then the annual period prevalence would be 365. By contrast, if the point prevalence were 20 but patients typically survived for 6 months or longer, then the annual period prevalence might be only 40. These two scenarios clarify how these two metrics—point prevalence and period prevalence—capture different perspectives on the nature and volume of the workload that a palliative care team would have to manage.

Fourth and finally, there is a relative lack of population-level data. There are to our knowledge no population-based assessments in the United States specifically designed to gather this information. A study based on primary data collection in the region around Bath, England, found an annual period prevalence of 1.2/1,000 children for conditions with a 50 percent chance or greater of causing death before age 40 while omitting patients with cancer or conditions that typically cause death within a month (Lenton et al., 2001). Another study, of all of England, based on analysis of health claims records and identifying cases on the basis of having diagnostic codes for conditions that are often the underlying conditions in patients receiving palliative care services, found an annual period prevalence of 3.2/1,000 children (Fraser et al., 2012).

With these caveats in mind, what can be offered as a range of estimates regarding the point and annual period prevalence of children with conditions that warrant palliative care? At one extreme, the data presented above regarding both the causes of death and age at the time of death strongly suggest that the point prevalence of pediatric patients living with life-threatening conditions on any given day is approximately equal to the annual number of deaths, or about 45,000. Why? Consider first the high proportion of all pediatric deaths represented by neonatal deaths and the short life span of many infants who die (1 day or 1 week). Consider second the high proportion of deaths beyond the neonatal period due to trauma (which often results in death immediately or within hours). Together, as stated above, these two observations imply that the point prevalence of infants and children living with life-threatening and life-shortening conditions may not be more than the annual cumulative incidence of pediatric deaths. The other end of the range of estimates—but also shifting from point prevalence to annual period prevalence—would be based on the English study of claims data, applying an annual prevalence of 3.2/1,000 to the population of infants, children, and adolescents in the United States (73.9 million) to estimate 236,480 potential pediatric palliative care patients over the course of 1 year (while also acknowledging that patients with these conditions might not warrant or want palliative care). A mid-range estimate would be based on the Bath study, adjusting a point prevalence of 1.2/1,000 upward by 100 percent to account for the omission of cancer patients and patients who died from acute conditions that typically cause death within 1 month, and so apply an estimated annual period prevalence of 2.4/1,000 to the U.S. pediatric age population. This approach would yield an annual period prevalence estimate of 177,360 children (but acknowledging that only 60 percent of the patients identified in the Bath study had pain).

Complex Chronic Conditions as a Cause of Pediatric Death

Amid the vast diversity of causes of pediatric deaths, a distinction can be drawn between life-threatening conditions that arise suddenly and most often unexpectedly (such as extreme premature birth, serious infections, and trauma) and complex chronic conditions (CCCs) that can be lethal. While many pediatric deaths are unexpected, those deaths attributed to these chronic conditions may have been foreseeable, providing an opportunity to provide palliative care and plan for end-of-life care.

CCCs have been defined as conditions likely to last 6 months or longer (unless death intervenes) and requiring care by pediatric subspecialists and often a period of hospital care. In turn, this definition can be used to classify ICD-9 codes indicative of CCC status, subcategorizing these diagnoses into organ- or system-based groups (Feudtner et al., 2000).

Among pediatric patients who died with a CCC diagnosis, the modal CCC categories are neonatal diagnoses, followed by cardiovascular and

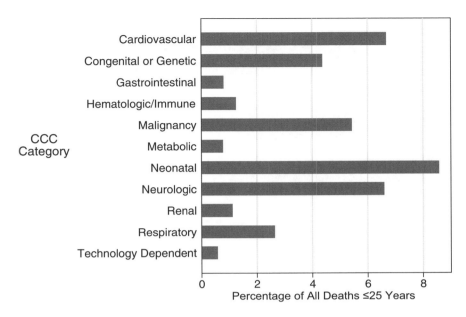

FIGURE F-4 Pediatric deaths involving complex chronic conditions.
SOURCE: Based on Multiple Cause of Death data 2010 from CDC WONDER online database.

neurologic conditions, and then malignancies (see Figure F-4). In other work, we have found that the proportion of all deaths due to CCCs is increasing because of the sharp declines in deaths due to trauma and other acute causes and the relative stability of rates of deaths due to CCCs.

Multiple Complex Chronic Condition Categories and Pediatric Deaths

In previous research, pediatric patients with a higher number of different categories of CCCs (e.g., cardiovascular and respiratory CCCs) have been found to have a heightened risk of readmission, more extensive health care utilization, and death. Among all pediatric deaths, one-third have CCCs, with 4.5 percent having two different categories of CCCs and 0.57 percent having three or more different categories (see Figure F-5).

Locations of Pediatric Deaths

Among all pediatric deaths (including trauma), the most common place of death for all persons aged 14 and younger is the hospital; this is the case

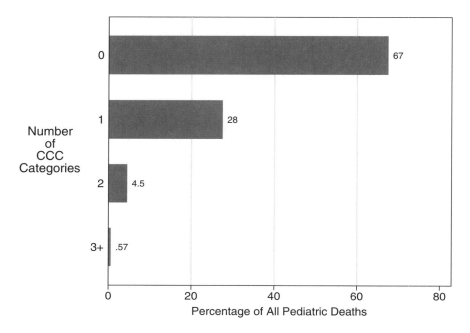

FIGURE F-5 Pediatric deaths involving multiple complex chronic conditions.
SOURCE: Based on Multiple Cause of Death data 2010 from CDC WONDER
online database.

especially for infants (74 percent of whom die in hospitals) (see Figure F-6).
EDs are also important sites of dying, as are homes.

Trajectories or Patterns of Experience of the Pediatric Dying Process

Based on the preceding data, as well as clinical experience, pediatric
patients who die typically experience one of four different patterns of illness trajectory: (1) sudden death (e.g., trauma, meningo-coccemia), (2) a
steady inexorable decline (e.g., unresectable brain tumor or Tay-Sachs), (3)
fluctuating decline (e.g., progressive diseases with intermittent crises, such
as worsening heart failure), and (4) constant medical fragility (e.g., "static"
neurologic impairment predisposing to crises due to infections or metabolic
decompensations) (see Figure F-7).

Good end-of-life care (illustrated by the shifts in the trajectories for
panels B, C, and D in Figure F-7, from black into the purple trajectories)
aims to improve quality of life and to prevent it from becoming so dominated by suffering that the patient descends to being in a worse-than-dead

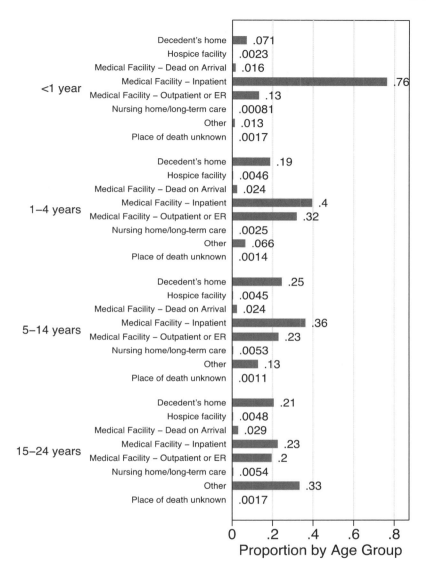

FIGURE F-6 Locations of pediatric deaths by age range.
SOURCE: Based on Multiple Cause of Death data 2010 from CDC WONDER online database.

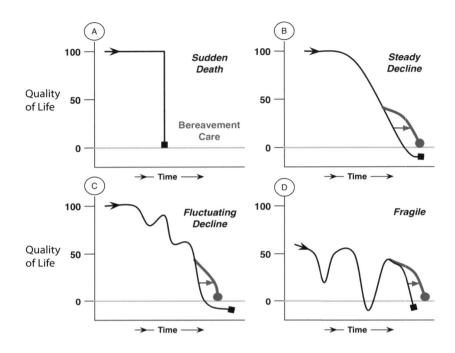

FIGURE F-7 Trajectories of pediatric dying.
SOURCE: A version of this figure appears in Feudtner, 2007. Reprinted with permission from Elsevier.

state (illustrated by the trajectories in the figure that fall below the grey line at zero quality of life). Interventions to improve or safeguard quality of life may have no impact on the patient's life span (as illustrated in panel B) or may shorten life span (panel C, illustrating the often-discussed "double effect" whereby medications designed to improve comfort may shorten life span) or lengthen life span (panel D, the "win-win effect"). Data with which to estimate which of these possibilities is most common are not available.

Although there are no precise epidemiologic data regarding the proportion of deaths that follow each trajectory, because many pediatric deaths follow trajectories A, C, or D, predicting death is either not appropriate (for trajectory A) or exceedingly imprecise (trajectories C and D). Furthermore, for trajectories C and D, patients and parents have often experienced previous serious medical crises from which the patient survived, which affects (accurately or inaccurately) the way they perceive a current health crisis.

Deaths Attributed to Complex Chronic
Conditions and Locations of Death

Again focusing on pediatric deaths attributed to CCCs (which is to say, deaths that may have been foreseeable and due to long-standing medical illness as opposed to trauma or sudden infectious illnesses), the number of such deaths declined overall from 1989 to 2006 (as shown previously for all pediatric deaths). Here we note a change in the locations of these deaths over time, with an increase in the number of deaths occurring at home (see Figure F-8).

Rising Proportion of Home Deaths Among Deaths
Attributed to Complex Chronic Conditions

The decline in deaths occurring in hospitals, combined with the rise in deaths occurring at home, has resulted in a significant increase in the proportion of all pediatric CCC-related deaths occurring at home (see Figure F-9). This increase may be due to a desire to have home be the place of death or to inadvertent deaths occurring to children who are medically

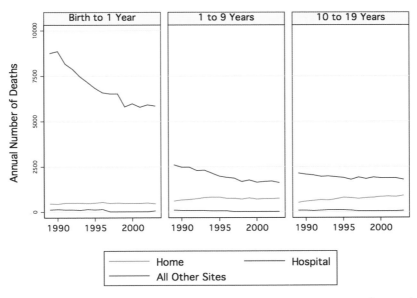

FIGURE F-8 Locations of death among deceased pediatric patients with complex chronic conditions.
SOURCE: Based on Multiple Cause of Death data from CDC; see Feudtner et al., 2007.

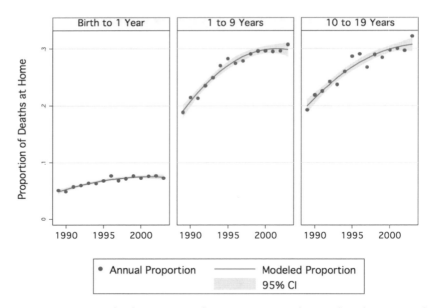

FIGURE F-9 Home deaths among pediatric patients with complex chronic conditions who died.
SOURCE: Based on Multiple Cause of Death data from CDC; see Feudtner et al., 2007.

fragile as a result of illness or dependence upon medical technology. Either way, this shift in location of death underscores the importance of having sufficient community-based capacity to provide care in the home for pediatric patients with CCCs, in the mode of either hospice or home nursing services, as well as the need for community-based bereavement services for families (parents, siblings, and others).

Rising Proportion of Home Deaths Beyond Infancy for Deceased Patients with Complex Chronic Conditions

The rise in the proportion of CCC-associated deaths that have occurred at home is observed for most of the CCC categories, with a much larger proportion and increase over time seen in patients beyond infancy (see Figure F-10).

Differences Across Race and Ethnicity in Location of Death

Across race and ethnicity categories, there are striking differences in the probability of dying at home among pediatric deaths attributed to CCCs

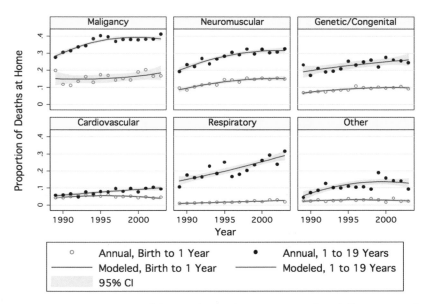

FIGURE F-10 Proportion of home deaths by age group for different complex chronic condition categories.
SOURCE: Based on Multiple Cause of Death data from CDC; see Feudtner et al., 2007.

(see Figure F-11). In other work focused on hospital care received by dying pediatric patients, we have not found such differences. This suggests that once a pediatric patient is hospitalized, care is fairly uniform across race and ethnicity categories, but access to home-based care (hospice or home nursing) may be limited because of either referral or supply or as the result of a culturally based preference not to be at home when death occurs.

State-Level Variation in Race and Ethnicity Disparities in Location of Death

The differences noted above also appear to depend upon where individuals reside. Examining the five largest states of residence in the United States (as illustrated in Figure F-12), marked state-level variation is evident even after stratification for specific underlying causes of death and specific age ranges: among these states, the baseline rates of death at home within each stratified group differ significantly. New York is observed to have had the lowest proportion of home deaths for all groups. White/non-Hispanic

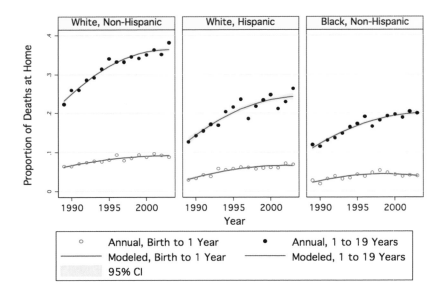

FIGURE F-11 Proportion of home deaths by age group for different race and ethnicity categories.
SOURCE: Based on Multiple Cause of Death data from CDC; see Feudtner et al., 2007.

children are observed to be more likely to have died at home than black/non-Hispanic and white/Hispanic children (with the exception of Florida for deaths due to neurologic CCCs among those aged 10-19). This geographic variability suggests that access to home-based services, in addition to any potential difference across race/ethnicity in preferences regarding palliative or end-of-life care, may be a major influence generating these differences.

Hospitalization During the Last Year of Life for Decedents with Complex Chronic Conditions

Hospitals are operationally important places in which to locate pediatric palliative care services. In multiple studies, the majority of patients whose deaths were attributed to a CCC were noted to have been hospitalized at some point during the last year of life. A study of Washington State data found that among deaths of pediatric patients with CCCs, 100 percent of infants and 84 percent of patients older than 1 year of age had been hospitalized prior to death, and many of these hospitalizations had

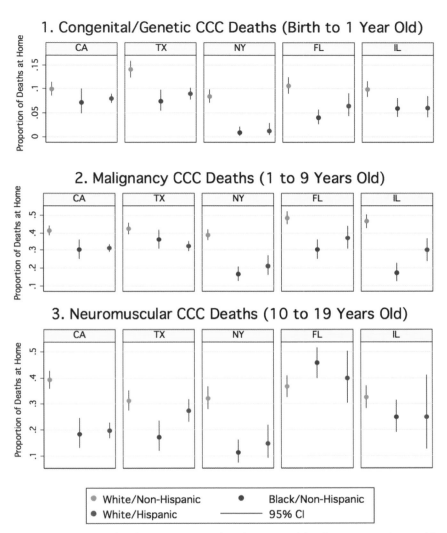

FIGURE F-12 State-level variation regarding location of death among patients with complex chronic conditions.
SOURCE: Based on Multiple Cause of Death data from CDC; see Feudtner et al., 2007.

occurred months prior to death (Feudtner et al., 2003). Hospital-based pediatric palliative care teams are thus positioned to introduce these patients
and their parents to palliative care during a hospitalization, including but
not limited to terminal hospitalizations.

At the same time, most patients spent the majority of their time outside
of the hospital. From the same study mentioned above, focusing on children with CCCs who were 1 year of age or older at the time of their death,
Figure F-13 shows the day-by-day prevalence of hospitalization among this
population of patients: as patients move closer to the time of death, a larger
proportion are residing in the hospital, but not until the final days are half
of the patients hospitalized. Thus, a robust system of pediatric palliative
care should be able to provide services both in hospitals and in homes. Because the vast majority of time during the last year of life is spent outside
of hospitals, mostly at home (and settings such as schools), the development
of community-based hospice or palliative care services for the delivery of
care in homes is vitally important.

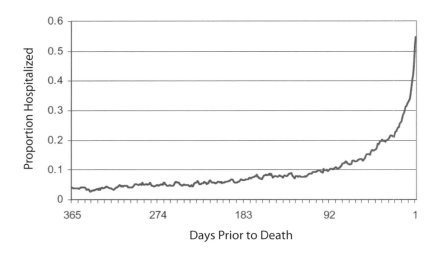

FIGURE F-13 Proportion hospitalized during the last year of life for pediatric patients >1 year of age with complex chronic conditions.
SOURCE: Based on data from Washington State; see Feudtner et al., 2003.

Terminal Hospitalization Lengths of Stay

Among pediatric patients who die during what proves to be a terminal hospitalization, the typical length of stay is a week or less, but with a very long tail of prolonged lengths of stay (see Figure F-14). Length of terminal hospitalizations does not vary substantially by patient age or race/ethnicity, but does vary based on the underlying diagnoses: these long lengths of stay are most common among patients with multiple CCCs, diagnosed either during that terminal hospitalization or during a previous hospitalization.

Intensity and Invasiveness of Terminal Hospitalization Care

Given that hospitals are where most pediatric deaths occur, examining the interventions received during terminal hospitalizations helps in assembling a portrait of pediatric end-of-life care (see Figure F-15). Most hospital deaths occur in intensive care unit (ICU) settings. Patients with no CCCs either quickly enter the ICU setting or remain outside of the ICU setting for the duration of their hospitalization. By contrast, patients with CCCs

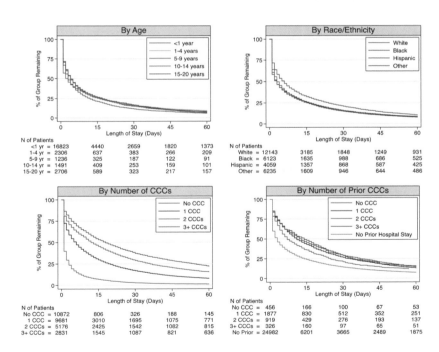

FIGURE F-14 Length of stay among pediatric patients who died in hospitals.
SOURCE: Based on PHIS and Premier data, 2007-2012.

appear to often decompensate during the course of a longer hospitalization and frequently require escalation of interventions and repeated transfers between the floor and the ICU. A similar pattern is observed for starting mechanical ventilation and undergoing the first surgery of a hospitalization

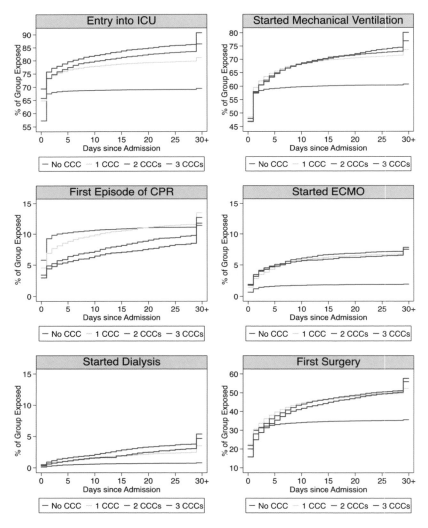

FIGURE F-15 Procedures to which pediatric patients who died in hospitals were exposed.
NOTE: ECMO = extracorporeal membrane oxygenation.
SOURCE: Based on PHIS and Premier data, 2007-2012.

(both of which are common interventions), as well as for the first episode of renal dialysis, cardiopulmonary resuscitation (CPR), or extracorporeal membranous oxygenation (ECMO).

Emergency Departments and Pediatric Deaths

As noted above, in addition to homes and hospitals, EDs are important locations of pediatric end-of-life care, with approximately 22 percent of pediatric deaths occurring in EDs in 2010 (Figure F-16 shows the age distribution of these deaths). Among an estimated (weighted sample) 29.6 million ED visits by pediatric patients (with a mean charge of $1,278), there were 9,699 deaths in EDs (with mean charges of $4,765), with another 4,449 deaths during a subsequent hospitalization (with mean ED charges for this group of $3,019). Among the ED deaths, 9.3 percent had CCCs. Among the ED patients who subsequently died in the hospital, 45 percent had CCCs. This suggests that most rapid demises that occur in EDs are due to acute processes, such as trauma or unexpected overwhelming infection, while patients with serious CCCs are stabilized in EDs and admitted to the

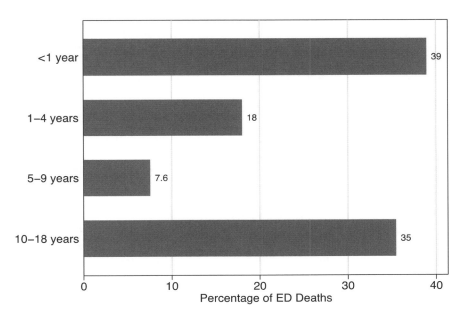

FIGURE F-16 Age distribution of pediatric deaths in emergency departments.
SOURCE: Based on data from NEDS, 2010.

hospital. Importantly, the care received by patients who died in EDs has not been characterized.

Pain and Symptoms Among Pediatric Patients Receiving Pediatric Palliative Care

In 2008, a 1-year cohort study conducted by six major hospital-based pediatric palliative care programs described the characteristics of pediatric patients receiving palliative care services (Feudtner et al., 2011). These patients experienced a broad array of impairments and symptoms, the most common being cognitive and speech impairment, fatigue and sleep problems, enteral intake, seizures, somatic pain, and dyspnea. While pain and dyspnea are prominent symptoms reported near the end of life for patients with cancer, this population includes many patients who are not near the end of life and who have conditions other than cancer, including many with neurologic or genetic conditions. Pediatric palliative care symptom management thus requires an extensive toolkit and considerable expertise. Unfortunately, research regarding pediatric symptom management is woefully lacking. This may be the single most important research priority.

Patterns of Survival Among Pediatric Palliative Care Patients

Pediatric patients receiving palliative care services have long (relative to common assumptions) life expectancies. In the cohort of 515 patients discussed in the previous section, 1-year survival was above 70 percent (Feudtner et al., 2011). This relatively long duration of survival (compared with adult patients receiving palliative care) means that pediatric palliative care services provide chronic care to patients with serious illness and are not limited to end-of-life care. Because many of these patients are hospitalized repeatedly, this also means that pediatric palliative care services often have very high daily census levels, consisting of new and ongoing patients.

Conceptual Models of Pediatric Palliative Care

Based on the findings presented thus far, with pediatric palliative care revealed as chronic care for pediatric patients with a broad array of serious and often complex illnesses, the ideal model of pediatric palliative care is not incompatible with so-called curative care (which often is not capable of effecting a cure as much as substantial life extension), nor does curative care have to be titrated down for palliative care to be titrated up (see Figure F-17). Instead, pediatric palliative care seeks to promote several modes of care simultaneously, including cure-seeking or life-extending care and quality-of-life and comfort-maximizing care, as well as support for family members and for health care staff.

Core Tasks of Pediatric Palliative Care

The core tasks of pediatric palliative care include the provision of effective interventions to enhance the well-being or comfort of patients, family, and staff; to assist in the logistical coordination of care across a variety of settings, including the hospital, home, and other facilities; and to support problem solving and decision making for patients, their surrogate decision makers, and health care staff (see Figure F-18).

1. Incompatable Domains of Curative Versus Palliative Care:

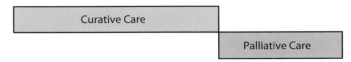

2. Competing Domains of Curative Versus Palliative Care:

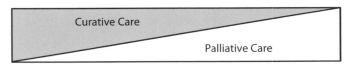

3. Complementary and Concurrent Components of Care:

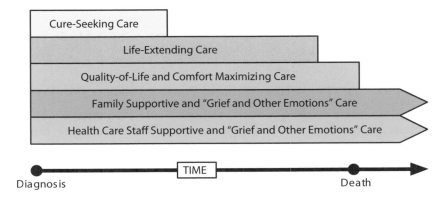

FIGURE F-17 Palliative care as patient-centered complementary and concurrent modes of care.
SOURCE: A version of this figure appears in Feudtner, 2007. Reprinted with permission from Elsevier.

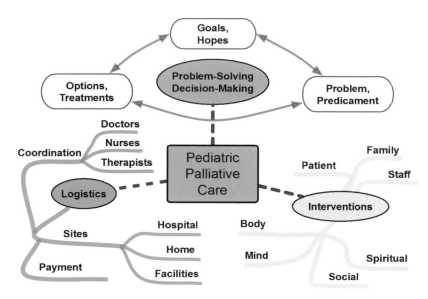

FIGURE F-18 Pediatric palliative care's three major tasks.
SOURCE: A version of this figure appears in Feudtner, 2007. Reprinted with permission from Elsevier.

Hospital-Based Pediatric Palliative Care Programs

Hospital-based pediatric palliative care programs are more common than was previously the case, arising across the United States. Figure F-19 shows programs identified by a 2012 survey of children's hospitals (Feudtner et al., 2013).

Establishment of New Hospital-Based Pediatric Palliative Care Programs

Most hospital-based pediatric palliative care programs are of recent vintage, having been established sometime after 2005; 12 new programs were established in 2008 alone, and another 10 were created in 2011 (Feudtner et al., 2013). These programs typically require substantial financial support from their hospital, given the relatively low rates of reimbursement for the kinds of services they provide. Ensuring the financial security of these programs is a major priority.

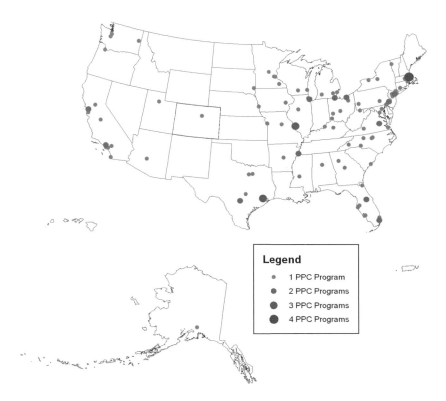

FIGURE F-19 Locations of hospital-based pediatric palliative care programs.
SOURCE: Feudtner et al., 2013. Reproduced with permission from Journal *Pediatrics*, Vol. 132, Page 1065, Coypright © 2013 by the AAP.

Staffing of Hospital-Based Pediatric Palliative Care Programs

Hospital-based pediatric palliative care programs are remarkably diverse in terms of staffing. Many programs subsist with a minimal staff, most commonly having less than a full-time equivalent (FTE) of physician time (Feutner et al., 2013). In the above-referenced survey of children's hospitals, more than half of surveyed programs had only one physician; of programs with more than one physician on staff, many had total physician staffing of less than one full-time equivalent. Staffing by nurses ranged from 0 to 6.6 FTE (with a mean overall FTE 0.8, and for advanced practice nurses in particular, a mean FTE of 0.4). While 66 percent of programs reported having a social worker, the mean social work FTE was only 0.29. All other members of the interdisciplinary team (including chaplains, child life specialists, bereavement specialists, music and art therapists, and psychologists) had mean FTE levels of 0.16 or less. This survey also demonstrated substantial differences in the clinical services provided by these programs. A major priority for both research and program development is to define and advance hospital-based pediatric palliative care program standards.

Hospital Charges for Pediatric Hospitalizations

We now turn to the financial aspects of pediatric end-of-life care. Ideally, we would be able to analyze cost data, including costs borne by patients, families, hospitals, and payers, but such data do not exist. We therefore focus here on hospital charges to illustrate and examine certain key issues, believing that this analysis can illuminate the financial aspects of pediatric end-of-life care.

We start with all pediatric hospitalizations. Among 8.6 million pediatric hospitalizations (which includes newborns) from 2007 to 2012 in the PHIS and Premier data, the median total charge was $8,167, and the mean was $28,654. The distribution of these charges fits the "Pareto principle" power law distribution almost exactly (see Figure F-20), with 78 percent of all hospital charges being concentrated among the top 20 percent of hospitalizations. Among the 0.5 percent of hospitalizations that ended with the death of the patient, the median charge was $68,279, and the mean was $290,416.

Correlation of Hospital Charges with Length of Stay in Children's Hospitals

Among all the above pediatric hospitalizations, the median length of stay was 2 days, with a mean of 3.6 days. The range of length of stay was from 0 to 877 days, with the 99th percentile at 35 days. Length of stay is the primary driver of total charges, with a correlation of 0.75 (see Figure F-21).

Long Lengths of Stay and Large Average Charges in Children's Hospitals

Reinforcing the fact that length of stay is a key driver of pediatric hospitalization charges, the average length of stay skyrockets among those patients with the largest hospital charges (see Figure F-22).

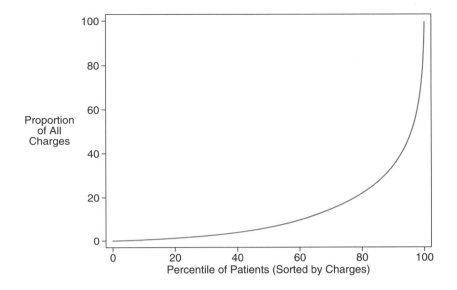

FIGURE F-20 Cumulative distribution of charges among hospitalized pediatric patients.
SOURCE: Based on data from PHIS and the Premier Perspective Database.

Prognosis and Predicted Probability of Death Among Hospitalized Pediatric Patients

Based on previous work, we implemented a prediction of mortality model, which we used as a tool for the subsequent analysis. In these data, the model is reasonably well calibrated. For example, patients with a predicted probability of dying of 0.5 were observed to have a proportion of death between 0.3 and 0.4 (see Figure F-23). Note that the calibration curve demonstrates that the predicted probability is biased upward, with those with the highest predicted probabilities of death never having an observed proportion of death as high as the predicted values.

Average Hospital Charges Across Predicted Probability of Death

Hospital charges are also associated with the probability of death, in a U-shaped function: some patients who die very soon after hospitalization incur relatively small charges, and patients with the largest charges have a much higher than average probability of having died (see Figure F-24).

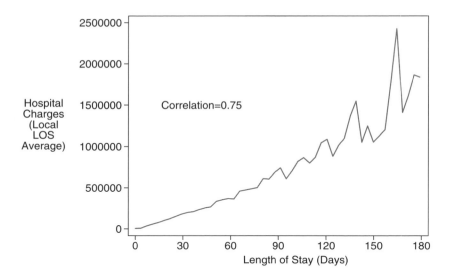

FIGURE F-21 Correlation of charges with length of stay (LOS) in children's hospitals.
SOURCE: Based on PHIS and Premier data, 2007-2012.

Note, though, that only 6 percent of those patients with the largest charges died. Stated differently, large hospital charges overwhelmingly are for children who survive.

Hospital Charges Across the Range of Predicted Probability of Death

If pediatric palliative care were to focus just on those patients with the highest probability of dying during that hospitalization, and this threshold could be set at a 50 percent predicted probability of dying (which, as was seen earlier, would translate into a slightly lower observed probability of dying), then the case mix would have a higher average hospital charge (approximately $500,000). These patients, though, account for only 4.7 percent of all charges (see Figure F-25). Furthermore, given that these large charges are accumulated over very long lengths of stay and that the probability of dying may have risen dramatically during the course of the hospitalization, the ability of pediatric palliative care to curtail these aggregate costs to a degree that would matter to the overall pattern of pediatric hospital expenditures is likely quite limited.

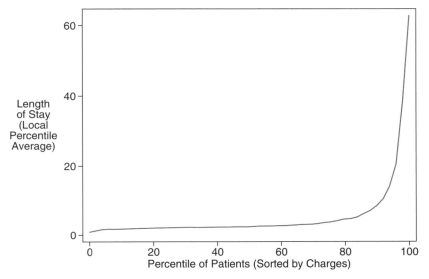

FIGURE F-22 Mean length of stay across the range of charges for patients in children's hospitals.
SOURCE: Based on PHIS and Premier data, 2007-2012.

This is not to say, however, that hospital-based pediatric palliative care is not cost-effective. With most pediatric palliative care programs requiring operating budgets of approximately $2 million per year, curtailing the length of stay of even a few long-stay terminal hospitalizations per year (or preventing terminal hospitalizations in the first place) would offset operating expenses.

Concurrent Care and Studies of Cost Implications

Beyond the analysis just presented, we used the following keywords and their combinations to search for publications on health care cost savings of pediatric palliative or hospice care: "pediatric or child," "palliative or hospice," "costs or (cost effectiveness) or spending or expenditure or savings," and "health care." We also checked the citations of some publications to look for other potential papers. This search revealed only three publications that focus on children and compare the cost before and after the initiation of palliative care:

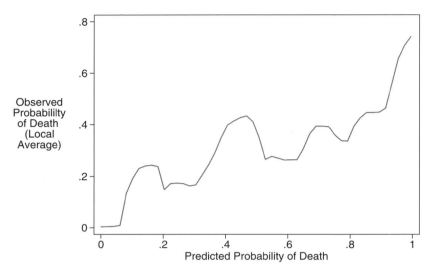

FIGURE F-23 Calibration of the predicted to the observed probability of death.
SOURCE: Based on PHIS and Premier data, 2007-2012.

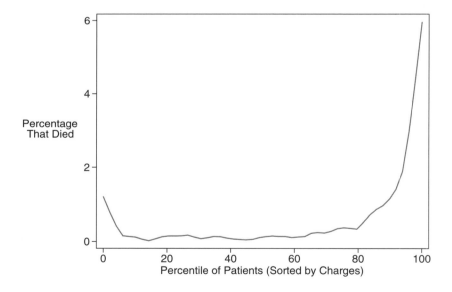

FIGURE F-24 Predicted probability of death across the range of hospital charges.
SOURCE: Based on PHIS and Premier data, 2007-2012.

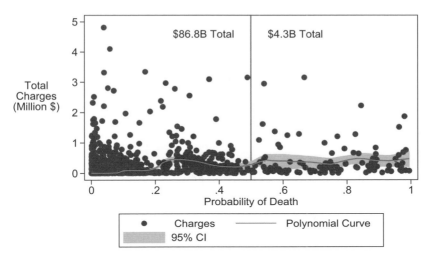

FIGURE F-25 Among patients in children's hospitals, the typical individual total charge across the range of the predicted probability of death.
NOTE: Total dollar sums are for patients who could be fitted in the model.
SOURCE: Based on PHIS and Premier data, 2007-2012.

- A small study (N = 66) from a children's hospital in Canada reports that providing respite care resulted in a mean decrease of $4,251.95 per month per patient (Pascuet et al., 2010).
- A California project shifted palliative care from hospital settings to in-home community-based care. The result was cost savings of $1,677 per child per month on average—an 11 percent decrease in spending on a traditionally high-cost population (Gans et al., 2012).
- Analyses involving data on Florida Medicaid children found that pediatric hospice users had higher inpatient (2.5 times), outpatient (1.1 times), ED (1.9 times), and pharmacy (2.3 times) expenditures than non-hospice users (a finding perhaps due to residual confounding by indication, whereby patients with greater ongoing need are referred to hospice more often than otherwise similar patients with less need). Black non-Hispanic and Hispanic children and children of other races incurred $730 to $880 less in hospice expenditures than whites (Knapp et al., 2009).

These mixed findings regarding the impact of pediatric palliative or hospice care on health care expenditures are consistent with the findings of a recent Cochrane Database Systematic Review focused on adult studies regarding the impact of home-based services. While receipt of such services is warranted based on symptom management and preferred place of dying, the cost implications are mixed (Gomes et al., 2013).

To assess the cost impact of pediatric palliative or hospice services, studies will have to ensure that any change in expenditures before and after exposure is due to exposure to the service, and not to a temporally confounded choice to pursue palliative or hospice care at the same time as the choice is made to forego or avoid further hospital-based or highly invasive forms of care.

Other Key Considerations Regarding Charge/Cost-Focused Evaluations of Pediatric End-of-Life Care

First, as argued above, while there may be greater certainty as death draws near (within hours or days), the potential cost savings that could arise from such prognostic knowledge would affect expenditures only from that point forward. And because large hospital bills are built on long lengths of stay, the marginal impact on the overall health care cost for hospital care may be more limited than is commonly hoped.

Second, many of the pediatric patients who consume the most resources are disabled, and they are vulnerable because of both disability-associated stigma and the impoverishment of families that can result from having a medically complex patient in the family. These patients are also protected by law from discrimination.

Gaps in Knowledge

Critical gaps exist in the knowledge and evidence base regarding many aspects of pediatric palliative care, including the follow six priority areas:

1. Comparative effectiveness studies of
    -   Symptom management approaches
        -   Pharmacologic
            -   Effectiveness of different medications and use of medications
            -   Potential problems of polypharmacy and drug-drug interactions
        -   Nonpharmacologic
    -   Different forms of providing decision support to patients and their surrogate decision makers
        -   How to communicate clearly regarding the patient's clinical situation

  – How to communicate effectively regarding potential benefits and harms of medical interventions
  – How to solicit, examine, and potentially adapt goals of care over time
  – How to support emotional as well as cognitive processing of this information
  – Different bereavement support interventions for family members and community peers

2. Descriptions of care
   • Received through hospice services and home nursing services, individually and in the concurrent care model
   • Received in different settings, including EDs, outpatient facilities, and long-term care facilities

3. Cohort studies examining the effect of receipt of palliative or hospice care
   • On patient-reported outcomes
   • On proxy reports by parents or others regarding patient experience
   • On outcomes defined using large clinically detailed datasets

4. Well-designed cost analyses regarding
   • The care received by pediatric patients with serious illness or complex chronic conditions
   • The impact of receipt of palliative care or hospice services

5. Studies of the impact of having a child with serious illness, while alive and after death
   • On parents
   • On siblings
   • On other family members, such as grandparents
   • On the patient's peer network of friends in school and elsewhere
   • Whether these impacts are modified if the patient or family is exposed to palliative or hospice care services

6. Studies of hospital-based pediatric palliative and community-based pediatric hospice services
   • How to best staff these services
   • How to optimize interdisciplinary team function
   • Best management practices
   • Financing challenges and best practices

REFERENCES

Feudtner, C. 2007. Collaborative communication in pediatric palliative care: A foundation for problem-solving and decision-making. *Pediatric Clinics of North America* 54(5):583-607.

Feudtner, C., D. A. Christakis, and F. A. Connell. 2000. Pediatric deaths attributable to complex chronic conditions: A population-based study of Washington State, 1980-1997. *Pediatrics* 106(1, Pt. 2):205-209.

Feudtner, C., D. L. DiGiuseppe, and J. M. Neff. 2003. Hospital care for children and young adults in the last year of life: A population-based study. *BMC Medicine* 1(1):3.

Feudtner, C., J. A. Feinstein, M. Satchell, H. Zhao, and T. I. Kang. 2007. Shifting place of death among children with complex chronic conditions in the United States, 1989-2003. *Journal of the American Medical Association* 297(24):2725-2732.

Feudtner, C., T. I. Kang, K. R. Hexem, S. J. Friedrichsdorf, K. Osenga, H. Siden, S. E. Friebert, R. M. Hays, V. Dussel, and J. Wolfe. 2011. Pediatric palliative care patients: A prospective multicenter cohort study. *Pediatrics* 127(6):1094-1101.

Feudtner, C., J. W. Womer, R. Augustin, S. S. Remke, J. Wolfe, S. Friebert, and D. E. Weissman. 2013. Pediatric palliative care programs in children's hospitals: A cross-sectional national survey. *Pediatrics* 132(6):1063-1070.

Fraser, L. K., M. Miller, R. Hain, P. Norman, J. Aldridge, P. A. McKinney, and R. C. Parslow. 2012. Rising national prevalence of life-limiting conditions in children in England. *Pediatrics* 129(4):e923-e929.

Gans, D., G. F. Kominski, D. H. Roby, A. L. Diamant, X. Chen, W. Lin, and N. Hohe. 2012. Better outcomes, lower costs: Palliative care program reduces stress, costs of care for children with life-threatening conditions. *Policy Brief (UCLA Center for Health Policy Research* (PB2012-3):1-8.

Gomes, B., N. Calanzani, V. Curiale, P. McCrone, and I. J. Higginson. 2013. Effectiveness and cost-effectiveness of home palliative care services for adults with advanced illness and their caregivers. *Cochrane Database of Systematic Reviews* 6:CD007760.

Knapp, C. A., E. A. Shenkman, M. I. Marcu, V. L. Madden, and J. V. Terza. 2009. Pediatric palliative care: Describing hospice users and identifying factors that affect hospice expenditures. *Journal of Palliative Medicine* 12(3):223-229.

Lenton, S., P. Stallard, M. Lewis, and K. Mastroyannopoulou. 2001. Prevalence and morbidity associated with non-malignant, life-threatening conditions in childhood. *Child: Care, Health and Development* 27(5):389-398.

Pascuet, E., L. Cowin, R. Vaillancourt, W. Splinter, C. Vadeboncoeur, L. G. Dumond, A. Ni, and M. Rattray. 2010. A comparative cost-minimization analysis of providing paediatric palliative respite care before and after the opening of services at a paediatric hospice. *Healthcare Management Forum* 23(2):63-66.

Appendix G

Committee Biographies

Philip A. Pizzo, M.D. (*Co-Chair*), served as dean of the School of Medicine and Carl and Elizabeth Naumann professor at Stanford University School of Medicine from 2001 to 2012. He is currently founding director of the Stanford Distinguished Careers College and David and Susan Heckerman professor of pediatrics and of microbiology and immunology at Stanford. Before joining Stanford, he was physician-in-chief of Children's Hospital in Boston and chair of the Department of Pediatrics at Harvard Medical School from 1996 to 2001. Dr. Pizzo is recognized for his contributions as a clinical investigator, especially in the treatment of children with cancer and HIV. He devoted much of his medical career to the diagnosis, management, prevention, and treatment of childhood cancers and the infectious complications that occur in children whose immune system is compromised by cancer and AIDS. He and his research team pioneered the development of new treatments for children with HIV infection, lengthening and improving their quality of life. Dr. Pizzo served as head of the National Cancer Institute's (NCI's) infectious disease section, chief of its pediatric department, and acting scientific director for its Division of Clinical Sciences between 1973 and 1996. He was elected to the Institute of Medicine (IOM) in 1997 and served on the IOM Council from 2006 to 2012. He has held numerous leadership positions, including chair of the Council of Deans of the Association of American Medical Colleges, and has received numerous honors and awards for his work and contributions. He received his undergraduate degree from Fordham University and his M.D. from the University of Rochester School of Medicine. He completed an internship and residency at Children's Hospital Medical Center in Boston.

David M. Walker (*Co-Chair*) founded and served as CEO of the Comeback America Initiative (CAI). In this capacity, he led CAI's efforts to promote fiscal responsibility and sustainability by engaging the public and assisting key policy makers on a nonpartisan basis to help achieve solutions to America's federal, state, and local fiscal imbalances. Previously, Mr. Walker served as the seventh comptroller general of the United States and was head of the U.S. Government Accountability Office (GAO) for almost 10 years (1998-2008). His previous government positions included serving as a public trustee for Social Security and Medicare and as assistant secretary of labor for pension and welfare benefit programs. He also has more than 20 years of private-sector experience, including approximately 10 years as a partner and global managing director of Human Capital Services for Arthur Andersen, LLP. He holds a B.S. in accounting from Jacksonville University and a senior management in government certificate in public policy from Harvard University's John F. Kennedy School of Government and is a certified public accountant.

Patricia A. Bomba, M.D., FACP, is vice president and medical director of geriatrics for Excellus BlueCross BlueShield. In this role, she serves as a geriatric consultant on projects and program development affecting seniors. She is a nationally recognized palliative care and end-of-life expert who designs and oversees the implementation of community projects. Prior to her work at Excellus BlueCross BlueShield, she was in private practice in internal medicine and geriatrics in Rochester, New York. Dr. Bomba is New York State's representative on the National POLST Paradigm Task Force, a multistate collaborative. In addition to serving as a New York State Delegate to the White House Conference on Aging, she served as a member of the Review Committee of the National Quality Forum's "Framework and Preferred Practices for a Palliative and Hospice Care Quality" project and the American Board of Internal Medicine's Primary Palliative Care Committee, and chaired the BlueCross and BlueShield Association's National Medical Management Forum. She chairs New York's MOLST Statewide Implementation Team, serves as eMOLST program director, and is a member of the Medical Society of the State of New York's Ethics Committee. Dr. Bomba earned a bachelor's degree from Immaculata College and graduated from the University of Virginia School of Medicine. She completed her residency in internal medicine at the University of Rochester and is board certified in internal medicine, with added qualifications in geriatric medicine.

Eduardo Bruera, M.D., is clinical medical director and department chair of palliative care and rehabilitation medicine at The University of Texas MD Anderson Cancer Center. He also holds the F.T. McGraw Chair in the Treatment of Cancer at The University of Texas. Dr. Bruera has been interested in the development of palliative care programs internationally, particularly in the developing world, where he helped in the establishment of numerous palliative care programs in the Latin American region, India, and throughout Europe. He served as president of the International Association of Hospice and Palliative Care for a period of 4 years ending in January 2006. He established the first academic fellowship in palliative care at the University of Alberta in Canada and one of the first academic palliative care fellowships in the United States at The University of Texas MD Anderson Cancer Center. He obtained his M.D. from the University of Rosario in Argentina. He trained in medical oncology and relocated to the University of Alberta in Edmonton, Canada, where he directed the clinical and academic palliative care programs until 1999.

Charles J. Fahey, M.S.W., M.Div., is a program officer with the Milbank Memorial Fund and a priest of the Diocese of Syracuse, New York. He previously served as an aging studies professor in the Fordham University Graduate School of Social Services. He was also a member of the National Commission on Quality in Long Term Care. He founded the Third Age Center at Fordham University in 1979. Msgr. Fahey was a charter member of the Federal Council on Aging, serving under Presidents Nixon, Ford, and Carter. He was a spokesperson for the Holy See at the 1982 World Assembly on Aging (Vienna); he served in leadership roles for the 1971, 1981, 1995 White House Conferences on Aging, and served as a delegate in 2005. He has been a board member and president of Catholic Charities USA, the American Association of Homes and Services for the Aging, and the American Society on Aging. He also has been a board member of the Catholic Health Association, the Daughters of Charity National Health System (Ascension), the Sisters of Mercy Health Care System, and Volunteers of America. He is currently a board member of ArchCare, the continuing care community of the Archdiocese of New York, and immediate past chair and board member of the National Council on Aging. He was ordained as a Roman Catholic priest in the Diocese of Syracuse, New York, and earned his master of social work degree from Catholic University in Washington, DC.

Pamela S. Hinds, Ph.D., R.N., FAAN, is director of the Department of Nursing Research and Quality Outcomes and associate director of the Center for Translational Science at Children's National Health System in Washington, DC. She has expertise in the care of children with cancer and in the development of effective team care to meet the immediate and long-term needs of children and their families. Her research focuses on decision making in pediatric oncology, coping and adolescents, the good parent concept in end-of-life care, and the experience of pediatric oncology nurses.

She was founding director of the Division of Nursing Research at St. Jude Children's Research Hospital, where she led the nursing research program for more than two decades. Dr. Hinds currently serves on NCI's Symptom and Quality of Life Scientific Committee and is co-director of the Patient-Reported Outcomes (PRO) Resource Center for the Children's Oncology Group. She is a member of the National Institute of Nursing Research's Ad Hoc Evaluation Advisory Committee for *End-of-Life and Palliative Care Science: A Needs Assessment of Federal and Private Research Funding Trends, Project Grants, and National Research Priorities.* She also served on the National Quality Forum's panel on palliative and end-of-life care in America and on the 2003 IOM Committee on Palliative and End-of-Life Care for Children and Their Families. Dr. Hinds received her undergraduate degree magna cum laude from the University of Vermont, Burlington, and her M.S.N. in psychiatric nursing (summa cum laude) and Ph.D. in clinical nursing research from the University of Arizona, Tucson.

Karla F. C. Holloway, Ph.D., M.L.S., M.A., is James B. Duke professor of English at Duke University. She also holds appointments in the Law School, Women's Studies, and African & African American Studies. She has been an affiliated faculty member with the Duke Institute on Care at the End of Life and the Trent Center for Bioethics and Medical Humanities. Her research and teaching interests focus on African American cultural studies, biocultural studies, gender, ethics, and law. Dr. Holloway serves on the Greenwall Foundation's Advisory Board in Bioethics and the Princeton University Council on the Study of Women and Gender. She is the author of more than 50 essays and eight books, including *Passed On: African-American Mourning Stories* (2002) and *Private Bodies, Public Texts: Race, Gender and a Cultural Bioethics* (2011). She has held fellowships from the Rockefeller Foundation (Bellagio Residency) and the Ford Foundation (DuBois Institute, Harvard University). Dr. Holloway was recently elected to the Hastings Center Fellows Association, a selected group of leading researchers who have made a distinguished contribution to the field of bioethics. She holds an M.L.S. from Duke University School of Law and an M.A. and a Ph.D. (English/linguistics) from Michigan State University.

Naomi Karp, J.D., is a senior policy analyst at the Consumer Financial Protection Bureau's (CFPB's) Office for Financial Protection for Older Americans, where she works on a range of issues, including elder financial exploitation, diminished capacity, financial education, retirement, and long-term planning. From 2005 to 2011, Ms. Karp was a senior strategic policy advisor at AARP's Public Policy Institute. She conducted research, developed policy positions, and supported advocacy efforts regarding elder abuse, guardianship, advance care planning, end-of-life care, probate, voting rights, and other legal rights issues. Her recent studies include protecting investors with diminished capacity, guardianship residential decision making, state implementation of the Physician Orders for Life-Sustaining Treatment (POLST) protocol for advanced illness care, power of attorney abuse, guardianship monitoring practices, and criminal background check screening in home care. Before joining AARP, she served as an associate staff director for the American Bar Association's Commission on Law and Aging. Ms. Karp has been a member of the Elder Justice Working Group, the Federal Partners Group of the National Council on Aging, the Department of Justice's Project Advisory Group for Elder Justice Roadmap Project, and the Ethics Committee of Washington Home and Hospices. She completed her undergraduate studies in English at the University of Michigan and holds a J.D. from the Northeastern University School of Law.

Jean S. Kutner, M.D., M.S.P.H., is Gordon Meiklejohn endowed professor of medicine and associate dean for clinical affairs at the University of Colorado School of Medicine and chief medical officer at the University of Colorado Hospital. She was the founding director of the University of Colorado Hospital Palliative Care Consult Service. She is board certified in internal medicine, geriatrics, and hospice and palliative medicine. Dr. Kutner developed the Population-based Palliative Care Research Network (PoPCRN) and is co-chair of the Palliative Care Research Cooperative (PCRC), a palliative care cooperative trials group funded by the National Institute of Nursing Research. These national networks of organizations providing palliative care facilitate the conduct of multisite studies of hospice and palliative care, addressing operational as well as clinical issues. Dr. Kutner's own research focuses on symptoms, care delivery, and family caregivers in hospice and palliative care. She received the Distinguished Service Award from the American Academy of Hospice and Palliative Medicine in 2010. Dr. Kutner received her M.D. from the University of California, San Francisco (UCSF), and completed residency training in internal medicine at UCSF. She completed a National Research Service Award (NRSA) primary care research fellowship, earning an M.S.P.H. degree with honors and a fellowship in geriatric medicine at the University of Colorado Denver.

Bernard Lo, M.D., is president of The Greenwall Foundation, whose mission is supporting bioethics research and young researchers in bioethics. He had been director of the Greenwall Faculty Scholars Program since 2001. He is professor emeritus of medicine and director emeritus of the Program in Medical Ethics at UCSF. Dr. Lo serves on the Board of Directors of the Association for the Accreditation of Human Research Protection Programs and on the Medical Advisory Panel of Blue Cross/Blue Shield. From 1996 to 2001, he served as a member of the National Bioethics Advisory Committee. From 1997 to 2001, he chaired the expert panel convened by the American College of Physicians to develop clinical, ethical, and policy recommendations regarding care near the end of life. He is a member of the IOM and previously served as chair of the Health Policy Board and as a member of the IOM Council. He chaired an IOM committee on Conflicts of Interest in Medical Research, Education, and Practice. Dr. Lo developed a course on responsible conduct of research taken by 120 UCSF postdoctoral fellows and junior faculty each year, and he is author of *Resolving Ethical Dilemmas: A Guide for Clinicians* (4th ed., 2010) and of *Ethical Issues in Clinical Research* (2010). He is a graduate of Stanford University Medical School, did his residency at both the University of California, Los Angeles, and Stanford, and completed a fellowship at Stanford as a Robert Wood Johnson Foundation clinical scholar.

Salimah H. Meghani, Ph.D., M.B.E., R.N., FAAN, is an associate professor in the Department of Biobehavioral Health Sciences and a member of the NewCourtland Center for Transitions and Health at University of Pennsylvania School of Nursing. Her research focuses on understanding sources of disparities in cancer pain and symptom outcomes among underserved and vulnerable populations. Dr. Meghani is chair of the American Pain Society's Pain Disparities Special Interest Group. She serves on the Editorial Board of *Pain Medicine*, the official journal of the American Academy of Pain Medicine, and on the Board of Directors of the Foundation for Ethics in Pain Care. Dr. Meghani has served on the Pennsylvania Department of Aging's statewide Task Force for Improving Quality at the End of Life for Pennsylvanians. She is a fellow of the American Academy of Nursing. She received her undergraduate degree in nursing summa cum laude from the Aga Khan University, Karachi. She holds an M.S.N. from the University of Pennsylvania School of Nursing and a Ph.D./M.B.E. (nursing/bioethics), both summa cum laude, from the University of Pennsylvania, Philadelphia. Her postdoctoral training is in health disparities research.

Diane E. Meier, M.D., is Director of the Center to Advance Palliative Care (CAPC), a national organization devoted to increasing access to quality palliative care in the United States. Under her leadership the number of palliative care programs in U.S. hospitals has more than tripled in the past 10 years. She is also co-director of the Patty and Jay Baker National Palliative Care Center; Vice-Chair for Public Policy and Professor of Geriatrics and Palliative Medicine; Catherine Gaisman Professor of Medical Ethics; and was the founder and Director of the Hertzberg Palliative Care Institute from 1997-2011, all at the Icahn School of Medicine at Mount Sinai in New York City. Dr. Meier is the recipient of the 2008 MacArthur Fellowship and the American Cancer Society's Medal of Honor for Cancer

Control in recognition of her leadership of the effort to bring nonhospice palliative care into mainstream medicine. She is a member of the IOM of the National Academy of Sciences. Dr. Meier has published more than 200 original peer review papers and several books. Her most recent book, *Meeting the Needs of Older Adults with Serious Illness: Challenges and Opportunities in the Age of Health Reform* was published by Springer in 2014. Dr. Meier received her B.A. from Oberlin College and her M.D. from Northwestern University Medical School. She completed her residency and fellowship training at Oregon Health Sciences University in Portland. She has been on the faculty of the Department of Geriatrics and Palliative Medicine and Department of Medicine at Mount Sinai since 1983.

William D. Novelli, M.A., is a professor in the McDonough School of Business at Georgetown University. He teaches in the M.B.A. program and has created and leads the Global Social Enterprise Initiative at the school. He is also co-chair of the Coalition to Transform Advanced Care (C-TAC), a national organization dedicated to reforming advanced illness care by empowering consumers, changing the health care delivery system, improving public policies, and enhancing provider capacity. Earlier, he was CEO of AARP, a membership organization of more than 40 million people aged 50 and older. Prior to that, he was president of the Campaign for Tobacco-Free Kids, whose mandate is to change public policies and the social environment, limit tobacco companies' marketing and sales practices to children, and serve as a counterforce to the tobacco industry and its special interests. He now serves as chairman of the board. Previously, Mr. Novelli was executive vice president of CARE, the world's largest private relief and development organization. Earlier, he co-founded and was president of Porter Novelli, now one of the world's largest public relations agencies. Porter Novelli was founded to apply marketing to social and health issues, and grew into an international marketing/public relations agency with corporate, not-for-profit, and government clients. Mr. Novelli received his B.A. from the University of Pennsylvania and his M.A. from the University of Pennsylvania Annenberg School for Communication.

Stephen G. Pauker, M.D., is professor of medicine and psychiatry at Tufts Medical Center and a faculty member of the Department of Medicine's Division of Clinical Decision Making, Informatics and Telemedicine at Tufts Medical Center. His research has focused on the application of decision analysis to clinical problems, cost-effectiveness and cost-benefit analyses, and medical informatics. His current interests include health policy and guidelines for cardiac disease, utility acquisition and comparison of health status measurement, expert systems for decision support in cardiovascular disease, inference and support of individual patients' decisions in genetics, neonatal screening programs, and decision analysis software. He is a long-standing member of the medical center's ethics committee. Dr. Pauker is a member of the IOM, the Association of American Physicians, and the American Society for Clinical Investigation. He is a past president of the Society for Medical Decision Making, now serving as its historian. He is a master of the American College of Physicians and a fellow of the American College of Medical Informatics, the American College of Cardiology, the American Society for Clinical Hypnosis, and the Society for Clinical and Experimental Hypnosis, of which he is immediate past president. He is also president of the American Board of Medical Hypnosis. He received his M.D. from Harvard Medical School and completed his postgraduate training at Boston City Hospital, Massachusetts General Hospital, and Tufts Medical Center. He is board certified in internal medicine, cardiology, and medical hypnosis.

Judith R. Peres, M.S.W., is currently an expert consultant in the areas of long-term care and palliative end-of-life care at Altarum Institute's Center for Elder Care and Advanced Illness. Her career spans more than four decades in both Medicare and Medicaid health policy, as well as direct clinical work. She maintains a private practice as a clinical social worker serving Medicare beneficiaries. Ms. Peres recently worked for 5 years with the U.S. Department of Health and Human Services (HHS) in the Office of the Assistant Secretary for Planning and Evaluation (ASPE) to develop the *Report to Congress on Advance Care Planning*. Previously, she was vice president for policy and advocacy of the former Last Acts Partnership and deputy director of the Last Acts National Program Office, funded by the Robert Wood Johnson Foundation to improve care and caring near the end of life. In those roles, she developed major policy pieces speaking to the need to improve end-of-life care in this country. Prior to her appointment at Last Acts, she served as director of health policy for the American Association of Homes and Services for the Aging, specializing in quality, reimbursement, and workforce issues. In addition, she had a distinguished career in Medicare and Medicaid reimbursement and financing policy for HHS. Her clinical practice also included employee assistance program work for the Sheppard Pratt Institute in Baltimore, Maryland, and work as a practicing psychotherapist for Kaiser Permanent, with a specialty in cognitive-behavioral therapy and mind/body health. Ms. Peres is a founding board member of the Social Work Hospice and Palliative Care Network. She holds a master's degree in social work from the University of Maryland, and received additional training at the Mind/Body Institute in Washington, DC, and in rational emotive behavioral therapy at the Albert Ellis Institute in New York.

Leonard D. Schaeffer is currently Judge Robert Maclay Widney chair and professor at the University of Southern California (USC) and a senior advisor to TPG Capital, a private equity firm. Mr. Schaeffer was chairman and CEO of WellPoint from 1992 to 2004 and continued as chairman through 2005. He was CEO of WellPoint's predecessor company, Blue Cross of California. Previously, he served as president and CEO of Group Health, Inc., executive vice president and chief operating officer of the Student Loan Marketing Association (Sallie Mae), and vice president of Citibank. Mr. Schaeffer has held appointments as administrator of the federal Health Care Financing Administration (now the Centers for Medicare & Medicaid Services); assistant secretary for management and budget of the federal Department of Health, Education, and Welfare; director of the Bureau of the Budget for the State of Illinois; chairman of the Illinois Capital Development Board; and deputy director of the Illinois Department of Mental Health. He was elected to the IOM in 1997 and as a member of the *Health Affairs* editorial board. He serves on the boards of various companies and organizations, including Amgen Inc.; the Brookings Institution; Harvard Medical School; RAND Corporation; Quintiles Transnational Corporation; USC; the Coalition to Transform Advanced Care; and the USC Schaeffer Center for Health Policy and Economics, which he established in 2009. Mr. Schaeffer is a graduate of Princeton University and was the Regent's lecturer at the University of California, Berkeley, and a Gilbert fellow at Princeton University.

W. June Simmons, M.S.W., is founding president and CEO of Partners in Care Foundation, formerly the Visiting Nurse Association (VNA) of Los Angeles, a nonprofit foundation that develops and tests health services innovations and works to ensure access to home and community care. In this role, she develops initiatives and proactive programs that meet the mutual needs of patient populations, providers, and health care delivery networks to encourage cost-effective, patient-friendly integration of care from hospital to home and community. Previously, she worked as an associate hospital administrator at Huntington Memorial Hospital, and before that she was founding director of Senior Care Network. Ms. Simmons is just completing a term as a member of the National Advisory Council to the National Institute on Aging. Among other professional memberships and experiences, she has contributed her expertise by serving on the Leadership Council of the National Council on Aging, the Executive Committee and National Board of the American Society on Aging, and the Advisory Board and Mentor Panel of the Practice Change Fellows. She is a founding member of the national Evidence Based Leadership Council and was founding chair of the National Chronic Care Consortium. In addition, Ms. Simmons has served on several local technical committees, panels, and advisory boards, including the L.A. County Long Term Care Strategic Planning Team, the Board of Councilors of the USC School of Social Work (chair), the Federal Hispanic Elders Project, and the USC Roybal Institute. She holds an M.S.W. from USC.

Christian T. Sinclair, M.D., FAAHPM, is assistant professor in the Division of Palliative Medicine at the University of Kansas Medical Center. Previously, he was a national hospice medical director at Gentiva Health Services, where he led physician support, education, and compliance for the North Central region of Gentiva Hospice. He has provided hospice and palliative care in nursing facilities, homes, hospitals, clinics, and stand-alone hospice units. Dr. Sinclair is serving his second term on the American Academy of Hospice and Palliative Medicine's Board of Directors and has experience as a palliative medicine fellowship director. He is the editor of the website Pallimed (www.pallimed.org), which discusses important research and media articles related to hospice and palliative care. He is highly active in social media for health care professionals, utilizing Facebook, Twitter, and other platforms to increase awareness of hospice and palliative care. Dr. Sinclair received his M.D. from the University of California, San Diego, and completed internal medicine residency training at Wake Forest University Baptist Medical Center. He completed his fellowship in hospice and palliative medicine at the Hospice and Palliative Care Center in Winston-Salem, North Carolina.

Joan M. Teno, M.D., M.S., is professor of health services, policy, and practice and associate director of the Center for Gerontology and Health Care Research at the Brown Medical School; she is also associate medical director at Home and Hospice Care of Rhode Island. She is a board-certified internist with added qualification in geriatrics and palliative medicine. Dr. Teno's research has focused on measuring and evaluating interventions designed to improve the quality of medical care for seriously ill and dying patients. She led the effort in the design of the Study to Understand Prognoses and Preferences for Outcomes and Risks of Treatments (SUPPORT) intervention analysis and was lead author of 12 publications resulting from that research effort, which ranged from addressing the role of advance directives to describing the dying experience of seriously ill and older adults. She was also lead investigator for a research effort to create a Toolkit of Instruments to Measure End-of-Life Care (TIME). She is a lead investigator for research examining health care transitions and the use of feeding tubes in persons with advanced cognitive impairment. Dr. Teno is a graduate of Hahnemann Medical University. She completed her internal medicine residency at Rhode Island Hospital in Providence and fellowships in geriatric medicine and health services research in gerontology at Brown University.

Also from Brown, she received her M.S. in community health, with a specialty in gerontology and chronic disease epidemiology.

Fernando Torres-Gil, Ph.D., is professor of social welfare and public policy at the University of California, Los Angeles (UCLA), adjunct professor of gerontology at USC, and director of the UCLA Center for Policy Research on Aging. He has served as associate dean and acting dean at the UCLA School of Public Affairs, and most recently as chair of the Social Welfare Department. His research focuses on such topics as health and long-term care, disability, entitlement reform, and the politics of aging. Dr. Torres-Gil was appointed to the Federal Council on Aging by President Jimmy Carter in 1978; he later was selected as a White House fellow and served under Joseph Califano, then secretary of the U.S. Department of Health, Education, and Welfare (HEW). He continued as a special assistant to the subsequent secretary of HEW, Patricia Harris. He was appointed (with Senate confirmation) by President Bill Clinton as the first-ever U.S. assistant secretary on aging in HHS. In 2010, he was appointed (with Senate confirmation) by President Barack Obama as vice chair of the National Council on Disability. He has written 6 books and more than 100 publications, including *The New Aging: Politics and Change in America* (1992). Dr. Torres-Gil earned his A.A. in political science at Hartnell Community College (1968), a B.A. with honors in political science from San Jose State University (1970), and an M.S.W. (1972) and a Ph.D. (1976) in social policy, planning, and research from the Heller Graduate School in Social Policy and Management at Brandeis University.

James A. Tulsky, M.D., is professor of medicine and nursing and chief, Duke Palliative Care at Duke University. His research focuses on clinician-patient communication, quality of life at the end of life, trajectories of patient experience, and the evaluation of interventions to improve the care of patients with serious illness. He has authored more than 150 publications on these topics, including a book titled *Mastering Communication with Seriously Ill Patients: Balancing Honesty with Empathy and Hope* (2009). He was a Project on Death in America faculty scholar; serves on the Advisory Council for the National Institute of Nursing Research; chairs the Greenwall Foundation Faculty Scholars Program Advisory Committee; and is a founding director of VitalTalk, a nonprofit dedicated to transforming the culture of communication throughout the medical community. He has received multiple awards for his work, including the 2002 Presidential Early Career Award for Scientists and Engineers; the 2006 American Academy on Hospice and Palliative Medicine Award for Research Excellence; and the 2013 George L. Engel Award from the American Academy on Communication in Healthcare for "outstanding research contributing to the theory, practice and teaching of effective healthcare communication and related skills." He is a graduate of the University of Illinois at Chicago School of Medicine, and he completed both his residency in internal medicine and a Robert Wood Johnson Foundation clinical scholar fellowship at UCSF.

Index

A

AARP, 96, 175, 299, 312
ACA (*see* Patient Protection and Affordable Care Act)
Accountable care organizations (ACOs)
    ACA and, 279-280, 310, 317-319
    Advance Payment Model, 317
    alternatives to, 320
    care management practices, 473
    defined, 317
    Medicare policies, 317, 318-319, 472
    outpatient care, 292
    palliative and hospice care, 292, 472-473, 479
    patient characteristics, 318
    performance measurement benchmark, 317, 472
    Pioneer program, 317, 318, 468, 471, 472, 473
    population-based payment model, 318
    proposed improvements, 318-319
    and quality of care, 84, 317, 318, 468, 469, 473
    reimbursement and payment approaches, 279-280, 317-318, 468, 471, 472, 479
    Shared Savings Program, 315, 317, 318, 468, 472, 473
    and social services, 310

Accreditation Council for Graduate Medical Education (ACGME), 14, 252, 417, 429
Activities of daily living (ADLs), assistance with, 9, 86, 144 n.20, 241, 248, 297, 302, 491-492, 501, 508, 509, 513
Acute Physiology and Chronic Health Evaluation (APACHE), 92
Adams, Lisa Bonchek, 365
Administration for Community Living, 279, 301
Administration on Aging, 299, 301, 311
Advance care planning
    ACA and, 12, 120, 132, 366-370
    age and, 126, 136
    autonomy principle and, 124-125, 152, 166, 181
    barriers and disincentives, 11, 12, 117, 125, 126-129, 141, 154-155, 213
    cancer context, 137, 140-141, 169, 170, 172, 214-215
    for children and youth, 68, 134, 136, 141-144, 146, 173, 184, 187, 188, 356, 425-426, 429, 432
    choice of health care agent, 129-132, 172
    chronic obstructive pulmonary disease context, 137, 212-213

clinician-patient communication, 2, 3,
    6, 11-13, 18, 50, 117, 118, 128-129,
    142, 146, 149-150, 152, 154, 155,
    157-172, 190-191, 212, 213, 237,
    345, 448
cognitive impairment/dementia context,
    119, 137, 145-146, 215-216
consultations and discussions, 118,
    128-129, 143, 155, 185-186, 190,
    211-212, 367, 510
Consumer's Toolkit for Health Care
    Advance Planning, 123-124
Conversation Project, 124, 125, 352-
    353, 354, 356-357, 360, 420
and costs of health care, 12, 18, 139-
    141, 369, 510
current state of, 118, 124-141
"death panels" controversy, 12, 120,
    132, 366-370
decision aids, 170-172
decision-making capacity, and methods
    of patients, 146, 167-172, 189
definitions, 120, 122, 385
demographic characteristics and,
    125-127
disability context, 145-147, 178
effects on health care agents and
    families, 2, 11, 136, 137-139, 367
elderly people, 136, 144-145
electronic health records and, 17, 181-
    185, 188, 331
family involvement in, 18, 128, 143,
    150, 152, 154, 164-166
financial planning considerations, 145,
    212
health care agents, 11, 18, 118, 122,
    124, 126, 129-132, 134, 135, 136,
    137-139, 142, 145, 147, 150, 157,
    158, 160, 164-166, 167, 173, 174,
    175, 176, 179, 183, 184, 185, 186,
    187, 189, 211, 212, 215, 216, 349,
    385, 386, 387, 389
health literacy and, 156-157
heart failure context, 137, 211-212
historical review, 120-124
homeless or "unbefriended" people,
    146-147
and hospice enrollment, 212
life cycle model (proposed), 185-187,
    189-190
literacy level and, 155-157

long-term care, 164, 172, 174, 179, 218
managed care and, 298 n.18
Medicare and, 121, 124, 139, 464, 510
model initiatives, 172-185
National Framework and Preferred
    Practices for Palliative and Hospice
    Care Quality, 172-173, 185, 425-426
nurses, 185, 186, 389, 448
nursing home residents, 126, 129, 132,
    151, 152, 171, 176, 177, 181, 182,
    188, 216, 286, 448, 468
palliative care consultation, 60, 66, 137,
    143, 155, 160-161, 169, 172-173,
    175, 215 n.13
and patient/caregiver satisfaction with
    care, 135-137
POLST paradigm, 17, 121, 123, 172,
    173-179, 180, 182, 183, 184, 187,
    188, 189-190, 217-219, 323, 331,
    358, 389, 448
preferences for care, 11, 12, 13, 18, 125-
    127, 141-157, 189, 369, 510
primary care and, 186
professional education and training, 181,
    225, 227, 237
public education and engagement, 18,
    19, 20, 32, 121-124, 125, 172-173,
    345, 346-347, 352-353, 354, 355,
    356-357, 358, 359, 360, 370, 371,
    420, 421
public support for, 368, 370
and quality of care, 78 n.13, 80, 135-
    137, 176-178
quality-of-life considerations, 147, 148
racial, ethnic, and cultural differences,
    11, 49, 125, 148-155, 188
recommendations, 12-13, 17, 19, 20,
    190-191, 330-331, 370, 371
reimbursement policies and financial
    incentives, 17, 117, 121, 188-189,
    320, 323, 331, 368, 369-370, 464,
    468
religion and, 147-149, 178-179, 212
research needs, 187-189, 432
Respecting Choices initiative, 179-181
and satisfaction with care, 135-137
shared decision making, 1, 4, 17, 136,
    138, 157, 166-172, 173, 174, 182,
    188, 326, 331
social workers and, 185, 186, 243
state policies and, 323

and longevity/survival, 136
system factors in, 11, 154-155
and utilization rates, 140
VA model, 146
Advance directives
adherence to, 11, 55, 56, 88, 132-135,
175, 180, 189-190, 323, 326, 369,
448
barriers to having, 126-127, 147, 155,
157
Caring Conversations® initiative, 123
for children, 134, 141-142, 143, 356,
426
clinician knowledge and training, 237
correlates of having, 126, 144, 148, 149,
151, 154
and costs of care, 139, 140, 510
default treatments, 169-170
definition of terms, 120, 122-123, 385,
387
do-not-hospitalize orders, 123, 152, 286
do not resuscitate (DNR), 60, 121, 123,
136, 146, 149, 152, 154-155, 174,
176, 184, 448
durable power of attorney for health
care, 118 n.1, 122, 124, 130, 145,
366 n.14, 386
effects on family and health care agent,
138
electronic storage of, 11, 17, 172, 180,
181-185, 331, 448
Five Wishes, 142, 356, 426
flexibility in interpreting, 134-135
homeless people, 146
Honoring Choices, 354, 356, 357, 421
incorporation into medical record, 121,
180, 181
and intensive care, 126, 151, 214, 216
legislation and legal implications,
88, 121, 124, 126, 134-135, 366,
369-370
living wills, 117, 120, 122, 124, 132,
133, 136 n.13, 147, 175, 181, 184,
366 n.14, 369, 385, 387
logistical/system challenges, 134, 212,
303, 426
physician concerns with, 133
POLST compared to, 175-176, 178
promotion of, 172-173, 179-181
racial and ethnic differences, 11, 49,
150, 151, 154, 155

Respecting Choices, 141, 143 n.19, 172-
173, 179-181, 212
shortcomings in, 11, 119-120
use outside the United States, 124
Advance Payment Model, 317
Advancing Palliative Care Research for
Children Facing Life-Limiting
Conditions, 431
Aetna, 53, 322, 408, 412, 476, 477
African Americans/Blacks
advance care planning, 129, 149, 151,
152-154
costs of care, 350, 495, 496, 497, 506,
507, 569
direct care workers, 249
hospice use, 152, 153, 154, 322, 569
insurance payor, 495
life expectancy, 34
literacy levels, 156
mortality data, 153
physicians, 240
preferences for end-of-life care, 60, 149,
153-154, 155, 322, 348, 364
site of death, 61-62, 152, 153, 553-554
treatment differences, 49, 153-154
trust issues, 153-154
utilization of services, 49, 506, 513
Age/aging (*see also* Children; Life
expectancy)
and advance care planning, 126, 136
and cause of death, 31, 34
and costs of end-of-life care, 494, 495,
499
demographic trends, 35-38
Agency for Healthcare Research and
Quality (AHRQ), 33, 79, 99, 211
n.36, 299 n.20, 537, 538
Aging with Dignity and *Five Wishes*, 352,
354, 356-357, 420
Aid to Capacity Evaluation, 145 n.22
Albom, Mitch, 352
Alliance for Excellence in Hospice and
Palliative Nursing, 243
Alternative Quality Contract (AQC), 468,
473-474
Alzheimer's disease, 36, 37, 38, 61, 165,
215, 295, 311, 444, 456, 509
Alzheimer's Disease Supportive Services
Program, 279
American Academy of Family Physicians, 51

American Academy of Hospice and
    Palliative Medicine (AAHPM), 78,
    84, 223, 410, 415, 417
American Academy of Pediatrics, 51, 52
American Association of Colleges of
    Nursing, 231, 232, 415
American Bar Association Commission on
    Law and Aging, 123, 124
American Board of Family Medicine, 239
American Board of Hospice and Palliative
    Medicine, 238, 417
American Board of Internal Medicine, 239
American Board of Medical Specialties
    (ABMS), 238-239, 240, 417, 429
American Cancer Society, 414
American College of Physicians, 51
American Geriatrics Society (AGS), 78 n.13,
    362-363
American Hospital Association, 173
American Indians, 152
American Medical Association, 33, 229
    Physician Consortium for Performance
        Improvement, 85
American Osteopathic Association, 51
American Public Health Association
    (APHA), 32-33
American Recovery and Reinvestment Act
    of 2009, 387
American Society of Clinical Oncology, 73,
    81 n.14
American Society of Health-System
    Pharmacists, 245-246
Anderson, Gloria, 152
Anxiety, 45, 48, 56, 96, 136, 145 n.21,
    157-158, 167, 213, 266, 284, 311,
    323
Approaching Death report
    progress since and remaining gaps,
        407-422
Asians/Pacific Islanders, 60, 152, 156
Assessing Care of Vulnerable Elders
    (ACOVE) initiative, 79, 84-85, 410
Associated Press-National Opinion Research
    Center, 127
Association of American Medical Colleges,
    222-223, 227
Association of Pediatric Hematology and
    Oncology Nurses, 67, 423
Association of Professional Chaplains, 247,
    418

Autonomy principle, 59, 78 n.13, 83, 124-
    125, 146, 150, 152, 166, 181, 316,
    362, 364-365

B

Bereavement services/support, 28, 58, 68,
    69, 72, 78-79, 96, 98, 165, 187, 233,
    241, 242, 244, 321, 411, 422, 423,
    424, 426, 428, 430, 431, 432, 453,
    535, 552, 564, 571
Biopsychosocial model of care, 62-63, 235
Bipartisan Policy Center, 269
Blacks (*see* African American/Blacks)
Board of Chaplaincy Certification Inc., 247,
    418
Board of Oncology Social Work
    Certification, 244
Board of Pharmacy Specialties (BPS), 246,
    418
Budget Neutrality Adjustment Factor, 319
    n.30, 413
Bundled Payments for Care Improvement
    Initiative, 316, 413, 471

C

California
    Advanced Illness Management program,
        322
    cessation-of-treatment conflict, 364
    Health-Care Partners Comprehensive
        Care Program, 313 n.28
    HealthCare Foundation, 127, 368
    home- and community-based care costs,
        300, 569
    Natural Death Act of 1976, 121
    palliative care education requirements,
        230, 232
    pediatric palliative care program, 68,
        427, 569
    POLST program, 123, 177
Campaigns, public education and
    engagement
    audiences, 358-360
    channels, 360-361
    evaluation, 361-362
    examples on health-related topics,
        378-383

Last Acts campaign, 33, 353, 361
  messages, 360
  sponsorship, 355, 358
Cancer care
  ACA and, 314 n.29
  advance care planning, 137, 140-141,
    169, 170, 172, 214-215
  advocacy groups, 64
  clinician-patient communication, 152,
    158, 159, 161, 165, 171-172, 214,
    237
  coordination of care, 51, 65, 67, 68
  costs of care, 37, 140-141, 275, 290,
    508, 510, 520
  and depression, 65, 67, 290
  eligibility for therapies, 65 n.8
  hospice care, 30, 61, 62, 65, 295, 393,
    465, 476, 520
  incidence, 37
  information preferences, 159
  longevity/survival, 62, 69, 215
  mortality data, 31, 34, 35, 36, 214, 456,
    546
  palliative care, 7, 62, 65, 67, 68, 69, 70,
    72, 73, 77, 171, 215, 228, 290, 294,
    414, 423, 519, 546, 560
  pediatric, 35, 38, 48, 67, 275, 423,
    545
  preferences for care, 55, 132, 133, 140,
    165, 171, 214, 215, 510
  prognostication, 30, 88, 89-90, 91, 294,
    466
  providers of care, 48, 51, 230, 232
  public engagement, 365
  quality of care, 77, 81, 82, 411
  quality of life, 72, 73, 290
  research on treatments, 99
  spiritual care, 140
  trajectories and symptoms, 46, 48, 515,
    534, 560
  and utilization of services, 519
Cardiopulmonary resuscitation (CPR), 24,
    78 n.13, 171, 173, 176, 216, 218,
    387, 558-559
Care Choices Model, 412, 476
Caregiver Action Network, 354 n.4
Caregivers, family
  bereavement services for, 96, 233, 424
  burdens on, 14, 96, 138, 266, 276, 297,
    452-453
  characteristics, 8, 46, 92-93, 94-95

complicated grief, 138
  and costs of care, 301
  delivery of care, 92-97, 102
  demand and supply, 8, 95, 102
  depression and anxiety, 213
  education and training, 2, 15, 53, 76,
    97, 138, 245, 311, 330
  financial toll, 94, 95
  hospice eligibility requirements, 294
  legislation protecting, 97
  meals and nutrition services, 287, 309,
    310, 312-313, 330
  Medicare benefit structure and, 296-297
  and palliative care, 58, 64, 67, 86, 95,
    245, 249
  prognosis and, 87
  research needs, 96, 98
  respite care, 97, 98, 243, 274, 292, 302,
    309, 310, 312-313, 330, 424, 427,
    450, 452, 464, 476, 539, 569
  responsibilities, 8, 14, 19, 53, 93
  suggestions for improving care, 450-451
  support needed for, 4, 9, 10, 15, 73
    n.12, 86, 97, 98, 233, 279, 304, 309,
    310-311
  and utilization of health services, 267,
    309
CARING (Cancer, Admissions ≥2,
    Residence in a nursing home,
    Intensive care unit admit with
    multiorgan failure, ≥2 Noncancer
    hospice Guidelines), 89-90, 91
Caring Conversations®, 123
Cash & Counseling program, 97, 313
Catholic Health Association, 178-179
Catholic Medical Association, 178
C-Change, 64
Center for Medicare & Medicaid
    Innovation, 81-82, 314
Center to Advance Palliative Care (CAPC),
    66, 78, 100, 223, 224 n.2, 234, 352,
    408, 419, 425
Centers for Disease Control and Prevention
    (CDC), 34, 383, 490-491, 499, 536,
    537, 540, 541, 542, 543, 544, 547,
    549, 551, 552, 553, 554, 555
Centers for Medicare & Medicaid Services
    (CMS) (*see also* Medicaid; Medicare)
  accountable care organization policies,
    317, 318-319, 472
  advance care planning policy, 369-370

Budget Neutrality Adjustment Factor,
    319 n.30, 413
Bundled Payments for Care
    Improvement Initiative, 316, 413,
    471
Community-based Care Transitions
    Program, 53
data collection suggestions for, 525
electronic health records promotion, 184
emergency services policy, 281
Financial Alignment Initiative, 315-316
hospice conditions of participation, 244
Hospital Readmissions Reductions
    Program, 53
integrating Medicare and Medicaid
    financing for dual-eligible individuals,
    474-475
National Health Expenditure estimates,
    488, 489
palliative medicine subspecialty
    approval, 417
policy advances, 33, 53, 315-316, 319,
    326
Quality Improvement Organization
    Program, 53, 79
quality-of-care measures and reporting
    requirements, 79, 83-84, 411, 469
Chaplains and chaplaincy services
certification, 14, 247-248, 250, 418
education and training, 15, 222, 228,
    230, 247-248, 252, 418
and hospital mortality rates, 247
hospital staffing, 564
and Medicare Hospice Benefit, 247
palliative care specialty, 8, 10, 67, 247-
    248, 418
and perceptions of quality of care, 247
scope of services, 4, 7 n.2, 8, 10, 27, 49,
    59, 67, 71, 101, 103, 221, 233, 237-
    238, 246-248, 251, 321, 385, 389,
    426, 428, 450
Children (see also Pediatric end-of-life care)
advance directives, 134, 141-142, 143,
    356, 426
age at death, 35, 540-542, 543
causes of death, 31, 35, 36, 542, 544,
    546-547
end-of-life trajectories and symptoms,
    47, 48
mortality rates, 34, 35, 536-537, 540-
    542, 551

pediatric age range defined, 535-536
site of death, 34, 61-62, 68, 547-548,
    549, 551, 552-554, 555
Children's Health Insurance Program, 412,
    424, 427, 477-478
Children's Hospital Boston, 68, 230, 423,
    428
Children's International Project on
    Palliative/Hospice Services, 429
Children's Oncology Group, 67, 423
Children's Program of All-Inclusive
    Coordinated Care for Children and
    Their Families, 422
Chronic obstructive pulmonary disease
    (COPD), 37, 70, 88, 133, 137, 170,
    212-213, 476, 500, 508, 509
City of Hope National Medical Center, 232
Clinician-patient communication
in advance care planning, 2, 3, 6, 11-13,
    18, 50, 117, 118, 128-129, 142,
    146, 149-150, 152, 154, 155, 157-
    172, 190-191, 212, 213, 237, 345,
    448
barriers to, 159-160
cancer care, 152, 158, 159, 161, 165,
    171-172, 214, 237
and costs of care, 25, 290
decision aids, 170-172
elements of good communication,
    351-352
emotional encounters with patients,
    161-162
family and health care agent
    involvement, 164-166
goals, 158
importance of conversations, 28,
    446-447
information preferences, 159
intensive care setting, 138, 165, 230,
    428
nurses, 129, 162, 226, 231, 235
nursing home residents, 216, 224
nurturing patients' hope, 162-163
palliative care, 64, 288, 290, 431
professional education and training, 225,
    226, 229, 230, 231, 232 n.11, 233,
    234, 235-237, 241, 250, 251-252,
    428, 451
prognosis discussions, 92, 160-161, 164-
    165, 212, 213
and quality of care, 79, 190, 283

racial, ethnic, and cultural
    considerations, 149-150, 152, 154,
    155, 522
recommendations, 12-13, 190-191
reimbursement issues, 452
and satisfaction with care, 158, 164,
    167, 290
shared decision making and patient-
    centered care, 166-172
spirituality and religion, 163
understanding patient decision-making
    methods, 167-170
Coalition to Transform Advanced Care, 227
Cognitive impairment (*see also* Dementias)
    and advance care planning, 119, 137,
    145-146, 215-216
    probability, 38
Coleman, Diane, 147
Colorado
    Evercare managed care model, 286
    pediatric palliative care program, 68,
    427
    POLST program, 123
    transitional care model, 53
Communication (*see* Clinician-patient
    communication)
Community-based Care Transitions
    Program, 53
Community-based services (*see* Home- and
    community-based services)
Community Conversations on
    Compassionate Care, 122, 172-173,
    354, 356, 358, 421
Community Living Assistance Services and
    Supports Act (CLASS), 315, 475
Community-State Partnerships to Improve
    End-of-Life Care, 33, 323
Community-Wide End-of-Life/Palliative
    Care Initiative, 358
Compassionate Friends, 354 n.4
CompassionNet, 68
Complex chronic conditions
    age and, 36
    children, 34, 546-547, 551-552, 554-
    559, 571
    contributing factors, 34-35
    coordination of care, 50-51
    and costs of care, 36, 266
    and delivery of care, 50
    hospitalizations, 266, 554, 556
    self-management, 156

site of death, 552, 555
VA Home Based Primary Care Program,
    72
Concurrent care
    ACA and, 319, 320, 412, 427, 475-476,
    477
    costs implications, 412, 477, 567-570
    demonstration projects, 319, 412, 427,
    475-476, 477
    financing, 278, 297, 319, 427, 475-478
    institutional long-term care and, 297
    and longevity, 72
    Medicare coverage, 154, 319, 412, 427,
    475-476, 477
    nursing home residents, 278
    palliative care and, 7, 58, 73, 277, 287,
    293, 295, 297-298, 321, 322
    pediatric, 319, 427, 477-478, 533-534,
    567, 569-570
    private-sector initiatives, 321-322, 476
    and quality of life, 72, 412
    recommendations of professional
    societies, 73
    satisfaction with, 322
Congestive heart failure, 46, 63, 70, 133,
    170, 476, 491, 493, 508, 509, 526
Congressional Budget Office, 284 n.10, 323,
    503
Consumer Assessments and Reports of End
    of Life (CARE) survey, 78, 80
Consumer's Toolkit for Health Care
    Advance Planning, 123-124
Continuity of care
    coordination of care and, 50-51
    hospitals, 68
    pediatric care, 68
    primary care and, 49-50, 68
    public testimony on, 448-451
    racial and ethnic differences, 155-156
    transitions between care settings and, 52
Conversation Project, 124, 125, 352-353,
    354, 356-357, 360, 420
Coordinated-Transitional Care (C-TraC),
    53-54
Coordination of care (*see also* Delivery of
    end-of-life care)
    across programs, 4, 25
    advance directive and, 134, 212, 303,
    426
    cancer care, 51, 65, 67, 68
    communication and, 50, 55

continuity of care and, 50-51
and costs of care, 4, 25
disease management programs, 54, 186, 212, 304, 305, 306
by family, 14
importance of, 46, 50, 86
incentive policies and, 17, 275-302, 329-330
interdisciplinary team approach, 7, 10, 13, 58, 68, 71-72, 79, 101, 102, 103, 226, 244, 424, 429, 563-564, 571
long-term care, 304-305, 308, 470
measurement of, 51 n.2, 81
medical homes, 51-52, 82, 302, 303, 314, 469
Medicare and, 304, 305, 308, 315-316, 330
multiple chronic conditions and, 50-51
palliative care and, 63, 68, 71, 84, 322
primary care and, 49-51, 68
public testimony on, 448-451
and quality of care, 31, 76, 81, 82, 265, 303-306
and satisfaction with care, 76
scenario of lack of, 55, 56-57
transfer of patient information across settings, 10, 17, 50, 103, 181-185, 188, 331
and transitions between care settings, 49-52, 53, 54, 100
and utilization of acute care services, 9, 50-51, 86
Costs of end-of-life care (see also Financing and organization of end-of-life care)
advance care planning and, 12, 18, 139-141, 369, 510
age and, 494, 495, 499
cancer patients, 37, 140-141, 275, 290, 508, 510, 520
changes over time, 4, 25, 504
chronic conditions and functional limitations and, 22-23, 36, 37, 266, 491-494, 516-517
clinician-patient communication and, 25, 290
concurrent care, 567-570
coordination across programs and, 4, 16, 25
data limitations and gaps, 517-518
dementias and, 37, 270, 303, 328, 509-510, 517
demographic characteristics, 506-507
delivery of care and, 16, 25
distribution and trends, 488-489
emergency services and, 281-282, 569
epidemiology of chronic conditions and, 499-501
family caregivers and, 301
fiscal challenges, 267-271
fragmentation of care and, 4, 25
geographic variations, 22, 305-307, 458-459, 510-512
goals of care discussions and, 510
health characteristics and, 508-510
hospice care, 292-295, 519-522
hospitalization, 22, 266, 280-281, 512-513, 564, 565-567, 568, 569
identifying high-cost patients, 525
identifying target population for cost-saving
informal care, 37, 38
interventions, 523-525
life expectancy and, 35-36
long-term care, 273, 274, 296, 300-301, 458, 502
magnitude and proportion, 502-503
Medicaid, 16, 268, 271, 273, 291, 298, 300-301, 302, 303, 312, 459, 495, 497, 498, 499, 502, 522
Medicare, 139, 268, 276, 279-280, 283-284, 451, 504, 519-523
nursing home population, 37, 272, 273, 277, 296, 310, 312, 457, 465, 489, 490, 492, 493, 494, 495, 496, 497, 498, 499, 501-502, 509, 514, 515, 517, 522
palliative care, 74, 264, 274, 287-292, 327, 329, 519
patient characteristics associated with, 505-513
by payor, 498-499
percent of gross domestic product, 15-16, 267, 268, 283-284, 308
populations with highest costs, 489-499, 513
preferences of patients and, 2, 15, 21, 510
public attitudes about, 3, 18, 451-452
and quality of care, 15, 22, 275-302
race/ethnicity and, 494-497

reimbursement policies and, 4, 16, 25, 137, 269 n.6, 276, 279-280, 318, 451-452, 473, 504-505, 508
and survival, 22
trajectories of illness and, 22, 513-517
utilization of services and, 456-458, 512-513, 525-526
variation among decedents, 504-505
Critical care (*see* Intensive care/critical care)
Critical Care End-of-Life Peer Workgroup, 77, 229, 231-232, 234, 323
Cruzan, Nancy Beth, 364

D

Dana-Farber Cancer Institute, 68
Data sources and methods, this study
additional activities, 393-394
commissioned papers, 394
committee description, 391-392
literature review, 392
public meetings, 392-393, 395-405
written public testimony, 443-454
Death and dying
Last Acts campaign, 33, 353, 361
perceptions of, 445-446
public venues for discussions of, 352-355
site of, 33-34, 54, 81, 119, 468
trajectories and symptoms, 22, 30-31, 46-48
Death Cafe, 352, 354, 420
Death over Dinner, 352, 354, 420
"Death panels" controversy, 12, 120, 132, 366-370
DeathWise, 352, 354, 420
Decision making by patients and families
aids, 170-172
biases and heuristics, 167-168
choice architecture, 168-169, 188
default choices on advance directives, 169-170
and patient-centered care, 166-172
research needs, 188
shared, 1, 4, 17, 80, 99, 118, 136, 138, 166-172, 173, 174, 182, 188, 320 n.32, 326, 331, 351
stages of change theory and, 188
video materials and, 171-172

Delivery of end-of-life care (*see also* Continuity of care; Coordination of care; Transitions between care settings; *specific services*)
ambulatory care environment, 282-285
for children, 67-69
communication and, 55-58
and costs of care, 16, 25
current situation, 46-55
family caregivers, 92-97, 102
hospice care, 46, 48-49, 50, 54, 56, 59, 60-62, 63, 65, 100, 101
hospital environment, 280-282
interdisciplinary team approach, 7, 10, 13, 58, 64, 67, 68, 71-72, 79, 86, 95, 101, 102, 103, 226, 234, 244, 245, 249, 424, 429, 563-564, 571
managed care environment, 285-287
multiple chronic conditions and, 50
in nonhospital settings, 69-70
palliative care, 7, 51-52, 55, 58-74, 97, 103, 287-292
preferences of family and patients and, 55, 56
primary care, 49-52, 70
prognosis problem, 47, 87-92, 101-102
providers, 48-49
public testimony on, 448-451
quality of care, 55-57, 74-87, 275-302
race/ethnicity and, 49, 60
recommendations, 10, 103-104
research needs and funding, 32, 97-100
strategy for changing, 40
trajectory and symptom challenges 46-48, 49
transitions between care settings, 49-52, 55, 100
unwanted care, 55-58
Dementias
advance care planning, 137, 171, 215-216
Alzheimer's disease, 36, 37, 38, 61, 165, 215, 295, 311, 444, 456, 509
challenges in end-of-life care, 49, 96, 266
chronic illness with, 48
costs of care, 37, 270, 303, 328, 509-510, 517
hospice care, 74, 81
hospitalizations, 54, 56-57, 298, 324, 328

managed care enrollees, 286, 412
nursing home residents, 54-55, 81, 249, 286, 303, 324, 328
palliative care, 54-55, 303
prognosis predictions, 88, 91
quality of care, 38, 49, 54-55, 56-57, 74, 79, 249, 286, 411, 412
racial and ethnic minorities, 49
training of caregivers, 249
trajectories and symptoms, 48
transitions for care, 54, 328
trends, 38, 144, 215
Depression, 35, 37, 45, 48, 54, 63, 65, 67, 71, 72, 73 n.12, 74, 96, 120, 136, 137 n.15, 138, 161, 162, 167, 213, 266, 284, 290, 311, 450, 499, 509
Direct care workers, 14, 248-249
Disease management programs, 54, 186, 212, 304, 305, 306
Do-not-hospitalize orders, 123, 152, 286
Do not resuscitate (DNR), 60, 121, 123, 136, 149, 152, 154-155, 174, 176, 184, 448
Dresser, Rebecca, 150
Dual eligibility, 271-272, 273, 278, 286, 287, 298, 302-303, 310, 315, 328, 386, 474-475, 522
Duchenne's muscular dystrophy, 147
Durable power of attorney for health care, 118 n.1, 122, 124, 130, 145, 366 n.14, 386

E

Early Periodic Screening, Diagnosis, and Treatment, 477-478
Educate, Nurture, Advise Before Life Ends (ENABLE), 73
Education and training (see Patient, family, or caregiver education; Professional education and development in end-of-life care; Public education and engagement)
    direct care workers, 14, 248-249
    family caregivers, 2, 15, 53, 76, 97, 138, 245, 311, 330
Education in Palliative and End-of-life Care (EPEC) Program, 222, 229-230, 251, 415, 428

Emergency department services
    and advance directives, 134, 179, 212, 426
    availability of alternatives, 467, 493, 519, 520, 569
    costs/expenditures, 281-282, 569
    database, 537-538
    deaths, 548, 559-560
    end-of-life care challenges, 49, 52, 57, 94
    palliative care providers, 243
    pediatric care, 98, 282, 304, 432, 559-560, 569, 571
    prevention, 309-310, 314, 321-322, 331, 526
    quality of care, 281-282, 453, 560
    reimbursement policies, 281-282, 296, 467
    research needs, 432, 526-527, 571
    utilization, 17, 52, 73, 74, 211, 264, 266, 267, 281-282, 290, 304, 314, 467, 519, 520
End-of-Life Nursing Education Consortium (ELNEC), 222, 231-232, 251, 415
    Pediatric Palliative Care curriculum, 429
End of Life/Palliative Education Resource Center, 222, 416
End-of-life trajectories and symptoms, 22, 30-31, 46-48
End-stage renal disease (ESRD), 64, 88, 471, 472, 547, 559
Engage with Grace, 352, 354, 420
EpicCare, 184
ePrognosis, 92
Evidence-based care, 1, 4, 6, 12, 19, 22, 28, 31, 64, 77, 84, 98, 190, 305, 310, 316, 362, 370, 410, 419
Excellus BlueCross BlueShield, 68, 127, 175, 320 n.31, 358
Expenditures for care (see Costs of end-of-life care; Financing and organization of end-of-life care; specific payors)

F

FACE Intervention, 143 n.19
Faculty Scholars Program, 222, 416
Family (see also Caregivers, family)
    advance care planning effects, 2, 11, 136, 137-139, 367

bereavement services/support, 28, 58,
    68, 69, 72, 78-79, 96, 98, 165, 187,
    233, 241, 242, 244, 321, 411, 422,
    423, 424, 426, 428, 430, 431, 432,
    453, 535, 552, 564, 571
  clinician communication with, 164-166
  defined, 28, 45-46
  financial considerations, 145, 212
  importance of, 45
  participation in advance care planning,
    18, 128, 143, 150, 152, 154,
    164-166
  social and support services, 68
Family and Medical Leave Act of 1993, 97,
    452
Federation of State Medical Boards of the
    United States, Inc., 413
Financing and organization of end-of-life
    care (see also Accountable care
    organizations; Costs of end-of-life
    care; Health insurance coverage,
    private; Medicaid; Medicare;
    Reimbursement policies and
    methods)
  ACA reforms, 4, 272, 314-321, 412
  concurrent care, 475-478
  Financial Alignment Initiative, 315-316
  home- and community-based services,
    315
  hospice and home care, 319
  impacts of, 455-456
  incentive policies and coordination of
    care, 275-302, 329-330
  integrated models, 466-467
  long-term care, 16, 266, 268, 271, 274,
    275, 278, 279, 287, 296-303, 306,
    315-316, 320, 327-328, 475, 478-
    479, 498, 499
  major programs, 271-275
  palliative care, 33, 59, 61, 68, 98, 287-
    292, 329
  payers, 459-460
  private-sector initiatives, 321-322
  and quality of care, 467-469
  recommendations, 16-17, 330-331
  reform impacts, 469-478
  research needs, 326-328
  social services integration, 309-314, 329
  state policy reforms, 322-323
  transparency and accountability, 324-
    326, 329

Five Wishes, 142, 356, 426
Florida
  hospice care, 74
  pediatric palliative care program, 68,
    427, 554, 569
  utilization and spending, 458, 569
Food and Drug Administration, 70 n.10,
    230, 381
Footprints Model, 143 n.19
Foundation for Advanced Education in the
    Sciences, 232-233
Functional limitations and disabilities
  aging and, 37
  and costs of care, 22-23, 36, 37, 266,
    491-494, 516-517
  disability rates, 37-38
  and end-of-life trajectory, 47
Futile care, 233, 288, 364-365, 359

G

George Washington University, 227
Geriatric care, 10, 50, 52, 227 n.5, 232,
    282
Geriatric Resources for Assessment and
    Care of Elders (GRACE), 313 n.28
Goodman, Ellen, 124
Gundersen Health System, 141

H

Hammes, Bernard, 181
Harvard Medical School Program in
    Palliative Care Education and
    Practice, 228
Health and Retirement Study (HRS), 38,
    47, 89-90, 91-92, 119, 144 n.20, 270
    n.7, 501, 502, 503, 504, 506, 508,
    509, 513, 514, 519
Health care agents, 11, 18, 118, 122, 124,
    126, 129-132, 134, 135, 136, 137-
    139, 142, 145, 147, 150, 157, 158,
    160, 164-166, 167, 173, 174, 175,
    176, 179, 183, 184, 185, 186, 187,
    189, 211, 212, 215, 216, 349, 385,
    386, 387, 389
Health Care Financing Administration, 33
Health Information Technology for
    Economic and Clinical Health
    (HITECH) Act, 184, 387

Health Information Technology Policy
    Committee, 184-185
Health insurance coverage, private (see also
    Medicaid; Medicare; Reimbursement
    policies and methods)
  ACA and, 419, 460
  concurrent care, 321-322, 476
  essential health benefits, 460
  programs and expenditures, 274
Health Insurance Portability and
    Accountability Act (HIPAA), 172, 247
Health literacy, 156-157
Health records
  advance directive incorporation, 121,
    180, 181
  electronic, 17, 181-185, 188, 331
Health Resources and Services
    Administration (HRSA), 81-82, 408
Healthcare Cost and Utilization Project,
    537-538
Healthcare Effectiveness Data and
    Information Set (HEDIS), 468
Heart Bypass Center Demonstration, 471
Heart disease/failure, 7, 30, 31, 34, 36, 37,
    38, 48, 54, 64, 70, 456, 500
Henry J. Kaiser Family Foundation, 367
Hispanics
  advance care planning, 60, 151, 154, 188
  costs of care, 497, 506, 507, 569
  direct care workers, 249
  hospice use, 153, 569
  insurance payor, 495, 507
  life expectancy, 34
  literacy levels, 156
  mortality data, 536, 537
  preferences for end-of-life care, 60, 149,
    154, 348
  site of death, 153, 553-554
  treatment differences, 49
  utilization of services, 506, 513
HIV/AIDS, 61, 62, 97, 142, 143, 356 n.5,
    444, 476
Hollywood Health and Society, 353
Home (see In-home care)
  site of death, 33, 34, 63, 73
Home- and community-based services, 94,
    298, 299-302, 312-313, 315, 316
Home health
  agencies, 49, 50, 61, 70, 71 n.11, 74,
    98, 246, 249, 306, 422, 424, 432,
    461-462

aides, 14, 248, 249, 251, 273, 296, 297,
    321, 386, 388
  hospices, 7, 63, 65, 75, 125, 294
  services, 75, 273, 299, 308, 323, 427,
    452, 456, 457, 458, 459-460, 461,
    462, 523, 525
Homeless people, 146-147, 300
Honoring Choices, 354, 356, 357, 421
Hopkins Competency Assessment Test, 145
    n.22
Hospice and Palliative Nurses Association,
    78, 84, 223, 242-243
Hospice and Palliative Nurses Foundation,
    242-243, 410
Hospice care (see also Palliative care)
  access to, 10, 30, 62, 103
  accountable care organizations and, 292,
    472-473, 479
  advance care planning and, 212
  cancer patients, 30, 61, 62, 65, 295,
    393, 465, 476, 520
  certification, 14, 48, 59 n.6, 100
  costs, 292-295, 519-522
  definitions, 18, 27, 60-61
  delivery of, 46, 48-49, 50, 54, 56, 59,
    60-62, 63, 65, 100, 101
  dementia patients, 54, 56, 74, 81
  growth of, 8, 20, 60-62, 100, 102-103
  hospital programs and referrals, 61,
    63
  in-home care, 7, 63, 65, 75, 125, 294
  interdisciplinary team approach, 101,
    102, 103
  life expectancy and eligibility, 8, 30,
    294, 321, 387, 388, 412, 426
  and longevity/survival, 30, 62, 73 n.12,
    74, 101
  Medicaid and, 62, 244, 298, 319,
    426-428, 460, 463, 465, 477-478,
    569
  Medicare benefit, 30, 59, 62, 83, 88, 96,
    102, 154, 238, 247, 273, 274, 277,
    285, 292-295, 388, 411, 412, 457,
    459, 460, 463-466, 470, 475-476,
    477, 478, 480, 522
  in nursing homes, 61, 65, 74, 81, 152-
    153, 278, 295, 298, 462, 465-466,
    479
  open-access, 522-523
  pediatric services, 61-62, 98
  in prisons, 62

professional education and development, 13, 14, 48, 221, 222, 224, 226-229, 232, 233, 237-247, 249-251
professional/provider support for, 32-33
prognosis and, 88, 90, 92, 102
public perceptions of, 50
and quality of care, 8, 50, 62, 65, 74, 77
quality-of-care measures and reporting, 7, 77-78, 79, 81, 83-85, 86, 411
and quality of life, 30, 63, 65
race/ethnicity and, 60, 61-62, 150, 153
recommendations, 10
referrals to, 8, 50, 54, 55, 60, 70, 86
reimbursement policies, 30, 59, 62, 83, 88, 96, 102, 154, 238, 247, 273, 274, 277, 285, 292-295, 319, 388, 408, 411, 412, 457, 459, 460, 462, 463-466, 470, 475-476, 477, 478, 480, 522
research needs, 97
satisfaction with care, 62, 74, 75, 80
and site of death, 33-34
specialty/specialists, 2, 7, 10, 13, 14, 20, 71
staffing, 10, 62
treatment approach, 2, 7, 8, 9, 18, 30, 60-61, 62, 63, 86
utilization of, 63
volunteers, 62
Hospice Experience of Care Survey, 83-84, 411
Hospice Item Set, 83, 411
Hospice Medical Director Certification Board, 240
Hospice Quality Reporting Program, 83, 411
Hospital at Home® project, 70, 523
Hospital environment (see Emergency department services; Hospitals/ hospitalization)
Hospital Readmissions Reductions Program, 53
Hospitals/hospitalization (see also Emergency department services; Intensive care/critical care)
accountability, 84
accreditation, 84
admissions, 17, 33, 74, 90
children's hospitals, 64, 68, 564-565, 569

complex chronic conditions and, 266, 554, 556
concurrent care, 72
continuity of care, 68
costs of care, 22, 266, 280-281, 512-513, 564, 565-567, 568, 569
deaths/dying in, 33, 69, 78, 81, 94
delivery environment, 280-282
hospice programs and referrals, 61, 63
lengths of stay, 73, 557, 564, 567
Medicare policies and, 52-53, 277, 280-281, 512-513, 520
nursing home residents, 52, 54, 281, 286, 297, 298, 307, 324, 462, 470, 501, 502
palliative care services, 7, 8, 15, 27, 59, 60, 61, 63-64, 65, 66, 68, 69, 71-72, 84, 85, 98, 100, 562-564
patient education interventions, 53, 73
pediatric care, 68, 98, 537-539, 554, 556-559, 562-567, 568, 569
prognosis and predicted probability of death, 90, 91, 92, 565-567, 568
quality of care, 57, 78, 81, 84, 85, 280-281
readmissions, 52, 53-54, 70, 304, 306, 314, 319, 471, 473, 520, 523, 547
reimbursement policies, 53, 277, 280-281, 319, 471
satisfaction with care, 56-57, 73, 74, 75
transitions between care settings, 52-53, 54, 57, 100
unwanted, uncoordinated care, 56-57, 266
Huntington's disease, 215-216

I

Implantable cardioverter defibrillator (ICD) deactivation, 78, 79, 80
In-home care (see also Caregivers, family)
communications technology and, 70
costs, 37, 38
hospice, 7, 63, 65, 75, 125, 294
Medicare and, 319, 523
nurses, 70, 273, 292, 294, 298 n.18, 321, 539, 552, 553, 571
palliative care, 70, 72, 73, 74, 290, 294, 320, 321-322, 328
preference for, 94

quality, 38, 65, 70
reimbursement policies, 97
satisfaction with, 70
Informed Medical Decisions Foundation,
    354 n.4
Initiative for Pediatric Palliative Care,
    429
Institute for Healthcare Improvement, 420
Instrumental activities of daily living
    (IADLs), 93, 248, 491-492
Intensive care/critical care
    admissions, 51
    advance directives, 126, 151, 214,
        216
    appropriateness of care, 130, 280-281,
        288, 557
    clinician communication, 138, 165, 230,
        428
    deaths, 68, 81, 520, 557
    dementia patients, 49
    family conferences, 164, 213, 236
    financial issues, 140, 267, 280-281, 288,
        289, 291, 329-330, 364-365, 458,
        506, 517
    futile care, 288, 364
    impacts on family, 138
    nurses/nursing, 232
    palliative/hospice care and, 63, 66, 73,
        74, 77, 187, 279, 289, 291, 329,
        457, 463, 473, 519, 520
    pediatric and neonatal, 68, 89, 230, 428,
        429, 542, 557
    and preferences of patients, 94
    primary care and, 51
    professional education and training,
        232
    and prognosis/survival status, 89, 90,
        92, 119, 165, 512
    quality of care measures, 77, 79
    race/ethnicity and, 49, 151, 506
    transitions between services and, 298
    utilization, 33, 214, 267, 279, 329-330,
        458, 512, 517, 519, 520, 557
Interdisciplinary team approach, 71-72,
    101
International Classification of Diseases
    (ICD) codes, 536, 537, 538, 546
Interprofessional collaboration, 226, 228,
    229, 230, 234, 252, 428

J

John A. Hartford Foundation, 227 n.5
Johns Hopkins University, 70, 523
Joint Commission, 84, 409
Josiah Macy Jr. Foundation, 234

K

Kids' Inpatient Dataset (KID), 537-538,
    539
Kubler-Ross, Elisabeth, 60

L

Last Acts campaign, 33, 353, 361
Liaison Committee on Medical Education,
    226, 231
Life Cycle Model of Advance Care
    Planning
    for children, 187
    in final year of expected life, 187
    at initial diagnosis, 186
    milestone specific, 185
    primary care setting, 186
    situation-specific, 186
    at worsening health, 186-187
Life expectancy (see also Prognosis)
    and assisted suicide, 363
    at birth, 30, 34, 35-36, 308
    and hospice eligibility, 8, 30, 294, 321,
        387, 388, 412, 426
    palliative care and, 62, 167, 560
    patient preferences for discussing,
        152
    and pediatric palliative care eligibility,
        424, 426
    predicting, 89, 91, 160
    race/ethnicity and, 34
LIVESTRONG Foundation, 414
Living Well at the End of Life poll, 347
Living wills, 117, 120, 122, 124, 132, 133,
    136 n.13, 147, 175, 181, 184, 366
    n.14, 369, 385, 387
Long-term care (see also Nursing home
    residents)
    acute care, 27, 48, 59-60, 306, 388-389,
        458
    advance care planning, 164, 172, 174,
        179, 218

and concurrent care, 297
coordination of services, 304-305, 308, 470
costs of care, 273, 274, 296, 300-301, 458, 502
coverage of services, 459-460
defined, 387-388
disability rates and, 37-38
dual-eligible individuals, 273, 278, 302-303, 457, 462, 522
environment, 296-303
family needs, 312-313
financing, 16, 266, 268, 271, 274, 275, 278, 279, 287, 296-303, 306, 315-316, 320, 327-328, 475, 478-479, 498, 499
home- and community-based, 94, 298, 299-302, 312-313, 315, 316
in hospice, 295-296, 462
institutional, 297-298, 310
insurance, 274, 315
interdisciplinary care teams, 102
Medicare and, 275, 287, 297-298, 459-460
need for, 37
palliative care, 27, 59, 69, 389
professional education and training, 229-230, 233, 247
quality of care, 247, 278
social services, 329
spiritual care, 247
Longevity/survival
advance care planning and, 136
cancer patients, 62, 69, 215
concurrent and, 72
cost of care and, 22
hospice care and, 30, 62, 73 n.12, 74, 101
palliative care and, 62, 68, 69, 72-73, 98, 101, 215, 322 n.33, 560

M

Managed care
and advance care planning, 298 n.18
for dual-eligible individuals, 286, 412
Massachusetts
hospice care, 74
Pediatric Palliative Care Network program, 68, 424, 425

Massachusetts General Hospital, 72
MD Anderson Cancer Center
Supportive and Palliative Care Service, 65, 67
Texas Community Bus Rounds program, 383
Meals and nutrition services, 287, 309, 310, 312-313, 330
Measuring What Matters initiative, 410
Medicaid (*see also* Centers for Medicare & Medicaid Services)
ACA and, 16, 268, 275, 315, 319, 412, 427, 469, 477-478
and advance directives and advance care planning, 121, 323, 464
age-related costs, 499
Cash & Counseling program, 97, 313
and concurrent care, 278, 319, 427, 477-478
costs and expenditures, 16, 268, 271, 273, 291, 298, 300-301, 302, 303, 312, 459, 495, 497, 498, 499, 502, 522
data for health services research, 525, 539
demonstration and waiver authority, 308
and direct care workers, 249
disease management programs, 305-306
dual eligibility, 271-272, 273, 278, 286, 287, 298, 302-303, 310, 315, 328, 386, 462, 474-475, 522
electronic health record incentives, 184
enrollees, 271-272, 273, 299, 459
financing, 269, 271, 315-316, 330, 412, 463-464, 467, 474, 522
health insurance coverage, 273, 275, 412, 426-427, 459-460, 477-478
Home and Community Based Services program, 298, 299-302, 315
home health, 279, 320, 459-460
hospice care, 62, 244, 298, 319, 426-428, 460, 463, 465, 477-478, 569
impacts of policies, 278-279, 298, 569
long-term-care/nursing home assistance, 10, 16, 54, 171, 264, 268, 271, 272, 273, 275, 277, 278-279, 285, 295, 296, 297-298, 302, 306, 307, 312, 324, 388, 448, 456, 457, 458, 459-460, 461, 462-463, 465, 470, 479, 498, 499, 501, 502, 503, 525
managed care, 285-286, 303, 323, 326

and mental health services, 284-285
nursing home care, 16, 273, 275, 277,
    278-279, 285, 457, 462
PACE program, 287, 302, 522
and palliative care, 68, 291, 295, 301-
    302, 427-428, 463, 519
racial difference in costs/payments, 495,
    497
reforms needed and proposed, 266-
    267, 270, 320-321, 426-428, 469,
    479
reimbursement policies, 263, 264, 278-
    279, 282, 283, 284-285, 298, 316,
    323, 329, 330, 464, 465, 474, 479
social services coverage, 309, 312
spending down for eligibility, 271-272,
    296
state policies, 323, 424, 427, 459-460
tax base, 269
transparency and accountability, 17,
    324
Medical Expenditure Panel Survey data,
    489, 490, 492, 493, 494, 495, 496,
    497, 499, 501, 503, 514, 515
Medical homes, 51-52, 82, 302, 303, 314,
    469
Medical orders, defined, 122
Medical Orders for Life-Sustaining
    Treatment (MOLST), 17, 123, 175,
    177, 179, 182, 183, 331, 358
Medical records (see Health records)
Medicare (see also Centers for Medicare &
    Medicaid Services)
    ACA-authorized changes, 314, 315-316,
        319, 469, 478
    accountable care organizations, 317,
        318-319, 472
    and advance care planning, 121, 124,
        139, 464, 510
    ancillary services, 284
    bundled payment model, 314, 316, 327-
        328, 455, 458-459, 469-475, 479
    burden of illness in eligible populations,
        16, 33, 36, 37, 52-53, 139, 265, 503,
        504-505
    Care Choices Model, 412, 476
    community-based services, 318
    concurrent care coverage, 154, 319, 412,
        427, 475-476, 477
    and coordination and continuity of care,
        304, 305, 308, 315-316, 330

and costs of care, 139, 268, 276, 279-
    280, 283-284, 451, 504, 519-523
deaths of covered population, 275
demographic characteristics related to
    spending, 506-507, 508
demonstration programs, 469-478
dual eligibility, 271-272, 273, 278, 285-
    286, 287, 298, 302-303, 310, 315,
    328, 386, 462, 474-475, 522
economic impacts, 269-270
and electronic health records, 184
enrollment/eligible population, 16, 36,
    271, 459-460, 503
expenditures, 16, 23, 36, 37, 139, 264,
    267, 268, 270-273, 275, 280-282,
    285, 289, 303, 304, 306-307, 457,
    458-459, 497, 498, 499, 502-503,
    504-512
family caregiver benefits, 296-297
fee-for-service policy, 16, 33, 36, 37,
    52-53, 139, 265, 269, 276, 277, 278,
    279-280, 282, 283, 285, 316, 317,
    318, 322, 327, 328-329, 386, 388,
    409, 461, 466, 467, 469, 470, 472,
    473, 503, 504-505, 523
financial incentives, 16, 184, 363
funding/tax base, 269, 271
geographic variation in spending, 306-
    307, 510-512
health characteristics related to
    spending, 508-510, 512, 516, 517,
    525
home care, 319, 523
hospice benefit, 30, 59, 62, 83, 88, 96,
    102, 154, 238, 247, 273, 274, 277,
    285, 292-295, 319, 388, 408, 411,
    412, 457, 459, 460, 462, 463-466,
    470, 475-476, 477, 478, 480, 522
and hospitalization, 52-53, 277, 280-
    281, 512-513, 520
limitations of payment approaches,
    460-466
long-term care, 275, 287, 297-298,
    459-460
managed care, 466-457 (see also
    Medicare Advantage)
mental health treatment, 284-285
out-of-pocket expenditures by
    beneficiaries, 458
PACE integrated model, 287, 467

palliative care financing, 412, 463-464, 476
physician services, 282-284, 464
and quality of care, 286-287, 293-294, 307, 324, 326
quality reporting requirements, 7, 77-78, 79, 81, 83-85, 86, 411
reform contexts, 265, 266-267, 329-330, 469-478
SEER-Medicare database, 51
Shared Savings Program, 315, 317, 318, 468, 472, 473
skilled nursing benefit, 272, 278, 297, 298, 306, 307, 324, 388, 457, 451, 457, 458, 459, 461, 462, 470, 479, 498, 499, 501, 502
sustainable growth rate, 283-284
traditional Medicare, 272-273, 388-389, 459, 461-463
training requirements for direct care workers, 349
transitions among services, 409
transparency and accountability, 17
and utilization of services, 16, 279, 280-281, 306-307, 408, 456-459, 501, 512-513
Medicare Advantage, 50-51, 53, 276, 278, 285-286, 309, 320, 321, 322, 326, 327, 388, 459, 466, 502
Medicare-Medicaid Coordination Office, 272, 315, 412
Medicare Modernization Act of 2003, 388
Medicare Payment Advisory Commission (MedPAC), 272, 286, 295, 320, 413, 465, 466, 479
Medicare Prescription Drug Improvement and Modernization Act of 2003 (MMA), 463-464, 466
Mental health services, 284-285
Methodist Hospital System, Houston, 247
Minnesota
    Honoring Choices series, 354, 356-357, 421
    hospice services, 74
    nursing home deaths, 33
    Rural Palliative Care Initiative, 408
Mortality data (*see also* Death and dying)
    age and causes of death, 31, 34
    cancer, 31, 34, 35, 36, 214, 456, 546
    pediatric, 31, 34, 536-537, 540-542, 551
Murray, Kenneth, 24

N

National Alliance for Caregiving, 96, 354 n.4
National Assessment of Adult Literacy, 155, 156
National Association for the Advancement of Colored People (NAACP), 33
National Association of Social Workers, 78, 243-244, 417
National Board for Certification of Hospice and Palliative Nurses, 241, 417
National Cancer Institute, 67, 158, 232, 423
National Center for Health Services Research (NCHSR), 299
National Center for Health Statistics, 367, 430, 536
National Commission on Fiscal Responsibility and Reform, 267
National Committee for Quality Assurance (NCQA), 82, 84-85
National Comprehensive Cancer Network, 73, 214
National Consensus Project for Quality Palliative Care (NCP), 9, 78, 79, 84, 85, 87, 214, 246, 410
National Council on Aging, 127
National Data Set, 430
National Family Caregiver Support Program, 97, 310
National Framework and Preferred Practices for Palliative and Hospice Care Quality, 61, 172-173, 185, 410, 425-426
National Healthcare Decisions Day, 124, 354, 356-357, 421
National Hospice and Palliative Care Organization, 67, 78, 84-85, 153, 175, 223, 352, 411, 421, 422, 424, 425, 428, 430, 521
National Institute of Nursing Research, 33, 39, 97, 418, 419, 431
National Institutes of Health (NIH), 33, 39, 98, 232-233, 418, 430, 535-536
National Long-Term Care Survey, 37
National Palliative Care Research Center, 78, 100, 419, 431
National Rural Health Association Technical Assistance Project, 408, 421, 425

National Quality Forum (NQF), 61, 77-78,
    79, 80, 81, 83, 84-85, 98, 172, 187,
    410, 411, 423, 425-426, 468-469
Nationwide Emergency Department Sample
    (NEDS), 537-538, 539, 559
New Mexico, 70, 363
New York State
    Community Conversations on
        Compassionate Care, 122, 358
    CompassionNet, 68
    MOLST program, 123, 175, 177, 178,
        179, 182, 183, 358
    PACE program, 177
    pediatric palliative care, 68, 427
    site of death, 553
    utilization and costs, 152-153, 291, 519,
        553
North Carolina, 68, 123, 421, 427
North Dakota, 68, 427, 458
Northeast Ohio Medical University, 227
Nurses/nursing
    advance care planning role, 185, 186,
        389, 448
    case/care managers, 53, 294, 304, 322,
        476
    certifications, 14, 15, 27, 48-49, 59,
        242, 252, 417, 429
    communication with patients, 129, 162,
        226, 231, 235
    delivery of care, 42, 50, 53, 70
    discharge advocate, 53
    education of patients and caregivers, 53,
        73
    faculty development, 222, 229-230, 231-
        232, 415, 416
    home visits, 70, 273, 292, 294, 298
        n.18, 321, 539, 552, 553, 571
    intensive care, 232
    interprofessional collaboration, 226,
        228, 229, 230, 234, 252, 428
    medical orders, 122, 175, 389
    palliative and hospice care, 8, 10, 14,
        27, 52, 59, 71, 85, 100, 101, 103,
        222, 223, 226, 231, 232, 237-238,
        240-243, 251, 252, 294, 321, 322,
        385, 389, 409, 417, 423
    primary care, 50, 286
    professional education and development,
        13, 14, 15, 221, 222, 223, 225, 226,
        228, 229-230, 231-232, 237-238,
        240-243, 251, 415, 416, 423, 428

scope-of-practice laws, 323
specialties, 240-243, 251, 389, 417, 429
spiritual care, 246
staffing of hospital-based pediatric
    palliative care programs, 563-564
transitional care, 52, 53, 54
Nursing Home Compare, 468, 480
Nursing home residents
    advance care planning and directives,
        126, 129, 132, 151, 152, 171, 176,
        177, 181, 182, 188, 216, 241, 286,
        448, 468
    alternative care for, 299, 301, 302, 303,
        310, 311, 312, 467, 522
    clinician communication with, 216, 224
    concurrent care, 278
    costs of care, 37, 272, 273, 277, 296,
        310, 312, 457, 465, 489, 490, 492,
        493, 494, 495, 496, 497, 498, 499,
        501-502, 509, 514, 515, 517, 522
    decision-making capacity, 119, 137, 189
    dementias/cognitive impairment in, 54,
        81, 216, 286, 295, 324, 328, 509
    hospice care, 61, 65, 74, 81, 152-153,
        278, 295, 298, 462, 465-466, 479
    hospitalizations, 52, 54, 281, 286, 297,
        298, 307, 324, 462, 470, 501, 502
    language barriers, 60
    long-term care insurance, 274, 498, 499
    managed care for dually eligible
        individuals, 286, 412
    Medicaid policies and payments, 16, 54,
        273, 275, 277, 278-279, 285, 312,
        324, 457, 462, 470, 498, 499
    Medicare policies and payments, 272,
        278, 297, 298, 306, 307, 324, 388,
        451, 457, 458, 459, 461, 462, 470,
        479, 498, 499, 501, 502
    palliative care, 7, 27, 55, 58, 59-60, 66,
        69-70, 72, 102, 243, 288, 479
    preferences for treatment, 16, 176, 177,
        216
    prognosis, 90, 91
    racial, ethnic, and cultural differences,
        152-153, 496, 497
    quality of care, 54-55, 74, 81, 247, 277,
        278, 286, 324, 326, 468, 480, 526
    research needs, 328, 526
    satisfaction with care, 74, 75
    shortage of care for, 37, 328
    site of death, 33, 54, 81, 119, 468

skilled nursing facilities, 10, 16, 171, 272, 277, 278, 297-298, 306, 307, 388, 448, 456, 457, 458, 459, 461, 462-463, 465, 479, 501, 502, 503, 525
social services for, 329
spiritual care, 247
standards of care, 54, 409
state regulation and oversight of facilities, 323
training of caregivers, 69-70, 248-249, 311
transitions to and from hospitals, 52, 54, 277, 281, 286, 297, 298, 328, 449
utilization of care, 306, 307, 456, 501

O

Office of the Assistant Secretary for Planning and Evaluation (ASPE), 299
Older Americans Act, 97, 275, 279, 309, 310, 312, 366 n.14
Open Society Institute, 222
Oregon
physician-assisted suicide, 349, 354, 363, 421
POLST program, 121, 123, 178, 217-219
Organisation for Economic Co-operation and Development (OECD), 308

P

Palliative care
access to, 4, 10, 50, 64, 86, 102, 103, 320-321
accountable care organizations and, 292, 472-473, 479
advance care planning, 60, 66, 137, 143, 155, 160-161, 169, 172-173, 175, 215 n.13
approach and components, 8, 9, 55, 58-60, 63, 65-67, 68, 85, 86, 560
basic, 7 n.2, 14, 20, 27, 52, 59, 70, 221, 224, 225-226, 229, 233, 235, 238, 251, 252, 385, 416
biopsychosocial model of care, 62-63
cancer patients, 7, 62, 65, 67, 68, 69, 70, 72, 73, 77, 171, 215, 228, 290, 294, 414, 423, 519, 546, 560

certification, 14, 48, 84, 100, 221, 228-229, 238-240, 241, 242, 243, 247-248, 250-251, 418
chaplains, 8, 10, 67, 247-248, 418
clinical competency domains, 225
communication skills and, 64, 226, 233, 235-237, 288, 290, 431
community-based, 70, 282, 292, 301-302
conceptual models of, 560-561
concurrent care, 7, 58, 73, 277, 287, 293, 295, 297-298, 321, 322
consultation and counseling on, 60, 61, 64, 66, 137, 143, 155, 160-161, 164, 167, 170, 172, 187
continuity of care, 68
coordination across settings, 63, 68, 71, 84, 322
core tasks, 561-562
cost savings and expenditures, 74, 264, 274, 287-292, 327, 329, 519
definitions, 27, 59, 67, 86, 389
delivery of, 7, 51-52, 55, 58-74, 97, 103, 287-292
demand for, 4, 25, 62-65, 70
dual eligibility and, 303
in emergency rooms, 243
evidence for effectiveness, 62, 72-74, 101
family support and role in, 58, 64, 67, 68, 69, 86, 95, 96, 245, 249
financing and policy, 33, 59, 61, 68, 98, 287-292, 329
gaps in knowledge, 8, 570-571
geriatric care and, 52
growth of specialty, 8, 60, 62-65, 100, 102-103, 221, 250
guidelines, 9, 67, 73, 78, 84, 87
home-based, 70, 72, 73, 74, 290, 294, 320, 321-322, 328
and hospice, 2, 7, 10, 18, 58, 59, 60-62, 70
hospital-based, 7, 8, 15, 27, 59, 60, 61, 63-64, 65, 66, 68, 69, 71-72, 84, 85, 98, 100, 290, 291, 292, 562-564
and intensive care, 63, 66, 73, 74, 77, 187, 279, 289, 291, 329, 457, 463, 473, 519, 520
interdisciplinary team approach, 7, 10, 13, 58, 64, 67, 68, 71-72, 79, 86, 95, 101, 102, 103, 226, 234, 244, 245, 249, 424, 429, 563-564, 571

long-term care settings, 27, 59, 69, 389
and longevity/survival, 62, 68, 69, 72-
73, 98, 101, 215, 322 n.33, 560
Medicaid and, 68, 291, 295, 301-302,
427-428, 463, 519
medical homes, 51-52
Medicare and, 412, 463-464, 476
in nonhospital settings, 7, 51-52, 59, 60,
69-70, 289-292
nurses/nursing, 8, 10, 14, 27, 52, 59, 71,
85, 100, 101, 103, 222, 223, 226,
231, 232, 237-238, 240-243, 251,
252, 294, 321, 322, 385, 389, 409,
417, 423
in nursing homes, 7, 27, 55, 58, 59-60,
66, 69-70, 72, 102, 243, 288, 479
palliative care, 74, 264, 274, 287-292,
327, 329, 519
pediatric, 67-69, 71 n.11, 98, 223-224,
232, 235-236, 292, 429, 535, 542-
543, 545-546, 560-564, 570-571
performance measures, 84
pharmacists, 14, 59, 245-246
physician specialists, 238-240
preferences for, 77, 169
professional education and development,
13, 14, 48, 221, 222, 224, 226-229,
232, 233, 237-247, 249-251
prognosis and, 89-90, 91, 92, 233
public awareness and engagement, 18,
347, 348-349, 351, 353, 358, 364,
368
quality of care, 7, 8, 72, 74, 76-87, 96,
211, 264, 325-326
and quality of life and mood, 1-2, 7, 30,
45, 46, 58, 59, 62, 65, 69, 72-73, 74,
98, 101, 233, 290
race/ethnicity and, 60, 240
recommendations, 10, 14-15, 103,
252-253
rehabilitation therapists, 14, 247
reimbursement policies, 283, 285, 287-
292, 294, 301-302, 320, 328
research needs and funding, 97, 98-99,
100, 228
satisfaction with care, 62, 64, 69, 70,
75, 290, 322
screening/assessment, 7-8, 65-68, 71, 77,
89, 92, 101
shortage of specialists, 224, 251
social services integration, 313-314, 330

social workers, 8, 10, 14, 15, 59, 222,
243-244
specialty/specialists, 2, 7, 13, 14, 15, 20,
27, 32-33, 48, 50, 52, 59, 61, 71, 74,
86, 100, 222, 224, 228, 233, 238-
240, 241, 242-243, 246, 247-248,
250, 251, 252-253, 289, 389, 415,
417, 418, 429, 533
spiritual care, 67, 163, 246-247
staffing, 59, 563-564
support for, 62-64, 65, 223
timeliness of referral, 7, 80, 81, 101
transparency and accountability, 74, 76,
84
and utilization of hospital/emergency
services, 69, 73, 74, 281, 290, 329
VA benefit, 61, 72, 274
Palliative Care Leadership Centers, 234-235
Palliative Care Research Cooperative
Group, 100, 419
Palliative Prognostic (PaP) score, 89-90, 91
Parkinson's disease, 37, 88, 295, 444
Partners Health System, 183
Patient, family, or caregiver education, 53,
73, 76, 184, 185, 305
Patient Aligned Care Team (PACT), 53
Patient-centered, family-oriented care (see
also Delivery of end-of-life care)
core values, 69
decision making by patients and families
and, 166-172
defined, 28, 31, 45
diversity of population and, 69
high-quality characteristics, 82-83
medical homes, 51-52, 82, 302, 303,
314, 469
primary care and, 68
Patient-Centered Outcomes Research
Institute (PCORI), 98-99, 419
Patient Protection and Affordable Care Act
(ACA), 25
accountable care organizations, 279-
280, 310, 317-319
and advance care planning, 12, 120,
132, 366-370
bundled payment approaches, 316, 327-
328, 469-475
and concurrent care, 319, 320, 412,
427, 475-476, 477
cost containment, 264, 265, 314,
315-316

"death panels" controversy, 12, 120, 366-370
and delivery of end-of-life care, 4, 97
and electronic medical records, 184
Financial Alignment Initiative, 315-316
financial and organizational changes under, 4, 272, 314-321, 412
gaps in, 319-321
home- and community-based services, 302-303, 315, 319
hospice care, 83, 295, 319, 320, 411, 412, 413, 469, 478, 480
insurance coverage, 419, 460
long-term care, 315, 320, 475
Medicaid expansion, 16, 268, 275, 315, 319, 412, 427, 469, 477-478
Medicare changes, 314, 315-316, 319, 469, 478
Medicare-Medicaid coordination, 412
palliative care services, 412
Patient-Centered Outcomes Research Institute, 98-99, 419
pay-for-performance, 319
proposed changes, 320-321
quality of care, 264, 265, 314, 327-328, 469
and research funding, 98-99, 419
training requirements for direct care workers, 249
transitions between care settings, 97
and transparency and accountability, 324, 329
Patient Self-Determination Act, 121
Pay-for-performance (P4P), 319, 474, 480
Payment systems (*see* Health insurance coverage, private; Medicaid; Medicare; Reimbursement policies and methods)
PEACE (Prepare, Embrace, Attend, Communicate, Empower) Project, 79, 84-85, 410
Pediatric Early Care program, 423
Pediatric end-of-life care (*see also* Children)
advance care planning, 68, 134, 136, 141-144, 146, 173, 184, 187, 188, 425-426, 429, 432
assessment scales, 67-68
clinical data, 538-539
complex chronic conditions, 34, 546-547, 551-552, 554-559

concurrent care, 319, 427, 477-478, 533-534, 567, 569-570
costs of care, 564-570
data sources and needs, 536-539
delivery of care, 67-69
emergency room visits, 98, 282, 304, 432, 559-560, 569, 571
gaps in knowledge, 570-571
geographic variations, 553-554, 555
guidelines, 67
hospice care, 61-62, 98
hospitalization, 68, 98, 537-539, 554, 556-559, 562-567, 568, 569
illness trajectories and clinical experience, 548, 550
intensity and invasiveness, 557-559
intensive care, 68, 89, 230, 428, 429, 542, 557
and longevity/survival, 68
multiple complex chronic conditions, 34, 547
pain and symptoms, 560
palliative care, 67-69, 71 n.11, 98, 429, 535, 542-543, 545-546, 560-564, 570-571
prognosis and predicted probability of death, 565-567, 568
race/ethnicity and, 552-554, 555
research needs, 98
social and support services, 68
terms and concepts, 534-536
When Children Die report recommendations, 422-432
Pediatric Health Information System (PHIS) data, 538, 539, 557, 558, 564, 565, 566, 567, 568, 569
Pediatric Palliative Care Network, 424, 425
Perceptions, public
clinician communication, 447
cost drivers, 487, 526
death and dying, 20, 30-31, 149, 445-446, 451
living wills, 117
politicization of end-of-life care and, 367, 446
and preference for care, 117, 149
prognosis, 164-165
public education and, 371, 451
quality of care, 20, 80, 21-22, 247
quality of life, 146, 147

racial, ethnic, and cultural differences,
149-150
shared decision making, 80
Performance measurement benchmark, 317,
472
Pew Research Center, 347, 352
Religion and Public Life Project,
148-149
Physician-assisted suicide, 362-363
Physician Data Query (PDQ®), 67, 423
Physician Orders for Life-Sustaining
Treatment (POLST) (see also Medical
orders, defined), 17, 121, 123, 172,
173-179, 180, 182, 183, 184, 187,
188, 189-190, 217-219, 323, 331,
358, 389, 448
Physicians (see also Clinician-patient
communication)
quality of end-of-life care, 282-284
treatment preferences of, 23-24
Pioneer accountable care organization
program, 317, 318, 468, 471, 472,
473
Practice-based research networks, 99
Preferences of patients and families
advance care planning and, 11, 12, 13,
18, 125-127, 144-155, 189, 369, 510
cancer and, 55, 132, 133, 140, 165,
171, 214, 215, 510
clinician discussion with family and
patients, 11, 13, 20, 350-352
and costs of care, 2, 15, 21, 510
delivery of care, 55, 56, 94
honoring, 31, 119
nursing home residents, 16, 176, 177,
216
palliative care, 77, 169
physician preferences compared to,
23-24
by population, 141-157
public education and, 19
public perceptions of death and dying
and, 117, 149
and quality of care, 2, 16-17, 22, 77,
307-314
quality of life, 11, 24
race/ethnicity and, 152-154
recommendations, 10, 16-17, 19
site of death, 33-34, 119
supportive care versus acute services,
22

Premier Perspective Database (PPD) data,
538-539, 565
Presbyterian Healthcare Services, 70
President's Council on Bioethics, 125, 150
Primary care
advance care planning, 186
basic palliative care, 7 n.2, 14, 20, 27,
52, 59, 70, 221, 224, 225-226, 229,
233, 235, 238, 251, 252, 385, 416
and coordination and continuity of care,
49-51, 68
defined, 49 n.1
delivery of, 49-52, 70
geriatrics, 10, 50, 52, 227 n.5, 232, 282
and hospital admissions, 51
pediatrics, 68
providers and roles, 49-50
Professional education and development in
end-of-life care
advance care planning, 181, 225, 227,
237
chaplains, 15, 222, 228, 230, 247-248,
252, 418
communication skills, 13-14, 225, 226,
229, 230, 231, 232 n.11, 233, 234,
235-237, 241, 250, 251-252, 428,
451
continuing medical education, 222, 229-
231, 239, 243, 244, 251, 415, 428
cross-cutting considerations, 233
curriculum, 13, 221-222, 223, 226-233,
234, 237, 245, 250, 251, 415, 416,
417, 428, 429, 451
domains of clinical competence, 225
faculty development, 13, 222, 228, 229-
230, 231-232, 236, 237, 415, 416,
431
funding/fellowships, 32, 221, 222, 226,
235, 238, 239, 240, 244, 415, 416,
417, 428
hospice care, 13, 14, 48
impediments to changing culture of care,
13, 225-237
infrastructure, 223, 251
interprofessional collaboration, 13, 226
knowledge base of palliative care, 223
licensure and certification, 14, 48, 59 n.6,
84, 100, 221, 228-229, 238-240, 241,
242, 243, 247-248, 250-251, 418
long-term care, 229-230, 233, 247

medical education, 222-223, 226-231, 238-240

nurses, 13, 14, 15, 221, 222, 223, 225, 226, 228, 229-230, 231-232, 237-238, 240-243, 251, 415, 416, 423, 428

palliative care, 13-15, 69-70, 102, 221-253

pharmacists, 14, 245-246

physician specialists, 238-240

progress and continuing needs, 221-225, 250

public health schools, 232-233

public testimony on importance, 451

recommendations, 14-15, 252-253

rehabilitation therapists, 14, 248

social workers, 14, 243-244

team roles and preparation, 13, 237-249, 251

undergraduate and graduate medical education, 226-229

Prognosis

APACHE tool, 92

cancer care and, 30, 88, 89-90, 91, 294, 466

CARING criteria, 89-90, 91

Cheng factors, 89-90, 92

clinician-patient communication, 92, 160-161

dementias, 88, 91

ePrognosis, 92

Health and Retirement Study, 91-92

hospitalization and predicted probability of death, 90, 91, 92, 565-567, 568

implications of, 30, 87-88

intensive care and, 89, 90, 92, 119, 165, 512

and Medicare Hospice Benefit, 88, 90, 92, 102

nursing home residents, 90, 91

and palliative care, 89-90, 91, 92, 233

PaP score, 89-90, 91

pediatric care and, 565-567, 568

predictive models, 89-92

public perceptions of, 164-165

research needs, 98

"surprise" question, 92

uncertainties in, 30, 47, 88-89, 92

Prognosis in Palliative Care Study (PIPS), 90, 91, 99

Program of All-inclusive Care for the Elderly (PACE), 177, 287, 302, 303, 467, 479, 522

Program to Enhance Relational and Communication Skills, 230, 428

Project Compassion, 352, 354, 420

Project on Death in America (PDIA), 32, 222, 244, 416

Public education and engagement (*see also* Campaigns, public education and engagement)

advance care planning, 18, 19, 20, 32, 121-124, 125, 172-173, 345, 346-347, 352-353, 354, 355, 356-357, 358, 359, 360, 370, 371, 420, 421

attitude trends, 347-348

and cancer care, 365

choices of care, 348-350

climate and venues for discussions of death and dying, 352-355

controversial issues, 362-370

knowledge about end-of-life care, 347-352

palliative care, 18, 347, 348-349, 351, 353, 358, 364, 368

preferences for care, 350-352

public testimony on importance, 451

recommendation, 19-20, 370-371

social media, 365-366

terminology and, 348-350

Q

Quality-adjusted life-year (QALY), 325 n.34

Quality Assessment and Performance Improvement Plan, 83, 411

Quality Improvement Organization Program, 53, 79

Quality Incentive Program, 471

Quality-of-care measurement and reporting

ACOVE initiative, 79, 84-85, 410

Carolinas Center for Medical Excellence, 79

Centers for Medicare & Medicaid Services requirements, 79, 83-84, 411, 469

current efforts, 77-79, 80-82

evidence-based performance measures, 84-85

feeding tubes in dementia patients, 79

hospice, 7, 77-78, 79, 81, 83-85, 86, 411

intensive care/critical care, 77, 79

limitations of current efforts, 76-77, 80-82

Measuring What Matters initiative, 84-85

Medicare requirements, 7, 77-78, 79, 81, 83-85, 86, 411

National Committee for Quality Assurance assessment, 82

National Consensus Project for Quality Palliative Care Clinical Practice Guidelines, 9, 78-79, 84, 85, 87, 214, 246, 410

National Quality Forum criteria, 77-78

opportunities for enhancing, 82-85

PEACE Project, 79, 84-85, 410

research needs, 98

satisfaction indicator, 80, 518

site-of-death measure, 81

transparency, 28

Quality of end-of-life care

ACA and, 264, 265, 314, 327-328, 469

accountable care organizations and, 84, 317, 318, 468, 469, 473

advance care planning and, 135-137, 176-178

ambulatory care environment, 282-285

approaches to improving, 76-77

cancer care, 77, 81, 82, 411

chaplains and chaplaincy services and, 247

in clinician-patient communication, 79, 190

coordination of care and, 31, 76, 81, 82, 303-306

costs of care and, 15, 22, 275-302

delivery of care and, 55-57, 74-87, 275-302

dementias and, 38, 49, 54-55, 56-57, 74, 79, 249, 286, 411, 412

emergency departments, 281-282, 453, 560

financing and organization of care and, 467-469

hospice, 8, 50, 62, 65, 74, 77

hospital environment, 57, 78, 81, 84, 85, 280-282

improvement approaches, 76-77

in-home care, 38, 65, 70

long-term care/nursing homes, 54-55, 74, 81, 247, 277, 278, 286, 324, 326, 468, 480, 526

managed care environment, 285-287

Medicare and, 286-287, 293-294, 307, 324, 326

palliative care, 7, 8, 72, 74, 76-87, 96

patient, family, or caregiver education and, 76

physician services, 282-284

preferences of patients and families, 2, 16-17, 22, 77, 307-314

proposed core components, 85-87

public perceptions of, 20, 21-22, 80, 247

public testimony on, 448-451

reimbursement policies and, 4, 16, 25, 137, 269 n.6, 276, 279-280, 318, 451-452, 473, 504-505, 508

Quality of life

advance care planning, 147, 148

cancer and, 72, 73, 290

concurrent care and, 72, 412

FACT-L scale, 72

hospice care and, 30, 63, 65

palliative care and, 1-2, 7, 30, 45, 46, 58, 59, 62, 65, 69, 72-73, 74, 98, 101, 233, 290

Quinlan, Karen Ann, 363-364

R

Racial, ethnic, and cultural differences (*see also specific populations*)

advance care planning, 11, 49, 125, 148-155, 188

clinician-patient communication and, 149-150, 152, 154, 155, 522

and continuity of care, 155-156

and costs of care, 494-497

delivery of care, 49, 60

diversity trends in the United States, 38

hospice patients, 60, 61-62, 150, 153

and intensive care utilization, 49, 151, 506

life expectancy, 34

Medicaid enrollees, 495, 497

nursing home residents, 152-153, 496, 497

palliative care, 60, 240

pediatric care, 552-554, 555

quality of care, 153

RAND Corporation, 79, 410
Recommendations
    advance care planning, 12-13, 17, 19,
        20, 32, 190-191, 370, 371
    clinician-patient communication, 12-13,
        190-191
    delivery of care, 10, 103-104
    financing care, 16-17, 330-331
    hospice and palliative care, 10, 14-15,
        103, 252-253
    professional education and training, 14-
        15, 252-253
    public education and engagement, 19-
        20, 370-371
Reimbursement policies and methods
    ACA reforms, 280, 315-316, 478
    accountable care organizations, 279-
        280, 317-318, 468, 471, 472, 479
    ancillary services, 284-285
    advance care planning, 17, 117, 121,
        188-189, 320, 323, 331, 368, 369-
        370, 464, 468
    bundled payment model, 314, 316, 327-
        328, 455, 458-459, 469-475, 479
    cancer treatments, 65 n.8
    capitation, 278, 279-280, 285-287,
        315-316
    in clinician-patient communication, 452
    and costs of care, 137, 269 n.6, 276,
        279-280, 318, 451-452, 473, 504-
        505, 508
    diagnosis-related group methodology, 461
    dual eligibility and, 271-272, 273, 278,
        286, 287, 298, 302-303, 310, 315,
        328, 386, 474-475, 522
    emergency services, 281-282, 296, 467
    fee-for-service policy, 16, 33, 36, 37,
        52-53, 139, 265, 269, 276, 277, 278,
        279-280, 282, 283, 285, 316, 317,
        318, 322, 327, 328-329, 386, 388,
        409, 461, 466, 467, 469, 470, 472,
        473, 503, 504-505, 523
    financial incentives and fragmentation of
        services, 17, 275-302, 329-330
    hospice care, 30, 59, 62, 83, 88, 96,
        102, 154, 238, 247, 273, 274, 277,
        285, 292-295, 319, 388, 408, 411,
        412, 457, 459, 460, 462, 463-466,
        470, 475-476, 477, 478, 480, 522
    hospital care, 53, 277, 280-281, 319,
        471

    in-home care, 97
    limitations of current approaches,
        460-469
    managed care, 285-287
    Medicaid, 263, 264, 278-279, 282, 283,
        284-285, 298, 316, 323, 329, 330,
        464, 465, 474, 479
    palliative care, 283, 285, 287-292, 294,
        301-302, 320, 328
    pay-for-performance, 319, 474, 480
    physician services, 282-284
    population-based payment model, 318
    public testimony on importance,
        451-452
    and quality of care, 266-267, 273, 275-
        302, 328-329, 409, 461
    and referrals to hospice, 276-277, 285
    and satisfaction with care, 316
    Shared Savings Program, 315, 317, 318,
        468, 472, 473
    and transitions between services, 52, 54,
        277, 281, 286, 297, 298, 328, 449
    and utilization of services, 279
Religion (*see also* Spirituality and spiritual
        support)
    and advance care planning, 147-149,
        178-179, 212
Research needs
    advance care planning, 187-189, 432
    delivery of care, 32, 97-100
    emergency services, 432, 526-527
    family caregivers, 96, 98
    financing care, 326-328
    funding, 28, 32, 39
    hospice care, 97
    "learning health care system" approach,
        99
    National Institutes of Health approval
        bodies (study sections), 39
    nursing home care, 328, 526
    palliative care, 97, 98-99, 100, 228
    pediatric care, 98
    practice-based research, 99
    quality of research, 99
Respecting Choices, 141, 143 n.19, 172-
        173, 179-181, 212
Respite care, 97, 243, 274, 292, 302, 309,
        310, 312-313, 330, 424, 427, 450,
        452, 464, 476, 539, 569
Rhode Island, nursing home deaths, 33
Rivlin, Alice, 265

Robert Wood Johnson Foundation, 32, 408
    Community-State Partnerships to
        Improve End-of-Life Care, 33
    Critical Care End-of-Life Peer
        Workgroup, 77, 229, 231-232, 234,
        323
    Last Acts initiative, 33, 353, 361

S

Satisfaction with care
    advance care planning and, 135-137
    clinician-patient communication and,
        158, 164, 167, 290
    coordination of care and, 76, 322
    concurrent care and, 322
    hospice care, 62, 74, 75, 80
    hospital care, 56-57, 73, 74, 75
    in-home care, 70, 322, 523
    indicators of, 75
    measuring, 80
    palliative care, 62, 64, 69, 70, 75, 290,
        322
    patient, family, or caregiver education
        and self-management and, 76
    quality-of-care measurement, 76, 78, 80,
        518
    reimbursement approaches and, 316
    social services and supports and, 138,
        309, 313
    transitions between services and, 76
Saunders, Cicely, 60
Schiavo, Teresa Marie, 364
Shared decision making, 1, 4, 17, 80, 99,
        118, 136, 138, 166-172, 173, 174,
        182, 188, 320 n.32, 326, 331, 351
Skilled nursing facility benefit, 10, 16, 171,
        272, 277, 278, 297-298, 306, 307,
        388, 448, 456, 457, 458, 459, 461,
        462-463, 465, 479, 501, 502, 503,
        525
Social Security Disability Income, 271
Social services and supports
    accountable care organizations and, 310
    bereavement, 28, 58, 68, 69, 72, 78-79,
        96, 98, 165, 187, 233, 241, 242,
        244, 321, 411, 422, 423, 424, 426,
        428, 430, 431, 432, 453, 535, 552,
        564, 571
    education and training of caregivers, 311
    essential services, 309-314

family caregivers, 4, 9, 10, 15, 73 n.12,
        86, 97, 98, 233, 279, 304, 309,
        310-311
    and health outcomes, 308-309
    home retrofitting, 311
    integrated approaches, 313-314, 329,
        330
    long-term care and, 329
    meals and nutrition services, 312
    Medicaid coverage, 309, 312
    nursing home residents, 329
    pediatric care, 68
    professional education and development
        in end-of-life care, 243-244
    respite care, 97, 243, 274, 292, 302,
        309, 310, 312-313, 330, 424, 427,
        450, 452, 464, 476, 539, 569
    and satisfaction with care, 138, 309, 313
    transportation, 313
Social Services Block Grant, 275
Social Work Hospice and Palliative Care
        Network, 223, 244, 416
Social Work Leadership Development
        Awards, 222, 416
Social Work Summits on End-of-Life and
        Palliative Care, 244
Social workers, 7, 10, 15, 27, 48, 49, 52,
        56, 57, 59, 60, 71, 101, 103, 185,
        186, 230, 237-238, 243-244, 246,
        251, 252, 289, 292, 321, 385, 409,
        428, 444, 450, 563-564
Soros Foundation, 32
Special Needs Plan, 50-51, 467
Spirituality and spiritual support, 28, 140,
        163, 247
State policies and programs
    advance care planning, 323
Stroke, 36, 37, 38, 46, 88, 456, 508, 509
Study charge and approach, 25-29
    guiding principles, 28
Study to Understand Prognoses and
        Preferences for Outcomes and Risks
        of Treatments (SUPPORT), 32, 510
Sulmasy, Daniel, 163
Supplemental Nutrition Assistance Program
        (SNAP), 300-301
Surveillance, Epidemiology, and End Results
        (SEER)-Medicare database, 51
Survey of Income and Program
        Participation, 38
Sutter Health Advanced Illness Management
        program, 140, 322, 408, 412

T

Texas, 74, 183, 237, 364, 414
  Community Bus Rounds program, 393
Thibault, George, 234
Toolkit of Instruments to Measure End-of-
  Life Care, 410
Transitional Care Model, 53
Transitions between care settings
  ACA and, 97
  and advance care planning
    documentation, 134
  Aetna Transitional Care Model, 53
  burdensome, 52-55
  communication across settings, 53
  and continuity and coordination of care,
    49-52, 53, 54, 100
  dementias and, 54, 328
  and hospital readmissions and ER visits,
    52-53, 54, 57, 100, 298
  and intensive care, 298
  Medicare nursing home policy and, 52,
    54, 277, 281, 286, 297, 298, 328, 449
  nurse managers, 52, 53, 54
  and reimbursement policies, 53
  and satisfaction with care, 76
Transparency and accountability, 10, 16,
  17, 28, 39-40, 82, 84, 103-104, 146,
  265, 269 n.6, 321, 324-325, 329,
  330, 365

U

Understanding Treatment Disclosure (UTD),
  145 n.22
University of California, Los Angeles,
  Medical Center, 79
University of California, San Francisco, 232
University of Rochester, 227, 232
University of Southern California's
  Annenberg School for
  Communication and Journalism, 353
University of Wisconsin, 414
Unwanted and unnecessary care, 12, 21,
  55-58, 266, 288, 298
U.S. Department of Health and Human
  Services (HHS), 82, 120-121, 126, 267,
  301, 324, 387, 475-476, 478, 480, 491
U.S. Department of Housing and Urban
  Development, 275

U.S. Department of Veterans Affairs (VA),
  17, 235, 275
  advance care planning model, 146
  Coordinated-Transitional Care (C-TraC),
    53-54
  Faculty Leader Project for Improved
    Care at the End of Life, 60-61, 72,
    222, 234 n.12, 274, 291, 330
  National Center for Patient Safety, 81
  palliative care benefit, 61, 72
  Patient Aligned Care Teams, 53
  Program of Comprehensive Assistance to
    Family Caregivers, 97
Utilization of services
  advance care planning and, 140
  cancer and, 519
  emergency department services, 17, 52,
    73, 74, 211, 264, 266, 267, 281-282,
    290, 304, 314, 467, 519, 520
  expenditures, 456-458, 512-513,
    525-526
  family caregivers and, 267, 309
  fragmentation of care and, 9, 50-51, 86
  geographic variations, 305-307, 458-459
  hospice, 63
  intensive care, 33, 214, 267, 279, 329-
    330, 458, 512, 517, 519, 520, 557
  nursing home residents, 306, 307, 456,
    501
  palliative care and, 69, 73, 74, 281, 290,
    329
  screening high-cost patients by patterns
    of, 525-526

V

Vulnerable populations, 28, 38-39

W

Warren Alpert Medical School of Brown
  University, 236
Washington State
  pediatric palliative care program, 68
  physician-assisted suicide, 362
  primary care, 50-51
  utilization and costs, 554-555
When Children Die report
  progress since and remaining gaps,
    422-432

Whites (non-Hispanic)
  advance care planning, 125, 128, 152,
    154-155
  costs of care, 495, 496, 497, 506, 507,
    569
  health literacy, 157
  hospice use, 153
  life expectancy, 34
  population distribution, 149
  preferences for end-of-life care, 148-149,
    322, 350

  site of death, 153, 553-554
  treatment differences, 49
  utilization of services, 506
Withholding/withdrawal of life support, 88
    n.17, 121, 147, 166, 363-364
Writers Project, 353
World Health Organization, 58, 67

Y

Yale School of Medicine, 237